PRINCIPLES OF HEALTH
Pain Management

PRINCIPLES OF HEALTH

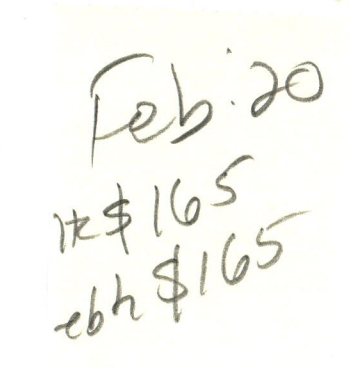

Pain Management

Editor
Michael A. Buratovich, PhD

SALEM PRESS
A Division of EBSCO Information Services, Inc.
Ipswich, Massachusetts

GREY HOUSE PUBLISHING

Cover photo: Man suffering from back pain. Image by ipopba. (Via iStock)

Copyright © 2020, by Salem Press, A Division of EBSCO Information Services, Inc., and Grey House Publishing, Inc.

Principles of Health: Pain Management, published by Grey House Publishing, Inc., Amenia, NY, under exclusive license from EBSCO Information Services, Inc.

All rights reserved. No part of this work may be used or reproduced in any manner whatsoever or transmitted in any form or by any means, electronic or mechanical, including photocopy, recording, or any information storage and retrieval system, without written permission from the copyright owner. For information, contact Grey House Publishing/Salem Press, 4919 Route 22, PO Box 56, Amenia, NY 12501.

∞ The paper used in these volumes conforms to the American National Standard for Permanence of Paper for Printed Library Materials, Z39.48 1992 (R2009)

Publisher's Cataloging-In-Publication Data
(Prepared by The Donohue Group, Inc.)

Names: Buratovich, Michael A., editor.
Title: Principles of health. Pain management / editor, Michael A. Buratovich, PhD.
Other Titles: Pain management
Description: [First edition]. | Ipswich, Massachusetts : Salem Press, a division of EBSCO Information Services, Inc.; Amenia, NY : Grey House Publishing, [2020] | Includes bibliographical references and index.
Identifiers: ISBN 9781642653878 (hardcover)
Subjects: LCSH: Pain. | Pain medicine.
Classification: LCC RB127 .P75 2020 | DDC 616/.0472–dc23

First Printing
PRINTED IN THE UNITED STATES OF AMERICA

Table of Contents

Publisher's Note vii
Editor's Introduction ix
List of Contributors xi

Pharmacological Treatments 1
   Acetaminophen 1
   Alpha-2 adrenergic agonists 2
   Analgesic 5
   Anesthesia 7
   Anti-inflammatory drugs 14
   Anti-nausea medications. 15
   Aspirin 17
   Baclofen 19
   Bismuth subsalicylate 20
   Carbamazepine. 21
   Carisoprodol 25
   Codeine. 26
   Corticosteroids 27
   Cyclooxygenase-2 (COX-2) inhibitors . . . 29
   Decongestants 30
   Dextromethorphan 32
   Fentanyl 33
   Gabapentin 34
   Hydrocodone 37
   Methadone 39
   Morphine 41
   Narcotics 42
   Nitrous oxide 48
   NMDA receptor antagonists 49
   Non-steroidal anti-inflammatory drugs (NSAIDs) . 51
   Opium 54
   Over-the-counter (OTC) drugs 55
   Over-the-counter (OTC) drugs: Cautions
      and precautions 60
   Oxycodone 62
   Pentazocine, butorphanol, nalbuphine . . . 65
   Pregabalin 66
   Prescription NSAIDs 67
   Sildenafil 68
   Tramadol 70
   Valium 71
   Vicodin and Norco 72

Non-Pharmacological Treatments 75
   Arthroplasty 75
   Astym® therapy 77

   Cervical epidural injection 80
   Chiropractic 82
   Deep brain stimulation 88
   Disk removal 89
   Epidural anesthesia in childbirth 92
   Exercise 94
   Exercise-based therapies 96
   Heat and cold therapy 99
   Hydrotherapy 100
   Massage therapy 102
   Neurosurgery 105
   Pain management during gestation . . . 109
   Progressive muscle relaxation 110
   Stone removal 113
   TENS machines 115
   Tooth extraction 117

Alternative Treatments 119
   Acupressure 119
   Acupuncture 121
   Biofeedback 136
   Boswellia 141
   Bromelain 143
   Capsaicin 145
   Comfrey 146
   Devil's claw 147
   Eucalyptus 149
   Feverfew 151
   Flaxseed 152
   Garlic 155
   Ginger 159
   Herbal medicine 162
   Hypnotherapy 164
   Integrative medicine 166
   Kratom 170
   Lavender 171
   Magnesium 173
   Magnet therapy 176
   Marijuana 185
   Medical marijuana 188
   Oregano oil 190
   Peppermint 192
   Rosemary 195
   Turmeric 196
   Valerian 198
   White willow 202

Witch hazel 204
Yoga 205

Death and Dying **211**
    Coping with a terminal illness 211
    Euthanasia 215
    Hospice 220
    Palliative care 224
    Palliative medicine 226

Psychological Pain **231**
    Antianxiety medications 231
    Antidepressants 233
    Antipsychotics 235
    Assimilative family therapy model 237
    Barbiturates 240
    Behavioral family therapy 243
    Benzodiazepines 246
    Bupropion 248
    Chronic pain management:
        psychological impact 249
    Cognitive behavior therapy (CBT) 253
    Companionship 257
    Coping strategies 258
    Couples therapy 262
    Dialectical behavioral therapy 266
    Equine-assisted therapy 269
    Faith healing 273
    Group therapy 274
    Ketamine 278
    Light therapy 279
    Meditation and relaxation 280
    Mirtazapine 285
    Music, dance, and theater therapy 287
    Pet therapy 291
    Play therapy 293
    Psychoanalysis 297
    Reminiscence therapy 301
    Serotonin-norepinephrine reuptake
        inhibitors 303
    Shock therapy 305
    Transcranial magnetic stimulation (TMS) . 309

Pain and Addiction **313**
    Anesthesia misuse 313
    Benzodiazepine misuse 314
    Center for Substance Abuse Treatment (CSAT) 317
    Narcotics and opioid misuse 318
    Prescription drug misuse 321
    Sedative-hypnotic misuse 325

Common Ailments **329**
    Conditions InDepth: Carpal tunnel syndrome 329
        Medications 329
        Lifestyle changes 331
        Surgical procedures 332
        Other treatments 333
    Conditions InDepth: Foot pain 334
        Medications 334
        Lifestyle changes 336
        Surgical procedures 338
        Other treatments 340
    Conditions InDepth: Headache 343
        Medications 344
        Lifestyle changes 348
        Surgical procedures 349
        Other treatments 350
    Conditions InDepth: Low back pain and sciatica . . 351
        Medications 352
        Lifestyle changes 354
        Surgical procedures 356
        Other treatments 358
    Conditions InDepth: Menopause 360
        Medications 361
        Lifestyle changes 365
        Other treatments 366
    Conditions InDepth: Osteoarthritis 366
        Medications 367
        Lifestyle changes 370
        Surgical procedures 371
        Other treatments 372
    Conditions InDepth: Sinusitis 374
        Medications 375
        Lifestyle changes 377
        Surgical procedures 377
        Other treatments 378

Appendices **381**
    Bibliography and Journals 383
    Glossary 423
    Organizations 431

Indexes **437**
    Category Index 439
    Subject Index 443

Publisher's Note

Salem Press is pleased to add *Principles of Health* to the *Principles of series* that includes *Principles of Science*, *Principles of Business*, and *Principles of Sociology*. *Pain Management* is the first *Principles of Health* volume.

This new resource introduces students and researchers to the fundamentals of pain management using easy-to-understand language for a solid background and a deeper understanding and appreciation of this important subject.

This work begins with a comprehensive Editor's Introduction to the topic of pain management written by Michael Buratovich, PhD.

Following the Introduction, *Principles of Health: Pain Management* includes 146 entries arranged in seven broad categories:

Pharmacological Treatments, includes both prescription and over-the-counter drugs used to manage pain.

Non-Pharmacological Treatments include procedures, surgeries, techniques, and prevention methods.

Alternative Treatments are those not commonly used in Western medicine, including herbs and supplements and techniques like acupuncture and yoga.

Death and Dying deals with end of life issues and includes entries on palliative care and euthanasia.

Psychological Pain deals with mental and behavioral health issues, including depression, anxiety, and post-traumatic stress disorder. Pain related to these disorders is often difficult to quantify, and can lead to physical issues as well.

Pain and Addiction deals with the use and misuse of prescription pain medications and related epidemics in the United States.

Common Ailments includes issues that most people will have to deal with at some point in their lives, such as Headache, Osteoporosis, and Sinusitis.

All entries include Category, System or Anatomy Affected, and References. Many entries also include Key Terms and images and photographs to illustrate concepts and treatments.

This work includes helpful appendixes, including:

- Bibliography;
- Glossary;
- Organizations;
- Category Index;
- Subject Index.

Salem Press extends appreciation to all involved in the development and production of this work. Names and affiliations of contributors to this work follow the Editor's Introduction.

Principles of Health: Pain Management, as well as all Salem Press reference books, is available in print and as an e-book. Please visit www.salempress.com for more information.

Editor's Introduction

Pain is a universal human experience. We fear it, prepare for it, and try to avoid it. Consequently, modern health care focuses heavily on pain relief, and pharmaceutical companies have invested enormous efforts into designing better, safer and cheaper pain relievers. As a physiological phenomenon, researchers have drilled substantial efforts into understanding the mechanisms behind feeling pain.

The physiology of pain is well understood. It can be artificially induced in laboratory animals without causing damage to the body. It can also be effectively relieved by a wide range of pharmaceutical agents and procedures, resulting in people living today with less pain than any of our predecessors. However, there is still much to be learned about pain. Why do people with no detectable damage to any organs, tissues, nerves, or blood vessels sometimes suffer from chronic, or even intractable pain? Why do some individuals experience horrific hardships and seemingly recover completely while others suffer near psychological collapse? Why do some people feel little pain while others are wracked with wrenching pain? While we do possess a deep understanding of pain receptors in the body, the neurotransmitters and neural pathways they use, and the areas of the brain that interpret and register painful sensations, we have little understanding of the variations in the experience of pain from one person to another.

To this end, this volume on pain and pain relief is designed for the curious, general reader who wishes to understand the phenomenon of pain more deeply. These articles will provide a foundation into this fascinating, but complicated, and, sometimes, intensely personal subject.

Principles of Pain Management begins with an examination of the available pharmaceutical agents commonly prescribed for pain relief. Such agents include opioids, nonsteroidal anti-inflammatory drugs, steroids and other anti-inflammatory drugs, muscle relaxants, NMDA receptor antagonists, alpha-2 receptor agonists, gabapentinoids, anti-nausea drugs, anti-inflammatory drugs, and over-the-counter pain killers. While not all agents work equally well for all types of pain, each plays some part in the collection of resources health care providers use to relieve pain in patients. The discussion includes the mechanisms by which these drugs work, what they are used for, and their potential side effects.

The section nonpharmaceutical treatments for pain includes those techniques for which there is reasonable evidence for efficacy. Some are used by physical therapists and athletic trainers to treat musculoskeletal injuries and other types of chronic pain. Some of these techniques have well understood mechanisms of action, while others do not, but are used regardless (e.g., Astym, TENS machines). Not all these techniques are equally well studied or effective, but they have their place in the array of possible pain-relief treatments.

Alternative treatments is next. While some of these alternative agents have been used for centuries, the analgesic properties of these agents are variable and sometimes difficult to access. We offer, however, solid information on these alternative treatments, many of which have been around for centuries, including information on the evidence base for their use, their history, and their potential risks.

Following alternative treatments, this volume tackles the difficult topic of pain relief during death and dying. Euthanasia and palliative medicine are both discussed in informative and sensitive manners that will provide useful information for any interested reader and may give care-givers working overviews of what they might expect as their loved ones face the end of their lives.

This volume addresses psychological pain. On this topic, the clinical trials become harder to interpret, finding reliable information becomes more tedious, and the researcher must exercise greater overall discernment. Nevertheless, *Principles of Pain Management* assembles a potent array of fine articles that address these topics in a subtle but authoritative manner. We also provide assessments of some of the less used, but potentially effective treatments, such as pet therapy, and others.

With powerful pain relievers that can induce euphoric states comes a risk of physiological or psychological dependence. Therefore, we also provide content that discusses the opioid abuse epidemic that has taken, or deleteriously affected, the lives of many people around the world. While simple, emotional narratives of this crisis peaks public interest and concern, they do little to increase our understanding of the crisis or help design strategies to address it. While it is convenient to scapegoat pharmaceutical companies or physicians for the opioid epidemic, such portrayals are inaccurate. Solving the opioid epidemic requires clear thinking and accurate representations of its multifaceted nature. The articles in this volume on the opioid epidemic offer level-headed assessments of the situation that might lead to concrete solutions.

Finally, several common ailments that may cause pain are addressed, specifically in terms of medications and other treatments for symptom relief. Each begins with a description of the illness, including carpal tunnel syndrome, osteoarthritis, and sinusitis. Prescription and over-the-counter drugs are listed with common brand names as well as potential side effects. Lifestyle changes and surgical options to relieve the pain associated with these ailments are also discussed.

Principles of Pain Management is designed to examine the common phenomenon of pain and its relief. We hope that you will benefit from these articles and their purview and that you will turn to it often, in good health or otherwise.

Michael A. Buratovich Ph.D.
Spring Arbor University
Spring Arbor, MI

List of Contributors

Christopher M. Aanstoos, PhD
University of West Georgia

Christine Adamec, BA, MBA
Independent Scholar

Charles N. Alexander
Maharishi International University

Bryan C. Auday, PhD
Gordon College

Mihaela Avramut, MD, PhD
University of Pittsburgh

Jimmy Bajaj, DO
Mount Sinai South Nassau

Grayson Baker, RN, BSN
Spring Arbor University

Iona C. Baldridge, EdD
Lubbock Christian University

Donald G. Beal, PhD
Eastern Kentucky University

Susan E. Beers, PhD
Sweet Briar College

Tanja Bekhuis, PhD, MS, MLIS, AHIP
University of Pittsburgh; TCB Research

Paul F. Bell, PhD
Heritage Valley Health System

Allison C. Bennett, PharmD
Duke University

Matthew Berria, PhD
Independent Scholar

Warren A. Bodine, DO, CAQSM
Greater Lawrence Family Health Center

James F. Breckenridge, ThD
Oral Roberts University

Christiane Brems, PhD
University of Alaska

Shauna Bumford, RN
Spring Arbor University

Michael A. Buratovich
Spring Arbor University

Josephine Campbell
Independent Scholar

Cristina Cesaro, DO
Mount Sinai South Nassau

Judith M. Chertoff, MD
Washington Baltimore Center for Psychoanalysis, Inc.

Andrea Chisholm, MD
Cody Regional Health

Rose Ciulla-Bohling, PhD
Independent Scholar

Nancy W. Comstock
Stanford University

Richard G. Cormack
Independent Scholar

James P. Cornell, MD
Glendale Adventist Medical Center

Liza Davis, RN
Spring Arbor University

LeAnna DeAngelo, PhD
Independent Scholar

Lillian Domingues, MD
Brown University

Stephanie Eckenrode, BA, LLB
Independent Scholar

Patricia Stanfill Edens, RN, PhD, FACHE
Independent Scholar

Marisela Fermin-Schon, RN
Hilltown Community Health Center

Ronald B. France, PhD
LDS Hospital, Salt Lake City

Robin Franck
Southwestern College

Cynthia McPherson Frantz, PhD
Amherst College

Katherine B. Frederich, PhD
Eastern Nazarene College

Rebecca J. Frey, PhD
Yale University

Christine Gamble
Mount Sinai South Nassau

Joanne R. Gambosi, BSN, MA
Independent Scholar

Jennifer L. Gibson, PharmD
Excalibur Scientific, LLC

Margaret Ring Gillock, MS
Independent Scholar

Lenela Glass-Godwin, MS
Independent Scholar

Jodi L. Guy, BSN, RN, CMSRN
Spring Arbor University

David Hernandez, ScB
Brown University

David L. Horn, MD, FACP
Mid-Atlantic Biotherapeutics

Mary Hurd
East Tennessee State University

Leah Jacob, MA
Independent Scholar

Mark E. Johnson, PhD
Pacific University

Cheryl Pokalo Jones
Independent Scholar

Karen Schroeder Kassel, MS, RD, Med
Independent Scholar

Mara Kelly-Zukowski, PhD
Felician College

Michael R. King, PhD
University of Rochester

Ernest Kohlmetz, MA
Independent Scholar

Patrice La Vigne
American Medical Writers Association

Martha Oehmke Loustaunau, PhD
New Mexico State University

Rimas Lukas, MD
University of Chicago

Arthur J. Lurigio, PhD
Loyola University Chicago

Maura S. McAuliffe
Independent Scholar

Marianne Moss Madsen, MS, BCND
University of Utah

Elizabeth A. Manning, PhD
Independent Scholar

Katia Marazova, MD, PhD
Yale University

Geraldine Marrocco, EdD, APRN, CNS, ANP-BC
Yale University

Michael R. Meyers, PhD
Independent Scholar

Briana Moglia
Independent Scholar

Michael Moglia
Independent Scholar

Virginia C. Muckler, CRNA, MSN, DNP
Duke University

Elizabeth Marie McGhee Nelson, PhD
Independent Scholar

Mary Nuckols, RN, BSN, CCM
Spring Arbor University

Kelly Owen, Esq.
Independent Scholar

Kimberly Ortiz-Hartman, PsyD, LMFT
Alliant International University

Terri Pardee. PhD
Spring Arbor University

Youngeun (Grace) Park
Gordon College

Kim J. Pearson, BSN, RN, CEN
Spring Arbor University

Nancy A. Piotrowski, PhD
University of California, Berkeley

Patricia Pitta, PhD, ABPP
St. John's University

Marie President, MD
Sequoia Hospital

R. Christopher Qualls, PhD
Emory and Henry College

Brian Randall, MD
Greater Lawrence Family Health Center

Douglas Reinhart, MD
University of Utah

Felix Rivera, MD
Mount Sinai South Nassau

David Sands, MD
Partnership for WellBEING

Jason J. Schwartz, PhD
Independent Scholar

Dwight G. Smith, PhD
Independent Scholar

Giri Sulur, PhD
The Janssen Pharmaceutical Companies of Johnson & Johnson

Leslie V. Tischauser, PhD
Prairie State College

Eugenia M. Valentine, PhD
Xavier University of Louisiana

Charles L. Vigue, PhD
University of New Haven

Gregory L. Wilson, PhD
Washington State University

George D. Zgourides, MD, PsyD
Z-MED Health Solutions

Richard M. Renneboog, MSc
Independent Scholar

Pamela Rose V. Samonte
Villanova University

Michelle Satava, BA
Gordon College

Rebecca Lovell Scott, PhD, PA-C
College of Health Sciences

Thomas L. Sevier, MD
Astym® Program

Manoj Sharma, MBBS, PhD
Jackson State University

Cathy Shell BSN, RN
Spring Arbor University

R. Baird Shuman, PhD
University of Illinois at Urbana-Champaign

Marcie L. Sidman, MD
North Shore Physicians Group

Candice N. Stevens, BSN, RN
Spring Arbor University

Rhea U. Vallente, PhD
Independent Scholar

Nicole M. Van Hoey, PharmD
Independent Scholar

Zhongqi Weng
Yale University

S. M. Willis, MS MA
Independent Scholar

Lynn D. Willis-Carr MSN, BSN-RN
Spring Arbor University

Michael Woods, MD, FAAP
Independent Scholar

Scott Zimmer, MLS, MS, JD
Alliant Internationa

Pharmacological Treatments

■ Acetaminophen

CATEGORY: NSAID; Over-the-Counter
ALSO KNOWN AS: Paracetamol and commercially as Tylenol and Panadol
ANATOMY OR SYSTEM AFFECTED: Musculoskeletal system, nervous system

KEY TERMS
- *analgesic*: a substance that reduces pain
- *antipyretic*: a substance that lowers body temperature
- *cyclooxygenase (COX)*: an enzyme in the synthesis of prostaglandins and thromboxanes
- *methemoglobinemia*: a condition where there is an elevated blood level of methhemoglobin where the iron is in a state which cannot carry oxygen
- *non-steroidal anti-inflammatory drugs*: drugs that do not have the steroid structure and reduce inflammation
- *thromboxane*: substance made by platelets that causes blood clotting and constriction of blood vessels

Structure and Functions

Acetaminophen is a non-steroidal anti-inflammatory drug (NSAID) that is a mild analgesic and antipyretic used to alleviate pain and reduce fever. It is the most widely used non-prescription drug in the general treatment of minor to moderate pain and fever reduction and is increasingly used to reduce osteoarthritic pain. For severe pain, acetaminophen is often used in combination with an opiate such as codeine.

Although the mechanism of action of acetaminophen is unclear, it may reduce the cyclooxygenase (COX) enzymes, COX-1 and COX-2, enzymes that synthesize prostaglandins and thromboxanes, within the central nervous system but not outside the central nervous system explaining its analgesic and antipyretic effect and non-effect on inflammation. Prostaglandins and thromboxanes have many physiological effects. Acetaminophen is not a direct inhibitor of either COX-1 or COX-2 but seems to reduce their amounts by inhibiting their oxidation to the active forms. Whether acetaminophen inhibits COX-3 is the subject of debate.

The therapeutic and inhibitory effect of acetaminophen toward the prevention of cataracts is currently under investigation.

Acetaminophen is increasingly used as treatment for osteoarthritis and has managed to maintain low gastrointestinal toxicity effects even at over-the-counter (OTC) doses. The widespread availability of the drug increased reports of self-overdosing and reports of severe liver damage and skin reactions. These complications are often seen when acetaminophen is used with alcohol, fasting, other drugs, and diet. The concerns of overdosing have continued to increase. The Food and Drug Administration has attempted to strengthen its messaging about the dangers of overdosing and limit the dose/tablet or capsule. Label warnings concerning liver damage and rare skin reactions were required in 2011, and further refinement was suggested in 2017. Acetaminophen is currently the leading NSAID with no significant contradictory reports to hinder consumers from continuing its use.

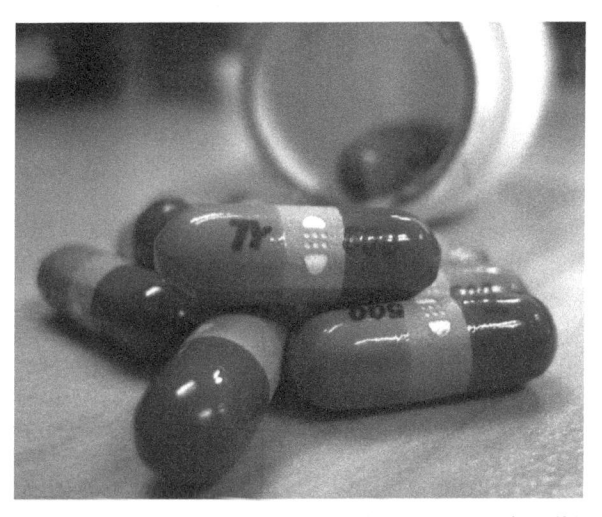

Tylenol 500 mg rapid-release capsules. (Katy Warner via Wikimedia Commons)

Perspective and Prospects

During the Middle Ages, typical antipyretic agents were derived from cinchona bark and white willow bark, more commonly known as the chemical family of salicins. The scarcity of the cinchona tree fueled the need for an alternative source for antipyretic agents. Harmon Northrop Morse first acetaminophen in 1877 at the Johns Hopkins University through the reduction of *p*-nitrophenol with tin in the presence of glacial acetic acid. Joseph von Mering first used acetaminophen in humans in 1887 and reported in 1893 that acetaminophen caused methemoglobinemia stimulating its discontinuation as a drug in humans. By 1948, scientists had demonstrated that acetaminophen is not toxic in humans and is an effective analgesic. The rediscovery of acetaminophen sparked public interest in the United States and was subsequently introduced to the market in 1950 as Triogesic, a combination with aspirin and caffeine. However, fears of agranulocytosis side effects, where the deficiency of white blood cells increases the vulnerability to infections, led to withdrawal of the drug from the market until it was reintroduced as a prescription drug in 1953 and as a single non-prescription analgesic in 1959. By the 1960s, acetaminophen proved its safety and reliability among its predecessors, particularly acetanilide and phenacetin, whose side effects included gastrointestinal ulceration and hemorrhage, among others.

—Pamela Rose V. Samonte
—Rhea U. Vallente, PhD
—Charles L. Vigue, PhD

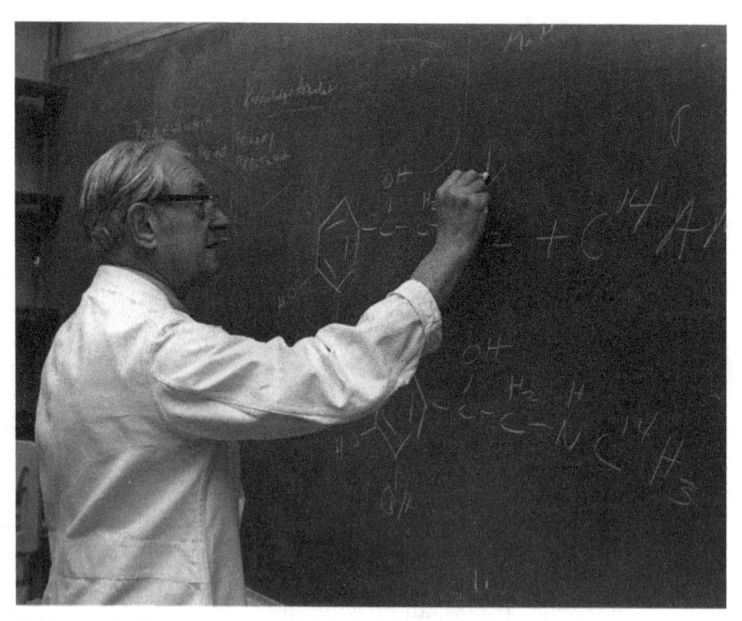

Julius Axelrod (pictured) and Bernard Brodie demonstrated that acetanilide and phenacetin are both metabolized to paracetamol, which is a better tolerated analgesic. (National Institutes of Health)

References

"Acetaminophen." *U.S. National Library of Medicine*, National Institutes of Health, 8 Aug. 2014, www.nlm.nih.gov/medlineplus/druginfo/meds/a681004.html.

"Acetaminophen Information." *U.S. Food and Drug Administration*, 14 Nov. 2017, www.fda.gov/drugs/information-drug-class/acetaminophen-information.

Javaherian, Atash, and Pasha Latifpour. *Acetaminophen: Properties, Clinical Uses and Adverse Effects*. Nova Science, 2012.

Liew, Zeyan, et al. "Acetaminophen Use During Pregnancy, Behavioral Problems, and Hyperkinetic Disorders." *JAMA Pediatrics*, vol. 168, no. 4, Apr. 2014, pp. 313–320., doi:10.1001/jamapediatrics.2013.4914.

Ogbru, Omudhome, and Jay W. Marks. "Acetaminophen Uses, Side Effects, and Dosage." *MedicineNet*, 19 June 2018, www.medicinenet.com/acetaminophen/article.htm.

"Use Only as Directed." *ProPublica*, 20 Sept. 2013, www.propublica.org/article/tylenol-mcneil-fda-use-only-as-directed.

■ Alpha-2 adrenergic agonists

CATEGORY: Class of Drug
ANATOMY OR SYSTEM AFFECTED: Cardiovascular system, Nervous system

KEY TERMS
- *adjuvant analgesic*: drugs with a primary indication other than pain that have analgesic properties in some painful conditions and are usually given in combination with other analgesics
- *analgesic*: a drug that relieves pain

- *hypertension*: high blood pressure; above 130 mm Hg (systolic) / 90 mmHg (diastolic)
- *hypotension*: low blood pressure; below 120 mm Hg (systolic) / 80 mm Hg (diastolic)
- *ion*: an atom or molecule with a net electric charge that results from the loss or gain of one or more electrons
- *ligand-gated ion channels*: transmembrane protein complexes that conduct ion flow through a channel pore in response to the binding of a neurotransmitter
- *locus coeruleus*: a cluster of neurons in the pons of the brainstem involved with physiological responses to stress and panic
- *nerve impulse*: signals transmitted along nerve fibers that consist of a wave of electrical depolarization that reverses the charge differential across the nerve cell membranes
- *neurotransmitters*: chemical substances released at the axon terminus, when a nerve impulse arrives there, and diffuses across the synapse and initiates a response in the target cell
- *synaptic cleft*: the space between neurons at a nerve synapse across which a nerve impulse is transmitted by a neurotransmitter; also called the synaptic gap

Alpha-2 adrenergic agonists have been in clinical use for decades to treat high blood pressure (hypertension), attention-deficit/hyperactivity disorder, various pain and panic disorders, the symptoms of alcohol, opiate, or benzodiazepine withdrawal, and cigarette craving. More recently, alpha-2 adrenergic agonists have been used in combination with sedatives to reduce the dosage of anesthetics.

Activation of alpha-2 adrenergic receptors inhibits the release of the neurotransmitter norepinephrine from presynaptic neurons. Because these receptors are found mainly on the surfaces of neurons in the central nervous system, their activation tends to result in system-wide effects, such as centrally-induced sedation, hypotension, and centrally-mediated pain modification.

How Alpha-2 Adrenergic Agonists Work
Nerve cells (neurons) communicate with each other by releasing neurotransmitters that bind to receptors on the cell surface of the neighboring neuron. These neurotransmitter-binding receptors also double as ion channels that allow ions to enter or leave the cell. Because these nerve cell-specific receptors open or close when bound by small molecules (ligands), they are referred to as "ligand-gated ion channels."

Neurons consist of a cell body that houses the nucleus, multiple extensions of the cell body known as dendrites, and a long extension that projects away from the cell body called an axon. The dendrites conduct nerve impulses toward the cell body and the axon conducts nerve impulses away from the cell body.

Ligand-gated channels are found on the cell body and dendrites of neurons. When the nerve impulse reaches the end of the axon, or axon terminus, the neuron releases its neurotransmitter. The neurons connect other neurons by means of a specialized cell-cell junction called a "synapse." The neurotransmitter released by the neuron floods the space between the two connected neurons (this space is called the "synaptic cleft") and binds to ligand-gated ion channels on the dendrites and cell body of the neighboring neuron. This neurotransmitter may activate or inhibit the adjacent neuron, depending on the receptor it binds, and the identity of the neurotransmitter.

One of the neurotransmitters released by specific neurons is norepinephrine. Neurons that primarily release norepinephrine are called "noradrenergic neurons." Although there are relatively few noradrenergic neurons in the brain, they project to multiple different areas of the brain and exert powerful effects on their targets. The most important cluster of noradrenergic neurons in the brain is the "locus coeruleus," which lies in the brainstem, and forms the lateral walls of the fourth ventricle, just in front of the cerebellum. Pain and other unpleasant stimuli stimulate the locus coeruleus. Additionally, the locus coeruleus sends projections to every significant part of the brain. Its activity regulates alertness, memory formation, and response to sensory inputs. Consequently, drug-induced suppression of the locus coeruleus has a powerful sedating effect on the body.

To properly regulate the release of this powerful neurotransmitter, noradrenergic neurons have norepinephrine receptors on their axon termini called alpha-2 adrenergic receptors. When activated, alpha-2 receptors decrease the release of norepinephrine from noradrenergic neurons, and act as an internal control to prevent overactivation of the targets of noradrenergic neurons.

Agonists are molecules that bind to receptors and activate them. Norepinephrine is an agonist for alpha-2 receptors, but other, synthetic molecules can also bind alpha-2 receptors and activate them. Alpha-2 receptor agonists are a class of drugs that bind to alpha-2 receptors and decrease norepinephrine neurotransmission. The three alpha-2 receptor agonists that have been used in pain relief include clonidine (Catapres and generics), tizanidine (Zanaflex), and dexmedetomidine (Precedex).

Clinical Uses of Alpha-2 Adrenergic Receptor Agonists

Cancer patients often have pain resulting from tissue damage or erosion by the tumor (e.g., cancer-induced fractures in patients with breast, lung, or prostate cancer and in patients with multiple myeloma), obstruction or perforation of internal organs (e.g., gastric cancers), bleeding within the tumor (e.g., hepatocellular carcinoma), or organ stretching (e.g., liver cancer). Oral tizanidine is used as an adjuvant analgesic for cancer patients whose pain is not entirely controlled by opioids. Adjuvant analgesics, or "coanalgesics," are drugs initially marketed for indications other than pain but successfully treat pain in patients when given in combination with other pain-relieving medications.

Tizanidine also treats painful spasms of the neck and shoulder. It not only relieves myofascial pain, but it also inhibits activation of motor neurons in the brain and spinal cord to prevent spasms of the head and neck.

Pain in postsurgical patients (perioperative pain) results from inflammation caused by tissue trauma, as in the case of surgical incision, dissection, or burns, or direct nerve injury (e.g., nerve transection, stretching or compression).

In surgical patients, clonidine, administered orally, intraspinally, or by means of a transdermal patch, or dexmedetomidine, administered by intravenous infusion reduce pain, especially if given in combination with opioid drugs. Clonidine is also an effective preoperative treatment that decreases postoperative pain and reduces the need for opioids. Dexmedetomidine is an anesthetic and a sedative for critically ill patients who require prolonged sedation and mechanical ventilation. It has two distinct advantages in that it does not produce respiratory depression and reduces the occurrence of delirium following outpatient anesthesia. Intranasal dexmedetomidine also sedates children who cannot tolerate intravenous medications for CT scans.

An additional benefit of clonidine is that it can manage the symptoms of opioid withdrawal. Discontinuing opioids after several months of daily use leads to a constellation of symptoms called abstinence syndrome elaborated in the table below.

Clinical Features of Opioid Withdrawal	
Changes in vital signs	Probable increases in blood pressure, respiratory rate, and heart rate
Gastrointestinal changes	Nausea, vomiting, and diarrhea
Neurological changes	Restlessness, seizures (in infants), tremor, yawning, irritability
Ophthalmologic changes	Lacrimation (eyes watering), mydriasis (dilation of the pupil)
Skin changes	Piloerection, sweating (diaphoresis)
Miscellaneous	Runny nose (rhinorrhea)

The cornerstone of medical therapy for opioid addiction is methadone, a long-acting opioid that blocks the euphoric effects of opioids and relieves opioid craving. The methadone dose is then gradually tapered to transition from opioid use to a drug-free status. Clonidine, or a combination of clonidine pluse methadone are alternative treatments to methadone alone for abstinence syndrome.

Clonidine treats children who suffer from sleeping problems due to restless legs syndrome (RLS). RLS is characterized by a strong urge to move the legs, typically accompanied by uncomfortable or unpleasant sensations in the legs, described as "itching," "burning," "tingling," or "like insects are crawling up their legs." Clonidine is the most commonly prescribed medication for sleep in children. It is especially useful when there are severe sleep onset problems due to RLS.

Side Effects

Since alpha-2 receptor agonists lower blood pressure, a common side effect of these drugs is hypotension (low blood pressure), and sedation. However, abruptly stopping these drugs can cause a steep rise in the patient's blood pressure (rebound hypertension). Therefore, patients should never stop taking these drugs without first consulting their physician.

The most commonly occurring side effects of dexmedetomidine are hypotension and low heart rate. However, when the patient stops receiving this medication, they may experience high heart rates (rebound tachycardia) or rebound hypertension. Some patients may experience constipation or nausea. Dexmedetomidine causes agitation in some patients, but dexmedetomidine seems to reduce the risk of postoperative delirium.

The mode of clonidine administration influences its side effect profile. Transdermally administered clonidine may cause rashes, blisters, or pigment changes in the skin. These side effects might be due to the patch itself rather than the drug. Oral and transdermal clonidine most frequently cause drowsiness, headache, fatigue, dizziness, dry mouth and abdominal pain. About 5% of children treated with clonidine experience vivid dreams or nightmares, but these side effects are dose-related.

Tizanidine most commonly causes drowsiness, dizziness, dry mouth, hypotension, and a condition called "asthenia," which refers to a physical weakness and lack of energy. Less frequently, patients have reported blurred vision, increased urinary frequency and urinary tract infections, nervousness, low heart rates, and constipation or vomiting.

—*Michael A. Buratovich Ph.D.*

References

Adams, Michael, Holland, Norman, and Carol Urban. *Pharmacology for Nurses: A Pathophysiologic Approach*, 5th edition. Pearson Education, 2017.

Giovannitti, Joseph, Sean Thoms, and James Crawford. "Alpha-2 Adrenergic Receptor Agonists: Review of Current Clinical Applications." *Anesthesia Progress*, vol 62, no. 1, 2015, pp. 31-38.

Miller, Ronald D., et al., eds. *Miller's Anesthesia*, 9th ed. Elsevier, 2019.

Malanga, Gerard, et al. "Tizanidine is Effective in the Treatment of Myofascial Pain Syndrome." *Pain Physician*, vol. 4, no. 4, 2002, pp. 422-432.

Prince, Jefferson, et al. "Clonidine for sleep disturbances associated with attention-deficit hyperactivity disorder: a systematic chart review of 62 cases." *J American Academy of Child and Adolescent Psychiatry*, vol 35, no. 5, 1996, pp. 599-605.

Semenchuk, Marilyn, and Scott Sherman. "Effectiveness of Tizanidine in Neuropathic Pain: An Open-Label Study." *Journal of Pain*, vol 1, no. 4, 2000, pp. 285-292.

Smith, Howard, and Jennifer Elliot. "Alpha(2) Receptors and Agonists in Pain Management." *Current Opinion in Anaesthesiology*, vol. 14, no. 5, 2001, pp. 513-518.

Streetz, Vonya, et al. "Role of Clonidine in Neonatal Abstinence Syndrome: A Systematic Review." *Annals of Pharmacotherapy*, vol. 50, no. 4, 2016, pp. 301–310. doi: 10.1177/1060028015626438

■ Analgesic

CATEGORY: Class of Drug
ANATOMY OR SYSTEM AFFECTED: Peripheral or central nervous system

An analgesic is a medication taken to alleviate pain. "Painkiller" is the common term for an analgesic. The outcome of taking an analgesic is analgesia, being without pain. Analgesia is not associated with loss of consciousness as in anesthesia. Most analgesics provide pain relief rather than reducing inflammation, although some varieties have an anti-inflammatory quality. Certain analgesics are available without a prescription and can be purchased over the counter at a pharmacy or local store. Others can only be obtained with a prescription provided by a doctor. The long-term use of an analgesic may result in a detrimental effect on body organs. While an analgesic may be safe under certain circumstances, in other instances it may not be.

Background

There are different types of analgesics, available either as over-the-counter or opioid analgesics. Over-the-counter analgesics do not require a prescription; these include brand names such as Tylenol (generic name acetaminophen). They may also be termed simple analgesics. Aspirin or paracetamol provide the generic makeup. An opioid analgesic can only be obtained through a licensed professional's prescription (MD, DO, APRN). When pain is severe, certain medications are available as a combination of acetaminophen and opioid analgesic. An analgesic is generally recommended to any person suffering from pain, with opioids often prescribed only for severe or acute pain. Often, chronic pain may also be treated by an opioid analgesic.

An opioid is also called a narcotic analgesic. Opioids contain opium or morphine derivatives. There is an increased risk of side effects when talking a narcotic. Moreover, the potential toward addiction of an opioid needs to be taken into account, particularly if the patient shows a propensity to addiction. Often when pain is severe and warrants an opioid, the practitioner has an assessment instrument to evaluate the diagnosis, intractability, risk and efficacy (DIRE). By means of a score system including what caused the pain, as well as the physical and psychological health of the patient, the adverse effects versus the benefits can be determined.

A non-steroidal anti-inflammatory drug (NSAID) is another type of analgesic. These medicines are generically known as ibuprofen, diclofenac sodium, or naproxen sodium. An NSAID is an analgesic drug that also acts as an anti-inflammatory. Aspirin, while primarily an analgesic, functions to reduce inflammation as well.

It is essential to follow the dosage and instructions for usage when taking an analgesic. The maximum amount for adults should not exceed 3,000 mg per day. This equals six 500 mg tablets or two tablets up to three times in a day. At times up to four times a day (4,000 mg) is permitted. The number of days one can continue taking the analgesic is clearly stated or will be advised by the doctor. Some stronger versions contain more than 500 mg, and this needs to be checked accordingly. In some instances, an analgesic is taken as needed, or at regular intervals as prescribed to control pain relief. With opioid analgesics, there is an added warning not to stop taking the medication abruptly to prevent withdrawal effects.

Overview

An analgesic creates pain relief by the medication blocking the pain signal on route to the brain. The inhibition of an enzyme, or diverting an interpretive message to the brain, may also be factors contributing to the modulation or alleviation of pain.

Simple analgesics and NSAIDs do not usually result in a dependency on the drug. Taking an opioid might. Over a period of time when taking an opioid, the body becomes tolerant to the drug. What transpires as a result is that the medication becomes less effective, and the person experiencing pain feels that he or she requires more medication. There is a cycle that occurs whereby the level of tolerance leads to a breakthrough withdrawal sensation. In this case, there is an increased degree of pain, often greater than when the analgesic was first taken. More medication is then consumed, and combined with the feeling that additional and more frequent use is required, a system of addiction sets in. Opioids create a physical dependency when used on a long-term basis. Checking that the dosage is not raised indiscriminately is crucial to avoid consumption overload. The problem with chronic pain is the requirement of regular analgesic use and the tolerance that comes about.

Side effects when taking analgesics may be mild or extremely severe. These effects depend largely on how much and how often the drug is taken. For instance, paracetamol may be considered a harmless drug, even when taken on a regular long-term basis. However, if too much paracetamol is taken, damage can occur to the liver and kidneys. Aspirin can likewise have an adverse effect on the renal system This type of analgesic is not indicated for children or during pregnancy. Anyone with asthma cannot take aspirin, nor should a person with stomach issues such as ulcers. NSAIDs can cause potentially serious or life-threatening side effects when taken in large doses or for a prolonged time. Circulatory or heart problems can occur, with the threat of a cardiac attack or stroke. The gastrointestinal system may be severely compromised. Bleeding or perforation may happen. Conditions such as these may result in fatalities. The elderly are at a higher risk. Damage to the kidneys is particularly pertinent regarding the use of analgesics. Over-the-counter analgesics, especially when medicines are mixed, can result in analgesic nephropathy (kidney damage). Acetaminophen and NSAIDs like aspirin or ibuprofen taken over a long duration can be responsible for this type of damage to the inner structures of the organ. When self-medicating and without following doctor's guidance, this is more likely to occur. An opioid analgesic may cause drowsiness or dizziness; other effects can include constipation, vomiting, blood pressure changes, or confusion, and even hallucinations. Driving when taking an opioid is not advised. Serious side effects are equivalent to other analgesics, in addition to the increased risk of tolerance and addiction.

Severe side effects often come about because of the mixture of medicines or taking more than the recommended daily dosage for a few years. A medical doctor will take into account the patient's history and other prescriptions in order to best ascertain the appropriate medicinal combination, where relevant. The reaction to incorrect usage or interactions with other medicines may be experienced immediately, or the damage may set in on an incremental basis. Interactions with other drugs or alcohol can be detrimental or fatal.

—*Leah Jacob, MA*

References

"Analgesics." *Arthritis Foundation*, www.arthritis.org/living-with-arthritis/treatments/medication/drug-guide/drug-class/analgesics.php.

Cazacu, Irina, et al. "Safety Issues of Current Analgesics: an Update." *Medicine and Pharmacy Reports*, vol. 88, no. 2, 15 Apr. 2015, pp. 128–136., doi:10.15386/cjmed-413.

Dugdale, David C. "Over-the-Counter Pain Relievers." *MedlinePlus*, U.S. National Library of Medicine, 12 Oct. 2018, medlineplus.gov/ency/article/002123.htm.

Yaksh, Tony L., et al. "Development of New Analgesics: An Answer to Opioid Epidemic." *Trends in Pharmacological Sciences*, vol. 39, no. 12, 1 Dec. 2018, pp. 1000–1002., doi:10.1016/j.tips.2018.10.003.

■ Anesthesia

CATEGORY: Class of Drug
ANATOMY OR SYSTEM AFFECTED: Brain, muscles, musculoskeletal system, nerves, nervous system, psychic-emotional system, skin, spine
SPECIALTIES AND RELATED FIELDS: Anesthesiology, critical care, dentistry, emergency medicine, general surgery, neurology, ophthalmology

KEY TERMS

- *epidural anesthesia*: anesthesia caused by injecting a local anesthetic between the vertebra and beneath the ligamentum flavum into the extradural space; also known as extradural anesthesia
- *local anesthesia*: anesthesia produced by injecting a local anesthetic solution directly into the tissues; also known as local block
- *local anesthetics*: drugs that produce a reversible blockade of nerve impulse conduction
- *regional anesthesia*: insensibility caused by the interruption of nerve conduction in a region of the body
- *spinal anesthesia*: anesthesia produced by injecting a local anesthetic around the spinal cord; also known as subarachnoid block

Indications and Procedures

Anesthetics are primarily used to prevent pain during surgical operations, though they are also used to reduce fear, relax tissues, and prevent a sympathetic nervous system response to surgery. Some believe, erroneously, that being "put to sleep" with a general anesthetic is the only way an operation can be performed pain-free.

General anesthesia is a type of anesthesia that causes total unconsciousness and affects the entire body. Regional anesthesia, on the other hand, does not cause unconsciousness but allows surgery to be performed without pain by producing loss of sensation in a region of the body through the interruption of nerve-impulse transmission from the area to be incised.

General anesthetics produce a neurophysiological state characterized by five primary effects: (1) unconsciousness, (2) amnesia, (3) analgesia, (4) inhibition of autonomic reflexes, and (5) skeletal muscle relaxation. No general anesthetic can

General Anesthetics		
Anesthetic	*Inhaled or intravenous (IV)*	*Comments*
Nitrous oxide	Inhaled	Gaseous anesthetic, incomplete anesthetic, rapid onset and recovery
Desflurane	Inhaled	Volatile anesthetic, low volatility; pungent, rapid recovery
Svoflurane	Inhaled	Volatile anesthetic, rapid onset and recovery
Isoflurane	Inhaled	Volatile anesthetic, medium rate of onset and recovery
Enflurane	Inhaled	Volatile anesthetic, medium rate of onset and recovery
Halothane	Inhaled	Volatile anesthetic, medium rate of onset and recovery
Dexmedetomindine	IV	Used for short-term sedation
Diazepam	IV	Barbiturate, intermediate-acting, has muscle-relaxation effects
Etomidate	IV	Minimal effects on heart rate and blood pressure, rapid recovery
Ketamine	IV	Analgesic activity, multiple modes of administration are possible
Lorazepam	IV	Barbiturate, slow onset and prolonged duration
Methohexital	IV	Barbiturate, short-acting and rapid onset of action
Midazolam	IV	Barbiturate, rapid onset but slow recovery
Propofol	IV	Rapidly turned over, fast recovery, well tolerated
Fospropofol	IV	Prodrug, converted to propofol in body, tends to cause paresthesias (including burning, tingling, stinging) and/or pruritus in the perineal region
Thiopental	IV	Rapid-onset, short-acting barbiturate

achieve all five of these primary effects by itself. Thus, patients receive a cocktail of general anesthetics drugs that are delivered both intravenously and by inhalation.

The goal is to induce rapid, smooth loss of consciousness that can be rapidly reversed and is safe. The composition of the anesthetic cocktail is determined by the type of procedure to be performed. For example, for minor superficial surgeries or invasive diagnostic procedures, oral or IV sedatives are administered in combination with local anesthetics (monitored anesthesia care). This technique retains the patient's ability to breathe on his/her own and respond to verbal commands. For more invasive surgical procedures, anesthesia can begin with oral or parenteral benzodiazepines prior to surgery, followed by intravenous anesthetics, such as thiopental or propofol to induce unconsciousness, which can be maintained during surgery with a combination of inhaled or intravenous drugs.

General anesthetics target neurons in the central nervous system. These drugs usually affect the connection between neurons known as the synapse. When neurons connect, one neuron is downstream of the synapse (presynaptic) and the other is upstream of the synapse (postsynaptic). In some cases, the presynaptic neuron generates stimulatory signals that activate the postsynaptic neurons. In other cases, the presynaptic neuron provides inhibitory signals that disable the postsynaptic neuron. General anesthetics seem to increase the inhibitory signals from presynaptic neurons to postsynaptic neurons or diminish the excitatory signals. The primary components of inhibitory signals include chloride ion channels (bound by the neurotransmitters gamma-aminobutyric acid or GABA and glycine) and potassium ion channels. The primary excitatory ion channels include those activated by acetylcholine, excitatory amino acids, and serotonin. All these ion channels are potential targets of general anesthetics. Benzodiazepines, for example, bind to GABA channels and potentiate their activity, inhibiting postsynaptic neurons. See the table below for examples of general anesthetics.

In regional anesthesia, the anesthetic agents are deposited either on the surface of the area to be anesthetized or near a specific nerve or pathway that lies between the area and receptors for painful stimuli that are part of the central nervous system. Thus, transmission of noxious stimuli to the brain is effectively blocked, allowing a surgical procedure to be performed without the patient feeling pain. Regional anesthesia is frequently referred to as regional nerve blockade.

Local anesthetics operate in several ways. Those injected near the nerves diffuse into the nerves and bind to receptors on their membranes. Once in the nerve sheath, local anesthetic agents prevent sodium from moving into the nerve interior by physically occluding sodium channels. Impulses traveling from the surgical area to the central nervous system are blocked so that nerves transmitting touch, temperature, and pain sensation are temporarily interrupted. Nerve impulses traveling from the central nervous system to the surgical area are also blocked, leading to an interruption of motor power to the surgical area. The number of nerves blocked depends on where the local anesthetic is deposited.

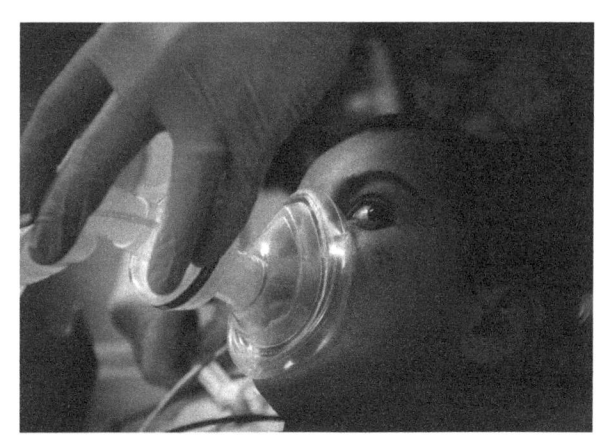

A child being prepared to go under general anesthesia. (ISAF Photo by U.S. Air Force Senior Airman Rylan K. Albright)

The duration of the nerve blockade depends on the type and dosage of local anesthetic injected as well as on the technique utilized. Diffusion of the local anesthetic out of the nerve and its absorption into the vascular bed causes the effect of the local anesthetic to be terminated. The blood flowing around the nerve removes the drug from the area. Decreasing the flow of blood to the area by adding vasoconstricting agents such as epinephrine to the local anesthetic to be injected is a common method used to prolong the duration of the nerve block.

Local anesthetics are weak bases whose structure consists of an aromatic moiety connected to a substituted amine through an ester or amide linkage. The two major families of local anesthetics are the amino amides and the amino esters. The clinical differences between the ester and amide local anesthetics involve their potential for producing adverse side effects and the mechanisms by which they are metabolized. Local anesthetics are also classified based on their potency and duration of action: a short duration of action (thirty to forty-five minutes), an intermediate duration of action (one to two hours), or a long duration of action (four to eight hours). The range in duration of nerve blockade is attributable primarily to two factors: the concentration of the drug used and the addition of vasoconstricting agents, such as epinephrine. Local anesthetics are listed in the table below.

Local and regional anesthetics are excellent ways of supplying surgical and postoperative analgesia (pain control). Local anesthetics are now being given in combination with narcotic

Local Anesthetics		
Drug	Potency relative to procaine	Duration
Procaine (Novocain)	1	Short
Prilocaine	2	Short
Chloroprocaine	2	Short
Tetracaine (Pontocaine)	8	Long
Benzocaine	Surface use only	
Lidocaine (Xylocaine)	4	Medium
Mepivacaine (Carbocaine, isocaine)	2	Medium
Bupivacaine (Marcaine) & Levobupivacaine (Charaxine)	8	Long
Ropivacaine	8	Long

analgesics (painkillers). Narcotics are almost always given in combination with local anesthetics and bind to narcotic receptors in the area and provide analgesia (pain relief) without interrupting nerve transmission. The combination of local anesthetic agents with narcotics is gaining popularity in postoperative pain control; the patient can experience longer durations of pain relief while avoiding the systemic side effects of intravenously administered narcotics.

There are six categories of regional anesthesia: topical anesthesia, local block and field block, nerve block, intravenous (IV) neural blockade, subarachnoid block (spinal anesthesia), and epidural anesthesia, including caudal block. These are primarily differentiated based on the size of the region that is anesthetized and the duration of the neural blockade.

Topical anesthesia. In this technique, also known as surface anesthesia, an anesthetic drug is sprayed or spread onto the area to be desensitized. This short-acting form of anesthesia blocks nerve endings in the skin as well as mucous membranes, such as those of the nasopharynx (nose and throat), mouth, rectum, and vagina. Topical anesthesia is employed in minor procedures such as eye or rectal examinations. The advantages of topical anesthesia include quick onset of action, ease of administration, and general nontoxicity. Disadvantages include lack of deeper-tissue anesthesia and lack of tissue relaxation. A frequently used topical anesthetic is the drug benzocaine, often utilized for the treatment of traumatic tissue pain secondary to sunburn.

Local blocks and field blocks. In local blocks, the local anesthetic is injected with a needle and syringe into the skin and tissues of an area to be incised. As a result, the nerves around the incision are blocked. Local blocks are used in short, minor operations and prior to the insertion of intravenous or spinal needles. A field block is another type of local block. In a field block, the area surrounding the incision is also injected with local anesthetics, preventing impulses transmitted from a larger area from reaching the central nervous system.

Nerve blocks. Nerve blocks interrupt the transmission of nerve impulses by nerves or by bundles of nerves that are further removed from the surgical site. Nerve blocks may be used to anesthetize a single finger or toe (digital nerve block), a foot (ankle block) or hand, or an entire arm (axillary, supraclavicular, and interscalene blocks) or leg (leg block). In each type of neural blockade, the physician or nurse anesthetist injects local anesthetic agents around the major nerves that supply the area to be incised. The number of injections depends on the location of the nerves to be blocked.

Some nerves may be blocked individually. An arm block can be accomplished by a single injection of a larger volume of local anesthetic into the axillary sheath or between the middle and anterior scalene muscles in the neck. Upper extremity blocks can be performed with a single injection because the brachial plexus (the nerves innervating the arm) is collectively encased in a sheath. Distal to the axillary area, the nerves innervating the arm are no longer encased in a sheath. Consequently, separate injections of the radial, median, and ulnar nerves are required to block the arm at the elbow or wrist.

Intercostal nerveblocks. Intercostal nerves innervate the outer and inner surfaces of the abdominal wall. Intercostal nerve blockade is utilized for postoperative pain control following thoracic or upper abdominal surgeries. A sterile needle is inserted into the skin over the lower margin of the rib along

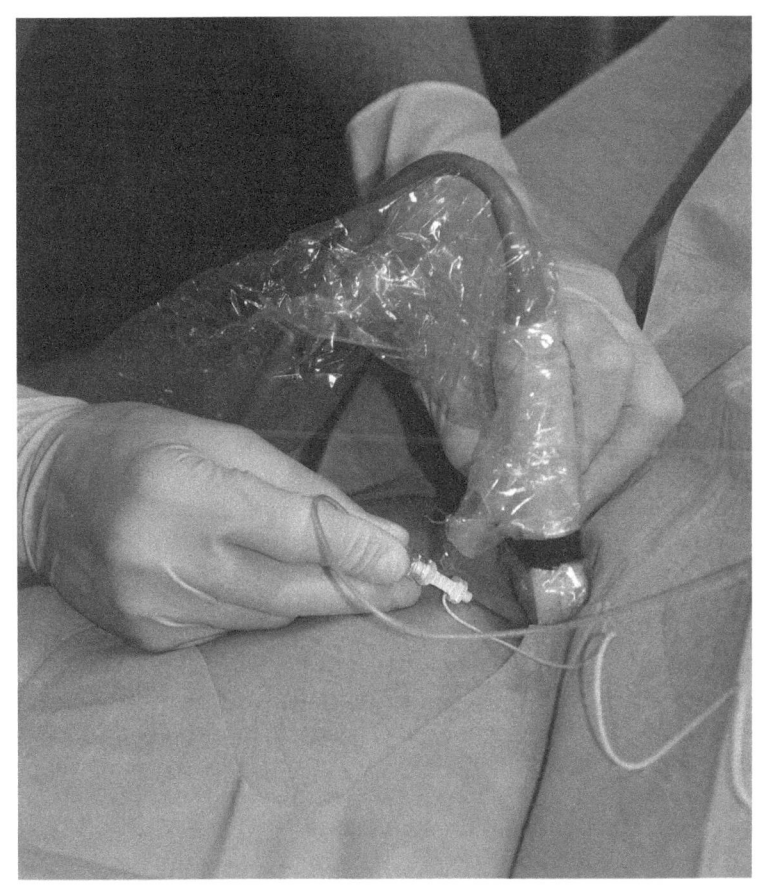

Sonography guided femoral nerve block. (Philipp N. via Wikimedia Commons)

the posterior axillary line. The needle is then directed toward the intercostal groove located inferior to the rib. A local anesthetic is injected into the intercostal space containing the intercostal nerve, vein, and artery. The anesthetic lasts from six to twelve hours and may be prolonged by the addition of epinephrine to the solution.

Intravenous neural blockade. Intravenous (IV) neural blockade was discovered by August Bier in 1908; he was also the first to routinely utilize spinal anesthesia. Today, IV regional neural blockade is also referred to as Bier blockade. With Bier blockade, the local anesthetic agent is injected into a leg or arm vein just below a tourniquet. Inflation of the tourniquet prevents the local anesthetic from being released into general circulation. This local anesthetic, thus contained in the extremity, travels to the major nerves in the limb and blocks neural transmission. The duration of the neural blockade is governed by the length of time that the tourniquet is inflated. Once the tourniquet is deflated, the local anesthetic enters the systemic circulation, the neural blockade recedes, and normal sensation and power to the extremity are rapidly returned. Intravenous regional blockade of the extremities has many advantages: ease of performance, rapid onset, controllable duration of action, and rapid recovery. The disadvantages include possible tourniquet discomfort, possible reaction to the local anesthetic when it is released into general circulation, and rapid return of sensation, including pain, upon removal of the tourniquet.

Spinal anesthesia. Spinal anesthesia, also called subarachnoid block, is a commonly utilized form of anesthesia. Spinal anesthesia can be used for almost any type of surgical procedure below the umbilicus, such as surgical procedures performed on the legs and hips, hysterectomies, appendectomies, and cesarean sections.

A lumbar puncture (spinal tap) is performed in the lower back, usually between the second and third lumbar vertebrae, the third and fourth lumbar vertebrae, or the fifth lumbar and first sacral vertebrae. The patient is placed on his or her side in a flexed position (or sometimes in a sitting position). The physician or nurse anesthetist, wearing sterile gloves, prepares the skin in the area to be punctured with a skin antiseptic, such as betadine, and drapes the area with a sterile towel. The anesthetist then infiltrates the area of the puncture with lidocaine, producing a local block. Once the skin is anesthetized, a needle is inserted through the intraspinous space into the subarachnoid space. The needle passes through the supraspinous ligament, intraspinous ligament, and ligamentum flavum. Proper placement of the needle is identified through an observation of freely flowing spinal fluid. A local anesthetic agent is then injected into the spinal fluid. Cerebrospinal fluid (CSF) is a clear, colorless ultrafiltrate of the blood that fills the subarachnoid space. The total volume of CSF is 100 to 150 milliliters; the volume contained in the subarachnoid space is 25 to 35 milliliters.

Once injected into the subarachnoid CSF, the local anesthetic agent spreads in both a cephalad (toward the head and anterior) and caudad (toward the feet and posterior) direction. Factors influencing this spread include the dose and volume of the agent used, patient position, and the specific gravity (weight) of the anesthetic solution relative to the CSF. One of three types of solutions—isobaric, hypobaric, or hyperbaric—can be used. Hyperbaric solutions are heavier than CSF; thus, placing the patient in Trendelenburg's position (with the head tilted downward) will increase the cephalad spread of the anesthetic. With the patient in Trendelenburg's position, hypobaric solutions (with a specific gravity less than that of CSF) of local anesthetic agents spread caudally. Spread of the local anesthetic in the subarachnoid space usually stops (fixation) within five to thirty-five minutes after injection. After fixation has occurred, patient position changes will not influence the spread of local anesthetic or the subsequent level of anesthesia. Within minutes after a subarachnoid injection of a local anesthetic, patients experience a warm sensation in their lower extremities, followed by a loss of sensation and inability to move the legs. The duration of the neural blockade is dependent on the type of local anesthetic utilized, as well as the addition of any vasoconstrictor.

Epidural anesthesia and caudal block. Like spinal anesthesia, epidural blockade can be used for the prevention of pain during surgery. It can also be used to relieve pain after surgery, chronic pain, or labor pains; to supplement a light general anesthetic; and to diagnose and treat autonomic nervous system dysfunction. The technique is excellent for operations performed on the lower abdomen, pelvis, and perineum; for laminectomies; and in obstetrics for the relief of labor pains.

As with spinal anesthesia, the patient is placed on his or her side in a flexed position (or sometimes in a sitting position). The physician or nurse anesthetist, wearing sterile gloves, prepares the skin around the puncture with an antiseptic such as betadine and drapes the area with a sterile towel. The anesthetist infiltrates the area of the puncture with lidocaine, producing a local block. Once the skin is anesthetized, an epidural needle is inserted between the appropriate lumbar vertebrae (occasionally between thoracic vertebrae). With epidural blockade, however, the needle is not advanced into the subarachnoid space. Instead, needle advancement is terminated when the needle tip is in the epidural space. Thus, the dura is not penetrated as in spinal anesthesia, and postdural puncture headache does not occur with a properly placed epidural needle. Once the epidural space has been identified, local anesthetic agents (in larger volumes than utilized with subarachnoid anesthesia) are injected through the needle or through a small catheter threaded through the needle. Placement of a catheter through the needle allows reinjection to take place without subsequent needle punctures. This is particularly desirable for long surgeries, postoperative pain control, and the control of labor pains. Local anesthetic agents injected through a catheter for postoperative or labor pain control are usually given at lesser concentrations so that nerve motor fibers are not interrupted.

Caudal block is another type of epidural anesthesia. In this case, the needle (with or without a catheter) is placed through the sacrococcygeal ligament just superior to the coccyx. The technique is gaining popularity as an adjunct to general anesthesia in children for postoperative pain control.

Uses and Complications

Regional anesthesia has several advantages over general anesthesia. The first is ease of administration. The agents used are injectable, the equipment required is minimal, and the costs are reasonable. Second is the relative safety of the technique. A localized area of the body can be operated upon without the patient experiencing most of the undesirable and potentially harmful side effects of general anesthesia, such as loss of consciousness and the depression of the cardiovascular and respiratory systems. In addition, advantages include excellent muscle relaxation, which is often required to facilitate surgical procedures; improved peripheral blood flow; an antithrombotic effect; a decreased loss of blood in some cases; and postoperative pain relief. Regional anesthesia is also utilized in combination with general anesthesia to increase the benefits of both while decreasing adverse side effects.

Yet regional anesthesia has some disadvantages. First, some operations, such as major surgical procedures involving the brain, heart, and lungs, cannot be performed under regional anesthesia. Second, some patients may be allergic to the local anesthetics. Local anesthetics of the amino ester type may result in allergic reactions because of the metabolite p-aminobenzoic acid. Local anesthetics of the amino amide class are essentially devoid of allergic potential. Many anesthetic solutions, however, contain methylparaben as a preservative, and this compound can produce an allergic reaction in persons sensitive to p-aminobenzoic acid. Third, some patients desire to be unaware of the operation and may be anxious at the thought of being "awake." They erroneously believe that the total unconsciousness produced by general anesthesia is the only method to produce unawareness. In most cases, patients who receive a regional anesthetic also receive intravenous sedation to decrease their level of awareness. Subsequently, many patients report having no recollection whatsoever of the surgical procedure. In addition, the advantages of spinal anesthesia, one of the most popular types of regional anesthesia, far outweigh the disadvantages, which include hypotension, a high required dosage of anesthesia, and postdural puncture headache. Hypotension is treated with intravenous fluids and, if necessary, the administration of vasoconstricting drugs. Postdural puncture headache (spinal headache) is thought to be caused from a loss of spinal fluid (which cushions the brain) through the dural hole produced by the spinal needle. Advances in the technique of spinal anesthesia administration, including the use of very small needles introduced in a manner that separates the dural fibers, have significantly decreased the incidence of postdural puncture headache. Should this complication arise, however, it is treated with analgesics, intravenous fluids, and, if necessary, an injection of saline (or a sample of the patient's own blood) around the site of the dural puncture, effectively "patching" the dural hole created by the spinal needle.

Perspective and Prospects
The first successful demonstration of anesthesia (diethyl ether) by William T. G. Morton occurred in 1846 at the Massachusetts General Hospital. The discovery of anesthesia occurred prior to the discovery of germ theory and aseptic techniques. Therefore, although anesthesia made surgery painless in the early nineteenth century, there was still a high rate of surgical morbidity and mortality because of infection. In the late 1860s, germ theory had evolved from the work of Robert Koch and Louis Pasteur, and Joseph Lister's subsequent work on principles of asepsis contributed significantly to a decline in surgical mortality from infection by the late 1880s. There remained, however, a high surgical mortality rate caused by anesthesia. At that time, general anesthetic agents were commonly utilized, and few, if any, practitioners specialized in the administration of anesthesia.

Regional anesthesia was first utilized in 1884 when a German physician named Carl Koller performed an operation to correct glaucoma using a local anesthetic. In this case, cocaine, an alkaloid obtained from the coca plant, was instilled into the eye. This successful operation brought significant acceptance to the principle of local anesthesia. The great advantage of local anesthesia was that it anesthetized only the part of the body on which the operation was to be performed. Patients could be spared the depressive effects of general anesthesia, especially on the cardiovascular and respiratory systems. By the 1930s, various regional anesthesia techniques had been developed, including subarachnoid block (spinal anesthesia), lumbar epidural, caudal epidural, intravenous, and brachial plexus anesthesia. The occurrence of these regional anesthetic techniques, along with the evolution of local anesthetic agents, allowed anesthetists to tailor the type and duration of regional anesthesia to the requirements of each patient. Thus, regional anesthesia has become a popular choice among surgeons, anesthetists, and patients.
—*Maura S. McAuliffe*
—*Michael A. Buratovich, PhD*

References
Cousins, Michael J., P. O. Bridenbaugh, et al., eds. *Neural Blockade in Clinical Anesthesia and Management of Pain*. 4th ed. J. B. Lippincott, 2008.
"General Anesthesia—Interactive Tutorial." Medline Plus, 2013. Katz, Jordan. *Atlas of Regional Anesthesia*. 4th ed. Appleton & Lange, 2010.
Hines, Roberta L., and Katherine Marschall. *Stoelting's Anesthesia and Co-Existing Disease*, 7th ed. Elsevier, 2017.
Kellicker, Patricia. "General Anesthesia." *Health Library*, 10 Sept. 2012.
Miller, Scott, and David Zieve. "Spinal and Epidural Anesthesia." *Medline Plus*, 28 Mar. 2011.
Sweeney, Frank. *The Anesthesia Fact Book: Everything You Need to Know Before Surgery*. Perseus, 2003.

Anti-inflammatory drugs

CATEGORY: Class of Drug
ANATOMY OR SYSTEM AFFECTED: All
SPECIALTIES AND RELATED FIELDS: Dermatology, endocrinology, family medicine, internal medicine, ophthalmology, orthopedics, otorhinolaryngology, rheumatology, vascular medicine.

KEY TERMS

- *arthritis*: a painful condition that involves inflammation of one or more joints
- *bursitis*: inflammation of the sac of lubricating fluid located between joints
- *hormone*: a substance made by the body that travels through the bloodstream to reach its target organ and have its effect
- *inflammation*: the body's response to injury that may include redness, pain, swelling, and warmth in the affected area
- *salicylates*: a group of drugs (including aspirin) derived from salicylic acid, used to relieve pain, reduce inflammation, and lower fever
- *steroids*: a class of hormones produced by the adrenal glands; can also be made synthetically
- *tendinitis*: inflammation of a tendon, a tough band of tissue that connects muscle to bone

Indications

Nonsteroidal anti-inflammatory drugs (NSAIDs), often referred to as aspirin, are utilized to relieve painful conditions such as arthritis, bursitis, gout, menstrual cramps, tendinitis, sprains, and strains. Additionally, aspirin is commonly prescribed to patients who have had one myocardial infarction (heart attack) to decrease the risk of a second. While some NSAIDs require a prescription, many are sold over the counter. Some common NSAIDs, with brand names in parentheses, are diclofenac (Voltaren), etodolac (Lodine), flurbiprofen (Ansaid), ibuprofen (Motrin, Advil, Rufen, Nuprin), nabumetone (Relafen), naproxen (Naprosyn or Aleve), and oxaprozin (Daypro). These drugs can come in the form of capsules, caplets, tablets, liquids, and suppositories.

Corticosteroids make up the second group of anti-inflammatory drugs used to ameliorate the symptoms associated with conditions such as asthma, lupus, arthritis, and allergic reactions. Like NSAIDs, corticosteroids are available in various forms including inhalants, creams, ointments, and oral (systemic) medications. Common corticosteroids are beclomethasone (Beconase, Vancensase, Vanceril), betamethosone (Diprolene, Lotrisone), hydrocortisone, mometasone (Elocon), prednisone (Deltasone, Orasone), and triamcinolone (Azmacort, Nasacort).

Complications

Although used across many medical specialties and for a plethora of reasons, NSAIDs are not without their dangers. Common side effects are mild and can include stomach pains or cramps, nausea, vomiting, indigestion, headache, and dizziness. Despite these relatively mild side effects, individuals currently taking other medications, women who are pregnant or who plan to become pregnant, women who are breastfeeding, and persons with stomach or intestinal problems, liver disease, heart disease, high blood pressure, bleeding diseases, diabetes, Parkinson's disease, or epilepsy should consult their physicians prior to taking NSAIDs. While side effects are rare, some can be life-threatening. In fact, research has shown that some NSAIDs can increase the risk of strokes and heart attacks. Any feelings of tightness in the chest, irregular heartbeat, swelling, or fainting are reasons to discontinue the use of NSAIDs and consult a physician. It is important to note that children should not be given aspirin if they are recovering from a viral infection as it can lead to Reye's syndrome -a potentially fatal condition that results in swelling of the liver and brain.

That said, there is research underway for new, anti-inflammatory painkillers that elicit fewer side effects. One example is licofelone, an NSAID that can inhibit both cyclooxygenase 1 and 2 (COX-1 and COX-2) as well as lipoxygenase (LOX), three of the enzymes involved in inflammation pathways. Licofelone is being tested on its ability to help in osteoarthritis management and is reported to be gentler on the stomach.

Corticosteroid therapy produces dramatic, immediate relief from pain, swelling, and inflammation due to arthritis. Small amounts of steroid may be injected directly into the inflamed joint or they can be taken by mouth. However, the beneficial effects tend to be temporary and long-term use can lead to the development of cataracts, increased blood sugar which can worsen a person's diabetes, reduced resistance to infections, as well as gastrointestinal ulcers and bleeding. It follows that the advent of other highly effective alternatives has led to less frequent use of steroids in the setting of arthritis.

Additionally, corticosteroids are a common treatment for persons suffering from more serious asthmatic conditions or when treatment with bronchodilators has not proven effective. Corticosteroids, which are not bronchodilators and do not open the airways, instead work to reduce inflammation to allow the lungs to function properly. They should be used regularly and for the complete course as prescribed to achieve full benefits. Corticosteroids may be sprayed into the nose for relief of stuffy nose, irritation, hay fever, or other allergies, while oral corticosteroids are used primarily for the prevention of asthma attacks.

Ophthalmic anti-inflammatory medicines can be used to reduce problems that occur during or following eye surgery, by alleviating eye inflammation. These can be obtained only with a doctor's prescription. Corticosteroids also serve to relieve inflammation of the temporal arteries, the blood vessels that run along the temples. Inflammation here can disrupt the blood supply and result in blindness, partial loss of vision, strokes, and even heart attacks.

Individuals who have medical conditions such as allergies, diabetes, pregnancy, osteoporosis, glaucoma, infections, thyroid problems, liver disease, kidney disease, heart disease, or high blood pressure should discuss these conditions with their physician before taking corticosteroids. If corticosteroids are used for a short time, development of side effects is rare. However, breathing problems or tightness in the chest, pain, rash, swelling, extreme exhaustion, irregular heartbeat, or wounds that do not heal should be reported to a physician. Steroids should not be stopped abruptly without consulting a physician, especially if the steroids have been taken for a long time, as the body requires a weaning process to adapt.

Perspective and Prospects

The bark of the willow tree, which contains salicylates, was known in 18th Century England to reduce fever and aches. In 1876, the first successful treatment of acute arthritis with sodium salicylate (aspirin) was reported. In the 1970s, pharmacologist John Vane amassed evidence of the effectiveness of NSAIDs.

The earliest demonstration of the importance of corticosteroids as anti-inflammatory agents occurred in the 1940s regarding rheumatoid arthritis. The challenge of corticosteroid therapy lies in achieving the desired results with a minimum of side effects.

—*Mary Hurd*
—*Lillian Dominguez, MD*

References

Davis, Jennifer S, et al. "Use of Non-Steroidal Anti-Inflammatory Drugs in US Adults: Changes over Time and by Demographic." *Open Heart*, vol. 4, no. 1, 2017, doi:10.1136/openhrt-2016-000550.

Liska, Ken. Drugs and the Human Body, with Implications for Society. 8th ed. Pearson/Prentice Hall, 2009.

Shmerling, Robert H. "Are You Taking Too Much Anti-Inflammatory Medication?" *Harvard Health Blog*, 23 Mar. 2018, www.health.harvard.edu/blog/are-you-taking-too-much-anti-inflammatory-medication-2018040213540.

Szalay, Jessie. "What Is Inflammation?" *LiveScience*, 19 Oct. 2018, www.livescience.com/52344-inflammation.html.

Yaksh, Tony L., et al. "Development of New Analgesics: An Answer to Opioid Epidemic." *Trends in Pharmacological Sciences*, vol. 39, no. 12, 1 Dec. 2018, pp. 1000–1002., doi:10.1016/j.tips.2018.10.003.

■ Anti-nausea medications

CATEGORY: Class of Drug
ALSO KNOWN AS: Antiemetics
ANATOMY OR SYSTEM AFFECTED: Gastrointestinal system

KEY TERMS

- *acathisia*: a condition of severe restlessness, in which the very thought of sitting still causes strong feelings of anxiety
- *cannabinoids*: compounds having molecular structures related to those of the compounds isolated from cannabis
- *dystonia*: prolonged periods of unusual muscle contractions exhibiting as limb twistings, repetitive movements, abnormal postures, or rhythmic jerks

Anti-nausea agents, or antiemetics, encompass a range of drug classes that act on the peripheral and central nervous systems to prevent nausea and vomiting. In patients with cancer, antiemetics are used to control acute, delayed, and anticipatory nausea and vomiting that result from chemotherapy.

Introduction

Nausea and vomiting are unpleasant, debilitating conditions even at the best of times. Few people have not experienced "motion sickness" while traveling or doing the rides at an amusement park, which are generally thought of as enjoyable pastimes. Illnesses such as "the flu" and food poisoning, not to mention "the morning after," are typically accompanied by violent bouts of vomiting. Pregnant women often experience "morning sickness." Poisoning is another frequent cause of nausea and vomiting, and the relationship between poisoning and certain courses of chemotherapy cannot be overlooked. Nausea and vomiting due to "simple" causes can generally be treated in a short time with rest and over-the-counter anti-nausea medications, but nausea and vomiting resulting from chemotherapy require a more stringent approach.

Anti-nausea medications are indirectly used in the treatment of many cancers to control nausea and vomiting associated with many chemotherapy regimens. The medications comprise a large group of different compound classes, including serotonin-3 antagonists, substituted benzamides, corticosteroids, phenothiazines, benzodiazepines, butyrophenones, cannabinoids, and neurokinin-1 antagonists. These may be administered to inpatients and outpatients as oral tablets, capsules, or liquids; as intravenous or solutions; or as rectal suppositories.

How Anti-nausea Medications Work

Nausea and vomiting, or emesis, are the most common chemotherapy-associated toxicities, affecting more than 75 percent of patients, especially with the development of combination regimens. The effective use of anti-nausea agents to improve chemotherapy tolerance is one of the most important advances of supportive cancer care. Among the first of agents to deter emesis was metoclopramide, a substituted benzamide that acts as a dopamine receptor antagonist and, at higher doses, as an additional serotonin receptor antagonist. Although the exact mechanisms of nausea and vomiting reflexes have not been determined, neurotransmitter blockade at dopaminergic, serotonergic, neurokinin-1, and other receptors in the central nervous system or peripherally in the gastrointestinal tract successfully controls the reactions. Like metoclopramide, phenothiazines such as chlorpromazine, and butyrophenones such as haloperidol, also prevent nausea and vomiting by dopaminergic blockade. Dopamine antagonism from these three subclasses provides relief of moderate emesis.

The more recently developed serotonin-3 (5HT-3) receptor antagonists work peripherally, especially in

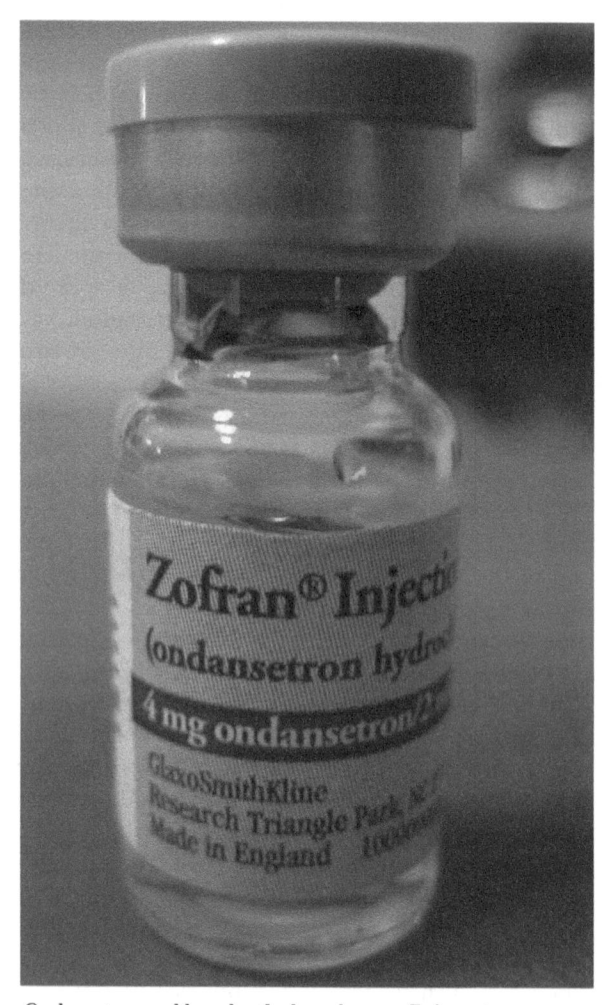

Ondansetron, sold under the brand name Zofran, is a common antiemetic. It is often used to treat morning sickness in pregnant women. (Intropin via Wikimedia Commons)

the small intestine, and are extremely effective for the treatment and prevention of acute emesis. Ondansetron, granisetron, and dolasetron are equivalent in efficacy and may provide total receptor blockade, as evidenced by their dose-related efficacy plateaus. *Palonosetron*, a newer agent, is longer acting than others in the subclass. Because acute emesis is associated with peripheral control and delayed emesis is associated with central control, 5HT-3 antagonists are more effective in treating acute nausea and vomiting, which occurs in the first twenty-four hours after chemotherapy is administered.

Benzodiazepines such as lorazepam have some activity by blocking cortical input to the emetic center but are more useful for their sedative and anxiolytic effects, which make the agents ideal for combination regimens. In addition, these drugs induce retrograde amnesia, which is successful in preventing anticipatory nausea and vomiting that may occur with repeat chemotherapy administration.

Neurokinin-1 (NK-1) receptors are more recently studied targets of nausea mechanisms; the only currently approved agent in the NK-1 antagonist class is aprepitant. Because NK-1 mediates substance P activation of NK-1 receptors in the brainstem, aprepitant's NK-1 receptor antagonism is useful for the treatment of delayed emesis, which is more centrally mediated. Although its efficacy alone is not yet confirmed, aprepitant successfully prevents acute and delayed nausea and vomiting when combined with serotonin antagonists and corticosteroids.

Corticosteroids, especially dexamethasone, methylprednisolone, and prednisone, have a confirmed effect, alone or in combination, against moderate nausea and vomiting, despite an unknown mechanism of action and a lack of receptor blockade. Corticosteroids are often the second drug in a combination regimen with dopamine, serotonin, or NK-1 receptor antagonists.

Lastly, cannabinoids such as dronabinol act centrally with psychotropic activity to provide limited but affirmed anti-nausea activity. They can be used for patients with moderate emesis and poor tolerance or response to other agents or for patients who need control of breakthrough pain.

Side Effects

Each subclass of anti-nausea agents is associated with different side effects; successful combination regimens provide greater efficacy without overlapping drug toxicities. Metoclopramide side effects are primarily related to dopamine antagonism and include extrapyramidal reactions, including acute dystonic reactions. Acathisia, or restlessness, is common and may persist for hours. Drowsiness and diarrhea are also possible. Phenothiazines and butyrophenones also cause dopamine-related drowsiness, diarrhea, and extrapyramidal reactions. In addition, constipation, dizziness, and hypotension have been noted. Lorazepam is associated with sedation in addition to amnesia, confusion, transient enuresis, and blurred vision. Serotonin antagonists all have similar side effects of mild to moderate headache in 20 to 30 percent of patients and mild, uncommon occurrences of constipation or diarrhea. Corticosteroids may cause insomnia, hyperglycemia, gastrointestinal upset, and, rarely, psychosis. NK-1 antagonism leads to fatigue, dizziness, headache, and gastrointestinal disturbances. Side effects of dronabinol include dysphoria, hallucinations, dizziness, dry mouth, sedation, and disorientation.

—*Nicole M. Van Hoey, PharmD*

References

Cafasso, Jacqueline, and Alan Carter. "Antiemetic Drugs." *Healthline*, 12 June 2017, www.healthline.com/health/antiemetic-drugs-list.

Check, Devon K., and Ethan M. Basch. "Appropriate Use of Antiemetics to Prevent Chemotherapy-Induced Nausea and Vomiting." *JAMA Oncology*, vol. 3, no. 3, 1 Mar. 2017, pp. 307–309., doi:10.1001/jamaoncol.2016.2616.

Encinosa, William, and Amy J. Davidoff. "Changes in Antiemetic Overuse in Response to Choosing Wisely Recommendations." *JAMA Oncology*, vol. 3, no. 3, Mar. 2017, p. 320., doi:10.1001/jamaoncol.2016.2530.

Parker, Linda A, et al. "Regulation of Nausea and Vomiting by Cannabinoids." *British Journal of Pharmacology*, vol. 163, no. 7, 2011, pp. 1411–1422., doi:10.1111/j.1476-5381.2010.01176.x.

Sanger, Gareth J., and Paul L. R. Andrews. "A History of Drug Discovery for Treatment of Nausea and Vomiting and the Implications for Future Research." *Frontiers in Pharmacology*, vol. 9, 4 Sept. 2018, p. 913., doi:10.3389/fphar.2018.00913.

Weant, Kyle A., et al. "Antiemetic Use in the Emergency Department." *Advanced Emergency Nursing Journal*, vol. 39, no. 2, 2017, pp. 97–105., doi:10.1097/tme.0000000000000141.

■ Aspirin

CATEGORY: NSAID; Over-the-Counter
ALSO KNOWN AS: acetylsalicylic acid
ANATOMY OR SYSTEM AFFECTED: nervous system, immunological system

KEY TERMS

- *antipyretic*: a substance that reduces body temperature
- *analgesic*: a substance that reduces pain
- *cyclooxygenase*: an enzyme in the synthesis of prostaglandins and thromboxanes
- *non-steroidal anti-inflammatory drug (NSAID)*: drugs that do have the steroid structure and reduces inflammation

- *prostaglandin:* hormones synthesized by many tissues that are vasodilators and inhibitors of platelet aggregation
- *Reye's syndrome:* an encephalopathy of unknown cause but is most commonly associated with aspirin use in children
- *thromboxane:* hormones synthesized by many tissues that are vasoconstrictors and stimulators of platelet aggregation

Structure and Functions

Aspirin is the commercial name of a drug developed by Bayer in the Nineteenth Century using an extract of the bark of the willow tree. Its active ingredient is acetylsalicylic acid. There is evidence in the archaeological record showing that willow tree bark has been used for medicinal purposes as far back as 2000 BCE.

Aspirin is a non-steroidal anti-inflammatory drug (NSAID) used to treat pain, inflammation, swelling and fever. It is commonly used to treat mild to moderate aches and pain such as what one would experience in a headache or muscle cramps, to reduce fever during mild infection, to reduce inflammation such as experienced in arthritis and to reduce blood clotting. Aspirin also seems to be able to prevent the development of colorectal cancer. The most common side effects are upset stomach and stomach ulcers in adults and Reye's syndrome in children. Occasionally, more severe side effects can occur.

In 1971, John Vane determined that aspirin functions by interfering with the synthesis of prostaglandins and thromboxanes by inhibiting cyclooxygenase (COX) enzymes which are also known as prostaglandinendoperoxide synthase. Prostaglandins and thromboxanes are synthesized by COX-1 and COX-2 enzymes. Prostaglandins and thromboxanes are produced by many cells and tissues and have many functions such as raising body temperature (pyretic), stimulating local muscle contraction (pain and cramps) and stimulating platelet aggregation (blood clotting), inhibiting platelet aggregation, constricting blood vessels and dilating blood vessels.

Aspirin can potentially prevent platelet aggregation and prevent heart attack and reduce pain and fever by inhibiting thromboxane and prostaglandin synthesis through its irreversible inhibition of COX-1. While the exact scope of its benefits as a preventative of heart attacks is still subject to debate, there is general agreement that aspirin does help reduce the risk of heart attacks.

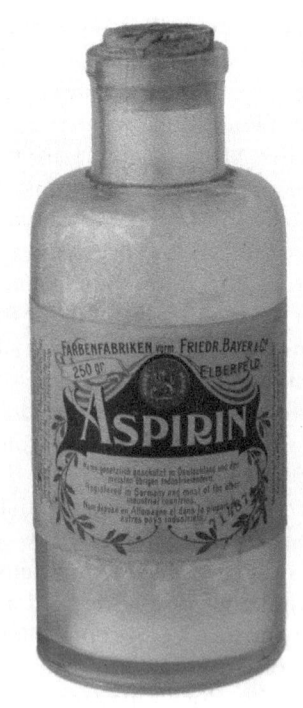

A bottle of Bayer aspirin from 1899. (Bayer AG via Wikimedia Commons)

Aspirin alters COX-2 so that it synthesizes lipoxins which have anti-inflammatory properties thus alleviating the symptoms of conditions such as rheumatoid arthritis.

Perspective and Prospects

Medical texts that date back to the ancient civilization of Sumer contain the oldest references to the beneficial effects of tea made from willow bark. The Egyptians were also aware of its beneficial properties, and the Greek and Roman civilizations were likewise familiar with it. During Europe's Middle Ages, physicians and folk healers remained aware of willow bark's uses. Finally, in the eighteenth century, scientific research was begun to determine the substance and the mechanism responsible for willow bark's effects. Several researchers were able to isolate the active ingredient and identify it as salicin by the early nineteenth century, and Charles Frederic Gerhardt synthesized a more stomach friendly "buffered" compound, acetylsalicylic acid, in 1853.

In 1899, drug manufacturer Bayer began selling its product, named Aspirin, for the treatment of fever and for pain relief. The drug quickly grew in popularity around the world, helped in part by the Spanish flu epidemic after World War I, which provided a venue for the drug to showcase its potency. Aspirin generated huge profits for drug companies all over the world, most of them producing the drug independently, without the authorization of Bayer. The trademarked name Aspirin soon came into the lexicon as the generic "aspirin," which is commonly listed as an ingredient in non-Bayer products.

Aspirin's popularity slowed in the 1950s and 1960s when alternatives to aspirin—acetaminophen and ibuprofen, most notably—entered the marketplace. These alternative drugs appealed primarily to the small portion of the population who experienced an allergic reaction or stomach irritation attributable to aspirin. In 1981, aspirin was also linked to Reye Syndrome in children, a potentially fatal complication following viral infections such as influenza or chickenpox. Aspirin came back into wide use not long after, however, as researchers noticed its ability to prevent blood clots that can block the flow of blood to various parts of the body, reducing the risk of stroke and heart attack. It is now common for doctors to prescribe one aspirin per day (often at 81mg strength, commonly called a 'baby aspirin.') for their patients who may be at risk for strokes and/or heart disease, since aspirin is unlikely to cause negative side effects and has been shown to reduce the incidence of heart attacks.

—*Scott Zimmer, MLS, MS, JD*
—*Charles L. Vigue, PhD*

References

"Aspirin and Your Heart: Many Questions, Some Answers." *Harvard Health*, 21 May 2018, www.health.harvard.edu/heart-health/aspirin-and-your-heart-many-questions-some-answers.

"Aspirin." *MedlinePlus*, U.S. National Library of Medicine, 15 Feb. 2018, medlineplus.gov/druginfo/meds/a682878.html.

"Daily Aspirin Therapy: Understand the Benefits and Risks." *Mayo Clinic*, Mayo Foundation for Medical Education and Research, 9 Jan. 2019, www.mayoclinic.org/diseases-conditions/heart-disease/in-depth/daily-aspirin-therapy/art-20046797.

Millard, Michael A., and Eduardo A. Hernandez-Vila. "What Do the Guidelines Really Say About Aspirin?" *Texas Heart Institute Journal*, vol. 45, no. 4, 2018, pp. 228–230., doi:10.14503/thij-18-6673.

Rooney, Steven M., and J.N Campbell. *How Aspirin Entered Our Medicine Cabinet*. Springer, 2017.

Williams, Craig D., et al. "Aspirin Use Among Adults in the U.S." *American Journal of Preventive Medicine*, vol. 48, no. 5, 2015, pp. 501–508., doi:10.1016/j.amepre.2014.11.005.

■ Baclofen

CATEGORY: Muscle relaxant
ALSO KNOWN AS: Lioresal
ANATOMY OR SYSTEM AFFECTED: Musculoskeletal system

History of Use

Baclofen was developed to control seizures in persons with epilepsy; however, its effectiveness for this treatment has been inadequate. Instead, baclofen has evolved into a treatment of choice for spasticity related conditions.

Baclofen was introduced as a possible addiction treatment when physician Olivier Ameisen self-treated his alcohol addiction with high-dose baclofen. His results were published in a self-case study report in the journal *Alcohol and Alcoholism* in 2005, prompting the public and the medical community to evaluate the use of baclofen to treat addiction.

Effectiveness

According to research, baclofen suppresses symptoms and cravings associated with alcohol dependence and reduces symptoms of alcohol withdrawal. Baclofen works by activating the gamma aminobutyric acid (B) receptors in the central nervous system. Baclofen is safe and effective, even in persons with alcohol-related liver damage. Baclofen possesses no misuse potential, has limited drug interactions, and causes fewer side effects than traditional medications used to treat alcohol dependence.

Baclofen is also being investigated as a treatment for cocaine- and opioid-dependence and misuse disorders. Large-scale clinical trials are needed to prove the long-term safety and effectiveness of baclofen in the treatment of substance misuse disorders.

Precautions

High doses of baclofen can cause excessive drowsiness, dizziness, psychiatric disturbances, and decreased muscle tone that may impair daily function. Overdoses of baclofen may precipitate seizures, slowed breathing, altered pupil size, and

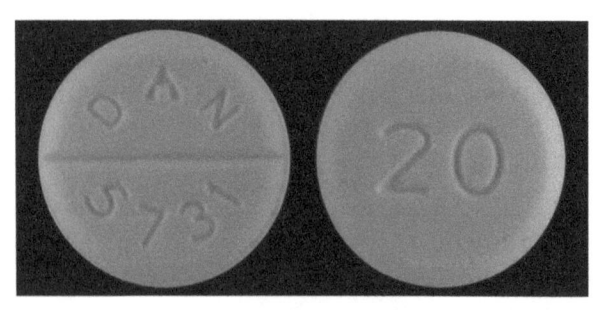

20mg of Baclofen. (National Library of Medicine)

coma. Abrupt discontinuation of baclofen can result in withdrawal symptoms, including hallucinations, disorientation, anxiety, dizziness, memory impairments, and mood disturbances.

Owing to increased publicity regarding baclofen as a potential treatment for addictions, some people have turned to illegally buying baclofen over the Internet in an attempt to control their addictions. As with any medication, baclofen should be used only under the guidance and supervision of a trained medical professional.

—*Jennifer L. Gibson, PharmD*

References

Ameisen, Olivier, and Hilary Hinzmann. *The End of My Addiction: How One Man Cured Himself of Alcoholism.* Piatkus, 2010.

"Baclofen." *MedlinePlus*, U.S. National Library of Medicine, 15 July 2017, medlineplus.gov/druginfo/meds/a682530.html.

Ghanavatian, Shirin, and Armen Derian. "Baclofen." *StatPearls*, 1 Oct. 2019.

Muzyk, Andrew, et al. "Clinical Effectiveness of Baclofen for the Treatment of Alcohol Dependence: a Review." *Clinical Pharmacology: Advances and Applications*, vol. 5, 2013, p. 99., doi:10.2147/cpaa.s32434.

■ Bismuth subsalicylate

CATEGORY: Salicylates, over the counter
ALSO KNOWN AS: Pepto-Bismol, Kaopectate, Maalox
ANATOMY OR SYSTEM EFFECTED: Gastrointestinal system

KEY TERMS
- *gastrointestinal tract*: organs which include mouth, esophagus, stomach and intestines
- *helicobacter pylori*: bacteria capable of causing intestinal damage and related symptoms

Diarrhea, nausea, and indigestion are common symptoms seen in patients who come to primary and ambulatory care clinics. Diarrhea and nausea can cause feelings of intense unease and restlessness. Many patients describe nausea as painless but miserable feeling. Diarrhea and nausea can be caused by disease processes, viruses and food poisoning. Bismuth subsalicylate effectively treats diarrhea and nausea before it leads to emesis (vomiting). Bismuth subsalicylate is used to manage pain and symptoms within the gastrointestinal tract. Certain conditions that persist within in the gastrointestinal tract can include heartburn, diarrhea, nausea and acid reflux. Bismuth subsalicylate is also used temporarily to control common symptoms related to the GI system such as *H. pylori* and ulcers caused by specific bacteria.

Mechanism of Action

Bismuth subsalicylate has multiple mechanisms of action. First, it has some antimicrobial effects and potentially increases the effects of antibiotics used to treat gastrointestinal infections. Second, bismuth subsalicylate inhibits local inflammation but also stimulates mucus and bicarbonate secretion in the stomach, which protects the stomach from acid- and enzyme-based damage. It also coats ulcers and erosions of the gastric or intestinal mucosae and creates a protective layer against further acid-based damage. In cases of traveler's diarrhea, bismuth subsalicylate binds to the toxins the infecting bacteria produce, which attenuates the effects of the disease. Finally, bismuth subsalicylate inhibits intestinal prostaglandin and chloride secretion, which effectively reduces stool frequency and liquidity in cases of infectious diarrhea.

Side Effects

Two very common albeit harmless, but potentially distressing, side effects of bismuth subsalicylate are black tongue and darker stools. Prolonged use of bismuth subsalicylate can lead to toxicity. Bismuth toxicity can present as imbalance, gait instability, tremors and cognitive deficits. Other side effects include constipation and hearing loss/ ringing in ears. Bismuth subsalicylate is an over-the-counter medication. In addition, there are many medications that interact with bismuth subsalicylate.

Risks

Adverse effects and severe risks include bismuth encephalopathy. Patients can present with symptoms such as discoloration of tongue and teeth, confusion and myoclonus. In addition, symptoms associated with seizures may present in patients treated with long term bismuth subsalicylate. In addition, children 12 and under should avoid treatment with bismuth subsalicylate due to Reye's syndrome.

—*Lynn D. Willis-Carr MSN, BSN-RN*

References

Borbinha, Cláudia, et al. "Bismuth Encephalopathy- a Rare Complication of Long-Standing Use of Bismuth Subsalicylate." *BMC Neurology*, vol. 19, no. 1, 29 Aug. 2019, doi:10.1186/s12883-019-1437-9.

Cohen, P. R. "Black Tongue Secondary to Bismuth Subsalicylate: Case Report and Review of Exogenous Causes of Macular Lingual Pigmentation." *Journal of Drugs in Dermatology*, vol. 8, no. 12, Dec. 2009, pp. 1132–1135.

Hogan, David B., et al. "Bismuth Toxicity Presenting as Declining Mobility and Falls." *Canadian Geriatrics Journal*, vol. 21, no. 4, 30 Dec. 2018, pp. 307–309., doi:10.5770/cgj.21.323.

National Center for Biotechnology Information. "Bismuth Subsalicylate." *PubChem Database*, U.S. National Library of Medicine, pubchem.ncbi.nlm.nih.gov/compound/Bismuth-subsalicylate.

Uygun, Ahmet, et al. "The Efficacy of Bismuth Containing Quadruple Therapy as a First-Line Treatment Option for Helicobacter Pylori." *Journal of Digestive Diseases*, vol. 8, no. 4, 2007, pp. 211–215., doi:10.1111/j.1751-2980.2007.00308.x.

■ Carbamazepine

CATEGORY: Anticonvulsant

ALSO KNOWN AS: Carbatrol, Epitol, Equetro, Novo-Carbamaz, Tegretol, Tegretol CR, Tegretol-XR, Teril

ANATOMY OR SYSTEM AFFECTED: Nervous system

KEY TERMS
- *complex seizure*: an epileptic seizure involving the whole body, accompanied by loss of consciousness
- *partial seizure*: an epileptic seizure that affects only one part of the body without loss of consciousness
- *polysynaptic*: pertaining to nerve pathways involving multiple synapses
- *post-tetanic potentiation*: the preparation of a muscle to undergo contraction again following relaxation from a tetanic convulsion
- *seizure*: a sudden attack of a debilitating condition, particularly of epilepsy
- *tetanic*: a convulsion characterized by constant contraction of the muscles
- *tonic-clonic*: refers to the prolonged and/or alternating contraction of muscles during seizures

Convulsions and Carbamazepine

A convulsion, or seizure, is the sudden onset of pain an illness, or the muscle contractions associated with epilepsy. A strong, uncontrollable muscular contraction is termed "tetanic," due to the similarity to characteristic muscle contractions associated with tetanus. Such convulsions may affect just one part of the body while the sufferer remains fully conscious, as in a partial seizure. A complex seizure will involve several parts and perhaps the entire body, with the sufferer losing consciousness as well. A seizure may be described as tonic, in which muscle tone is maintained throughout the seizure. Alternatively, a seizure that involves alternating periods of muscle tension and relaxation is termed clonic.

Carbamazepine is an anticonvulsant agent used primarily for the control of seizures, including tonic-clonic, complex partial, and mixed seizures. It is sometimes also used in the treatment of trigeminal neuralgia, or pain arising from the trigeminal nerves, and in the treatment of bipolar disorder. Its exact mechanism of action is unknown, but appears to involve decreasing polysynaptic responses and blocking of post-tetanic potentiation. It should not be used during pregnancy or while using tricyclics. It is known to interact with a broad variety of other herbal preparations and medications. It can be administered as chewable tablets, oral suspensions or capsules of different dosages. Other drugs in this class include phenobarbital, phenytoin, primidone and valproic acid.

Interactions

Ginkgo: The herb ginkgo (*Ginkgo biloba*) has been used to treat Alzheimer's disease and ordinary age-related memory loss, among many other conditions. This interaction involves potential contaminants in ginkgo, not ginkgo itself. A natural nerve toxin present in the seeds of *Ginkgo biloba* that may have made its way into standardized ginkgo extracts prepared from the leaves is associated with convulsions and death in laboratory animals. The detected amounts of this toxic substance are considered harmless. However, given the lack of satisfactory standardization of herbal formulations in the United States, it is possible that some batches of product might contain greater amounts of the toxin depending on the season of harvest. In light of these findings, taking a ginkgo product that happened to contain significant levels of the nerve toxin might theoretically prevent an anticonvulsant from working as well as expected.

Glutamine: The amino acid glutamine is converted to glutamate in the body. Glutamate is thought to act as a neurotransmitter (a chemical that enables nerve transmission). Because anticonvulsants work (at least in part) by blocking glutamate pathways in the brain, high dosages of the amino acid glutamine might theoretically diminish an anticonvulsant's effect and increase the risk of seizures.

Grapefruit juice: Grapefruit juice slows the body's normal breakdown of several drugs, including the anticonvulsant carbamazepine, allowing it to build up to potentially dangerous levels in the blood. This effect can last for three days or more following the last glass of juice. Because of this risk, if one uses carbamazepine, the safest approach is to avoid grapefruit juice altogether.

Ipriflavone: Ipriflavone, a synthetic isoflavone that slows bone breakdown, is used to treat osteoporosis. Test-tube studies indicate that ipriflavone might increase blood levels of the anticonvulsants carbamazepine and phenytoin when they are taken therapeutically. Ipriflavone was found to inhibit a liver enzyme involved in the body's normal breakdown of these drugs, thus allowing them to build up in the blood. Higher drug levels increase the risk of adverse effects. Because anticonvulsants are known to contribute to the development of osteoporosis, a concern is that the use of ipriflavone for this drug-induced osteoporosis could result in higher blood levels of the drugs with potentially serious consequences. Persons taking either of these drugs should use ipriflavone only under medical supervision.

Hops, kava, passionflower, valerian: The herb kava (*Piper methysticum*) has a sedative effect and is used for anxiety and insomnia. Combining kava with anticonvulsants, which possess similar depressant effects, could result in "add-on" or excessive physical depression, sedation, and impairment. In one case report, a fifty-four-year-old man was hospitalized for lethargy and disorientation, side effects attributed to his having taken the combination of kava and the anti-anxiety agent alprazolam (Xanax) for three days.

Other herbs having a sedative effect that might cause problems when combined with anticonvulsants include ashwagandha (*Withania somnifera*), calendula (*Calendula officinalis*), catnip (*Nepeta cataria*), hops (*Humulus lupulus*), lady's slipper (*Cypripedium* species), lemon balm (*Melissa officinalis*), passionflower (*Passiflora incarnata*), sassafras (*Sassafras officinale*), skullcap (*Scutellaria lateriflora*), valerian (*Valeriana officinalis*), and yerba mansa (*Anemopsis californica*). Because of the potentially serious consequences, one should avoid combining these herbs with anticonvulsants or other drugs that also have sedative or depressant effects, unless advised by a physician.

Nicotinamide: Nicotinamide (also called niacinamide) is a compound produced by the body's breakdown of niacin (vitamin B3). It is a supplemental form that does not possess the flushing side effect or the cholesterol-lowering ability of niacin. Nicotinamide appears to increase blood levels of carbamazepine and primidone, possibly requiring a reduction in drug dosage to prevent toxic effects. Carbamazepine blood levels have been observed to increase in children with epilepsy after they were given nicotinamide, but the fact that the children were on several anticonvulsant drugs clouds the issue somewhat. Similarly, nicotinamide given to children on primidone therapy increased blood levels of primidone. It is thought that nicotinamide may interfere with the body's normal breakdown of these anticonvulsant agents, allowing them to build up in the blood.

Dong quai and St. John's wort: St. John's wort (*Hypericum perforatum*) is primarily used to treat mild to moderate depression. The herb dong quai

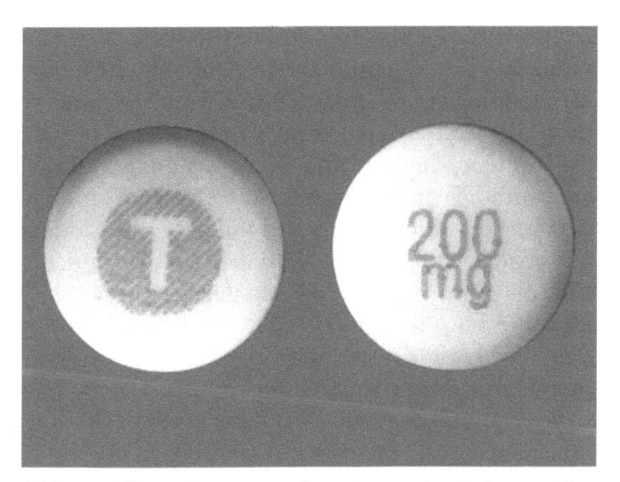

200 mg of Tegretol, a common brand name for Carbamazepine. (National Library of Medicine)

(*Angelica sinensis*) is often recommended for menstrual disorders such as dysmenorrhea, premenstrual syndrome (PMS), and irregular menstruation. The anticonvulsant agents carbamazepine, phenobarbital, and valproic acid have been reported to cause increased sensitivity to the sun, amplifying the risk of sunburn or skin rash. Because St. John's wort and dong quai may also cause this problem, taking them during treatment with these drugs might add to this risk. It may be a good idea to use sunscreen or wear protective clothing during sun exposure if one takes one of these herbs while using these anticonvulsants.

Biotin: Supplementation with biotin is possibly helpful, but should be taken at a different time of day than anticonvulsant medications. Anticonvulsants may deplete biotin, an essential water-soluble B vitamin, possibly by competing with it for absorption in the intestine. It is not clear, however, whether this effect is great enough to be harmful. Blood levels of biotin were found to be substantially lower in people with epilepsy on long-term treatment with anticonvulsants compared with untreated people with epilepsy. The effect occurred with phenytoin, carbamazepine, phenobarbital, and primidone. Valproic acid appears to affect biotin to a lesser extent than other anticonvulsants. A test-tube study suggested that anticonvulsants might lower biotin levels by interfering with the way biotin is transported in the intestine. Biotin supplementation may be beneficial if one is on long-term anticonvulsant therapy. To avoid a potential interaction, one should take the supplement two to three hours apart from the drug. It has been suggested that the action of anticonvulsant drugs may be at least partly related to their effect of reducing biotin levels. For this reason, it may be desirable to take enough biotin to prevent a deficiency, but not an excessive amount.

Folate: Folate (also known as folic acid) is a B vitamin that plays an important role in many vital aspects of health. Carbamazepine appears to lower blood levels of folate by speeding up its normal breakdown by the body and also by decreasing its absorption. Other antiseizure drugs can also reduce levels of folate in the body. Low folate can lead to anemia and reduced white blood cell count, and folate supplements have been shown to help prevent these complications of carbamazepine treatment. Adequate folate intake is also necessary to prevent neural tube birth defects, such as spina bifida and anencephaly. Because anticonvulsant drugs deplete folate, babies born to women taking anticonvulsants are at increased risk for such birth defects. Anticonvulsants may also play a more direct role in the development of birth defects. The low serum folate caused by anticonvulsants can raise homocysteine levels, a condition hypothesized to increase the risk of heart disease. However, the case for taking extra folate during anticonvulsant therapy is not as simple as it might seem. It is possible that folate supplementation itself might impair the effectiveness of anticonvulsant drugs, and physician supervision is necessary.

Calcium: Supplementation with calcium is possibly helpful, but should be taken at a different time of day than anticonvulsant medications. Anticonvulsant drugs may impair calcium absorption and, in this way, increase the risk of osteoporosis and other bone disorders. Calcium absorption was compared in people on anticonvulsant therapy (all taking phenytoin and some also taking carbamazepine, phenobarbital, and/or primidone) and the same number of other people who received no treatment. Calcium absorption was found to be 27 percent lower in the treated participants. An observational study found low calcium blood levels in 48 percent of people taking anticonvulsants. Other findings in this study suggested that anticonvulsants might also reduce calcium levels by directly interfering with parathyroid hormone, a substance that helps keep calcium levels in proper balance. A low blood level of calcium can itself trigger seizures, and this might reduce the effectiveness of anticonvulsants. Calcium supplementation may be beneficial for people taking anticonvulsant drugs. However, some studies indicate that antacids containing calcium carbonate may interfere with the absorption of phenytoin and perhaps other anticonvulsants. For this reason, one should take calcium supplements and anticonvulsant drugs several hours apart if possible.

Carnitine: Carnitine is an amino acid that has been used for heart conditions, Alzheimer's disease, and intermittent claudication. Intermittent claudication is a possible complication of atherosclerosis, in which impaired blood circulation causes severe pain in calf muscles during walking or exercising. Long-term therapy with anticonvulsant agents, particularly valproic acid, is associated with low levels of carnitine. However, it is not clear whether the anticonvulsants cause the carnitine deficiency or whether it occurs for other reasons. It has been hypothesized that low carnitine levels may contribute to valproic acid's damaging effects on the liver. The risk of this liver damage increases in children younger than twenty-four months, and carnitine supplementation may be protective. However, in double-blind crossover studies, carnitine supplementation produced no real improvement in well-being as assessed by parents of children receiving either valproic acid or carbamazepine. L-carnitine supplementation may be advisable in certain cases, such as in infants and young children (especially those younger than two years) who have neurologic disorders and are receiving valproic acid and multiple anticonvulsants.

Vitamin D: Anticonvulsant drugs may interfere with the activity of vitamin D. As proper handling of calcium by the body depends on vitamin D, this may be another way that these drugs increase the risk of osteoporosis and related bone disorders. Anticonvulsants appear to speed up the body's normal breakdown of vitamin D, decreasing the amount of the vitamin in the blood. A survey of forty-eight people taking both phenytoin and phenobarbital found significantly lower levels of calcium and vitamin D in many of them compared with thirty-eight untreated persons. Similar but lesser changes were seen in thirteen people taking phenytoin or phenobarbital alone. This effect may be apparent only after several weeks of treatment. Another study found decreased blood levels of one form of vitamin D but normal levels of another. Because there are multiple forms of vitamin D circulating in the blood, the body might be able to adjust in some cases to keep vitamin D in balance, at least for a time, despite the influence of anticonvulsants. Adequate sunlight exposure may help overcome the effects of anticonvulsants on vitamin D by stimulating the skin to manufacture the vitamin. Of 450 people on anticonvulsants residing in a Florida facility, none were found to have low blood levels of vitamin D or evidence of bone disease. This suggests that environments providing regular sun exposure may be protective. Persons regularly taking anticonvulsants, especially those taking combination therapy and those with limited exposure to sunlight, may benefit from vitamin D supplementation.

Vitamin K: Supplementation with vitamin K is possibly helpful for pregnant women. Phenytoin, carbamazepine, phenobarbital, and primidone speed up the normal breakdown of vitamin K into inactive byproducts, thus depriving the body of active vitamin K. This can lead to bone problems, such as osteoporosis. In addition, use of these anticonvulsants can lead to a vitamin K deficiency in babies born to mothers taking the drugs, resulting in bleeding disorders or facial bone abnormalities in the newborns. Mothers who take these anticonvulsants may need vitamin K supplementation during pregnancy to prevent these conditions in their newborns.

—*Richard M. Renneboog, MSc*
—*EBSCO CAM Review Board*

References

"Carbamazepine." *MedlinePlus*, U.S. National Library of Medicine, 15 Apr. 2019, medlineplus.gov/druginfo/meds/a682237.html.

Chen, Chia-Hui, and Shih-Ku Lin. "Carbamazepine Treatment of Bipolar Disorder: a Retrospective Evaluation of Naturalistic Long-Term Outcomes." *BMC Psychiatry*, vol. 12, no. 1, 23 May 2012, doi:10.1186/1471-244x-12-47.

Gierbolini, Jaime, et al. "Carbamazepine-Related Antiepileptic Drugs for the Treatment of Epilepsy - a Comparative Review." *Expert Opinion on Pharmacotherapy*, vol. 17, no. 7, 21 Mar. 2016, pp. 885–888., doi:10.1517/14656566.2016.1168399.

Koliqi, Rozafa, et al. "Prevalence of Side Effects Treatment with Carbamazepine and Other Antiepileptics in Patients with Epilepsy." *Materia Socio*

Medica, vol. 27, no. 3, 2015, p. 167., doi:10.5455/msm.2015.27.167-171.

Tolou-Ghamari, Zahra, et al. "A Quick Review of Carbamazepine Pharmacokinetics in Epilepsy from 1953 to 2012." *Journal of Research in Medical Studies*, vol. 18, no. Suppl1, Mar. 2013, pp. S81–S85.

Woods, Bernadette A. *Carbamazepine: Indications, Contraindications and Adverse Effects*. Nova Science Publishers, 2017.

■ Carisoprodol

CATEGORY: Addiction Risk; Muscle relaxant
ALSO KNOWN AS: Carisoma; Soma, sanoma; sopradol; vanadom
ANATOMY OR SYSTEM AFFECTED: Musculoskeletal system

History of Use

Since the mid-1950s, the North American market for tranquilizing medications has been enormous. Most tranquilizers developed at this time were designed to overcome specific problems that had become apparent in earlier medications. For example, carisoprodol (brand name Soma) was developed because of problems with meprobamate, an older anxiolytic medication that had both high potential for dependence and difficult withdrawals.

The brand name "Soma" refers both to the drink of the gods in Hindu religious literature and to a fictional medication in the dystopic novel *Brave New World* (1932) by Aldous Huxley. Since the late 1950s, the medical and scientific communities have come to recognize that although Soma is an effective skeletal-muscle relaxant, it also has a high potential for misuse, dependence, and illegal purchase.

Effects and Potential Risks

How Soma works in the brain is not well understood, although studies have suggested that it stimulates the receptors for gamma-aminobutyric acid, which in turn prompts overall relaxation of skeletal muscles and then sedation. Because of these two effects, Soma has been frequently prescribed along with anti-inflammatory medications as an aid for muscle sprains.

However effective in the short-term, Soma has significant potential risks. Some users have experienced anterograde amnesia after taking large doses, during which they have driven vehicles or engaged in other dangerous behaviors. Like other tranquilizing medications, Soma can cause dependence; predictably, those who become dependent tend to take larger doses to achieve desired effects, which in turn substantially increases the subsequent risk of cardiac problems, coma, and death. Withdrawal from Soma also proves difficult, as its symptoms include increased sensitivity to pain and anxiety, jitteriness, hallucinations, memory loss, agitation, depression and bizarre behavior.

In addition to the potential for dependency is the recreational use and misuse of Soma. More medical professionals have recently recognized the addictive properties of the drug and believe it to be more significant than originally anticipated: especially as a combination drug with alcohol, Xanax and Oxycodone (Soma combined with Oxycodone and Xanax referred to the "Holy Trinity" among recreational drug users). Recreational users seek its muscle relaxing and euphoric effects, and it is particularly popular with opioid users, who use Soma to combine with other narcotics for a more intense high, as well as to prevent withdrawals from opioid use.

—*Michael R. Meyers, PhD*
—*Kelly Owen, Esq.*

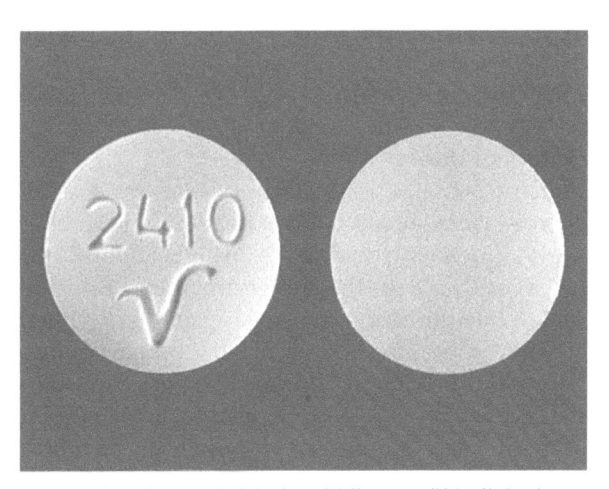

350mg of Carisoprodol. (National Library of Medicine)

References

"Addiction to Muscle Relaxers: Carisoprodol (Soma)." *American Addiction Centers*, 17 Oct. 2019, americanaddictioncenters.org/prescription-drugs/soma-addiction.

"Carisoprodol." *MedlinePlus*, U.S. National Library of Medicine, 15 Oct. 2018, medlineplus.gov/druginfo/meds/a682578.html.

Chou, Roger, et al. "Comparative Efficacy and Safety of Skeletal Muscle Relaxants for Spasticity and Musculoskeletal Conditions: a Systematic Review." *Journal of Pain and Symptom Management*, vol. 28, no. 2, 2004, pp. 140–175., doi:10.1016/j.jpainsymman.2004.05.002.

Horsfall, Joseph T., and Jon E. Sprague. "The Pharmacology and Toxicology of the 'Holy Trinity.'" *Basic & Clinical Pharmacology & Toxicology*, vol. 120, no. 2, 2016, pp. 115–119., doi:10.1111/bcpt.12655.

Paul, Gunchan, et al. "Carisoprodol Withdrawal Syndrome Resembling Neuroleptic Malignant Syndrome: Diagnostic Dilemma." *Journal of Anaesthesiology Clinical Pharmacology*, vol. 32, no. 3, 2016, p. 387., doi:10.4103/0970-9185.173346.

Reeves, Roy R., et al. "Carisoprodol." *Southern Medical Journal*, vol. 105, no. 11, 2012, pp. 619–623., doi:10.1097/smj.0b013e31826f5310.

■ Codeine

CATEGORY: Addiction Risk; Opioid
ALSO KNOWN AS: Methylmorphine; morphine methylester; 3-methylmorphine
ANATOMY OR SYSTEM AFFECTED: Nervous system

History of Use

Codeine was isolated from opium by French chemist Pierre-Jean Robiquet in 1832 and was used in the nineteenth century for pain relief and diabetes control. Near the end of the nineteenth century, codeine was used to replace morphine, another substance found in the opium poppy, because of the highly addictive properties of morphine. Codeine has effects similar to, albeit weaker than, morphine and was not thought to be addictive. Codeine was subsequently used in treatment for withdrawal from morphine.

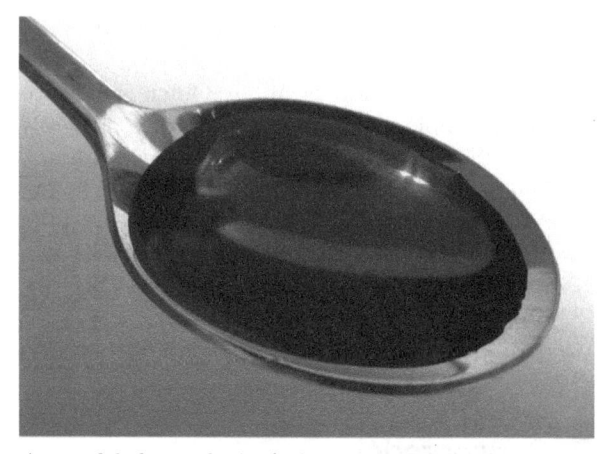

A spoonful of promethazine/codeine syrup showing the characteristic purple color. "Purple drank" is a recreational drug created by combining prescription-grade cough syrup with a soft drink and hard candy. Effects include mild euphoric side effects as well as lethargy, drowsiness, and dissociative feelings. (Stickpen via Wikimedia Commons

The first detailed report of codeine addiction is thought to be from 1905, and reports by others followed. In the 1930s, concern over the widespread misuse of codeine in Canada was noted. Codeine misuse in the United States was evaluated more fully in the 1960s, leading to inclusion of codeine as a schedule II controlled substance. Schedule II drugs have a high potential for misuse.

Subsequently, among substance misusers, prescription cough syrups containing codeine began to be mixed with soft drinks and candy (in a combination known as lean syrup, sizzurp, or purple drank). The combination remains a substance of concern.

Effects and Potential Risks

Codeine primarily exerts its medicinal effects by being metabolized by liver enzymes to substances that bind to specific receptors in the central and peripheral nervous systems. One of the most potent of these substances is morphine. The codeine metabolites can effectively block the transmission of pain signals to the brain and can inhibit the cough reflex. The metabolites also contribute to the usefulness of codeine in treating diarrhea by affecting, among other things, the contraction of gastrointestinal tract muscles.

Short-term use of codeine provides pain relief and euphoric effects. Some of the more common side effects of codeine ingestion include itching, constipation, dizziness, sedation, flushing, sweating, nausea, vomiting, and hives.

Long-term use of codeine can lead to tolerance, necessitating higher doses to achieve the same euphoric effect. Endorphin (natural painkiller) production may be slowed or stopped, causing increased sensitivity to pain if codeine is not used. More serious side effects include respiratory depression, central nervous system depression, seizures, and cardiac arrest.

—*Jason J. Schwartz, PhD*

References

Benini, Franca, and Egidio Barbi. "Doing without Codeine: Why and What Are the Alternatives?" *Italian Journal of Pediatrics*, vol. 40, no. 1, 11 Feb. 2014, doi:10.1186/1824-7288-40-16.

Bhandari, Monika, et al. "Recent Updates on Codeine." *Pharmaceutical Methods*, vol. 2, no. 1, 2011, pp. 3–8., doi:10.4103/2229-4708.81082.

Carney, Tara, et al. "A Comparative Analysis of Pharmacists' Perspectives on Codeine Use and Misuse – a Three Country Survey." *Substance Abuse Treatment, Prevention, and Policy*, vol. 13, no. 1, 27 Mar. 2018, doi:10.1186/s13011-018-0149-2.

"Codeine." *MedlinePlus*, U.S. National Library of Medicine, 15 Mar. 2018, medlineplus.gov/druginfo/meds/a682065.html.

Smith, Cooper. "Codeine: Drug Effects, Addiction, Abuse and Treatment - Rehab Spot." *RehabSpot*, 9 July 2019, www.rehabspot.com/opioids/codeine/.

■ Corticosteroids

CATEGORY: Class of Drug; Anti-inflammatory
ANATOMY OR SYSTEM AFFECTED: All

KEY CONCEPTS
- *steroids*: a class of organic molecules having a common framework structure consisting of four fused six-membered rings and one five-membered ring
- *virilization*: the acquisition of physical characteristics typical of males

Structure and Functions

Corticosteroids are steroid hormones produced by the cortex of the adrenal glands. They have several physiological actions, including regulation of glucose, lipid and protein metabolism, regulation of inflammation and the immune response, maintenance of homeostasis during stress, and control of water and electrolyte balance and blood pressure. Corticosteroids that have their primary effects on glucose metabolism are glucocorticoids, whereas those that have the control of electrolyte and water balance as their main functions are mineralocorticoids. Cortisol is the primary glucocorticoid, although significant amounts of corticosterone and cortisone are secreted. Aldosterone is the primary mineralocorticoid.

Glucocorticoids promote an increase in blood glucose by stimulating the synthesis of glucose (gluconeogenesis). They also stimulate the catabolism of lipids and proteins. Thus, glucocorticoids increase blood glucose and are antagonistic to insulin.

The synthesis of corticosteroids is controlled by adrenocorticotropic hormone (ACTH) produced by the pituitary gland. Corticotropin-releasing hormone (CRH) produced by the hypothalamus controls the secretion of ACTH. A feedback loop exists so that when cortisol levels are high, the release of CRH and ACTH is inhibited, and when cortisol levels are low, CRH and ACTH are released. Aldosterone is primarily responsible for the control of salt and water balance by promoting the excretion of potassium and the retention of sodium and water. Through its effect on salt and water balance, aldosterone can increase blood pressure. Plasma levels of aldosterone are controlled by a variety of mechanisms, including plasma volume and potassium ion concentration.

Disorders and Diseases

The condition known as Addison's disease results from adrenal insufficiency (hypocortisolism). Although most cases are caused by a disorder of the adrenal glands (primary adrenal insufficiency), some cases are caused by a disorder of the pituitary gland (secondary adrenal insufficiency). An autoimmune disorder that destroys the adrenal cortex is the major cause of primary adrenal insufficiency. Secondary adrenal insufficiency is usually caused by a lack of ACTH. Pituitary tumors, surgical removal of the pituitary, and loss of blood flow to the pituitary are the major causes of secondary adrenal insufficiency. Major symptoms of adrenal insufficiency include loss of appetite, weight loss, fatigue, muscle weakness, and hypotension. Addison's disease can be diagnosed by administering ACTH and monitoring the adrenal gland's response by measuring serum and urine cortisol levels. Adrenal insufficiency is treated by oral administration of hydrocortisone, a synthetic form of cortisol. If aldosterone is also deficient, then fludrocortisone is administered.

Adrenal insufficiency is often caused by a mutation in one of the enzymes synthesizing cortisol. These cases are referred to as congenital adrenal hyperplasia (CAH). Since serum cortisol is low or absent, the pituitary gland stimulates the adrenal gland to produce more cortisol. The precursor steroids and their metabolic products that accumulate can cause varying degrees of virilization of female fetuses and infants. Replacement therapy is the treatment of choice. Surgery to reconstruct the genital organs may be necessary in severe cases.

Hypercortisolism can lead to Cushing's syndrome. Major symptoms include obesity, osteoporosis, fatigue, hypertension, hyperglycemia, and amenorrhea (absence of menstruation). Cushing's syndrome may be caused by prolonged use of glucocorticoids or by an overproduction of glucocorticoids by the adrenal glands. The major causes of an overproduction of glucocorticoids are pituitary and adrenal tumors. Diagnosis of Cushing's syndrome is most commonly made by determining the amount of cortisol in the urine. Cushing's syndrome can be treated by reducing administered glucocorticoids or by treatment of the tumor causing the disease through surgical removal, radiation, and/or chemotherapy.

Hypoaldosteronism is a condition in which the adrenal cortex does not produce an adequate amount of aldosterone, which results in an inability to control and regulate blood volume and blood pressure. Blood pressure can fall to dangerously low levels.

Synthetic corticosteroids such as prednisone, prednisolone, methylprednisolone, hydrocortisone, and dexamethasone have an immunosuppressive effect and are used to treat a variety of chronic autoimmune and inflammatory diseases. They can reduce the pain, swelling, itching, inflammation, and redness associated with arthritis, bursitis, asthma, dermatitis, eczema, psoriasis, lupus erythematosus, Crohn's disease, and various ear, eye, and skin infections and allergic reactions.

Corticosteroid Drug	Treatment for
Betamethasone	Dermatitis
Budesonide	Asthma Nasal polyposis Noninfectious rhinitis
Cortisone	IgE-mediated allergies
Dexamethadone	Inflammation Rheumatoid arthritis
Hydrocortisone	Dermatitis
Methylprednisolone	Arthritis Bronchial inflammation
Prednisolone	Asthma Crohn's disease Rheumatoid arthritis Ulcerative colitis
Prednisone	Asthma Bell's palsy Dermatitis Systemic lupus erythematosus
Triamcinolone	Diabetic retinopathy Eczema

Prolonged use of corticosteroids can lead to medically induced Cushing's syndrome, suppression of the immune system, hypertension, hypokalemia (low serum potassium), and hypernatremia (high serum sodium).

Interactions

Interactions between hormones and other drugs and materials can be very complex and difficult to determine. Corticosteroid hormones are known to be affected in either a positive sense or a negative sense by the presence of certain other materials.

Calcium and vitamin D. Interference with the function of both calcium and Vitamin D by corticosteroids is believed to result in the acceleration of osteoporosis. Calcium and vitamin D supplements are definitely beneficial for fighting ordinary osteoporosis. In addition, there is good evidence that they also protect against osteoporosis brought on by corticosteroids.

Aloe and licorice in topical applications. Aloe and licorice are two herbs sometimes used topically for skin problems. Preliminary evidence suggests that each one might help topical corticosteroids, such as hydrocortisone, work better.

Dehydroepiandrosterone (DHEA). There are theoretical reasons (but little direct evidence) to believe that persons taking corticosteroids, such as prednisone, might be protected from some side effects by taking DHEA at the same time.

Chromium. Long-term, high-dose corticosteroid treatment can cause diabetes, at least partly caused by chromium deficiency. A very preliminary study found treatment with corticosteroids caused increased loss of chromium in the urine. Another preliminary study found that persons with corticosteroid-induced diabetes could improve blood sugar control by taking chromium supplements.

Creatine. Long-term use of corticosteroids, whether orally or possibly by inhalation can slow a child's growth. Animal studies suggest that use of the supplement creatine may help prevent this side effect.

Ipriflavone. The supplement ipriflavone is used to treat osteoporosis. There is worrisome evidence that ipriflavone can reduce white blood cell count in some people. For this reason, anyone taking medications that suppress the immune system should avoid using ipriflavone except under a physician's supervision.

Licorice (internal). When taken by mouth, the herb licorice appears to enhance some actions of oral corticosteroids but to interfere with others. Because of the unpredictable nature of this interaction, persons using oral corticosteroids should avoid licorice.

Perspective and Prospects

In 1855, Thomas Addison became the first physician to describe the clinical symptoms of adrenal insufficiency. In the early 1930s, Frank Hartman, Wilbur Swingle, and Joseph Pfiffner were the first to prepare active adrenal extracts capable of treating the symptoms of adrenal insufficiency. By the mid-1930s, Pfiffner, Edward Calvin Kendall, Oskar Wintersteiner, and Tadeus Reichstein had isolated and crystallized some of the adrenal hormones. In 1944, Lewis Sarett became the first to synthesize cortisone. In the late 1940s, Philip Showalter Hench discovered that the administration of cortisone could alleviate the symptoms of arthritis.

In recent years, it has been shown that corticosteroids express their effect by modulating the expression of a variety of genes involved in many physiological functions, including metabolism and the immune or inflammatory response.

—*Charles L. Vigue, PhD*
—*EBSCO CAM Review Board*

References

Ando, Hironori. *Handbook of Hormones: Comparative Endocrinology for Basic and Clinical Research.* Academic Press Inc, 2015.

"Corticosteroids." *Cleveland Clinic,* 16 Mar. 2015, my.clevelandclinic.org/health/drugs/4812-corticosteroids.

Liu, Dora, et al. "A Practical Guide to the Monitoring and Management of the Complications of Systemic Corticosteroid Therapy." *Allergy, Asthma & Clinical Immunology,* vol. 9, no. 1, 2013, p. 30., doi:10.1186/1710-1492-9-30.

Ramamoorthy, Sivapriya, and John A. Cidlowski. "Corticosteroids." *Rheumatic Disease Clinics of North America,* vol. 42, no. 1, 2016, pp. 15–31., doi:10.1016/j.rdc.2015.08.002.

Ramsahai, J Michael, and Peter Ab Wark. "Appropriate Use of Oral Corticosteroids for Severe Asthma." *Medical Journal of Australia,* vol. 209, no. S2, 17 July 2018, doi:10.5694/mja18.00134.

Russo, Emilio, et al. "Corticosteroid-Related Central Nervous System Side Effects." *Journal of Pharmacology and Pharmacotherapeutics,* vol. 4, no. 5, 2013, pp. 94–98., doi:10.4103/0976-500x.120975.

Waljee, Akbar K, et al. "Short Term Use of Oral Corticosteroids and Related Harms among Adults in the United States: Population Based Cohort Study." *Bmj,* 12 Apr. 2017, doi:10.1136/bmj.j1415.

■ Cyclooxygenase-2 (COX-2) inhibitors

CATEGORY: NSAID
ANATOMY OR SYSTEM AFFECTED: All

KEY TERMS

- *colorectal*: refers to cancers of the lower digestive tract consisting of the colon and the rectum
- *expression*: the action of cell biochemistry to produce and release a particular hormone in response to a stimulus

- *prostaglandins*: a large group of biologically active unsaturated, twenty-carbon fatty acids that represent some of the metabolites of arachidonic acid

How COX-2 Inhibitors Work

The cyclooxygenase, or COX, enzymes catalyze the production of hormones called prostaglandins, which stimulate cells to produce inflammatory responses. COX-1 is always expressed and is found in many tissues. Its inhibition can reduce inflammation but may also cause serious gastrointestinal side effects. In contrast, COX-2 is expressed only in response to stimulation signals and is present in a limited number of tissues. COX-2 is overexpressed, however, in several cancers, correlating with poorer overall survival. Therefore, COX-2 inhibitors are being investigated for the treatment and prevention of cancer.

COX-2 contributes to tumor growth by enhancing tumor cell proliferation and survival, inhibiting the body's immune response to cancer, and inducing the development of new blood vessels that feed a tumor and help it spread to other parts of the body. Because the active sites of the COX enzymes differ, COX-2 inhibitors can form tight complexes with COX-2 that dissociate slowly, thereby blocking enzyme activity. These inhibitors only loosely and reversibly bind to COX-1, however, with no effect on its activity. Blocking only COX-2 may reduce tumor cell growth and survival, and improve immune responses against tumor cells without the risk of severe gastrointestinal complications as seen with COX-1 inhibition.

Side Effects

The major side effects of COX-2 inhibitors are cardiovascular, such as increased risks of blood clots, heart attack, stroke, and high blood pressure. This has led to two drugs, Vioxx (rofecoxib) and Bextra (valdecoxib), being removed from the market by the Food and Drug Administration (FDA). COX-2 inhibitors may also cause indigestion, stomach bleeding, ulcers, and perforation of the stomach or intestines. Long-term administration may result in kidney toxicity and (rarely) liver toxicity. Allergic skin rashes may also occur with celecoxib (Celebrex).

—*Elizabeth A. Manning, PhD*

References

"How to Spell Pain Relief in the Wake of COX-2 Problems." *Harvard Health*, Harvard Medical School, Mar. 2014, www.health.harvard.edu/newsletter_article/How_to_spell_pain_relief_in_the_wake_of_COX-2_problems.

Katz, Jeffrey A. "COX-2 Inhibition: What We Learned—A Controversial Update on Safety Data." *Pain Medicine*, vol. 14, no. suppl 1, 23 Dec. 2013, doi:10.1111/pme.12252.

Mathew, Sam T., et al. "Efficacy and Safety of COX-2 Inhibitors in the Clinical Management of Arthritis: Mini Review." *ISRN Pharmacology*, 2011, pp. 1–4., doi:10.5402/2011/480291.

Ogbru, Omudhome. "Cox-2 Inhibitors Side Effects, List, Uses & Dosage." *MedicineNet*, 28 Feb. 2019, www.medicinenet.com/cox-2_inhibitors/article.htm.

Phend, Crystal. "FDA Advisors Weigh COX-2 Inhibitor Safety." *MedPage Today*, Everyday Health Group, 25 Apr. 2018, www.medpagetoday.com/painmanagement/painmanagement/72522.

Seliger, Corinna, et al. "Use of Selective Cyclooxygenase-2 Inhibitors, Other Analgesics, and Risk of Glioma." *Plos One*, vol. 11, no. 2, 12 Feb. 2016, doi:10.1371/journal.pone.0149293.

Solomon, Daniel H. "Overview of COX-2 Selective NSAIDs." *UpToDate*, 30 Mar. 2019, www.uptodate.com/contents/overview-of-cox-2-selective-nsaids?topicRef=35&source=see_link.

■ Decongestants

CATEGORY: Class of Drug
ANATOMY OR SYSTEM AFFECTED: Circulatory system, ears, nose, respiratory system, throat
SPECIALTIES AND RELATED FIELDS: Family medicine, otorhinolaryngology

KEY TERMS

- *adjunctive*: referring to the treatment of symptoms associated with a condition, not the condition itself
- *contraindication*: a condition that makes a particular treatment not advisable; contraindications may be absolute (should never be used) or relative (should be

used only with caution when the benefits outweigh the potential problems)
- *evidence-based medicine*: a method of basing clinical medical practice decisions on systematic reviews of published medical studies
- *systemic*: affecting the entire body; systemic treatments may be administered orally, directly into a vein, into the muscle, or through mucous membranes
- *topical*: referring to treatments applied directly to the skin or mucous membranes that affect primarily the area in which they are applied
- *upper respiratory tract*: the nose, sinuses, throat, ears, Eustachian tubes, and trachea

Indications and Procedures

Decongestants are used to shrink inflamed mucous membranes, promote drainage, or open collapsed Eustachian tubes. They are often used for the temporary relief of congestion caused by an upper respiratory tract infection (a cold), a sinus infection, or hay fever and other nasal allergies by promoting both nasal and sinus drainage. They are also often used as adjunctive therapy in the treatment of middle-ear infection (otitis media) to decrease congestion around the openings of the Eustachian tubes, and they may relieve the ear pressure, blockage, and pain experienced by some people during air travel. Careful scientific evaluation of the effectiveness of decongestants, however, has shown somewhat contradictory results.

The action of decongestants is accomplished primarily through stimulation of specific receptors in the smooth muscle of the upper respiratory tract, which in turn leads to constriction of the blood vessels and shrinkage of the mucous membranes. This improves air flow through the upper respiratory tract and relieves the sensation of stuffiness.

Uses and Complications

Decongestants may be applied topically, as sprays or drops, or taken by mouth. Commonly used decongestants include ephedrine, epinephrine, naphazoline, oxymetazoline, phenylephrine, pseudoephedrine, tetrahydrozoline, and xylometazoline. Some of these drugs are available over the counter and some by prescription only.

Oral preparations must be used with caution in elderly persons, children, and people with high blood pressure or other cardiac problems. If used as directed, decongestants do not usually cause excessive increases in blood pressure, overstimulate the heart, or change the distribution of blood in the circulatory system. The topical preparations are somewhat safer, because they are less likely to cause side effects, but they must also be used with caution.

The major advantage of oral decongestants is their long duration of action. Topical decongestants work more quickly but last a shorter period of time and are more likely to cause irritation of the tissues to which they are applied. If used too often or for too long a period of time (more than three to five days), nasal preparations may lead to a condition called rhinitis medicamentosa or rebound congestion, in which the congestion may be worse than before the person started using the medication.

People who take a certain type of antidepressant medication called a monoamine oxidase inhibitor (MAOI) and those with severe high blood pressure or heart disease should not take decongestants at all. People with thyroid disease, diabetes mellitus, glaucoma, or an enlarged prostate gland should take these drugs only after consulting a health care professional. Specific decongestants are contraindicated in infants and children.

People who take excessive doses of decongestants or who take them with other drugs that stimulate the central nervous system may experience insomnia, restlessness, dizziness, tremors, or nervousness. Overdose or long-term use of high doses may lead to hallucinations, convulsions, cardiovascular collapse, or even death.

Perspective and Prospects

Although decongestants have been widely used for decades, evidence-based medicine reveals few good studies indicating that decongestants do, in fact, treat illnesses. Systematic and careful reviews of the scientific studies available in the medical literature suggest that a single dose of a decongestant may relieve the stuffiness associated with the common cold in adults, but that no evidence exists for the usefulness of repeated doses. In people with a cough, a combination decongestant-antihistamine provides some relief in adults but not in children. In children with otitis media, there is a small statistical benefit from use of a combination decongestant-antihistamine, but it is not clear that the children benefit clinically. An evidence-based medicine review suggests that they not be used in children, especially given the increased risk of side effects from these medications in this age group.

—*Rebecca Lovell Scott, Ph.D., PA-C*

References

BMJ. "Do Not Give Decongestants to Young Children for Common Cold Symptoms." *ScienceDaily*, 11 Oct. 2018, www.sciencedaily.com/releases/2018/10/181011103628.htm.

Deckx, Laura, et al. "Nasal Decongestants in Monotherapy for the Common Cold." *Cochrane Database of Systematic Reviews*, vol. 2016, no. 10, 17 Oct. 2016, doi:10.1002/14651858.cd009612.pub2.

"Decongestants: OTC Relief for Congestion." *Familydoctor.org*, American Academy of Family Physicians, 16 Nov. 2017, familydoctor.org/decongestants-otc-relief-for-congestion/.

"Don't Let Decongestants Squeeze Your Heart." *Harvard Health Publishing*, Harvard Medical School, 3 Apr. 2019, www.health.harvard.edu/heart-health/dont-let-decongestants-squeeze-your-heart.

Kiefer, Dale, et al. "Decongestants to Treat Allergy Symptoms." *Healthline*, 11 Mar. 2016, www.healthline.com/health/allergies/decongestants#1.

Terrie, Yvette C. "A Guide to the Proper Use of Nonprescription Decongestant Products." *Pharmacy Times*, 17 Nov. 2018, www.pharmacytimes.com/publications/issue/2018/november2018/a-guide-to-the-proper-use-of-nonprescription-decongestant-products.

■ Dextromethorphan

CATEGORY: Addiction Risk; Decongestant
ALSO KNOWN AS: CCC; DXM; poor man's PCP; robo; skittles; triple C
ANATOMY OR SYSTEM AFFECTED: Nervous system

History of Use

Familiar since the 1950s to people with coughs and colds, dextromethorphan (DXM) was originally developed as a safer alternative to the codeine cough syrups that were then common. DXM was long considered devoid of any potential for misuse, even though it is an opioid derivative. When taken at higher than recommended doses, however, DXM

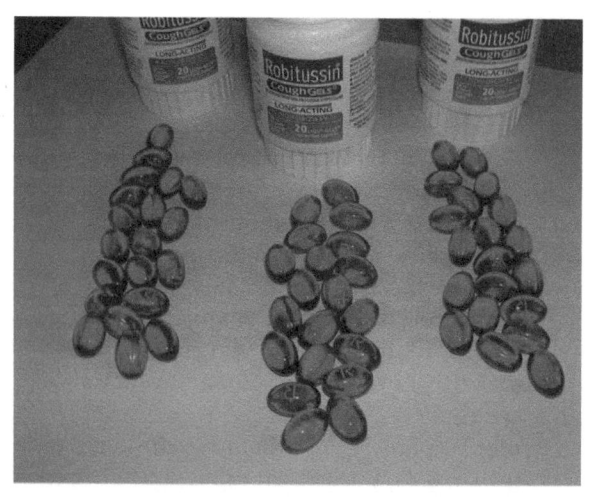

Dextromethorphan is an active ingredient in the expectorant Robitussin. (Psychonaught via Wikimedia Commons)

produces dissociative hallucinogenic effects. As a result, since the 1990s, misuse of over-the-counter (OTC) medications, including DXM, has grown. In 2011, only alcohol, tobacco, and cannabis were misused more frequently than OTC medications.

Effects and Potential Risks

DXM acts in the brain and spinal cord to inhibit receptors for N-methyl-d-aspartate (NMDA). As such, DXM—along with other NMDA antagonists—alters distribution of the neurotransmitter glutamate throughout the brain, in turn altering the user's perception of pain, the user's understanding of the environment, and the user's memory. Subjective effects include euphoria, hallucinations, paranoid delusions, confusion, agitation, altered moods, difficulty concentrating, nightmares, catatonia, ataxia, and anesthesia. The typical clinical presentation of DXM intoxication involves hyperexcitability, lethargy, ataxia, slurred speech, sweating, hypertension, and nystagmus.

Misusers of DXM describe the following dose-dependent plateaus: mild stimulation at a dosage between 100 and 200 milligrams (mg); euphoria and hallucinations begin at a dosage of between 200 and 400 mg; between 300 and 600 mg, the user will experience distorted visual perception and loss of motor coordination; and between 500 and 1,500 mg, the user will experience dissociative sedation. These effects are experienced only when a person has consumed vastly more DXM than recommended for normal therapeutic use.

This consumptive practice is particularly dangerous when DXM is combined with other active ingredients, such as pseudoephedrine, acetaminophen, or guaifenesin. Health risks associated with abusing these latter substances include increased blood pressure (pseudoephedrine), potential liver damage (acetaminophen), and central nervous system toxicity, cardiovascular toxicity, and anticholinergic toxicity (antihistamines).

—*Michael R. Meyers, PhD*

References

"Dextromethorphan." *MedlinePlus*, U.S. National Library of Medicine, 15 Feb. 2018, medlineplus.gov/druginfo/meds/a682492.html.

Martinak, Bridgette, et al. "Dextromethorphan in Cough Syrup: The Poor Man's Psychosis." *Psychopharmacology Bulletin*, vol. 47, no. 4, Sept. 2017, pp. 47–51.

Reissig, Chad J., et al. "High Doses of Dextromethorphan, an NMDA Antagonist, Produce Effects Similar to Classic Hallucinogens." *Psychopharmacology*, vol. 223, no. 1, 2012, pp. 1–15., doi:10.1007/s00213-012-2680-6.

Taylor, Charles P., et al. "Pharmacology of Dextromethorphan: Relevance to Dextromethorphan/Quinidine (Nuedexta®) Clinical Use." *Pharmacology & Therapeutics*, vol. 164, 2016, pp. 170–182., doi:10.1016/j.pharmthera.2016.04.010.

Weinbroum, Avi A., et al. "The Role of Dextromethorphan in Pain Control." *Canadian Journal of Anesthesia/Journal Canadien D'anesthésie*, vol. 47, no. 6, 2000, pp. 585–596., doi:10.1007/bf03018952.

■ Fentanyl

CATEGORY: Addiction Risk; Opioid

ALSO KNOWN AS: Apache; the bomb; China girl; China white; dance fever; friend; goodfella; jackpot; murder 8; perc-a-pop; poison; tango and cash; TNT

ANATOMY OR SYSTEM AFFECTED: Nervous system

History of Use

Fentanyl was first synthesized in a medical drug research laboratory in Belgium in the late 1950s. The original formulation had an analgesic potency of about eighty times that of morphine. Fentanyl

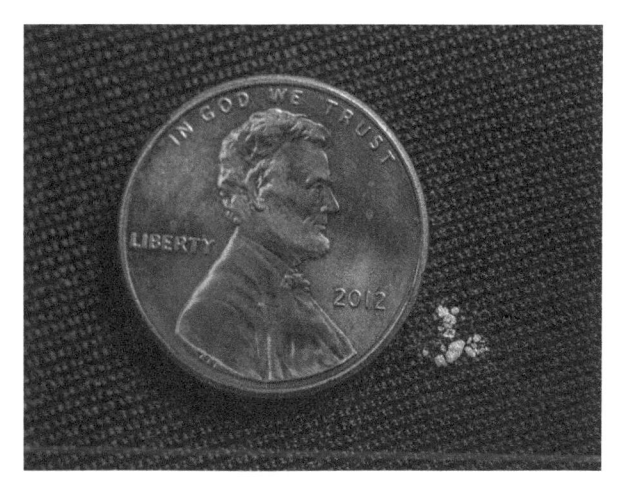

2 milligrams of fentanyl, a lethal dose for most people. (U.S. Drug Enforcement Administration)

was introduced into medical practice in the 1960s as an intravenous anesthetic. Subsequently, two other fentanyl analogs were developed for medical applications: alfentanil, an ultrashort-acting analgesic (of 5–10 minutes), and sufentanil, an exceptionally potent analgesic (5–10 times more potent than fentanyl) for use in heart surgery. Fentanyls are used now for anesthesia and analgesia. The most widely used formulation is a transdermal patch for relief of chronic pain.

Illicit use of fentanyl first occurred within the medical community in the mid-1970s. Among anesthesiologists, anesthetists, nurses, and other workers in anesthesiology settings, fentanyl and sufentanyl are the two agents most frequently misused. Potential misusers have ready access to these agents in liquid formulations for injection and can divert small quantities with relative ease. Transdermal patches cannot be readily adapted for misuse. The fentanyl lozenge has been diverted to illegal use. On the street, the lozenge is known as perc-a-pop.

More than one dozen analogs of fentanyl have been produced clandestinely for illegal use outside the medical setting. Since the mid-2000s, fentanyl misuse has emerged as a serious public health problem. Fentanyl-laced heroin or cocaine powders have become the drugs of choice for some addicts. In the 2010s, fentanyl played a major part in the drastic spike in overdose deaths due to opioid misuse, as the drug was often mixed with heroin or cocaine. Its potency means that users who are unaware of the mixture can easily overdose. Beginning around 2013 and accelerating in 2014 and

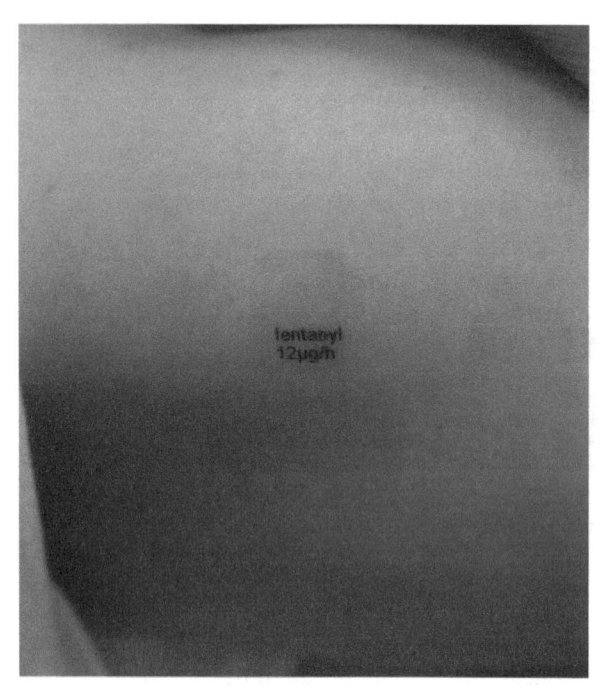

Fentanyl sticker at a release rate of 12 micrograms per hour, affixed to the skin. (Daniel Tahar via Wikimedia Commons)

2015, the sharp rise of fentanyl-related overdose deaths contributed to the growing opioid crisis. In 2016 the National Institute on Drug Abuse (NIDA) estimated that over 20,000 deaths were caused by overdoses of fentanyl analogs.

Effects and Potential Risks

The biological effects of fentanyl are indistinguishable from those of heroin, with the exception that illicit fentanyl analogs may be hundreds of times more potent. Short-term effects of fentanyl misuse include mood changes, euphoria, dysphoria, and hallucinations. Anxiety, confusion, and depression also may occur. High doses or long-term use may impair or interrupt breathing due to respiratory depression. Unconsciousness and even death can occur.

The 2000s and 2010s have seen a sharp increase in fentanyl use, as well as related overdoses and deaths. For example, in 2014 twenty-eight people died over a span of two months in Philadelphia due to the use of fentanyl-laced heroin. Police seizure of illegal drugs containing fentanyl tripled between 2013 and 2014; there were 942 fentanyl-related cases in 2013, compared with 3,344 in 2014. In 2015 the Drug Enforcement Administration (DEA) issued an alert about the spike in fentanyl-laced heroin. The problem was originally thought to be concentrated on the East Coast, but in April 2016 a spate of overdoses in the Sacramento area of California (thirty-six overdoses with nine deaths in a single week) showed that the problem was nationwide and growing. Notably, the drug used as a painkiller was responsible for the April 2016 death of the musician Prince.

With the rise of the opioid crisis, law enforcement and health care organizations began to press for wider availability of the overdose medication naloxone, also known as Narcan. The medication is effective in reversing the effects of overdose, though some critics claim it encourages drug users to use more recklessly, as they know they can be revived in case of overdose.

—*Ernest Kohlmetz, MA*

References

Dima, Delia, et al. "The Use of Rotation to Fentanyl in Cancer-Related Pain." *Journal of Pain Research*, vol. 10, 2017, pp. 341–348., doi:10.2147/jpr.s121920.

"Fentanyl." *MedlinePlus*, U.S. National Library of Medicine, 15 Oct. 2019, medlineplus.gov/druginfo/meds/a605043.html.

NIDA. "Fentanyl." *National Institute on Drug Abuse*, 6 June 2016, www.drugabuse.gov/drugs-abuse/fentanyl.

Ramos-Matos, Carlos F., and Wilfredo Lopez-Ojeda. "Fentanyl." *StatPearls*, 3 Oct. 2019.

Stanley, Theodore H. "The Fentanyl Story." *The Journal of Pain*, vol. 15, no. 12, 2014, pp. 1215–1226., doi:10.1016/j.jpain.2014.08.010.

Westhoff, Ben. *Fentanyl, Inc.: How Rogue Chemists Are Creating the Deadliest Wave of the Opioid Epidemic.* Atlantic Monthly Press, 2019.

■ Gabapentin

CATEGORY: Class of Drug
ALSO KNOWN AS: Gralise, Gralise Starter, Neurontin
ANATOMY OR SYSTEM AFFECTED: Nervous system

KEY TERMS

- *action potential*: a fast, sudden, transient, and propagating change of the resting membrane potential of excitable cells

- *ataxia:* a neurological sign characterized by a lack of voluntary coordination of muscle movements that may include gait abnormality, speech changes, and abnormalities in eye movement
- *depolarization:* the first part of an action potential during which there is less negative charge inside the cell, resulting in a more positive membrane potential.
- *ligand-gated ion channels*: a group of transmembrane ion-channel proteins that open to allow the passage of ions or close to prevent the passage of ions into cells in response to the binding of a neurotransmitter
- *membrane potential*: a difference in electrical potential across the cell membrane that results from a disparity in the concentration of ions on either side of the cell membrane
- *Neurotransmitters*: small molecules released from axon termini of neurons that diffuse across the synapse and initiate or prevent an action potential in the target cell.
- *off-label prescribing*: when a health provider prescribes a drug that the U.S. Food and Drug Administration (FDA) approved to treat a condition different from your condition
- *repolarization*: the second part of an action potential, after depolarization, in which positive potassium ions leave the cell and the membrane potential is returned to a negative value
- *voltage-gated ion channels*: a class of transmembrane proteins that form ion channels that open or close in response to changes in the membrane potential near the channel

Gabapentin is an established treatment for seizures and non-cancer neuropathic pain, including diabetic neuropathy, postherpetic neuralgia and central neuropathic pain. It is also used off-label for alcohol use disorder, alcohol and marijuana withdrawal, chronic refractory cough, fibromyalgia, intractable hiccups, postoperative pain, chronic pruritis (itching), restless legs syndrome, social anxiety disorder, and vasomotor symptoms associated with menopause. It is a relatively well-tolerated medicine that is safe at many different doses. Unfortunately, gabapentin has been somewhat overprescribed by physicians in place of opioids. Consequently, its greater availability has resulted in increased diversion and misuse by substance abusers in the community and penal system.

How Gabapentin Works

All animal cells use energy-linked ion pumps to expel positively-charged sodium and calcium ions from the cell and bring potassium ions into the cell. This active movement of positively-charged ions causes the cell interior to be more negatively charged than the cell exterior. This charge differential across the cell membrane constitutes the "membrane potential." Most cells cannot change the magnitude of their membrane potential. However, so-called "excitable cells," like neurons and muscle cells, can vary their membrane potential to communicate with other cells (neurons), or contact (muscle cells).

Neurons conduct nerve impulses by creating "action potentials." An action potential is a fast, sudden, transitory, and propagating change in the membrane potential of an excitable cell. Providing excitable cells with adequate stimuli raises their membrane potential and initiates an action potential if the membrane potential reaches a level known as the "threshold." Resting nerve cells usually have a resting membrane potential of -70 to -90 millivolts (mV). The threshold level is usually somewhere around -50 to -55 mV. When the neuron reaches threshold, voltage-gated ion channels in the axon open and positively-charged sodium ions rush into the cell, which makes the cell interior more positively charged and raises the membrane potential from a negative to a positive value (usually around +30 mV). This abrupt rise in the membrane potential is called "depolarization." Depolarization causes voltage-gated sodium channels to close and voltage-gated potassium channels to open. Because cells pump sodium from the cell and potassium into the cell, sodium levels are high outside cells but low inside cells, whereas potassium levels are high inside cells and low outside cells. Therefore, when potassium channels open, potassium ions leave the cell, which makes the cell interior more negative and lowers the membrane potential. The return of the membrane potential to a negative value is called "repolarization."

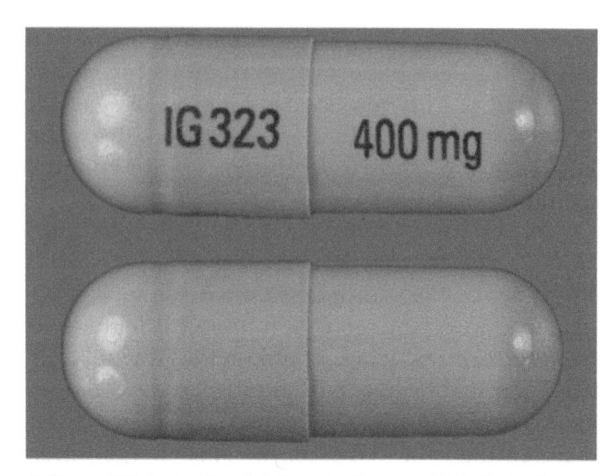

400mg of Gabapentin. (National Library of Medicine)

Depolarization begins as a local phenomenon in neurons, but it spreads from a local area to the rest of the cell. Neurons have an extension called an "axon," and the axon forms a connection to another neuron or some other target cell. When the action potential moves down to the axon, it comes to the axon terminus. At the axon terminus, depolarization of the axon causes voltage-gated calcium channels to open and flood the axon terminus with calcium. Calcium is an internal signal for vesicles loaded with neurotransmitters beneath the membrane to fuse with the membrane and dump large quantities of neurotransmitters into the space between the two neurons (synaptic cleft). Neurotransmitters bind to ligand-gated channels, which causes them to open and allow ions to move into the postsynaptic neuron, thus depolarizing it.

Some neurotransmitters may cause negatively-charged ions to enter the neuron, which prevents it from depolarizing, or they may cause ion channels to close. Therefore, some neurotransmitters are stimulatory and induce depolarization in postsynaptic cells, while other neurotransmitters are inhibitory and prevent depolarization of postsynaptic neurons.

Gabapentin binds to the alpha-2-delta subunit of the voltage-gated calcium channel and inhibits it from opening. Consequently, gabapentin ultimately inhibits the release of neurotransmitters by presynaptic neurons. Its ability to prevent neurotransmitter release means that gabapentin can potentially impede the function of pain-transmitting neurons, and, subsequently, relieve pain.

Clinical Uses of Gabapentin

Gabapentin is an effective treatment for chronic neuropathic pain or pain caused by a lesion or disease of the somatosensory nervous system that lasts three months or longer. Chronic neuropathic pain compromises function and quality of life and contributes to sleep disorders and mood disorders, such as anxiety and depression. Gabapentin is FDA-approved for postherpetic neuralgia, a complication of shingles attacks in which the pain of shingles remains even after resolution of the lesions. Although not FDA-approved for diabetic neuropathy, clinical trials have demonstrated the efficacy of gabapentin as a treatment for this condition and gabapentin is routinely prescribed off-label for it. Diabetic neuropathy is the most common complication of diabetes and leads to the gradual loss of integrity of the long sensory nerve fibers that service the toes and feet. This sensory nerve loss increases the risk of foot ulcers, and amputations. As these nerves die off, they can cause burning or stabbing foot pain that affects movement and quality of life. Off-label gabapentin includes distal symmetric peripheral neuropathy, which is associated with HIV infections.

There are many other conditions for which gabapentin is prescribed off-label. Alcohol withdrawal syndrome affects people with alcohol use disorder who sharply reduce or abruptly stop alcohol consumption. Although usually treated with benzodiazepines, gabapentin is an effective alternative treatment for mild alcohol withdrawal syndrome that is better tolerated than benzodiazepines. Gabapentin also effectively treats the symptoms of cannabis withdrawal and it is used off-label for this indication. Other off-label uses of gabapentin include the treatment of alcohol use disorder, but the evidence of its efficacy is equivocal.

Opioids, such as codeine, effectively treat chronic cough, but gabapentin is a viable alternative treatment, especially for those cases in which the health care provider wishes to avoid prescribing opioids.

Gabapentin effectively treats persistent, intractable hiccups in dying patients or recovering stroke patients.

Persistent itching (pruritus) may be associated with neuropathic disorders, and gabapentin may be an effective treatment for neuropathic-based pruritis, although evidence for this is limited. Uremic pruritus is a common and bothersome symptom among patients with end-stage kidney disease, and gabapentin effectively treats it.

Gabapentin is a first-line treatment for restless legs syndrome in children and an effective treatment in adults.

Several clinical trials have demonstrated that gabapentin is an effective treatment for hot flashes associated with menopause, and is prescribed, off-label for this indication.

Gabapentin is prescribed, off-label, as a treatment for fibromyalgia, but there is little evidence that it effectively treats fibromyalgia.

Gabapentin has been evaluated in several clinical trials as a treatment for postsurgical pain. However, unless the patient is already suffering from neuropathic pain, these studies have failed to demonstrate that gabapentin is an effective treatment for postsurgical pain.

Social anxiety disorder, or social phobia, is a condition marked by an extreme fear of situations that involve possible scrutiny by others. Patients with social phobia are afraid of public embarrassment or humiliation, so they avoid public situations or endure them with intense anxiety. In Europe, gabapentin is approved as a treatment for anxiety. However, in clinical trials, gabapentin shows only modest effectiveness as a treatment for social phobia.

Side Effects

The most common adverse effects of gabapentin include dizziness, drowsiness (somnolence), fatigue, and dry mouth, but almost all these side effects are dose-dependent. The immediate-release formulation of gabapentin may cause adverse effects not observed in patients who take other formulations. For example, nausea is more common in patients who take the immediate-release formulation. Children who take the immediate-release formulation show fever or increased incidence of viral infections. Adults on the same formulation may notice an increase in hostility or emotionalism or may have tremor or weakness (asthenia). Some patients who take gabapentin experience weight gain, but this is uncommon.

Though originally considered to have no potential for misuse, gabapentin has emerged as a drug of abuse. Because of the opioid abuse epidemic, gabapentin was increasingly prescribed, off-label, as a cheap, alternative pain treatment, which greatly increased its availability. From 2006 to 2016, gabapentin prescriptions in the U.S. increased from 18 million per year to over 45 million per year. Current estimates suggest that approximately one percent of the general population misuses gabapentin, as do 15-22% of people who misuse opioids. 40-65% of patients prescribed gabapentin abuse it. At high doses, gabapentin increases the respiratory depression caused by opioids, which makes co-misuse of these two drugs particularly disconcerting. In the U.S. and U.K., gabapentin abuse and diversion within the prison system are well documented.

—*Michael A. Buratovich Ph.D.*

References

Brody, Jane E. "Millions Take Gabapentin for Pain. But There's Scant Evidence It Works." *The New York Times*, Section D, May 21, 2019, Page 7.

Jordan, Roberta, Mulvey, Matthew, and Michael Bennet. "A Critical Appraisal of Gabapentinoids for Pain in Cancer Patients." *Current Opinion in Supportive and Palliative Care*, vol. 12, no. 2, 2018, pp. 108-117.

Modesto-Lowe, Vania, Barron, Gregory, Aronow, Benjamin, and Margaret Chaplin. "Gabapentin for Alcohol Use Disorder: A Good Option, or Cause for Concern?" *Cleveland Clinic Journal of Medicine*, vol 86, no. 12, 2019, pp. 815-823.

Moore, Jerrel, and Chloe Gaines. "Gabapentin for Chronic Neuropathic Pain in Adults." *British Journal of Community Nursing*, vol. 24, no. 12, 2019, pp. 608–609.

Morrison, Emma, Sandilands, Euan, and David Webb. "Gabapentin and Pregabalin: Do the Benefits Outweigh the Harms?" *The Journal of the Royal College of Physicians of Edinburgh*, vol 47, no. 4, 2017, pp. 310-313.

Pop-Busui, R, et al. "Diabetic Neuropathy: A Position Statement by the American Diabetes Association." *Diabetes Care*, vol. 40, no. 1, 2017, pp. 136-154.

Stahl, Stephen. *Stahl's Illustrated Chronic Pain and Fibromyalgia*. Cambridge University Press, 2009.

■ Hydrocodone

CATEGORY: Addiction Risk; Opioid
ALSO KNOWN AS: Dihydrocodeinone; Lortab; Vicodin
ANATOMY OR SYSTEM AFFECTED: Nervous system

History of Use

Hydrocodone was first synthesized in Germany in 1920 by Carl Mannich and Helene Löwenheim. The first report of euphoria and habituation was

Side effects of Hydrocodone

Central
- Drowsiness
- Dizziness
- Lightheadedness
- Fuzzy thinking
- Anxiety
- Abnormally happy or sad mood

Pupils
- Narrowing

Throat
- Dryness

Skin
- Rash
- Itching

Respiratory
- Slowed or irregular breathing
- Chest tightness

Gastric
- Nausea
- Vomiting

Intestinal
- Constipation

Urinary
- Difficulty urinating

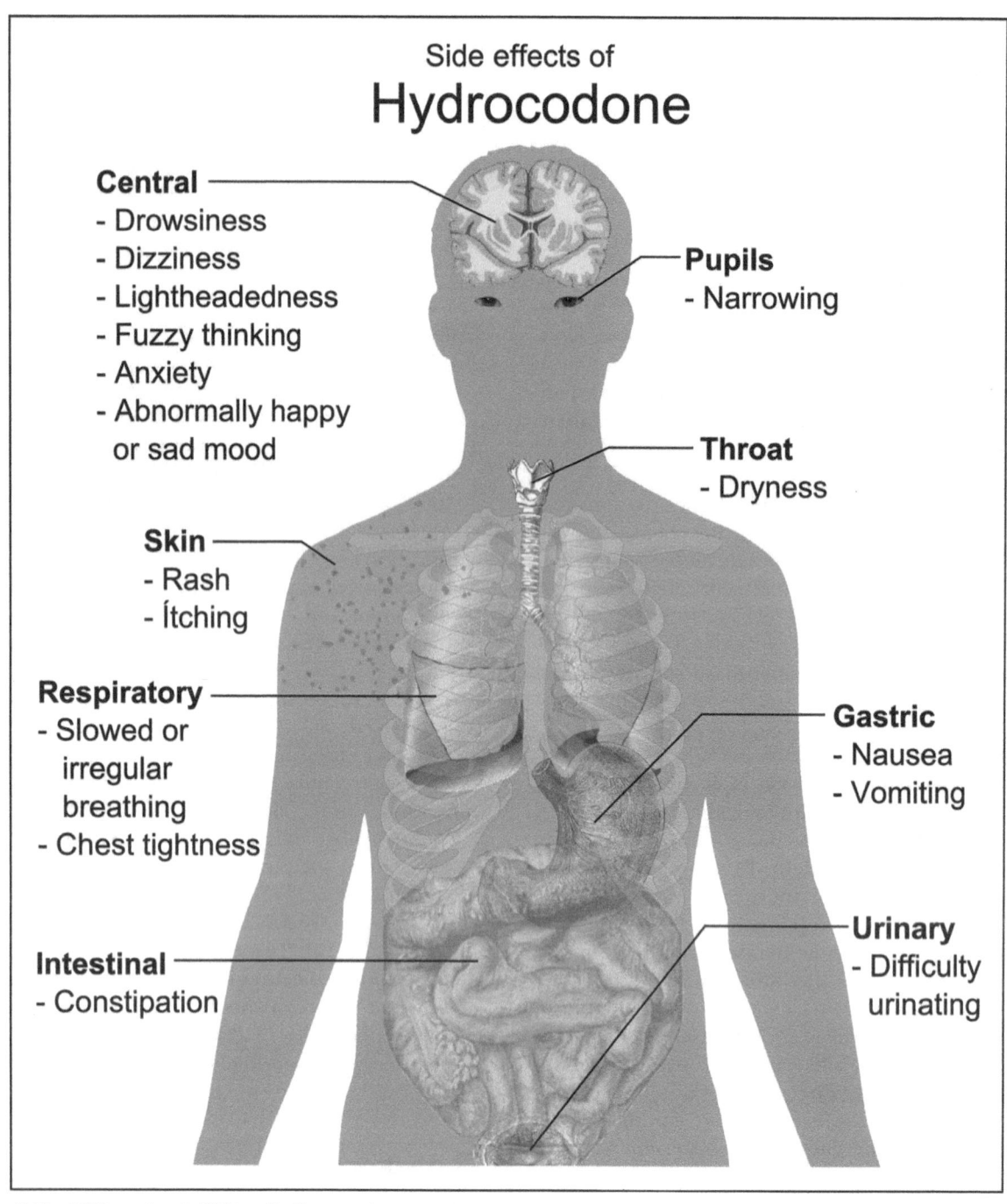

(Mikael Häggström via Wikimedia Commons)

published in 1923, and the first report of dependence and addiction was published in 1961. Hydrocodone was approved by the US Food and Drug Administration in 1943 for sale in the United States.

Hydrocodone relieves pain by changing the way the brain and nervous system respond to pain, that is, by binding to the opioid receptor sites in the brain and spinal cord. It is not usually produced illegally; diverted pharmaceuticals are the primary source for misuse. Misuse comes in the form of fraudulent call-in prescriptions, altered prescriptions, theft, and illicit purchases

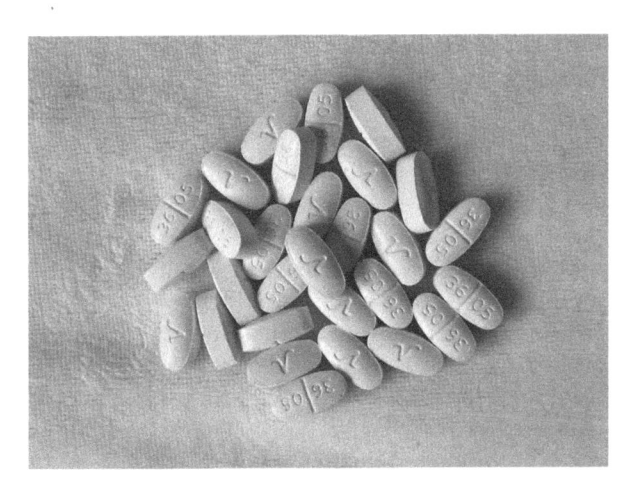

Hydrocodone-acetaminophen tablets, 7.5mg/325mg. (INeverCry via Wikimedia Commons)

online. Diversion and misuse have been increasing. In 2008, hydrocodone was the most frequently encountered opioid in drug evidence submitted to state and local forensics laboratories, as reported by the National Forensic Laboratory Information System.

Effects and Potential Risks

Short-term effects are improvement of mood, reduction of pain, euphoria, sedation, light-headedness, and changes in focus and attention. Side effects include nausea, vomiting, constipation, anxiety, dry throat, rash, difficulty urinating, irregular breathing, and chest tightness. When inhaled, burning in nose and sinuses usually occurs. A newborn of a woman who was taking the medication during pregnancy may exhibit breathing problems or withdrawal symptoms.

Symptoms of overdose include cold and clammy skin, circulatory collapse, stupor, coma, depression, respiratory depression, cardiac arrest, and death. Mixing hydrocodone with other substances, including alcohol, can cause severe physical problems or death.

Misuse of hydrocodone is associated with tolerance, dependence, and addiction. There is no ceiling dose for hydrocodone in users tolerant to its effects. Acetaminophen carries the risk of liver toxicity with high, acute doses (of around 4,000 mg per day).

—*Stephanie Eckenrode, BA, LLB*
—*Marianne Moss Madsen, MS, BCND*

References

"Hydrocodone." *MedlinePlus*, U.S. National Library of Medicine, 15 March 2018. https://medlineplus.gov/druginfo/meds/a614045.html

Cardia, Luigi, et al. "Preclinical and Clinical Pharmacology of Hydrocodone for Chronic Pain: A Mini Review." *Frontiers in Pharmacology*, vol. 9, 1 Oct. 2018, p. 1122., doi:10.3389/fphar.2018.01122.

Godman, Heidi, and Zara Risoldi Cochrane. "Understanding Hydrocodone Addiction." *Healthline*, 8 Jan. 2019, www.healthline.com/health/understanding-hydrocodone-addiction.

Trescot, Andrea, et al. "Extended-Release Hydrocodone – Gift or Curse?" *Journal of Pain Research*, vol. 6, 2013, p. 53., doi:10.2147/jpr.s33062.

■ Methadone

CATEGORY: Addiction Risk; Opioid; Treatment
ALSO KNOWN AS: Dolophine; methadose
ANATOMY OR SYSTEM AFFECTED: Nervous system

History of Use

Methadone hydrochloride is a synthetic opioid with mu (μ) agonist properties. It was developed in the 1930s in Germany, and by the 1950s methadone began to be used by the US government, specifically the Public Health Service, in the treatment of opioid abstinence syndrome.

Methadone acts on the same brain receptor as heroin and other opioids, producing similar effects. For this reason, it is used to help bridge users from more hazardous drugs. In the treatment of addiction in the United States, methadone is used primarily for the treatment of heroin addicts. Persons who stop taking heroin without taking medication for withdrawal, such as methadone, naltrexone, or buprenorphine, can experience severe withdrawal symptoms. These symptoms include agitation, anxiety, sweating, flu-like symptoms, and dehydration potentially leading to hospitalization or death.

When beginning therapy with methadone, those treated may experience common adverse effects, including constipation, dizziness, sedation, gastrointestinal distress (nausea and vomiting), and possibly itching, headache, and hypotension. More serious adverse reactions include cardiac and pulmonary complications and respiratory depression. Patients are monitored and undergo a complete medical history assessment to identify any significant medical conditions that may increase risks of developing complications from methadone.

Opioid Detoxification
Methadone is one of several possible drugs used for opioid detoxification, for treating opioid addiction, and for maintaining treatment for opioid addiction as part of a medication-assisted treatment (MAT) plan. Methadone is available orally in 5 and 10 milligram (mg) tablets and as a solution and in suspension. Patient response to methadone is highly variable, in part because of its broad range of bioavailability, because of the time to peak plasma concentration, and because of the drug's half-life. Knowing methadone's half-life's variability is critical because respiratory depression, which occurs with methadone and other opioids as a class, generally lasts longer than pain control. Respiratory depression from methadone and other opioids can be severe and fatal.

Starting doses of methadone are generally between 20 and 30 mg and are gradually increased until withdrawal symptoms are controlled. This taper usually occurs during the first week of treatment. The typical maintenance dose is 80 to 120 mg, once daily. However, it is not uncommon for higher doses to be required.

Treatment generally continues for one year or more, followed by a slow taper. Tapering off methadone requires dose reductions of less than 10 percent within ten to fourteen days, often requiring an extended period before a patient is completely weaned off the methadone.

Patients also generally require a combination of psychosocial and behavioral counseling to be successful at staying free of opioids. During the first week of therapy and until the medication and side effects are fully realized, patients are advised to avoid activities requiring mental alertness. Additionally, while being treated with methadone, patients should avoid ingesting other central nervous system depressants (including alcohol and other medications) and should avoid discontinuing the medication abruptly.

Authorized Treatment
Methadone used for the treatment of opioid dependence can be provided only by authorized opioid treatment programs (OTPs), which are certified by the federal Substance Abuse and Mental Health Services Administration. Providers must meet specific criteria, including board certification in addiction specialties, to legally prescribe methadone for opioid dependence treatment. However, if a patient on methadone is admitted as an inpatient for reasons other than opioid addiction, therapy can be continued with provider certification if it can be verified that the patient is receiving treatment at an OTP.

—*Allison C. Bennett, PharmD*

References

Chou, Roger, et al. "Methadone Safety: A Clinical Practice Guideline From the American Pain Society and College on Problems of Drug Dependence, in Collaboration With the Heart Rhythm Society." *The Journal of Pain*, vol. 15, no. 4, 2014, pp. 321–337., doi:10.1016/j.jpain.2014.01.494.

D'hotman, Daniel, et al. "Methadone for Prisoners." *The Lancet*, vol. 387, no. 10015, 2016, p. 224., doi:10.1016/s0140-6736(16)00044-1.

Fei, Joni Teoh Bing, et al. "Effectiveness of Methadone Maintenance Therapy and Improvement in Quality of Life Following a Decade of Implementation." *Journal of Substance Abuse Treatment*, vol. 69, 2016, pp. 50–56., doi:10.1016/j.jsat.2016.07.006.

"Methadone." *MedlinePlus*, U.S. National Library of Medicine, 15 Oct. 2019, medlineplus.gov/druginfo/meds/a682134.html.

"Methadone." *Substance Abuse and Mental Health Services Administration*, 30 Sept. 2019, www.samhsa.gov/medication-assisted-treatment/treatment/methadone.

Rajan, J, and J Scott-Warren. "The Clinical Use of Methadone in Cancer and Chronic Pain Medicine." *BJA Education*, vol. 16, no. 3, 2016, pp. 102–106., doi:10.1093/bjaceaccp/mkv023.

"What Is a Methadone Clinic? MedMark's Guide to Methadone Clinics." *MedMark Treatment Centers*, medmark.com/resources/comprehensive-guide-to-methadone-clinics/.

Morphine

CATEGORY: Addiciton Risk; Opioid; Treatment
ALSO KNOWN AS: Dreamer, Emsel, First Line, God's Drug, Hows, MS, Mister Blue, Morpho, Unkie
ANATOMY OR SYSTEM AFFECTED: Nervous system

History of Use

Morphine was first isolated in the early nineteenth century by Friedrich Sertürner in Germany. The word *morphine* is derived from the term *morphium*, for Morpheus, the Greek god of dreams. Within twenty years, morphine was available across Europe as an agent for treating pain and for many other uses, including treating alcohol misuse.

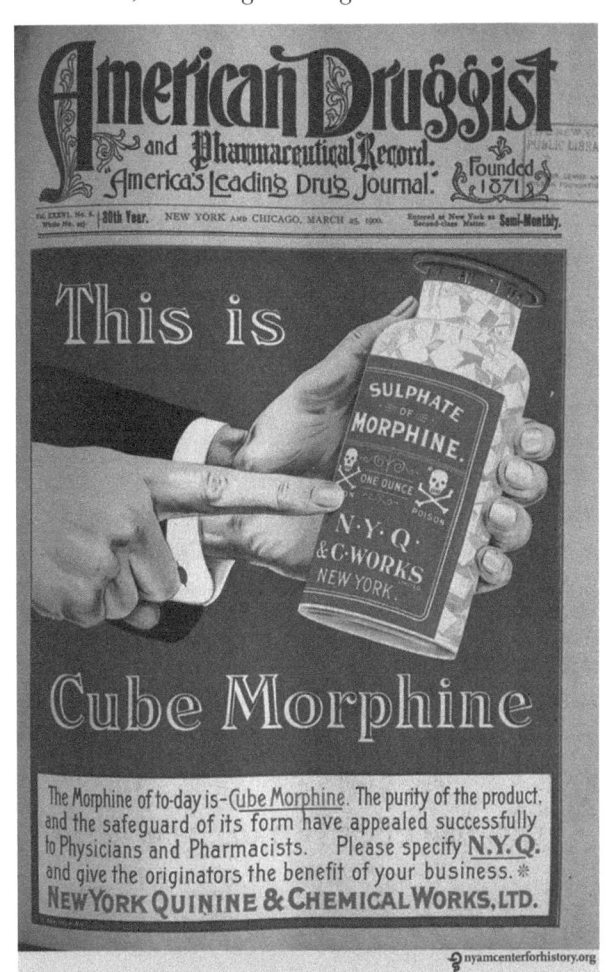

By 1900, use of narcotics was at its peak for both medical and non-medical purposes. Advertisements promoting opium- and cocaine-laden drugs saturated the newspapers; morphine seemed more easily obtainable than alcohol. (New York Academy of Medicine)

In the United States, morphine became a controlled substance in 1914 under the Harrison Narcotics Tax Act. Morphine is now the gold-standard by which other analgesics are measured. The drug is used for treating moderate and severe pain, both acute and chronic. Many available painkillers, such as codeine, are chemically related to morphine.

Illicit opioid use, including the use of morphine, is more common now than the use of cocaine, heroin, or methamphetamine (as reported by the 2008 National Survey of Drug Use and Health). Studies have shown that up to 40 percent of people who report misusing opioids have tried intravenous injection of opioids. Intravenous injection produces the fastest onset both of euphoric and of negative effects, including respiratory depression and central nervous system (CNS) effects. Oftentimes these prescription opiates are legally prescribed for a friend or family member and then obtained by the drug misuser. Because of the legitimate pain-relieving properties of morphine, the drug is highly prescribed and used. This high level of use increases opportunities for diversion and misuse.

Effects and Potential Risks

Decreased respiratory rate and sedation are two common adverse effects of morphine, effects experienced even in patients treated with normal doses and dosing regimens. However, these normal adverse effects can become extremely problematic and even fatal in acute morphine overdoses or with chronic administration. Respiratory depression occurs more commonly in elderly patients and in patients with underlying respiratory conditions, and it occurs to a higher extent with intravenous administration. Respiratory complications and sedative effects are also much more common in patients who are opioid naïve.

Like other mu (µ) opioid agonists (such as oxycodone and hydrocodone), morphine causes a feeling of euphoria, which can lead to psychological dependence. Following intravenous administration, euphoria can occur within five minutes, and although the physiological effects can last for greater than six hours, the feeling of euphoria generally dissipates sooner. This can

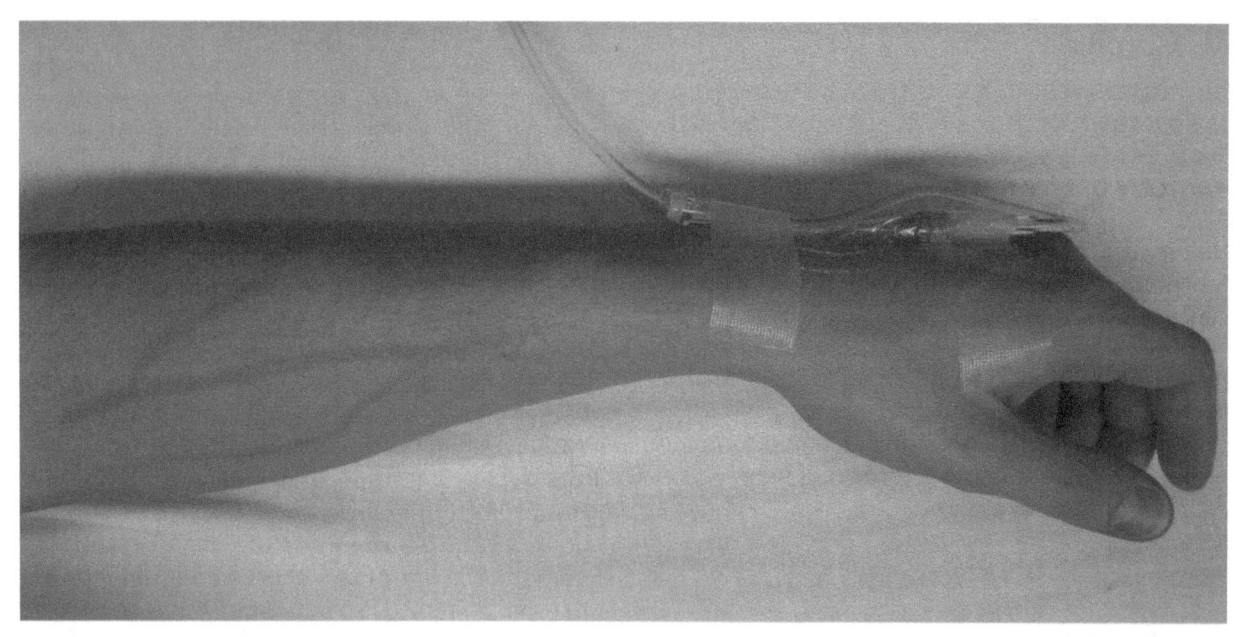

A localized side effect of morphine due to histamine release in which the veins become red. (James Heilman, MD via Wikimedia Commons)

lead a misuser to re-inject the medication at a time when his or her body is still reacting to the respiratory and CNS effects of the initial dose of morphine; this can lead to death. Intravenous injection also increases the risk of infection and vessel occlusion, both of which can have serious and fatal consequences.

Chronic morphine users who abruptly stop use can experience withdrawal. Signs and symptoms of withdrawal include nausea and diarrhea, profuse sweating, twitching muscles, and temperature disturbances, all of which can persist up to two weeks in some persons.

—*Allison C. Bennett, PharmD*

References

Gulur, Padma, et al. "Morphine versus Hydromorphone: Does Choice of Opioid Influence Outcomes?" *Pain Research and Treatment*, 1 Nov. 2015, pp. 1–6., doi:10.1155/2015/482081.

Jeurgens, Jeffrey, and Theresa Parisi. "Morphine Addiction and Abuse." *AddictionCenter*, 12 Sept. 2019, www.addictioncenter.com/opiates/morphine/.

Kuebler, Karen M. "Using Morphine in End-of-Life Care." *Nursing*, vol. 44, no. 4, 2014, p. 69., doi:10.1097/01.nurse.0000444548.72595.ac.

"Morphine." *MedlinePlus*, U.S. National Library of Medicine, 15 Oct. 2019, medlineplus.gov/druginfo/meds/a682133.html.

■ Narcotics

CATEGORY: Class of Drug
ANATOMY OR SYSTEM AFFECTED: Brain, spinal cord and peripheral nerves
SPECIALTIES AND RELATED FIELDS: Pharmacology

KEY TERMS
- *agonist*: a drug that mimics the effects of a hormone or neurotransmitter normally found in the body
- *analgesia*: relief of pain; analgesics are compounds that stop the neurotransmission of pain messages
- *antagonist*: a drug that acts to block the effects of a hormone or neurotransmitter normally found in the body
- *brainstem*: the region between the brain and spinal cord that controls vital functions such as breathing and heart rate
- *central nervous system*: the brain and spinal cord
- *dependence*: a craving for a drug

- *endogenous*: something naturally found in the body, such as neurotransmitters
- *exogenous*: something originating outside the body and administered orally or by injection
- *neurotransmitter*: a chemical substance released by one nerve cell to stimulate or inhibit the function of an adjacent nerve cell; a chemical message released from a neuron
- *opioids*: endogenous or exogenous substances (opiates) that relieve pain and cause euphoria
- *opiates*: drugs synthetically made from the opium flower, such as opium, morphine, and codeine
- *neuron*: a nerve cell that can conduct electrical impulses from one region of the body to another; it is capable of releasing neurotransmitters
- *tolerance*: diminished effect of a drug over time due to its chronic use
- *withdrawal*: the body's response, both physical and mental, when an addictive substance is reduced or not given to the body

The Effects of Narcotics

Narcotics are drugs commonly used to treat pain (analgesics), suppress coughing, control diarrhea, and aid in anesthesia. These drugs are some of the oldest and most commonly used agents in medicine. They have psychoactive effects on the body which either block (an antagonist) or mimic (an agonist) the effects of naturally occurring chemicals. Researchers have studied the many effects of opiates, such as morphine, codeine, and heroin in comparison to the body's own endogenous opioids. Naturally occurring opioids, such as endorphins, dynorphins, and enkephalins, act as neurotransmitters, which send chemical signals throughout the human nervous system to relieve pain and increase euphoria.

To understand how opioids affect the body's response to pain, one must first understand the physiology of pain. When tissues are damaged, they release chemical substances into the space outside of the damaged cell, known as the extracellular space. Sensory neurons that have the ability to detect these chemicals are known as pain neurons. Once the chemicals bind to receptors on a pain neuron, the neuron is stimulated to send an ascending electrical message from the peripheral nerve, to the spinal cord and eventually to the brain. One type of neurotransmitter that transfers this message is called substance P. Once released and transmitted, two actions occur when the message arrives to the brain. The first is an immediate initiation of a reflex, which attempts to remove the tissue from the source of injury. For example, when one accidentally places an arm on a hot stove, a neural reflex causes the muscles of the limb to retract the arm from the burner. This is accomplished when the pain neuron releases a descending chemical message (neurotransmitter) from the brain to the spinal cord which then stimulates peripheral neurons that control the muscles of the affected limb. The second action of sensory pain occurs in terms of memory where appropriate behavioral modification can take place. For example, one may become more cautious around the kitchen after burning one's arm on the stove.

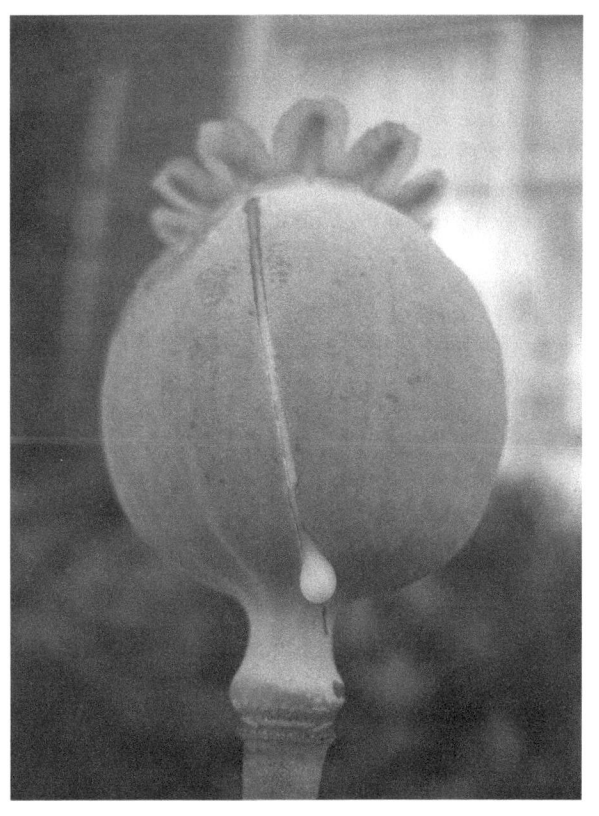

Capsule of Papaver somniferum *showing latex (opium) exuding from incision.* (via Wikimedia Commons)

Regulation of pain occurs via neurotransmitters such as 5-hydroxytryptamine (5-HT) receptors, glycine, gamma-aminobutyric acid (GABA), and opioids. Morphine acts as an exogenous opioid, dampening the transmission of pain messages at various sites in the nervous system. One of the most clinically important places is within the spinal cord at the region where the pain neurons release substance P. Opioids are known to reduce the amount of substance P that is released and thereby decreasing the stimulatory message in the neural pathway to the brain. If the pain impulses traveling to the brain are reduced, so is one's perception of pain. The second area of the nervous system known to be involved in regulating the perception of pain is a dense area of neurons located between the brain and spinal cord referred to as the brainstem. When researchers stimulated a particular region of the brainstem, pain impulses traveling to the brain were reduced by the modulation of endogenous opioids.

Considering exogenous opioids mimic endogenous opioids, one may wonder why there is a need for narcotic drugs if the body already produces opioids such as endorphins and enkephalins. The answer is that every individual has a different degree of pain tolerance. How much pain one can endure also changes with certain circumstances. For example, one hardly notices the pain of a cut when participating in an exciting outdoor game. If the same wound occurs while one's attention is focused on it, however, the cut becomes noticeably painful. Perhaps the best explanation for the differing interpretation of pain during these activities and among different people is the endogenous opioid system. It is postulated that the analgesic effects of acupuncture are a result of stimulating neurons to release endorphins, enkephalins, and

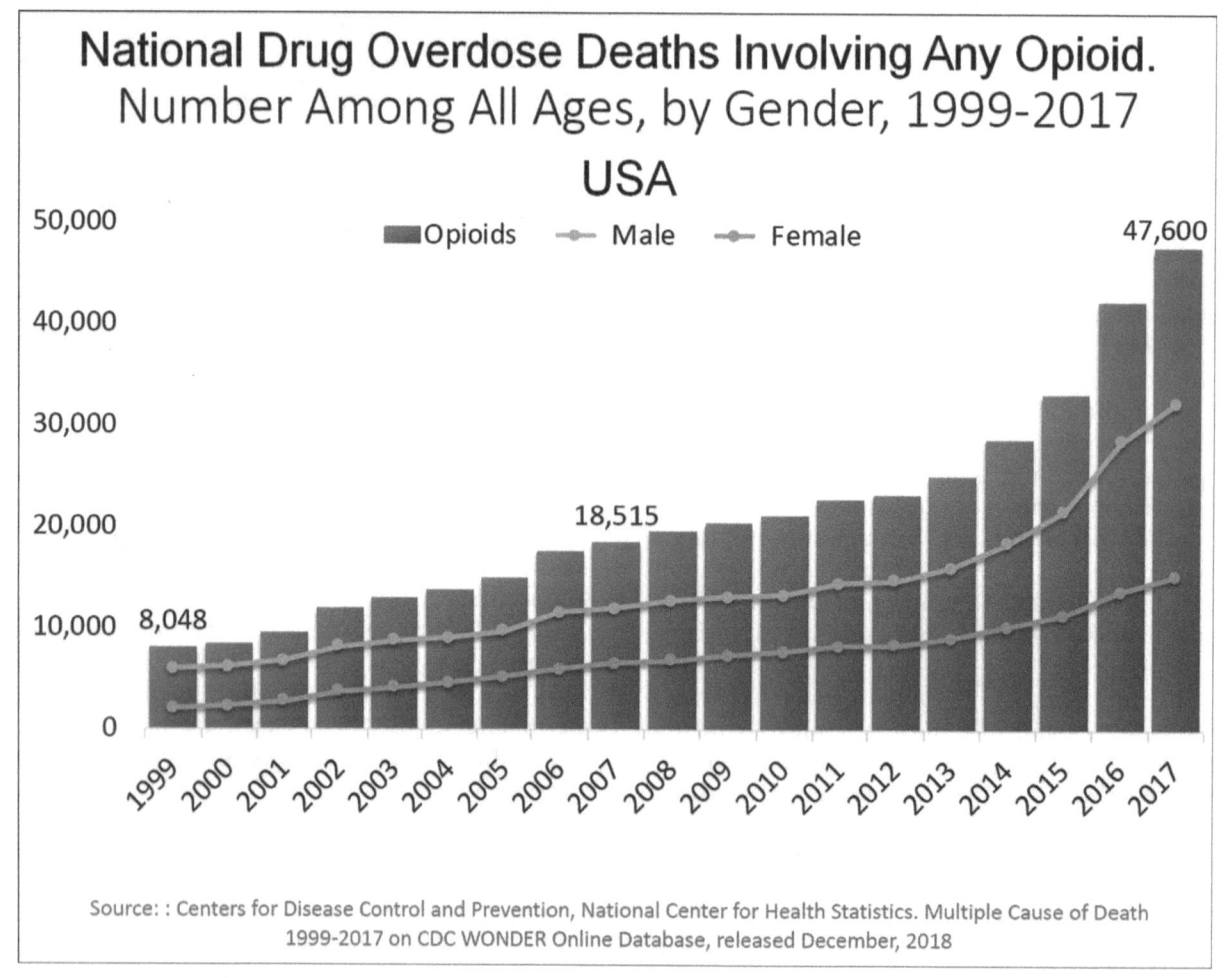

National Drug Overdose Deaths Involving Any Opioid. Number Among All Ages, by Gender, 1999-2017
USA

Source: Centers for Disease Control and Prevention, National Center for Health Statistics. Multiple Cause of Death 1999-2017 on CDC WONDER Online Database, released December, 2018

"Any Opioids" includes prescription opioids (and methadone), heroin and other synthetic narcotics (mainly fentanyl). Drug overdose deaths rose from 8,048 in 1999 to 47,600 in 2017. (CDC / National Institute on Drug Abuse)

dynorphins. In the same way, with the administration of narcotics, one artificially increases the amount of opioids in the body in order to block pain impulses.

Opioids also act on the brainstem to modulate other pathways not associated with pain. They suppress coughing in a way that is similar to their effect on neural signals to decrease pain messages to the brain. Narcotics appear to inhibit the release of neurotransmitters responsible for the cough reflex. Unfortunately, opiates can simultaneously activate other areas of the brainstem responsible for nausea and vomiting. This unwanted side effect is related to the dose and type of drug used. Therefore, physicians can usually diminish the vomiting response with appropriate treatment selections. Perhaps the most dangerous problem with opioid usage is the effect on the brainstem's regulation of respiration. When the brainstem senses that the level of carbon dioxide is too high, breathing is increased to rid the body of this excess gas. Narcotics decrease the responsiveness of the brainstem to carbon dioxide. Therefore, breathing rates tend to be inappropriately low, causing a buildup of carbon dioxide.

Constriction of the pupils of the eyes is a very common side effect of opiates on the visual system. In fact, this constriction serves as an important diagnostic clue in examining a patient who has taken an overdose of a narcotic.

Opiates have a constipating effect, indirectly through the central nervous system and directly through their influence on the intestines. Opiates cause a decrease in peristalsis, concerted muscular contractions of the intestinal wall that would normally move food toward the anus.

Most opiate analgesics have no direct effect on the heart and blood vessels. Thus, they do not alter heart rate or blood pressure to any significant degree. The only noticeable effect on the cardiovascular system is a flushing and warming of the skin because of a slight increase in blood flow. Occasionally, this is accompanied by sweating. Kidney function tends to be depressed by opiates, which may be attributable to a decrease in the amount of blood that is filtered through the kidneys. There is also a decrease in the ability to urinate, as these drugs increase contraction of the muscle that prevents urine from leaving the bladder.

Uses and Complications

Medical personnel utilize narcotics to alter the body for the patient's advantage. Narcotics such as opiates are used for the relief of pain and anxiety, adjuncts for anesthesia, reduction of coughing, and control of diarrhea.

Opiate analgesics are among the most effective and valuable medications for the treatment of acute and chronic pain. They are often used to treat pain in the postoperative period, in which they effectively reduce or eliminate the short-term pain from tissue trauma that is caused by surgery. When pain is reduced, patients tend to eat, sleep, and recover much more rapidly. Physicians often prescribe narcotics such as morphine or codeine for an as-needed basis ("PRN"). By doing so, the patient, who knows firsthand the effectiveness of the drug, can control the frequency of analgesic administration. In fact, patients are usually advised to administer a small dose before the pain becomes too intense, thus decreasing the pain message before it reaches a higher level, requiring a higher dosage for relief.

A painful sensation consists of the neural response to the tissue damage and the patient's reaction to the stimulus. The analgesic properties of narcotics are related to their ability to diminish both pain perception and the reaction of the patient to pain. These drugs effectively raise the threshold for pain, perhaps because of the euphoria experienced by patients given opioids. For example, a patient in pain who is given morphine experiences a pleasant floating sensation with a great reduction in distress and anxiety. It is interesting to note, however, that some subjects do not experience euphoria when given morphine. In fact, they tend to have an unpleasant response known as dysphoria, which often includes restlessness and a feeling of general discomfort.

Physicians and other health care workers must achieve a delicate balance between alleviating pain from known causes and masking pain as a warning signal from unexpected sources. For example, a patient having abdominal surgery would likely require relatively high doses of analgesics to reduce the postoperative pain. Yet the administration of an analgesic could mask the pain from an unexpected abdominal infection. Therefore, if used excessively, narcotics may prevent the early recognition of complications.

In addition to their analgesic effects, opiates tend to have a sedative effect and are often used as an adjunct to anesthesia. Potent opiates are used in relatively large doses to achieve general anesthesia, particularly in patients undergoing heart surgery. These narcotics are also commonly used during other surgeries in which it is important that heart function be affected only minimally. Examples of narcotic agents used in anesthesia include fentanyl (Sublimaze), sufentanil, alfentanil, and propofol.

Suppression of the cough reflex is a clinically useful effect of opiates. Therapeutic doses needed to reduce coughing are much lower than doses to achieve analgesia. The opioid derivatives most commonly used to suppress the cough reflex are codeine, dextromethorphan, and noscapine. The exact mechanism of action is unknown; however, it is thought to act on the brainstem.

Diarrhea from almost any cause can be controlled with opiates. Diphenoxylate (Lomotil) and loperamide (Imodium) are commonly used to treat diarrhea and do not possess analgesic properties. These drugs appear to act on the nerves within the intestinal tract to decrease muscular activity.

Like all drugs, narcotics have both beneficial and undesired effects. The toxic effects of an opioid depend on the dosage, the agent used, the clinical condition in which it is used, and an individual patient's response to the drug. Some of the more common unwanted side effects include restlessness and hyperactivity instead of sedation, respiratory depression, nausea and vomiting, increased pressure within the brain, low blood pressure, constipation, urinary retention, and itching around the nose. Most of these conditions are of short duration and resolve after the drug has been discontinued.

Patients on chronic opiate therapy may develop tolerance and become physically and mentally dependent upon these agents. Many people abuse narcotics in high dosages in order to experience euphoric effects. With chronic use, the euphoric effects diminish and the user eventually requires higher doses to achieve the same euphoria. Physiological adaptation to the long-term use of opioids (two to three weeks) causes the development of tolerance towards these drugs.

Exogenous opioids take the place of endogenous ones. Therefore, the nervous system and other physiological systems attempt to bring the levels of these neurotransmitters back to normal. First, the liver speeds up its metabolism of the drugs to eliminate them from the system more rapidly. Second, the regions of the nervous system that respond to opioids become desensitized by reducing the number of neural receptors that are available. Finally, after a few weeks of high levels of opiates, changes in other areas of the brain attempt to compensate for the rising opioid levels. Individuals who abruptly stop taking the drugs enter a period of withdrawal in which they experience symptoms similar to a bad case of influenza. Morphine and heroine withdrawal symptoms usually start within twelve hours of the last dose. Peak symptoms of narcotic withdrawal occur after one to two days. Most symptoms gradually subside and resolve after one week. It should be emphasized that, under a physician's direction, the abuse potential of narcotics is very low.

There are certain clinical conditions in which opiates should not be used or should be used with extreme caution. Because of the potential for respiratory depression with opiate treatment, these drugs should not be administered to patients with head injuries or impaired lung function. Most opioid drugs can cross the placenta and therefore should be avoided during pregnancy; with long-term use, the infant can be born addicted to narcotics.

Fortunately, some drugs can reverse the effects of narcotics when required. Three commonly used opioid antagonists are nalmefene, naloxone (Narcan), and naltrexone (Trexan). When these agents are given in the absence of an opioid agonist, they have no noticeable effect. When administered to a morphine-treated patient, however, they completely reverse the opioid effects almost immediately. These narcotic antagonists are particularly useful in treating patients who have taken an overdose of opiates. Such patients often arrive in the hospital emergency room with severe respiratory depression or in a coma. These antagonists will normalize respiration, restore consciousness, and counteract other opioid effects. Interestingly, individuals who have become tolerant to and dependent upon opioids will immediately experience withdrawal symptoms when given naloxone or naltrexone.

Perspective and Prospects

Narcotic drugs were originally found in the opium poppy five thousand years ago. Opium is obtained from the milky fluid of the unripe seed capsules of the poppy plant. The juice is dried in the air and forms a brown, sticky substance. With continued drying, the mass can be pulverized into powder. It is this powder that opiates are derived from. Morphine, codeine, and papaverine are the natural opiates that are used clinically. Most other narcotics are chemically derived.

The opium poppy, *Papaver somniferum*, was named after the Roman god of sleep, Somnis. Ancient Egyptian medical texts listed opium as a cure for illness and as a poison. Although opium was used extensively, the abuse potential was low because the poppy has a very bitter taste. Smoking opium became popular in eighteenth century China as a treatment for severe diarrhea and was also a socially acceptable drug used mainly for its euphoric effects.

The opium poppy contains more than twenty distinct agents with a variety of potencies and unwanted side effects. In 1806, a pharmacist refined opium into one active substance, morphine, which was found to be ten times as potent. Morphine was named after Morpheus, the Greek god of dreams, because of its powerful sedative effects. The discovery of other medically active agents quickly followed. Codeine and papaverine were identified next and found to be slightly less potent than morphine. At this time, clinicians used these purified products rather than the crude opium juice.

Shortly after purified narcotics became available, so did the widespread use of hypodermic needles. This allowed physicians to administer narcotics directly into the bloodstream. The injected opioids would rapidly travel via the blood to the brain and exert its effects. In the United States, morphine found widespread use as an analgesic for wounded soldiers during the Civil War. It was one of the most powerful painkillers available to physicians, but its unrestricted availability created great potential for addiction with long-term use.

Opioid derivations became so popular that hundreds of medications became available to the public in many different forms. Tonics promised to cure everything from "tired blood" to common aches and pains. Their widespread unregulated usage allowed for potential addiction. At the beginning of the twentieth century, the U.S. government attempted to address this issue by making it illegal to buy any opiate-containing compound without a prescription. Chemists then tried to synthesize compounds with morphine-like characteristics but without the addictive effects.

Physicians now have a vast selection of narcotics with different pharmacological properties to choose from. For example, there are drugs without addictive, euphoric, or sedative properties that can treat coughing or diarrhea. Narcotic analgesics can only be prescribed and administered under the direction of a physician. With proper medical supervision, the benefit of narcotics can be maximized and the side effects, including addiction, can be minimized. Morphine is still used as a potent pain reliever, and when used appropriately, there is less potential for addiction. With further research into opioids and pain pathways, the potential for further medical usage remains an endless possibility.

—*Matthew Berria, Ph.D.*
—*Cristina Cesaro, D.O.*
—*Jimmy Bajaj, D.O.*

References

Bonnie, Richard J., et al. "Pain Management and Opioid Regulation: Continuing Public Health Challenges." *American Journal of Public Health*, vol. 109, no. 1, Jan. 2019, pp. 31–34., doi:10.2105/ajph.2018.304881.

"CDC Guideline for Prescribing Opioids for Chronic Pain." *Centers for Disease Control and Prevention*, 28 Aug. 2019, www.cdc.gov/drugoverdose/prescribing/guideline.html.

Inaba, Darryl S., William E. Cohen, and Michael E. Holstein. Uppers, Downers, All Arounders: Physical and Mental Effects of Psychoactive Drugs. 8th ed. CNS, 2014.

Jones, Mark R., et al. "A Brief History of the Opioid Epidemic and Strategies for Pain Medicine." *Pain and Therapy*, vol. 7, no. 1, 24 Apr. 2018, pp. 13–21., doi:10.1007/s40122-018-0097-6.

Klimas, Jan, et al. "Strategies to Identify Patient Risks of Prescription Opioid Addiction When Initiating Opioids for Pain." *JAMA Network Open*, vol. 2, no. 5, 3 May 2019, doi:10.1001/jamanetworkopen.2019.3365.

"Narcotics (Opioids)." *United States Drug Enforcement Administration*, U.S. Department of Justice, 16 Sept. 2019, www.dea.gov/taxonomy/term/331.

Nelson, Harry. *The United States of Opioids: a Prescription for Liberating a Nation in Pain*. Ingram Pub Services, 2019.

"Opioid Overdose Crisis." *National Institute on Drug Abuse*, National Institutes of Health, 22 Jan. 2019, www.drugabuse.gov/drugs-abuse/opioids/opioid-overdose-crisis.

Wood, Evan, et al. "Pain Management With Opioids in 2019-2020." *Jama*, 10 Oct. 2019, doi:10.1001/jama.2019.15802.

Nitrous oxide

CATEGORY: Analgesic, Anxiolytic
ALSO KNOWN AS: Laughing gas, nitrous, N₂O
ANATOMY OR SYSTEM EFFECTED: Respiratory, Central Nervous System

KEY TERMS
- *agonist*: a biochemical substance that, when bound to a receptor, initiates a physiologic response
- *antagonist*: a biochemical substance that opposes the function an agonist
- *endogenous*: a substance that originates naturally within the organism
- *peptides*: short chains of amino acids that, when released, carry out functions in other areas of the body

Nitrous oxide has been used as an analgesic and anxiolytic for more than 150 years. It is commonly referred to as "laughing gas" and is best known for its use in minor dental procedures. Nitrous oxide can also be used as an inhaled anesthetic for minor medical procedures and acute pain. It is administered as a gas through a facemask with the typical dosing of 50% oxygen and 50% nitrous oxide. In the United States, nitrous oxide is most commonly used to reduce pain and anxiety during labor for pregnant women and in dental procedures such as filling a cavity or removing a tooth.

Mechanism of Action

When inhaled, nitrous oxygen travels into the lungs and into the alveoli where the gas molecules are absorbed into the cardiovascular system. The nitrous oxide then travels to the central nervous system, where it begins to produce its analgesic effects. The exact mechanism of action is unknown, but it is hypothesized that nitrous oxide functions either as a partial agonist to opioid receptors or by stimulating the release of endogenous opioid peptides. This hypothesis is supported because its effects are quickly reversed with the use of the opioid antagonist naloxone. It is estimated that inhaled nitrous oxide has a similar analgesic effect to 10-15 mg of morphine.

Nitrous oxide begins to work almost immediately after it is inhaled and has a peak effect after about 2-5 minutes. Similarly, the medication wears off rapidly when the facemask is removed, making it ideal for procedures. It is believed that only 1% of nitrous oxide is metabolized by the body with 99% being exhaled without absorption. While nitrous oxide is administered, patients commonly describe a reduction in pain and anxiety while also experiencing a euphoric sensation. Unlike other anesthetics, nitrous oxide does not cause patients to become unconscious.

Uses and Applications

Nitrous oxide is best used to reduce pain and anxiety during various procedures. It is commonly used in dental offices for root canals, cavity fillings, and tooth extractions. Nitrous oxide can be especially helpful in reducing fear and anxiety in pediatric patients who are undergoing common painful procedures such as IV starts, wound dressing changes, or suture removal.

Women who are in labor or giving birth may also benefit from nitrous oxide administration. Studies have demonstrated favorable analgesic and anxiolytic effects, while also being safe for the mother and baby. Nitrous oxide is an inexpensive and safe intervention that may be used as an alternative to an epidural for pain control during labor.

Nitrous oxide is also useful in the emergency medicine setting. For patients who are transported via emergency medical services, nitrous oxide can safely provide rapid pain and anxiety relief. In patients who are experiencing a myocardial infarction, severe burn, or musculoskeletal trauma, paramedics can administer nitrous oxide until stronger analgesic medications can be provided in an emergency department.

Finally, nitrous oxide is useful in the primary care setting for a variety of procedures. It can be used as an analgesic and anxiolytic for procedures like wound debridement, removing staples, obtaining skin biopsies, and drain removal. Unfortunately, there is no evidence to support the use of nitrous oxide in the treatment of chronic pain.

Risks

When used appropriately, nitrous oxide has proven to be a safe medication. Long-term exposure to nitrous oxide has been shown to cause spontaneous abortion, infertility, and neurologic deficits. There is also a risk of abuse due to the euphoric sensation it causes. Nitrous oxide is contraindicated in people with altered mental status, respiratory distress, maxillofacial abnormalities, and those who have experienced chest or abdominal trauma.

—*Grayson Baker, RN, BSN*

References

Becker, Daniel E., & Morton Rosenberg. "Nitrous oxide and the Inhalation Anesthetics." *Anesthesia Progress*, vol. 55, no. 4, 2008, pp. 124-131. doi: 10.2344/0003-3006-55.4.124

Collins, M. R., Starr, S. A., Bishop, J. T., & Baysinger, C. L. (2012). "Nitrous Oxide for Labor Analgesia: Expanding Analgesic Options for Women in the United States." *Reviews in Obstetrics and Gynecology*, vol. 5, no. 3-4, 2012, p. e126.

Emmanouil, Dimitris E., & Raymond M. Quock. "Advances in Understanding the Actions of Nitrous Oxide." *Anesthesia Progress*, vol. 54, no. 1, 2007, pp. 9-18. doi: 10.2344/0003-3006(2007)54[9:AIUTAO]2.0.CO;2

Gregory, Julie. "Using Nitrous Oxide and Oxygen to Control Pain in Primary Care." *Nursing Times*, vol. 98, no. 46, 2008, pp. 28–29.

Oglesbee, Scott. "Using Nitrous Oxide to Manage Pain." *Journal of Emergency Medical Services*, vol. 39, no. 4, 2014, pp. 34-37.

Judith P. Rooks. "Safety and Risks of Nitrous Oxide Labor Analgesia: A Review." *Journal of Midwifery & Women's Health*, vol. 56, no. 6, 2011, pp. 557-565. doi:10.1111/j.1542-2011.2011.00122.x

Turan, A., et al. (2015). "Nitrous Oxide for the Treatment of Chronic Low Back Pain." *Anesthesia & Analgesia*, vol. 121, no. 5, 2015, pp. 1350-1359. doi: 10.1213/ANE.0000000000000951.

■ NMDA receptor antagonists

CATEGORY: Class of Drug
ALSO KNOWN AS: N-methyl-D-aspartate receptor antagonists
ANATOMY OR SYSTEM AFFECTED: nervous system

KEY TERMS

- *AMPA receptor*: a subtype of ionotropic glutamate receptor that modulates the glutamate-mediated stimulation of neurons by allowing the influx of calcium and sodium ions
- *glutamate*: a naturally occurring amino acid that is the most abundant stimulatory neurotransmitter in the nervous system
- *glycine*: the simplest naturally occurring amino acid that is a constituent of most proteins and one of the two main inhibitory neurotransmitters in the central nervous system, mainly in the spinal cord
- *neurotransmitter*: chemicals released by neurons that transmit an impulse or inhibit a target cell
- *NMDA receptor*: glutamate-gated cation channels that are highly permeable to calcium ions and play several important roles in the neurobiology of animals.
- *signal transduction pathway*: A cascade of biochemical reactions inside cells that culminate in a specific cellular response, and are set in motion when a signaling molecule, such as a hormone or growth factor, binds receptors inside the cell or on the cell surface

Healthcare providers use NMDA receptor antagonists to treat dementia (memantine), cough (dextromethorphan), pain (ketamine and methadone), and depression, and as anesthetics (ketamine). Drug abusers also use NMDA receptor antagonists as drugs of abuse.

How NMDA Receptor Antagonists Work

In the nervous system, neurons communicate with each other by releasing small molecules called neurotransmitters. Neurotransmitters bind to specific receptors in the membranes of other neurons called "ligand-gated ion channels." When neurotransmitters bind to ligand-gated ion channels, they regulate the opening or closing of those channels. The entrance of positively-charged ions into neurons can activate them, or the entry of negatively-charged ions into neurons can inhibit them. Therefore, neurotransmitters can be stimulatory or inhibitory.

The most prevalent stimulatory neurotransmitter in the central nervous system is the amino acid glutamate. There are two different categories of glutamate receptors: 1) ionotropic glutamate receptors, which are ligand-gated ion channels that open in response to glutamate binding; and 2) metabotropic glutamate receptors that activate a signal transduction pathway within cells when bound by glutamate that elicits specific cellular responses. There are three types of ionotropic glutamate receptors; NMDA, AMPA, and kainite receptors. Of these, NMDA receptors have the most critical role in pain modulation.

NMDA receptors usually exist in combination with AMPA receptors. When bound by glutamate,

AMPA receptors tend to cause rather rapid, though short-lived stimulations of the neuron. Glutamate binds NMDA receptors, but as long as the membrane potential of the neuron remains negative, magnesium ions (Mg^{2+}) block the NMDA receptor. If the neuron is sufficiently stimulated by the AMPA receptors so that the membrane potential becomes positive, then the Mg^{2+} ions are displaced from the NMDA receptors and they bind glutamate and another amino acid called glycine, which opens them. Open NMDA receptors admit sodium and calcium ions into the neuron, which drives two significant events in the neuron: 1) calcium ions cause phosphorylation of the AMPA receptor, which sensitizes it to glutamate and increases stimulation of the neuron; and 2) calcium influx also increases the number of AMPA receptors in the neuronal membrane, which further increases the stimulation of the neuron. This leads to a long-term stimulation of the neuron that is called "long-term potentiation," which plays a significant role in learning and memory, and other neurological functions.

Neurons that relay pain signals also have NMDA receptors in their cell membranes. Several different types of neurons release glutamate in response to noxious peripheral stimuli, and prolonged release of glutamate by sensory neurons that transmit pain signals activates the NMDA receptor. Consequently, NMDA receptor antagonists can provide pain relief.

Clinical Uses of NMDA Receptor Antagonists

Commonly found in over-the-counter cough medications, dextromethorphan relieves persistent cough and neuropathic pain.

Methadone is an opioid that also acts as an NMDA receptor antagonist. It is the first-line treatment for opioid dependence and withdrawal. However, methadone also relieves neuropathic pain (pain that results from nerve damage), cancer pain, and pain in critically-ill patients.

Ketamine is an NMDA antagonist and a weak opioid with potent pain relief activity. Ketamine treats severe pain during surgical operations (intraoperative pain), cancer pain, pain in newborn babies, refractory pain at the end of life, and is also effective for treatment-resistant depression. It is also used off-label as an anesthetic.

Two other NMDA receptor agonists, amantadine and memantine have little to no pain-relieving activities.

Side Effects

Methadone has a variable drug half-life (from 12 hours to almost one week) and carries the highest risk among the opioids of accumulation and overdosage. The consequences of methadone overdose are the same as that for other opioids: depressed consciousness, respiratory depression, hallucinations and delirium, nausea and vomiting, itching, ileus (intestinal blockage), and urinary retention. Methadone, however, can also cause heart arrhythmias (prolongation of the QTc interval), and methadone recipients should have their heart ECG regularly monitored.

Ketamine can cause hallucinations, delirium, confusion, a dream-like state, excitement, irrational behavior, and vivid dreams. It can also increase heart rate and raise blood pressure. Because of its ability to induce euphoria, illusions, dream-like states, and out-of-body experiences, ketamine is a drug of abuse. Ketamine overdose can cause coma, but at lower doses, ketamine abuse typically impairs consciousness. In others, ketamine may cause fear, agitation, and psychiatric disturbance. Prolonged ketamine abuse can permanently damage the bladder.

The reported side effects of dextromethorphan are light-headedness, dizziness, drowsiness, restlessness, nausea, and nervousness, but if used at the recommended doses, these adverse effects are infrequent and not severe. Rarely, some people are allergic to dextromethorphan. Drug users also divert over-the-counter dextromethorphan for illicit recreational use. Dextromethorphan overdose produces behavioral changes (e.g., euphoria, hallucinations, inappropriate laughing, psychosis with dissociative features, agitation, and coma), dilated pupils, tachycardia (abnormally high heart rate), nystagmus (involuntary, rapid, and repetitive movements of the eyes), sweating (diaphoresis), and a "zombie-like" ataxic gait. In young children, dextromethorphan poisoning causes respiratory depression and, rarely, coma.

—*Michael A. Buratovich Ph.D.*

References

Chizh, B, and P. M. Headley. "NMDA Antagonists and Neuropathic Pain - Multiple Drug Targets and Multiple Uses." *Current Pharmaceutical Design*, vol. 11, no. 23, 2005, pp. 2977-2994. doi:10.2174/1381612054865082.

Collins, Susan, et al. "NMDA Receptor Antagonists for the Treatment of Neuropathic Pain." *Pain Medicine*, vol. 11, no. 11, 2010, pp. 1726–1742. doi:10.1111/j.1526-4637.2010.00981.x

Dellwo, Adrienne. "NMDA Receptors and How They're Involved in Disease." *Verywell Health*, 28 Sept 28, 2019. https://www.verywellhealth.com/nmda-receptors-and-how-they-re-involved-in-disease-4151196.

Jamero, Dana, et al. "The Emerging Role of NMDA Antagonists in Pain Management." *US Pharmacist*, vol. 35, no. 5, 2011, HS4-HS8.

Quibel, Rachel, et al. "Ketamine." *Journal of Pain and Symptom Management*, vol. 41, no. 3, 2011, pp. 640-649.

Thompson, Trevor, et al. "NMDA Receptor Agonists and Pain Relief: A Meta-Analysis of Experimental Trials." *Neurology*, vol. 92, no. 14, 2019, e1652-e1662. doi:10.1212/WNL.0000000000007238

■ Non-steroidal anti-inflammatory drugs (NSAIDs)

CATEGORY: Class of Drug
ANATOMY OR SYSTEM AFFECTED: Any area of inflammation or pain throughout the body
SPECIALTIES AND RELATED FIELDS: Primary care, internal medicine, family medicine, orthopedic surgery, rheumatology, nurse practitioner, physician assistant

KEY TERMS
- *arachidonic acid*: an omega-6 unsaturated fatty acid the body requires to function properly; when broken down in the body, prostaglandins are produced
- *COX-1 AND COX-2*: cyclooxygenase 1 and 2 (COX-1 and COX-2) are important enzymes in the function of the human body; they both convert arachidonic acid to prostaglandins, and are implicated in pain, inflammation, cell multiplication, and other key biologic responses
- *NSAIDs*: nonsteroidal anti-inflammatory drugs (NSAIDs) are medications that are used to control pain and inflammation in the body
- *osteoarthritis*: a progressive disorder of the joints caused by gradual loss of cartilage that can result in the development of bone spurs and cysts at the margins of joints
- *prostaglandins*: one of a number of hormone-like substances that participate in a wide range of body functions such as the contraction and relaxation of smooth muscle, the dilation and constriction of blood vessels, control of blood pressure, and modulation of inflammation
- *Reye syndrome*: a rare but serious disease that most often affects children ages 6 to 12 years old; can cause brain swelling and liver damage; may be related to using aspirin to treat viral infections

Indications

Enzymes known as COX-1 and COX-2 are produced by cells in the body and are responsible for the creation of substances called prostaglandins from a fatty acid called arachidonic acid. Arachidonic acid is generated by the degradation of membrane phospholipids by enzymes called phospholipases A2, which are activated when cells are damaged in any way. Prostaglandins are responsible for many functions in the body and can foster inflammation, pain, and fever. Nonsteroidal anti-inflammatory drugs (NSAIDs) are used to inhibit the activity of the COX-1 AND COX-2 enzymes, which cause the pain and inflammation.

The most well-known NSAIDs are aspirin, ibuprofen, and naproxen, but there are many other NSAIDs including the following generic drugs: ketoprofen, sulindac, fenoprofen, diclofenac, flurbiprofen, ketorolac, piroxicam, indomethacin, mefenamic acid, meloxicam, nabumetone, oxaprozin, famotidine, meclofenamate, tolmetin, and salsalate.

NSAIDs are used to reduce fever and inflammation and for pain control. Currently, they are among the most commonly prescribed medications used for inflammation and pain control, particularly for osteoarthritis, joint pain, or muscle strain.

NSAIDs are commonly indicated for use in the following conditions: joint pain and inflammation from osteoarthritis and rheumatoid arthritis; gout (build-up of uric acid causing pain in the extremities); headaches; pain after surgery; pain from an injury such as sprains or strained muscles; and pain from kidney stones.

Many NSAIDs also have an anti-clotting effect. Preventing clotting can have an effect on reducing strokes and other cardiovascular issues, however,

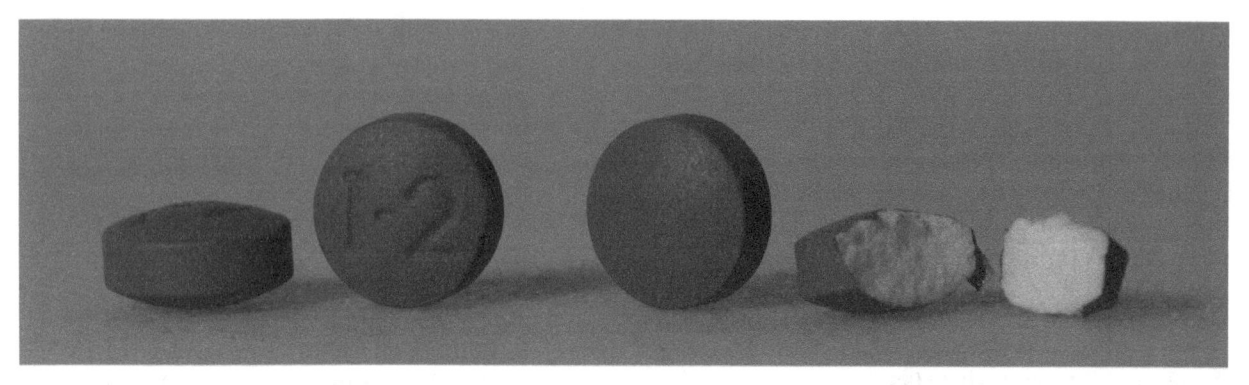

Coated 200 mg tablets of generic ibuprofen, a common NSAID. (Ragesoss via Wikimedia Commons)

NSAIDs are not generally taken to prevent cardiovascular disease. A common side effect of NSAIDs is high blood pressure (hypertension), which offsets the anti-platelet action.

However, low-dose aspirin (81 mg.) is often recommended to patients who have already been diagnosed with cardiovascular disease to reduce the chances of heart attack and stroke. Many people also take low-dose aspirin as a preventative measure, but researchers are still unsure whether or not it is helpful for a healthy individual to take low-dose aspirin as a preventative treatment against heart attack or stroke.

Uses and Complications

Although NSAIDs are generally safe, it is reported that as many as 30-35% of individuals who take NSAIDs experience some side effects or adverse drug reactions. Various NSAIDs may affect individuals differently.

The most common reported side effects of NSAIDs are gastrointestinal problems. Usually, the reactions are mild, but sometimes they can result in more serious problems. The following gastrointestinal side effects may include nausea, indigestion, excess gas, vomiting, stomach ulcers or intestinal bleeding.

To lessen the chance of gastrointestinal side effects, many over-the-counter NSAIDs are produced with a special coating called an enteric coating, but to date there is no evidence that coating the medication is effective in reducing the possibility of digestive side effects.

NSAIDs carry an increased risk of cardiovascular disease. Some research implies that the occurrence of serious cardiovascular disease such as heart attacks and stroke can be twice as likely in people using NSAIDs, even if there is no pre-existing heart disease.

As mentioned in the Indications section, low-dose aspirin is an exception to this adverse reaction, and it is often used to reduce the risk of further heart attack and stroke among those who have a pre-existing condition.

Kidney problems can also be a side effect of using NSAIDs, especially when these drugs are combined with use of other drugs such as those used to treat high blood pressure. Sometimes NSAIDs can also affect the kidneys' filtering ability, leading to water retention and high blood pressure. Recent studies have suggested that routine increased use of NSAIDs by athletes, for example, ultrarunners, to decrease pain from muscle soreness or stiffness and pain, may lead to increasing the chance of them developing acute kidney injury.

If an individual using NSAIDs experiences pain in the kidneys, a reduction in the amount of urine produced, or changes in the urine color, etc., they should let their healthcare provider know immediately.

The use of NSAIDs has been linked to erectile dysfunction, but it is not understood exactly why this is the case. Men—particularly middle-aged men—regularly taking NSAIDs are up to 2.4 times more likely to suffer from erectile dysfunction.

Less common side effects of taking NSAIDs may also include an allergic skin reaction to sunlight (rash).

A positive effect of NSAIDs, however, is its use in colon cancer increased survival. A recent study at Fred Hutchinson Cancer Research Center in Seattle, Washington, concluded that the use of NSAIDs improved survival for certain colorectal cancer patients. In the study, NSAIDs were associated with about a 25 percent reduction in all-cause mortality.

However, the benefit versus increased risk of cardiovascular issues needs to still be determined.

Aspirin and other NSAIDs are also thought to prevent the growth of intestinal polyps that can precede the development of colorectal cancer. Aspirin and other NSAIDs activate cell suicide pathways found in intestinal stem cells that can carry a certain mutated and dysfunctional gene known as APC and make the cells dysfunctional. NSAIDs activate the early auto-destruction of cells that could lead to precancerous polyps and tumors, according to the 2014 study at the Pittsburgh Cancer Institute (UPCI) and the School of Medicine.

Precautions

NSAIDs are not recommend to be taken during pregnancy, especially the last trimester of pregnancy. These drugs can affect the infant's developing heart and kidneys, and may also contribute to premature birth and miscarriage. Also, NSAIDs should not be used in individuals with kidney disease, congestive heart failure, or liver cirrhosis to prevent the kidneys from failing (acute renal failure).

NSAIDs should not be given to an individual who is taking an anti-clotting medication (other than low-dose aspirin if prescribed by their healthcare provider) since this may increase the risk of bleeding.

The use of aspirin for viral infections in children or teens should not be given because of the risk of Reye's syndrome.

NSAIDs are not recommended for individuals with uncontrolled diabetes, active congestive heart failure, nasal polyps, or in phenylketonuria (an inherited disorder that prevents the disposal of the amino acid phenylalanine), ulcerative colitis, and gastroesophageal reflux disease (GERD).

It is important for an individual to let their healthcare provider about any other medications that they are taking since some drug combinations should not be used with NSAIDs. When taken with some kidney and blood pressure medications, for example, NSAIDs may cause those medications to work less effectively.

The use of NSAIDs should always be discussed with an individual's healthcare provider. Usually, treatment with higher doses of NSAIDs is used to control pain and reduce inflammation, e.g., in osteoarthritis, a sprain, etc. A prescription from a healthcare provider is needed for the higher doses to be taken at regular intervals throughout the day as prescribed. For temporary conditions to relieve pain, like back pain for example, over-the-counter doses of NSAIDs are adequate.

The Federal Drug Administration (FDA) suggests individuals obtain medical attention right away if any of the following occur: chest pain, shortness of breath, trouble breathing, slurred speech, or weakness on one side or part of the body.

—*Joanne R. Gambosi, BSN, MA*

References

Davis, Abigail, and John Robson. "The Dangers of NSAIDs: Look Both Ways." *British Journal of General Practice*, vol. 66, no. 645, Apr. 2016, pp. 172–173., doi:10.3399/bjgp16x684433.

Felson, David T. "Safety of Nonsteroidal Antiinflammatory Drugs." *New England Journal of Medicine*, vol. 375, no. 26, 29 Dec. 2016, pp. 2595–2596., doi:10.1056/nejme1614257.

Flores, Diane. *Nonsteroidal Anti-Inflammatory Drugs (NSAIDs): Common Uses, Risks and Effectiveness.* Nova Biomedical, 2017.

Fookes, C. "Nonsteroidal Anti-Inflammatory Drugs." *Drugs.com*, 22 Mar. 2018, www.drugs.com/drug-class/nonsteroidal-anti-inflammatory-agents.html.

Hertz, Sharon. "The Benefits and Risks of Pain Relievers: Q & A on NSAIDs." *U.S. Food and Drug Administration*, 24 Sept. 2015, www.fda.gov/consumers/consumer-updates/benefits-and-risks-pain-relievers-q-nsaids-sharon-hertz-md.

Ho, Kok Yuen, et al. "Nonsteroidal Anti-Inflammatory Drugs in Chronic Pain: Implications of New Data for Clinical Practice." *Journal of Pain Research*, vol. 11, 2018, pp. 1937–1948., doi:10.2147/jpr.s168188.

Osafo, Newman, et al. "Mechanism of Action of Nonsteroidal Anti-Inflammatory Drugs." *Nonsteroidal Anti-Inflammatory Drugs*, 23 Aug. 2017, doi:10.5772/68090.

Solomon, Daniel H. "Patient Education: Nonsteroidal Antiinflammatory Drugs (NSAIDs) (Beyond the Basics)." *UpToDate*, 21 Feb. 2019, www.uptodate.com/contents/nonsteroidal-anti-inflammatory-drugs-nsaids-beyond-the-basics.

Wong, Rebecca S. Y. "Role of Nonsteroidal Anti-Inflammatory Drugs (NSAIDs) in Cancer Prevention and Cancer Promotion." *Advances in Pharmacological Sciences*, vol. 2019, 31 Jan. 2019, pp. 1–10., doi:10.1155/2019/3418975.

Opium

CATEGORY: Addiction Risk; Opioid
ALSO KNOWN AS: Aunti, Aunti Emma, Big O, Black pill, Chandu, Chinese Molasses, Dopium, Dream Gun, Fi-do-nie, Gee, Guma, Midnight Oil, Zero
ANATOMY OR SYSTEM AFFECTED: Nervous system

History of Use

Opium is processed in a manner that has changed little from fifth-century methods. Ancient peoples too used the plant to alleviate pain and anxiety and to perform minor surgeries. Early civilizations wrote about the healing powers of opium, as did such early physicians as Dioscorides, Galen, and Avicenna. Throughout these times, written records indicate that opium was considered primarily a healing tool and not a recreational drug.

China was the next great civilization to be introduced to the opium plant through trade with the Islamic world around the fifteenth century. The Chinese also used opium for medicinal purposes, but as opium use spread, people began to find a new use for the plant. The gummy rolled-up balls of the poppy plant, which resemble clay, were smoked in special pipes that circulated air under the opium balls. The result was a euphoric and hallucinogenic experience. While smoking opium was by no means epidemic, it was popular and highly addictive.

By 1900, Friedrich Sertürner had isolated morphine from opium, Pierre Jean Robiquet had discovered codeine, and opium and opium derivatives were becoming the most popular medicines in the United States. Produced by Bayer, Heroin (the brand name) was given to children as a cough syrup. Laudanum, a tincture of opium, was one of the most highly prescribed medicines, primarily to middle-class women for menstrual pains, creating countless addicts. Soon, the Harrison Act of 1914 was passed to regulate opiate use in the United States.

Opiates now are integrated into medicine as necessary tools for pain control. However, physicians are facing more and more regulation in prescribing opiates. Strict regulation of opioid drugs has gained support due to the rising rates of misuse by a small group of physicians and by the alarming rates of prescription medication misuse. This regulation has affected patient care, as physicians, especially those who care for persons with chronic pain and those who provide end-of-life or palliative care, often fear prescribing opiates. However, studies have shown that the first group, people in chronic pain, has little to no risk of becoming addicted to pain medications. For the second group, those needing palliative care, physicians argue that denying dying patients pain medicine for fear they will get addicted goes against the Hippocratic oath. Even physicians who do not treat patients needing such care tend to underprescribe pain medications. Studies show that about 50 percent of patients report that they are not receiving adequate treatment for their pain.

By the second decade of the twenty-first century, opioid misuse had steadily increased to the point where opioid overdose was considered an epidemic by organizations such as the Centers for Disease Control and Prevention (CDC) and the US Department of

Naturally derived opium from opium poppies has been used as a drug since before 1100 BCE. (Erik Fenderson via Wikimedia Commons)

Health and Human Services (HHS). By 2015, deaths resulting from drug overdose had become the leading cause of death from injury in the United States, and that same year, the HHS launched an initiative targeting this epidemic. Opioid misuse and overdose were of greatest concern because, according to the CDC, more than six out of ten drug overdose deaths involved an opioid as of 2015, with an estimated ninety-one Americans dying each day after overdosing on the drug, including heroin. Health officials had grown particularly concerned over the increased misuse of prescription opioids, especially among younger populations.

Effects and Potential Risks

Opiates work by disrupting the signals of pain sent to the brain from various channels. Some signals move through the nervous system. Other signaling systems are chemical and involve a biochemical cascade. One of the reasons why opiates are so effective is that they can block pain at many of these points.

Opiates are quick acting: A patient in severe pain will feel instant relief through the aid of intravenous morphine, for example. Oral medication takes about twenty to thirty minutes before acting but is extremely effective at controlling pain.

The most common side effects of opiates are constipation, sedation, nausea and vomiting, respiratory distress, tolerance, and addiction. For persons with cardiac or pulmonary disease, careful monitoring is necessary to check the patient's breathing. This is especially relevant in hospice care, where patients may be receiving high doses of morphine, which can severely impair breathing.

Detoxification from any opiate, whether a street drug like heroin or a legally prescribed medication, is extremely difficult and can, for some people, be life threatening if not performed under medical supervision. Any person taking large doses of an opiate who attempts to detox can suffer seizures, prolonged insomnia, severe depression, suicidal thoughts, anxiety, and panic attacks. Physical symptoms include vomiting, shaking, anorexia, fever, and chills. It is recommended that a person who needs help with any kind of opium addiction seek the help of a physician.

—*S. M. Willis, MS MA*

References

Batmanabane, Gitanjali. "Why Patients in Pain Cannot Get 'God's Own Medicine?'." *Journal of Pharmacology and Pharmacotherapeutics*, vol. 5, no. 2, 2014, p. 81., doi:10.4103/0976-500x.130040.

Berridge, Virginia. "Opium through History." *The Lancet*, vol. 379, no. 9834, 2012, p. 2332., doi:10.1016/s0140-6736(12)61005-8.

Blistein, David, and John Halpern. *Opium: How an Ancient Flower Shaped and Poisoned Our World*. Hachette Books, 2019.

Brazil, Rachel. "Pain Relief: Designing Better Opioids." *The Pharmaceutical Journal*, vol. 300, no. 7912, 19 Apr. 2018, doi:10.1211/pj.2018.20204708.

Kamangar, Farin, et al. "Opium Use: an Emerging Risk Factor for Cancer?" *The Lancet Oncology*, vol. 15, no. 2, 2014, doi:10.1016/s1470-2045(13)70550-3.

Shad, Bijan, et al. "Does Opium Have Benefit for Coronary Artery Disease? A Systematic Review." *Research in Cardiovascular Medicine*, vol. 7, no. 2, 2018, p. 51., doi:10.4103/rcm.rcm_12_17.

■ Over-the-counter (OTC) drugs

CATEGORY: Over-the-Counter
ANATOMY OR SYSTEM AFFECTED: All

KEY CONCEPTS

- *self-diagnosis*: determining the nature of an ailment and the method of treating it without the aid of a physician; should always be based on sound experience and education rather than on hearsay and guesswork

Indications and Procedures

Drugs or medications that can be purchased directly, without a prescription, are called over-the-counter (OTC) medications or drugs. These medications may be suggested by physicians or simply purchased for consumption as a result of self-diagnosis and self-prescription. Most of the common OTC medications are used to treat common ailments such as cold and fever symptoms, headache, coughs, and similar complaints. Such self-treatment may be initiated at will and discontinued at any time.

Dozens of pharmaceutical companies produce and market hundreds of drugs for sale as over-the-counter medications, but they fall into only a few categories. The basic types of OTC medications, along with some brand examples, include analgesics (Advil, Tylenol), antacids (Milk of Magnesia), antidiarrheal medications (Imodium), antifungal agents (Tinactin), antihistamines (Benadryl), anti-acne treatments (Clearasil), anti-inflammatory drugs (Motrin), decongestants (Sudafed), motion sickness (Mcclizinc), laxatives (Metamucil, Dulcolax), dandruff treatments (Selsun Blue), expectorants (Robitussin), hair growth formulas (Rogaine), and sleep aids (L-Tryptophan).

The most frequently used category of OTC medications is analgesics, which are more popularly known as painkillers. Analgesics include a diverse group of drugs that are used to relieve soreness, general body pain, and headaches. Probably the most common analgesic is aspirin, which is part of a group of medications termed nonsteroidal anti-inflammatory drugs (NSAIDs) that chemically affect the central and possibly the peripheral nervous system by leading to a decrease in prostaglandin production. Many analgesics are used in combination with other drugs such as vasoconstriction drugs that contain pseudoephedrine, which is especially important for the relief of sinus congestion, and in combination with antihistamine drugs, which relieve the worst symptoms of allergy.

Decongestants must certainly rank as the second most common category of OTC medications. Generally, decongestants are taken to relieve nasal congestion and allied symptoms of colds and flu by acting to reduce swelling of the mucous membranes of the nasal passageways. A recurring problem with most nasal decongestants is that they increase hypertension, but this effect is lessened by including one or more antihistamines in the preparation. The brand name drug Dimetapp, for example, is both an antihistamine and a decongestant, while various Tylenol products may contain drugs that collectively work to soothe sore throat, relieve nasal congestion, or suppress coughing.

Despite the fact that over-the-counter drugs are available to everyone, their marketing and use is restricted by the Food and Drug Administration (FDA) in the United States, by Health Canada and similar government agencies with regulatory powers in many other countries. The FDA mandates ingredients and labeling of OTC drugs and specifies rigid testing and safety standards that must be met prior to marketing. Pharmaceutical companies must apply to the New Drug Agency (NDA) for the approval of drugs. The NDA specifies testing requirements prior to issuing a license for the sales and marketing of the proposed new drug. Following approval, the FDA regularly reviews and maintains the right to remove or restrict marketing and sales of OTC drugs that create adverse side effects or are potentially addictive.

Following discovery, testing, and FDA approval of a new drug, it is given a unique trade name or brand name. The pharmaceutical company is awarded an exclusive patent to manufacture and market the drug for a specified period of time, usually seventeen years in the United States but of variable length in other countries. At the end of this time, the company no longer has proprietary rights to the drug, which may then be manufactured and marketed by other pharmaceutical companies. These drug companies may choose to market the drug under a new brand name of their choosing but not under the original label, which may still be manufactured by the original pharmaceutical company that designed and patented the drug. Spin-off products of these companies must still pass rigid FDA quality control standards to demonstrate that their product contains sufficient amounts of the active ingredients to promote bioequivalence before it can be marketed as an OTC medication; in other words, the new drug has to be the therapeutic equal of the original drug.

Drugs manufactured by other pharmaceutical companies following patent expiration are typically called generic drugs and are strictly regulated by the US Drug Price Competition and Patent Term Restoration Act (also known as the Hatch-Waxman Act), which was enacted in 1984. Tylenol, for example, is the exclusive brand name of an analgesic over-the-counter medication that contains the active chemical ingredient acetaminophen. Following the release of its patent, many other pharmaceutical companies started marketing pain relief drugs containing products for pain relief under the their own trade name or brand name. These copies are considered generic drugs and provide the consumer with a wide choice of the most popular drugs, usually at greatly reduced cost.

Manufacture and marketing of a generic drug by new companies usually means that their product costs considerably less, partly because of competition but mostly because the new drug companies did not bear the initial costs of development, marketing, and promotion that were part of the original financial investment of the parent company. Furthermore, manufacturers of generic drugs enjoy all the benefits of prior marketing, public acceptance, and possibly dependence on the most popular OTC medications. Generally, however, the parent company enjoys a certain competitive advantage of brand name recognition that promotes continued use of their marketed product, thereby reducing the impact of cheaper competition.

Over-the-counter medications may take the form of packets, tablets, capsules, pills, drops or droplets, ointments, inhalants, lotions, creams, suppositories, or syrups. Except for creams and topical ointments, OTC medications are administered orally, in contrast to drugs that are taken by injection. This mode of delivery places natural limits on their therapeutic effectiveness in several ways.

After being swallowed, OTC medications pass down the esophagus, through the stomach, and into the small intestine, where they are digested and absorbed. This mode of delivery requires a certain time interval between oral intake of the drug and its arrival in the bloodstream that transports it to target cells, tissues, and organs, thus delaying the effects of the drug. Tablets or capsules sometimes get stuck in the back of the mouth or on the lining of the esophagus, where they start to dissolve. When this happens, the ingredients may cause irritation, nausea, and sometimes vomiting, and the therapeutic value is lost. Furthermore, a certain amount of each key ingredient will be destroyed by the digestive enzymes of the gastrointestinal system, may be metabolized by cells of the intestinal epithelia, or may simply pass through the gut without being absorbed. Even following absorption into the blood, a certain amount of the drug may be lost because liver and other body cells set about removing foreign substances in the blood almost as soon as they are detected, generally by metabolizing the ingredient into a harmless chemical that will be excreted into the bile or be removed by the kidneys. This process explains why all drugs, including OTC medications, must be taken in repeated doses at regularly prescribed intervals in order to obtain maximum therapeutic value.

A final factor complicating delivery efficiency and thus the therapeutic value of OTC medications involves their packaging. Capsules, tablets, and pills in particular all contain substances in addition to the chemical ingredient, such as coatings, fillers, stabilizers, and often color additives. These substances, called excipients, do not contribute to the actual working of the drug itself, but they often modify both the rate and the extent of dissolution of the drug as it travels the gastrointestinal tract. While most excipients ultimately reduce the overall degree of delivery, some have important functions of permitting them to transit through the stomach, which has limited absorption ability, and into the small intestine, where chemical dissolution and absorption occurs at an optimum rate. For some drugs, the natural limits placed on delivery efficiency by gastrointestinal processes and excipient components can be sharply reduced by placing the capsule or tablet directly under the tongue, thus entirely bypassing the alimentary tract.

Uses and Complications
Primarily because of liability issues, all OTC medications include labels that are sometimes extensive. Label components typically consist of a list of one or more symptoms addressed by the medication, active ingredients contained in the drug, warnings, directions for use, and the date after which the medication should be discarded. For example, the label on a common OTC medication used to treat severe colds notes that it is to be used to relieve symptoms of nasal congestion, cough, sore throat, runny nose, headache and body ache, and fever. Directions for use are specific as to number of times a day, hours between use, and factors involving taking the medication, such as with or without glasses of water prior to or following administration and limits regarding food intake.

Most labels also carry prominent warnings regarding use with respect to age, alcohol consumption, sedatives or tranquilizers, and combinations of medications. Most over-the-counter medications also state that use should be continued only for a specified time and that, if symptoms persist, the user should stop taking the medication and consult

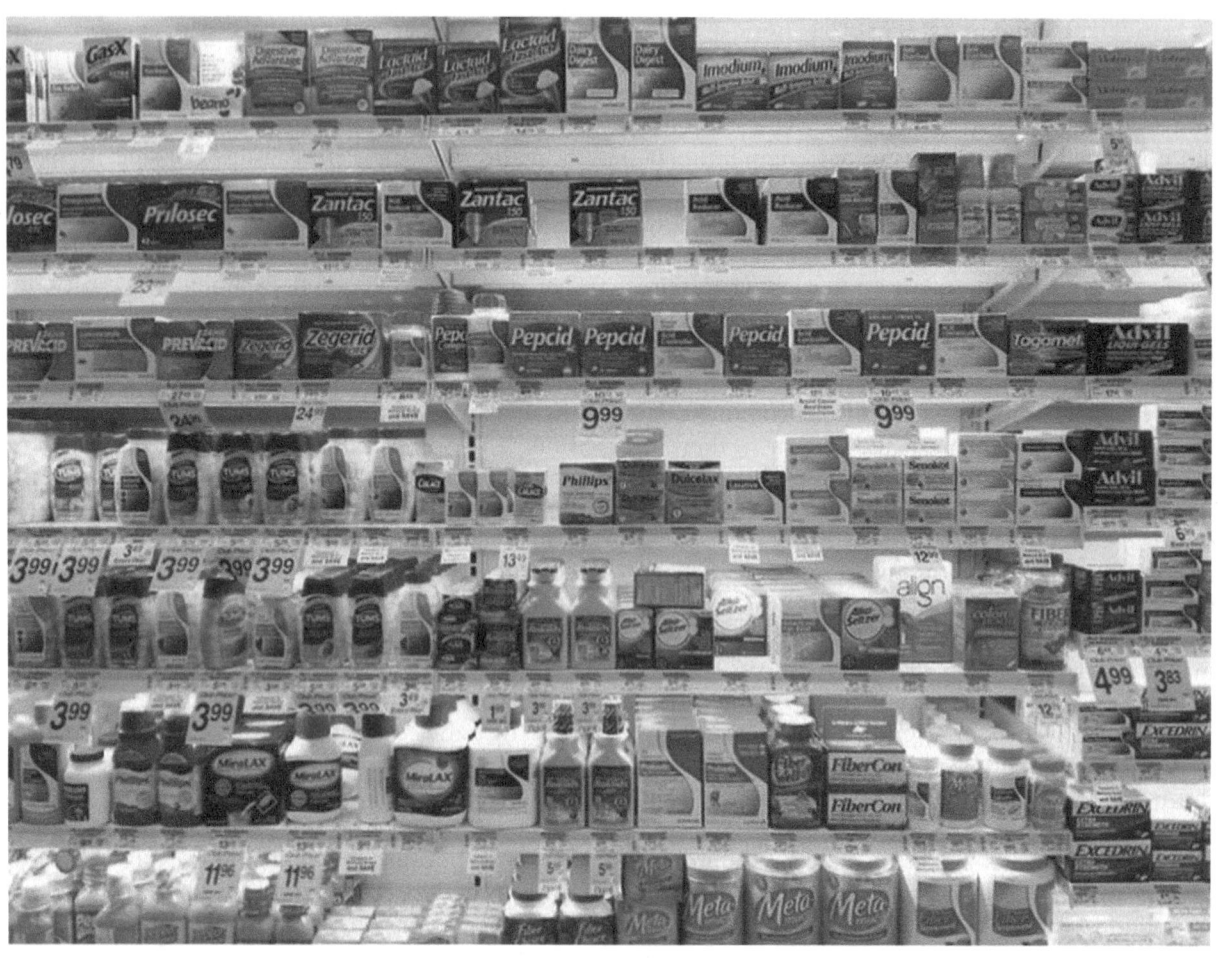

Shelves of over-the-counter drugs, mostly digestive-tract products, at a Safeway grocery store in Wheaton, Maryland. (Ben Schumin via Flickr)

a physician. Finally, the user is usually cautioned to stop taking the OTC medication immediately if headache, rash, nausea, or similar symptoms appear. Despite these warnings, even commonly used OTC medications pose certain health hazards, and the user is advised to take these medications with full recognition of potential problems.

In the United States, while the FDA periodically issues warnings regarding OTC medications, their actual use by consumers normally is not regulated, documented, or monitored. This has led to a number of concerns regarding real and potential overuse of OTC drugs, particularly for reasons unrelated to their medicinal intent. It has also led directly to the modification of certain OTC medications to engineer drugs that are highly addictive.

Because their use is unregulated—or, more correctly, cannot be regulated—over-the-counter medications can be deliberately abused. Overdosing with certain types of painkillers, for example, has become a frequent method of suicide attempt. The use of Tylenol in suicide attempts is increasing. Tylenol overdosing causes the destruction of liver cells that synthesize blood coagulants. Loss of these blood coagulants results in uncontrolled bleeding, most evidently through the eyes, nose, and mouth but also internally. Internal bleeding continues until death occurs, usually within a few days following onset.

Perhaps the most egregious misuse of OTC medications is to induce or achieve temporary "highs" that parallel those obtained by use of street or hard drugs. Cough suppressants that contain the drug dextromethorphan, for example, affect the central nervous system and can be used as mood-altering drugs that cause brain damage and even death at high doses. An even more serious abuse is the cooking of common drugs to obtain the highly addictive drug methamphetamine, popularly called meth. Also known as ice or speed, meth is a highly addictive drug that is often devastating and sometimes deadly. In some regions of the United States, it ranks with heroin and cocaine as the popular drug of choice. Record growth in use and the ability to cook meth from readily obtained OTC drugs has led to the creation of National Methamphetamine Awareness Day to draw attention at all levels to this problem.

This cooking process involves the conversion of certain OTC medications into meth. Some other sources for cooking meth include diet aids, tincture of iodine or other iodine solutions, and household cleaning solutions. In response to the widespread home manufacture of meth, a national federal law was enacted to require pharmacies to check photo identification and keep records of over-the-counter sales of cold medications that contain pseudoephedrine and ephedrine, which are the two popular ingredients in many cold medications. By-products of in-home meth cooking labs are garbage cans filled with Sudafed packages and a distinct odor of cat urine. The cooking process itself releases potentially harmful toxic chemicals that can pose serious health hazards to lungs and the respiratory system and also poses the risk of fire.

Perspective and Prospects

Originally, OTC medications were available for purchase only at pharmacies, along with physician-prescribed drugs. Today, a varied selection of OTC medications is available at many retail outlets, including supermarkets, food stores, and even convenience stores, although pharmacies still continue to offer the greatest selection. This can lead to a confusion of terms, as such medications or drugs are often no longer sold "over the counter" but instead can be found on shelves alongside other items for sale.

To complicate matters, certain drugs are offered as OTC medications at low dosages but must be obtained by prescription at higher dosages. For example, the popular analgesic ibuprofen (Advil, Motrin) can be purchased as an OTC medication at dosages of less than 200 milligrams, but higher dosages can be obtained only via prescription. Similarly, the antidiarrheal medication Imodium, an opiate, is available as an OTC medication in liquid form, while tablets of Imodium are available only by prescription.

The status of over-the-counter medications may change over time, depending on effectiveness and safety issues. While some OTC drugs are removed from the general market following various concerns regarding safety, other drugs are transferred from prescription drugs to OTC medications. Examples include the antihistamine drug Benadryl, which is used to relieve symptoms of allergy and guard against allergic reactions, and the painkiller ibuprofen, both of which were, until recently, sold as prescription drugs only but are now available as OTC medications.

While the distribution and sale of over-the-counter medications is strictly regulated by state and federal laws in the United States, certain drugs that are deemed harmless may be offered for sale as medical cures for many ailments and thereby compete with OTC medications. These so-called miracle drugs have become increasingly popular because of the Web, which opens the door to purchases without prescription. Media promotions also sometimes offer these medications, complete with testimonials that dramatically describe their success as a cure-all for ailments. These types of medications are often labeled "quack" drugs. They pose a threat to users of prescription and OTC medications in several ways. First, they are generally useless, offering a nonexistent cure for health problems. Second, they are manufactured without regard to quality control measures that legitimate drug manufacturers must follow. Third, time may be lost in using the quack drug, especially if the condition is chronic and the symptoms need to be treated immediately. Finally, while some may be harmless, other quack drugs contain chemical ingredients that are potentially dangerous when used in combination with genuine over-the-counter medications.

—*Dwight G. Smith, PhD*

References

Chang, Jongwha, et al. "Prescription to over-the-Counter Switches in the United States." *Journal of*

Research in Pharmacy Practice, vol. 5, no. 3, 2016, pp. 149–154., doi:10.4103/2279-042x.185706.

Eaves, Emery R. "'Just Advil': Harm Reduction and Identity Construction in the Consumption of over-the-Counter Medication for Chronic Pain." *Social Science & Medicine*, vol. 146, 19 Oct. 2015, pp. 147–154., doi:10.1016/j.socscimed.2015.10.033.

Kenny, Kathleen. "OTC Pain Medications: The Pros and Cons." *Pharmacy Times*, 30 Apr. 2017, www.pharmacytimes.com/publications/issue/2017/august2017/otc-pain-medications-the-pros-and-cons.

"Over-the-Counter Medicines." *MedlinePlus*, U.S. National Library of Medicine, 23 Oct. 2019, medlineplus.gov/overthecountermedicines.html.

"Over-the-Counter Pain Relievers." *MedlinePlus*, U.S. National Library of Medicine, 12 Oct. 2018, medlineplus.gov/ency/article/002123.htm.

Sirois, Jay, and Stefanie P. Ferreri. "OTC Combination Products in Pharmacistassisted Self-Care." *Pharmacy Today*, vol. 19, no. 6, June 2013, pp. 49–53., doi:10.1016/s1042-0991(15)31306-2.

"Understanding Over-the-Counter Medicines." *U.S. Food and Drug Administration*, 16 May 2018, www.fda.gov/drugs/buying-using-medicine-safely/understanding-over-counter-medicines.

■ Over-the-counter (OTC) drugs: Cautions and precautions

CATEGORY: Over-the-Counter
ANATOMY OR SYSTEM AFFECTED: All

Regulation and Advertising

In the United States, OTCs have been regulated by the FDA since Congress passed the Federal Food, Drug, and Cosmetic Act (FFDCA) of 1938. This legislation was introduced after a tragic mass poisoning in the fall of 1937, in which more than one hundred people died after taking a sulfanilamide medication that had been made with diethylene glycol, a solvent that is poisonous to humans. The then-new medication had not been tested on animals before being sold, even though diethylene glycol was known at the time to be poisonous. The FFDCA replaced the Pure Food and Drug Act of 1906, which did not require companies to submit safety data to the FDA before marketing and selling their products.

Manufacturers of drugs seeking FDA approval for sale as nonprescription items must follow one of two main paths. The first path is to state that the OTC complies with an existing FDA monograph (set of rules) for a specific category of OTC. According to the FDA, these monographs, which are published in the *Federal Register*, "state [the] requirements for categories of non-prescription drugs, such as what ingredients may be used and for what intended use." Examples of OTCs covered by FDA monographs include sunscreen, acne soap and cream, and dandruff shampoo. FDA monographs also cover OTCs that were in use long enough before the 1938 passage of the FFDCA to be considered "generally recognized as safe and effective" when used as directed. This phrase, taken from the FFDCA, is abbreviated as GRAS or GRAS/E. Aspirin is an example of an OTC that is considered GRAS/E.

The other path to FDA approval for an OTC is obtaining a new drug application, or NDA. The manufacturer or sponsor of the proposed drug must show that it is safe and effective and that its benefits outweigh any risks. An NDA must be obtained if the product does not fit within any of the existing FDA monographs for OTCs.

The NDA system is also used to move drugs that were first approved as prescription-only into the OTC category. In addition to determining that OTCs are safe and effective when consumers use them according to package directions, the FDA has the authority to decide that drugs formerly available only with a prescription can be safely sold to consumers as an OTC. This change, which the FDA calls an Rx-to-OTC ("Rx" meaning "prescription") switch, has made available about 700 new drugs as OTCs since 1980. Acid reducers and antihistamines are recent examples of the Rx-to-OTC switch.

The major difference between FDA oversight of prescription drugs and its oversight of OTCs is a matter of advertising. In the case of prescription drugs, the FDA regulates advertising and approval for use. Advertising of nonprescription drugs, however, is regulated by the Federal Trade Commission.

An important aspect of FDA regulation of OTCs is labeling. Each OTC approved for sale in the United States must carry a "Drug Facts" label on the product or its package. The label has a

> ### Over-the-Counter Labeling
>
> *The US Food and Drug Administration mandates that all over-the-counter, nonprescription drugs and therapies must be labeled with certain facts and information for consumers. The label is standardized and must display the facts in the following order:*
>
> - Product name
>
> - Active ingredient (therapeutic substance or substances in the product, including the amount in each dosage unit)
>
> - Purpose (product category, such as antihistamine, antacid, or cough suppressant)
>
> - Uses (symptoms or diseases the product treats or prevents)
>
> - Warnings (when not to use the product, when to stop taking it, when to see a doctor, and possible side effects)
>
> - Directions (when, how, and how often to take the product)
>
> - Other information (e.g., how to best store the product)
>
> - Inactive ingredients (substances such as binders, colors, or flavoring; helps avoid allergic reactions)
>
> *Source:* Adapted from the US Food and Drug Administration

standard format and must be clearly and simply written. It has the following parts: product name, active ingredient or ingredients, purpose, uses, warnings, directions, inactive ingredients, and other information.

Safety

Although the FDA's definition of OTCs includes the assurance that OTCs are "safe and effective," this assurance assumes that the medications are used correctly by consumers. There are several steps consumers should follow to make sure that they are using nonprescription medications correctly. These steps include the following:

Read the Drug Facts label carefully. It is especially important to note the active ingredients in the medicine, particularly when using two or more OTCs to treat the same condition or illness, such as the common cold. It is possible to take an accidental overdose of the active ingredients in cough and cold medicines because many of these preparations contain several active ingredients. The Drug Facts label will also contain important warnings about drug interactions (particularly interactions with alcohol), activities to avoid while taking the medicine (usually driving and operating heavy equipment), and dosage instructions.

Persons should never take more than the recommended dosage or take the medicine more often than recommended. If one's symptoms do not improve within a few days, that person should see a doctor. Persons should also consult a doctor or pharmacist if they have any questions about the medication, particularly its possible side effects or possible interactions with other drugs.

Check for tampering. Before purchase, one should check the tamper-evident packaging (TEP) features, such as internal plastic seals or blister packaging, to ensure the medication has not been tampered with. TEPs are safety features that were mandated by the FDA in 1983 following a still-unsolved crime in which seven people in Chicago died after taking a pain reliever that had been poisoned with potassium cyanide. If the package or the contents look suspicious in any way, the consumer should return the OTC to the store or pharmacy where it was purchased.

Store medication in a childproof cabinet or medicine chest. Also, one should keep all medicines away from children. OTCs should never be left on counter tops or tables where curious children can open and use them. Medications should always be kept in their original containers so that no one in the household can take the wrong drug by accident. Expiration dates should be checked periodically; medicines with expired dates should be discarded safely.

OTC Abuse

The purchase of some OTCs is restricted in the United States because these medications have been abused or have been used illegally. The purchaser may be required to show proof of age before buying the product or may have to ask a registered pharmacist for the product.

The two major types of OTCs in this category are cold and allergy medications containing ephedrine or pseudoephedrine, which are decongestants, and cough medicines containing dextromethorphan (DMX), a cough suppressant. Ephedrine and pseudoephedrine can be used to make methamphetamine, a dangerous drug of abuse. To prevent the illicit production of methamphetamine from OTCs, the US Congress passed the Combat Methamphetamine Epidemic Act, or CMEA, in 2005. The CMEA sets monthly limits on the amount of these products that consumers can purchase and requires that consumers show proof of identity to a pharmacist before purchase.

Cough medicines containing DMX have been abused by teenagers and others who consume large amounts of the preparations to get intoxicated. According to the CHPA, about 6 percent of teenagers in the United States abuse cough syrups containing DMX. Although there is no federal legislation controlling the sale of medications containing DMX, some states require proof that a would-be purchaser is eighteen years of age or older at the time of sale.

Impact

Over-the-counter medications represent a considerable portion of the money spent on health care in the United States. In the first decade of the twenty-first century, sales of OTCs for minor health conditions came to $20 billion per year, with dietary supplements accounting for another $12 billion. Nonprescription drugs are also widely available for purchase on the Internet and in supermarkets and other retail outlets that do not have pharmacies. OTCs can be purchased at more than 750,000 locations in the United States.

The widespread availability of nonprescription products and the ongoing transfer of some classes of prescription drugs into the OTC category make it easier for consumers, particularly older adults, to take a more active part in their health care. The FDA notes that increased access to nonprescription drugs is beneficial to people age sixty-five years and older, 80 percent of whom have some type of chronic health problem that can be managed effectively with OTCs. In terms of infectious diseases, however, it is unlikely that many anti-infective drugs will be switched into the OTC category because of concern about the potential overuse of antibiotics, commonly used for bacterial infections, and concern about the risk of developing even more drug-resistant disease organisms.

—*Rebecca J. Frey, PhD*

References

Lee, Chun-Hsien, et al. "Inappropriate Self-Medication among Adolescents and Its Association with Lower Medication Literacy and Substance Use." *Plos One*, vol. 12, no. 12, 14 Dec. 2017, doi:10.1371/journal.pone.0189199.

"OTC Drug Facts Label." *U.S. Food and Drug Administration*, 5 June 2015, www.fda.gov/drugs/drug-information-consumers/otc-drug-facts-label.

"OTC Medicines: Know Your Risks and Reduce Them." *Familydoctor.org*, 23 May 2018, familydoctor.org/otc-medicines-know-your-risks-and-reduce-them/.

Rojas, Katia M., and Huiyang Li. "Adverse Events and Over-the-Counter (OTC) Drugs: Is Inappropriate Labeling the Problem? - The Case of Acetaminophen." *Proceedings of the Human Factors and Ergonomics Society Annual Meeting*, vol. 61, no. 1, 2017, pp. 676–680., doi:10.1177/1541931213601656.

Sansgiry, Sujit, et al. "Abuse of over-the-Counter Medicines: a Pharmacist's Perspective." *Integrated Pharmacy Research and Practice*, vol. 6, 2016, pp. 1–6., doi:10.2147/iprp.s103494.

■ Oxycodone

CATEGORY: Addiction Risk; Opioid
ALSO KNOWN AS: Blue; hillbilly heroin; kicker; OC; OX; oxy; oxycotton, Perc, Roxy
ANATOMY OR SYSTEM AFFECTED: Nervous system

History of Use

Oxycodone was first synthesized in 1916 at the University of Frankfurt in Germany. It was developed as a non-addictive substitute for opioids including morphine, heroin, and codeine. Oxycodone initially became available in the United States in 1939 but its misuse potential was not recognized until the 1950s, when Percodan, an oxycodone and aspirin combination, was introduced. As a result, all oxycodone-containing products are classified as schedule II controlled substances, the strictest classification

Side effects of Oxycodone

Red color - more serious effect

Central:
- Hallucination
- Confusion
- Fainting
- Dizziness
- Loss of appetite
- Lightheadedness
- Drowsiness
- Headache
- Mood changes

Mouth, tongue or lips:
- Swelling
- Dryness

Eyes:
- Swelling
- Smaller pupil
- Redness

Face:
- Swelling

Throat:
- Hoarseness
- Swelling
- Difficulty swallowing

Skin:
- Hives
- Rash
- Flushing
- Sweating
- Itching

Heart:
- Fast or slow heartbeat

Respiratory:
- Difficulty breathing
- Slowed breathing

Muscular:
- Seizures
- Weakness

Gastric:
- Nausea
- Vomiting

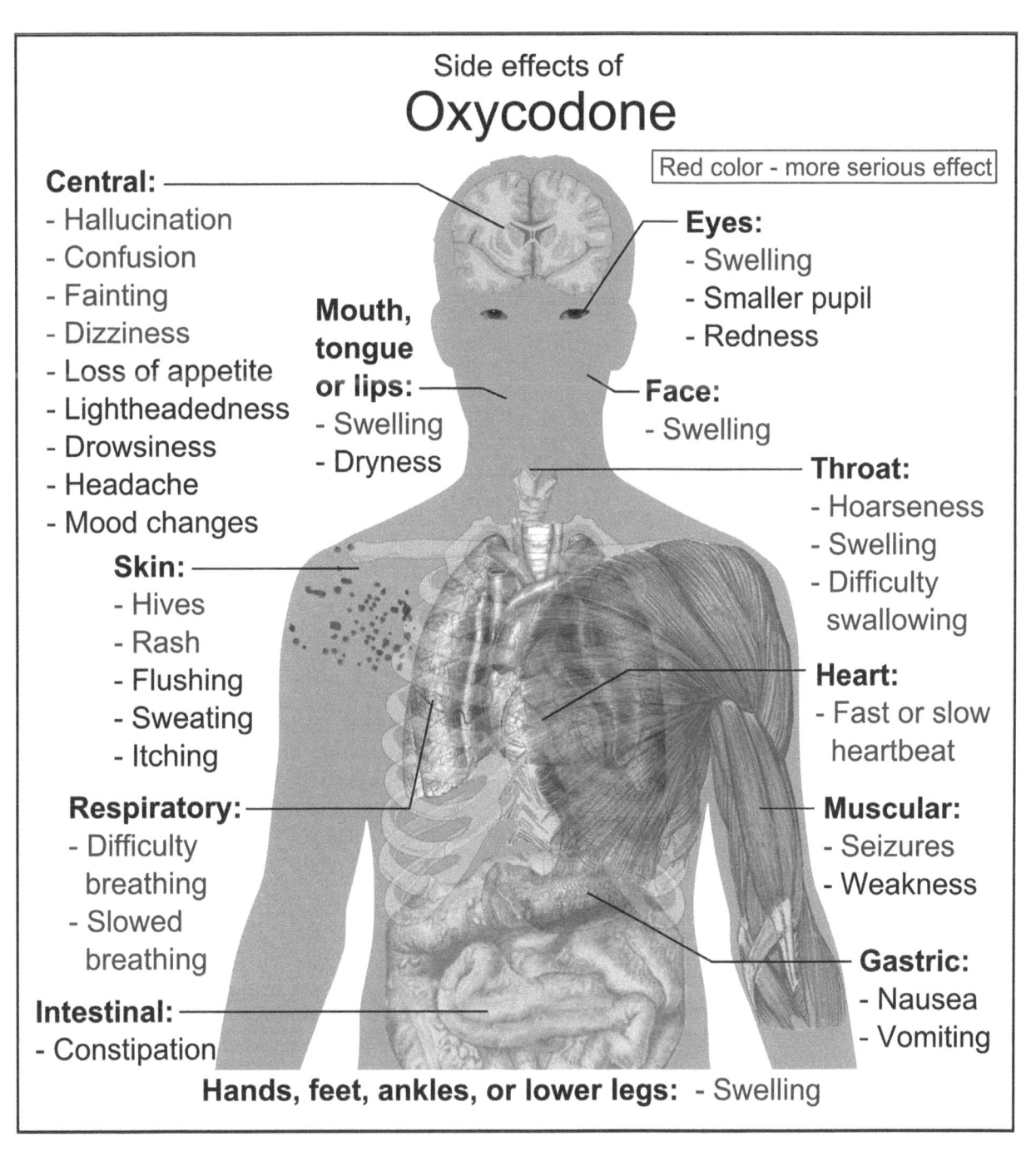

Intestinal:
- Constipation

Hands, feet, ankles, or lower legs: - Swelling

(Mikael Häggström via Wikimedia Commons)

for legal medications. Schedule II drugs are those with a high misuse potential and a legitimate medical use.

The illicit misuse of oxycodone dramatically increased in 1996 in the United States after the marketing by Purdue Pharma of OxyContin, the controlled-release prescription form of oxycodone. OxyContin, consumed for its relaxing and euphoric effects, became the best-selling narcotic pain reliever on the market.

Although oxycodone is not as potent as heroin, it remains one of the most highly addictive and

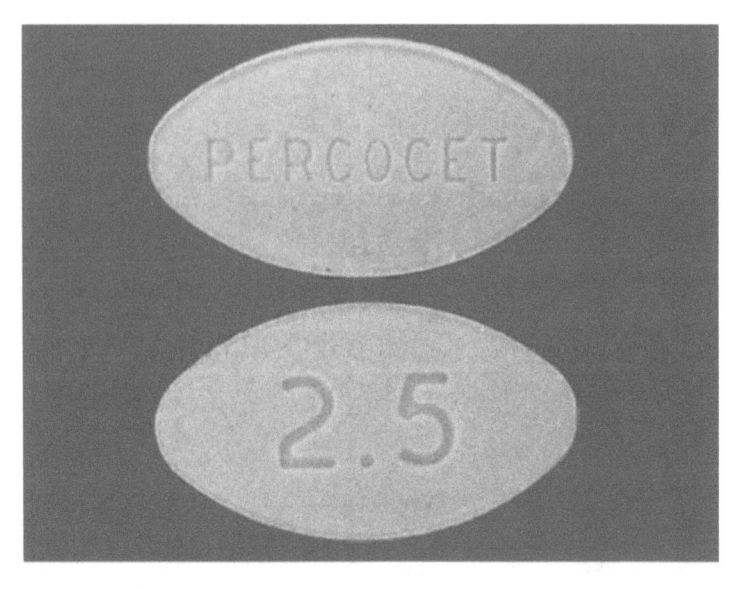

Percocet pills containing 2.5mg of oxycodone hydrochloride and 325mg acetaminophen. (National Library of Medicine)

widely misused prescription drugs of all time and has served as a gateway for many to heroin addiction. Despite numerous efforts to curb the illegal use of oxycodone-containing products, its misuse remains a major concern in the United States.

Effects and Potential Risks

Oxycodone is structurally similar to codeine and hydrocodone but pharmacologically resembles morphine. It acts through opioid receptors to alter the brain's response to pain, lessening pain sensations. Like other opiates, oxycodone elevates dopamine levels, the neurotransmitter linked to pleasurable experiences. Physiological effects include pain relief, respiratory depression, sedation, constipation, cough suppression, and in combination with acetaminophen, may cause liver damage. Oxycodone's short-term effects include a rush of euphoria and joy leading to a dreamy relaxed state. Negative short-term effects include nausea, vomiting, constipation, dizziness, and sedation.

Many people use oxycodone to achieve an opiate-like high, while others use it to minimize withdrawal symptoms of morphine and heroin addiction. Oxycodone users achieve the greatest high by bypassing OxyContin's controlled-release mechanism, consuming the entire dose at once. Typically, pills are either chewed or crushed and snorted or mixed with a liquid and injected.

Oxycodone leads to dependency and addiction and must be used with extreme caution and supervision. Individuals with a previous history of alcohol or drug addiction are more likely to become addicted to oxycodone. Long-term misuse may affect brain functioning because of hypoxia (low blood-oxygen levels) in the brain that results from repeated respiratory depression. Oxycodone addiction often requires professional intervention and treatment to help individuals overcome addiction. Greater emphasis is being placed on the illegal use of oxycodone, including the legal prosecution of over-prescribing by physicians.

—*Rose Ciulla-Bohling, PhD*
—*Patricia Stanfill Edens, MS, MBA, PhD, RN, LFACHE*

References

Jeurgens, Jeffrey, and Theresa Parisi. "Oxycodone Addiction and Abuse." *AddictionCenter*, 16 July 2019, www.addictioncenter.com/opiates/oxycodone/.

Joseph, Andrew. "New Details Revealed about Purdue's Marketing of OxyContin." *STAT*, 18 Jan. 2019, www.statnews.com/2019/01/15/massachusetts-purdue-lawsuit-new-details/.

Moradi, Mohammad, et al. "Use of Oxycodone in Pain Management." *Anesthesiology and Pain Medicine*, vol. 1, no. 4, 2012, pp. 262–264., doi:10.5812/aapm.4529.

"Oxycodone." *MedlinePlus*, U.S. National Library of Medicine, 15 Oct. 2019, medlineplus.gov/druginfo/meds/a682132.html.

Raffa, R.b., et al. "Oxycodone Combinations for Pain Relief." *Drugs of Today*, vol. 46, no. 6, 2010, p. 379., doi:10.1358/dot.2010.46.6.1470106.

Raleigh, M. D., et al. "Safety and Efficacy of an Oxycodone Vaccine: Addressing Some of the Unique Considerations Posed by Opioid Abuse." *Plos One*, vol. 12, no. 12, 2017, doi:10.1371/journal.pone.0184876.

Schmidt-Hansen, Mia, et al. "Oxycodone for Cancer-Related Pain." *Cochrane Database of Systematic Reviews*, 2017, doi:10.1002/14651858.cd003870.pub6.

Pentazocine, butorphanol, nalbuphine

CATEGORY: Opioid; Narcotic
ANATOMY OR SYSTEM AFFECTED: Central nervous system

KEY TERMS
- *agonist*: A drug that activates certain receptors.
- *antagonist*: A drug that blocks a certain receptor by attaching to it and preventing activation of it

Pain is an unpleasant sensation generated from the central nervous system in response to bodily injury, disease, or inflammation. Regardless of the origin, there are a variety of medications that can be used in the treatment of pain. Partial opioid agonists are used to treat moderate to severe pain. While full opioid agonists elicit the full effect of opioids, partial opioids elicit only a partial effect of the opioid drug by activating the receptors to a lesser degree. There are also a group of drugs that are considered agonists-antagonists, since they act an agonist or partial agonist at one receptor, and as an antagonist at another receptor.

Pentazocine, butorphanol, and nalbuphine are categorized as partial opioid agonists and mixed agonists, or agonist-antagonists. These three medications are used in the treatment of moderate to severe pain, mostly in the acute hospital setting, as either an intramuscular or intravenous injection. They are also used as a supplement to general anesthesia during surgical procedures both preoperatively and postoperatively for pain control.

How Partial Opioid Agonists Work

Opioid receptors are found throughout the body and they function to express pain transmission impulses to the brain. Skin, muscles, joints, and the gastrointestinal system are some of the areas in which opioid receptors are positioned throughout the body. The four types of opioid receptors that have been identified are mu, delta, kappa, and opioid-receptor like-1 (ORL-1). The type of receptor that is activated will determine the effect the drug has on a person.

When an opioid receptor is activated, it inhibits intracellular synthesis of the second messenger molecule cyclic AMP (cAMP), which elicits a decrease in the intracellular levels of potassium and calcium ions. This leads to a more negatively-charge cell interior, a condition called hyperpolarization, and neurons that are in a hyperpolarized state are prevented from signaling to other neurons. Consequently, pain impulses are no longer transmitted to the brain, decreasing pain sensation.

Pentazocine is a partial agonist of mu receptors and an agonist of kappa receptors. Butorphanol is an antagonist of mu receptors and a partial agonist of kappa receptors. Nalbuphine is an antagonist of mu receptors and an agonist of kappa receptors.

The effect a medication has will be determined by the receptor that it is formulated to target. Since pentazocine is a partial agonist on the mu receptor, it will produce analgesia, euphoria, respiratory depression, and physical dependence and since it is a partial agonist, these effects will be to a lesser degree. Butorphanol, being a partial agonist on kappa receptors, will produce effects of analgesia, dysphoria, and diaphoresis. It also has an antagonist effect on mu receptors, meaning it blocks the mu receptors from being activated by substances capable of activating them. Nalbuphine will produce effects of analgesia, dysphoria, and diaphoresis because it is an agonist on kappa receptors but, being an antagonist on mu receptors, will also block the mu receptors from being activated.

Side Effects

The side effects of pentazocine, butorphanol, and nalbuphine are all very similar. All three have a high risk for addiction and/or abuse, as well as withdrawal, and possibly death. Common side effects of these partial opioid agonists include, but are not limited to, respiratory depression, tachycardia, hypotension, hallucinations, dizziness, lightheadedness, confusion, euphoria, syncope, disorientation, nausea, vomiting, dry mouth, constipation, diarrhea, blurry vision, heart palpitations, allergic reaction, difficulty breathing, wheezing, and swelling of the face or throat.

—*Kim J. Pearson, BSN, RN, CEN*

References

Hoskin, P.J. and G. W. Hanks, G.W. "Opioid Agonist-Antagonist Drugs in Acute and Chronic Pain States." *Drugs*, vol. 41, no. 3, 1991, pp. 326-344. Retrieved from doi:10.2165/00003495-199141030-00002

Fudin, Jeffery. "Opioid Agonist, Partial Agonists, Antagonists: Oh My!". *Pharmacy Times*, 6 Jan 2018. https://www.pharmacytimes.com/contributor/jeffrey-fudin/2018/01/opioid-agonists-partial-agonists-antagonists-oh-my

Pathan, H., & Williams, J. Basic opioid pharmacology: an update. British *Journal of Pain*, vol. 6, no. 1, 2012, pp. 11–16. doi:10.1177/2049463712438493

Pregabalin

CATEGORY: Anti-convulsant
ALSO KNOWN AS: *Lyrica*
ANATOMY OR SYSTEM AFFECTED: Nervous system

Pregabalin (*Lyrica*) is classified as an anticonvulsant and miscellaneous analgesic. It received Food and Drug Administration (FDA) approval on December 30, 2004 and was originally created for use as an epileptic drug (anticonvulsant). Pregabalin diminished the impulses in the brain that cause seizures. Later Lyrica was released for use to treat a variety of nerve related pain conditions including; fibromyalgia, nerve pain in people with diabetes (diabetic neuropathy), herpes zoster (postherpetic neuralgia), or spinal cord injuries to name a few. Some off-label uses have developed in the last 10 years as well including; panic disorder, migraine prophylaxis, social phobia, mania, bipolar disorder, and alcohol withdrawal.

Mechanisms of Action

Pregabalin affects the central nervous system (CNS) without interaction with benzodiazepine or GABA receptors of the brain. Its mechanism of action is related to its connection with the alpha/delta subunit of the voltage-dependent calcium channel in the CNS. Pregabalin subtly decreases the synaptic release of several neurotransmitters, by binding to and inhibiting alpha2-delta subunits. This possibly accounts for its actions to reduce neuronal excitability and seizures. Pregabalin is rapidly absorbed with at least 90% of dose being used in action. Pregabalin does not bind to plasma proteins and is excreted virtually unchanged by the kidneys. Pharmacokinetics are linear and predictable across the therapeutic dose range of pregabalin (150-600 mg/ day).

Side Effects

Pregabalin has varied side effects. Many side effects are related to the decrease in synaptic release created by the action of Lyrica. Common side effects include; ataxia, blurred vision, constipation, diplopia, dizziness, drowsiness, fatigue, headache, peripheral edema, tremor, weight gain, visual field loss, accidental injury, and xerostomia. Other rarer side effects include; abnormal gait, abnormality in thinking, amnesia, arthralgia, asthenia, cognitive dysfunction, confusion, edema, neuropathy, sinusitis, speech disturbance, vertigo, visual disturbance, myasthenia, amblyopia, increased appetite, and twitching.

Risks

Antiepileptic medications have been associated with an increased risk of suicidal thinking and behavior. Persons considering the use of antiepileptic drugs need to assess this risk with their clinical need. Patients who are at high risk should be closely observed for clinical worsening, suicidal thoughts, or unusual changes in behavior when started on therapy. Signs of concern include; thoughts about suicide or dying, attempts to commit suicide, new or worse depression, new or worse anxiety, feeling agitated or restless, panic attacks, trouble sleeping (insomnia) new or worse irritability, acting aggressive, being angry, or violent, acting on dangerous impulses, an extreme increase in activity and talking (mania), other unusual changes in behavior or mood.

Patients should be educated on somnolence and dizziness as possible side effects; therefore, their ability to drive or operate machinery may be impaired. Additionally, the use of alcohol or central nervous system (CNS) depressants while taking Lyrica can potentiate the sedation induced by pregabalin and creates increased risk of adverse effects.

—*Candice N. Stevens, BSN, RN*

References

Entringer, Sophia. "Lyrica." *Drugs.com*, 5 Jan. 2019, www.drugs.com/lyrica.html.

Lowther, Chadrick. "Pregabalin (Lyrica®): Part II." *Pharmacotherapy Update*, vol. 8, no. 6, 2005.

Ogbru, Omudhome. "Lyrica (Pregabalin) Side Effects (Weight Gain), Uses & Dosage." *MedicineNet*, 14 Nov. 2019, www.medicinenet.com/pregabalin_lyrica/article.htm.

"Pregabalin." *MedlinePlus*, U.S. National Library of Medicine, 15 Sept. 2019, medlineplus.gov/druginfo/meds/a605045.html.

Taylor, Charles P., et al. "Pharmacology and Mechanism of Action of Pregabalin: The Calcium Channel α2–δ (alpha2–Delta) Subunit as a Target for Antiepileptic Drug Discovery." *Epilepsy Research*, vol. 73, no. 2, 2007, pp. 137–150., doi:10.1016/j.eplepsyres.2006.09.008.

Prescription NSAIDs

CATEGORY: NSAID, Anti-Inflammatory
ANATOMY OR SYSTEM AFFECTED: Kidneys; Gastrointestinal system; Blood platelets

KEY TERMS
- *NSAID*: non-steroidal anti-inflammatory drugs
- *cyclooxygenase*: enzymes that catalyze the initial reactions that culminate in the synthesis of prostaglandins
- *platelets*: blood cells that help your body form clots to stop bleeding

Many people worldwide deal with pain caused by chronic inflammatory conditions like arthritis or musculoskeletal problems and receive significant benefits from NSAIDs to manage their pain. NSAIDs are a type of anti-inflammatory analgesic medication used to treat mild to moderate pain, which can be short or long term in nature. They can also be used to assist in bringing down a fever. NSAIDs are not opioids and do not have addictive properties. They are relatively inexpensive and accessible, but it is crucial to understand how to use them properly. There are over 20 different brands of NSAIDs that can be purchased over-the-counter such as aspirin, *Advil*, or *Motrin* (ibuprofen), and *Aleve* (naproxen sodium). Many other NSAIDs are prescription medications prescribed by health care providers. Examples of prescription NSAIDs include *Mobic* (meloxicam) and *Celebrex* (celecoxib). Health care providers prescribe NSAIDs to patients who deal with chronic pain to help them manage their pain more effectively. For unknown reasons, patients differ in response to different NSAIDs, so if one isn't working, another in the same class may work much better.

How NSAIDs Work

Oral NSAIDs work within one hour of taking the medication, and their effects usually last from 4-12 hours depending on whether they are short- or long-acting. Patients typically experience the maximum anti-inflammatory effects of NSAIDs after they have taken them for about two weeks.

NSAIDs inhibit cyclooxygenase enzymes (or COX enzymes) from working inside the body. These enzymes catalyze the formation of small molecules called "prostaglandins," which activate pain receptor nerve endings, thus causing a sensation of pain, and mediate tissue inflammation. Prostaglandins also protect the gastrointestinal mucosa, regulate blood flow to the kidneys, and help with platelet aggregation. NSAIDs inhibit COX enzyme activity, which relieves pain. There are two subtypes of COX enzymes, COX-1 and COX-2. Most NSAIDs block the action of both COX-1 and COX-2, but usually specific NSAIDs inhibit one type of COX enzyme more than the other. Celebrex is the FDA-approved medication that specifically inhibits COX-2. The reduction of COX-1 enzymatic activity concomitantly reduces pain and inflammation. Unfortunately, blocking COX-1 also diminishes the gastric protective properties of prostaglandins and, therefore, causes damage to the mucosa of the gastrointestinal tract and increases the risk of gastrointestinal bleeding. Pharmaceutical companies developed new NSAIDs that specifically target COX-2 in hopes of assisting with inflammation and pain without the undesired gastrointestinal and bleeding effects. However, blocking COX-2 causes a greater risk of forming blood clots and having a heart attack or stroke.

Uses and Applications

NSAIDs are used for many types of pain, including; toothaches, strains and sprains, joint pain, muscle pain, earaches, headaches, and menstrual cramps, to name a few. Providers can prescribe NSAIDs in the form of pills, gels, or creams. Gels and creams are applied directly on the skin over the area of pain and provide similar benefits as the pill forms for arthritis and back pain. For some, the topical form may be safer than pill forms. The doses of prescription NSAIDs are higher than their over-the-counter versions.

Side Effects

In general, NSAIDs are relatively safe medications and benefit many individuals. Common side effects of NSAIDs may include dizziness, heartburn, constipation, epigastric pain, nausea, rash, tinnitus, edema, fluid retention, headache, or vomiting.

Those who are already at higher risk for gastrointestinal, cardiovascular or renal adverse effects will have an increased risk for adverse effects. Side effect profiles of specific NSAIDs depends on their selectivity for COX-1 or COX-2. Those NSAIDs that are relatively nonselective for COX-1 or COX-2, such as aspirin, have more gastrointestinal side effects such as nausea, heartburn, indigestion, and potentially peptic ulcers. However, at low doses, aspirin is cardioprotective. NSAIDs that are slightly more selective for COX-2 than COX-1, such as ibuprofen and naproxen, have a low risk of cardiovascular events, but a higher risk of gastrointestinal side effects, though not as high as aspirin. Those NSAIDs that are even more selective for COX-2, such as meloxicam, diclofenac, etodolac, indomethacin, piroxicam, nabumetone, and sulindac, should be used with caution in patients with increased risk for cardiovascular side effects, but have a lower risk for gastrointestinal side effects. Celecoxib, marketed as Celebrex, is entirely selective for COX-2 and carries the lowest low risk of gastrointestinal side effects, but the highest risk of blood clots, heart attacks, or stroke (in rare cases).

Patients on NSAIDs should take the lowest dose that achieves the desired effects. Such a strategy reduces the risk of adverse effects. Long-term NSAID use has serious side effects when taking high doses. Patients can prevent the gastrointestinal adverse effects of NSAIDs by taking medications such as proton pump inhibitors (PPIs) with the NSAID. Those with high blood pressure need to use caution when taking NSAIDs, as they can further increase their blood pressure. Patients with cardiovascular disease should exercise care when taking NSAIDs since they may increase the risk of cardiac events. Likewise, patients with chronic renal failure should also avoid NSAIDs since they can harm the kidneys. Pregnant women should not use NSAIDs during the last three months of pregnancy. As with any drug, there is also a risk of an allergic reaction.

—*Jodi L. Guy, BSN, RN, CMSRN*

References

Goroczyca, Pamela, et al. "NSAIDs: Balancing the Risks and Benefits." *US Pharmacist*, vol. 41, no. 3, 2016, pp. 24-26.

Hecht, Marjorie. "Side Effects from NSAIDs." *Healthline*, 23 July 2019, https://www.healthline.com/health/side-effects-from-nsaids#7-side-effects

Perry, Laura, et al. "Cardiovascular Risks Associated with NSADs and COX-2 Inhibitors." *US Pharmacist*, vol. 39, no. 3, 2014, pp. 35-38.

Underwood, M., et al. "Advice to Use Topical or Oral Ibuprofen for Chronic Knee Pain in Older People: Randomized Control Trial and Patient Preference Study." *British Medical Journal*, vol. 336, no. 138, 2007, pp. 1-12. doi:10.1136/bmj.39399.656331.25

Shah, Seema, and Vivek Mehta. "Controversies and Advances in Non-Steroidal Anti-Inflammatory drug (NSAID) Analgesia in Chronic Pain Management." *Postgraduate Medical Journal*, vol. 88, no. 1036, 2012, pp. 73-78.

■ Sildenafil

CATEGORY: Vasodilator
ALSO KNOWN AS: Viagra, Revatio
ANATOMY OR SYSTEM AFFECTED: Genitourinary, pulmonary, cardiovascular systems

KEY TERMS

- *angina pectoris*: Chest pain caused by partial blockages of the arteries that feed blood to the heart
- *corpus cavernosum*: The spongy tissue which runs along both sides of the penis and fills with blood to produce an erection
- *dyspepsia*: Upset stomach/indigestion
- *hypertension*: High blood pressure
- *interstitial cystitis*: Chronic inflammation of the bladder and urinary tract
- *ischemia*: Inadequate blood supply to an organ or part of the body
- *primary dysmenorrhea*: Pelvic pain which occurs with any underlying infection, condition, or syndrome
- *priapism*: A prolonged and painful erection
- *suppository*: A solid, conical-shaped medication preparation designed to be placed into the rectum or vagina and allowed to dissolve to deliver localized medication
- *vasoconstriction*: narrowing of blood vessels (arteries and veins)

Originally developed to treat both hypertension and angina pectoris, sildenafil has become the medication commonly known as "the little blue pill." During clinical trials, sildenafil (Viagra) failed to insufficiently prevent or reduce the symptoms of angina pectoris and hypertension. However, it was highly effective at producing penile erections. After this discovery, sildenafil was rebranded and marketed as a treatment for erectile dysfunction. Once considered to be a strictly psychological condition, oral sildenafil could effectively treat erectile dysfunction, which helped restore function and satisfaction to millions of men worldwide.

Health care providers use sildenafil primarily to treat erectile dysfunction and pulmonary hypertension. Emerging research suggests that sildenafil can also relieve pain related to primary dysmenorrhea and interstitial cystitis with lower urinary tract symptoms (LUTS). In such cases, sildenafil, prepared in suppository form, is placed inside the vagina and left to dissolve. The slow, localized release of the medication helps to decrease or prevent pain associated with primary dysmenorrhea and interstitial cystitis. Administering sildenafil in this manner also lessens the occurrence of side effects. Studies have shown that 100 mg of sildenafil, administered as a vaginal suppository, effectively reduces pain related to primary dysmenorrhea. A similar study found that a daily low dose (25 mg) of oral sildenafil effectively reduces pain from interstitial cystitis. These two studies provide hope for those individuals who suffer from chronic pain related to primary dysmenorrhea and interstitial cystitis and those who have already failed more conservative/traditional methods of pain control or have a contraindication to those same treatment modalities.

How Sildenafil Works
Sildenafil inhibits an enzyme called "phosphodiesterase-5" (PDE-5). When taken for erectile dysfunction, and in the presence of sexual stimulation, sildenafil blocks the breakdown of the second messenger cyclic guanosine monophosphate (cGMP) by PDE-5. Increased cGMP concentrations induce smooth muscle relaxation in the corpus cavernosum, which increases blood flow to the corpus cavernosum, resulting in an erection. Sexual stimulation causes increased production of nitric oxide (NO), which in turn activates the enzyme guanylyl cyclase. Guanylyl cyclase synthesizes cGMP from guanosine triphosphate (GTP).

The mechanism by which sildenafil relieves pain in primary dysmenorrhea slightly differs from how it treats erectile dysfunction. During normal menstruation, the uterus produces small molecules called "prostaglandins" that induce uterine contraction, increase uterine pressure, and assist with the shedding of the uterine lining. However, patients who suffer from primary dysmenorrhea produce excess quantities of prostaglandins, which leads to constriction of blood vessels and abnormal uterine contractions. Insufficient blood flow deprives the uterus of oxygen and nutrients (i.e., tissue ischemia), which causes debilitating generalized lower abdominal pain. Sildenafil inhibits the breakdown of cGMP, which induces smooth muscle relaxation, increases blood flow, and augments the activity of NO. Increased NO activity reduces blood vessel constriction, thus increasing uterine blood flow, and alleviating pain.

With regards to interstitial cystitis with LUTS, the mechanism by which PDE-5 inhibitors reduce pain remains inconclusive.

Side Effects
The side effects of the oral and intravenous forms of sildenafil are well documented and include headache, flushing (redness) of the skin, dyspepsia, and nasal congestion. Some patients complain of disturbances in color vision and changes to hearing, but these side effects are rare. Delivering sildenafil as a vaginal suppository significantly reduces its adverse effects. Infrequent complaints of mild headaches were the only reported side effect, but the long-term effects of vaginal sildenafil remain unknown.

—*Adam M. Farnum BSN, RN*

References
Chen, Hongde, et al. "Efficacy of Daily Low-Dose Sildenafil for Treating Interstitial Cystitis: Results of a Randomized, Double-Blind, Placebo-Controlled Trial—Treatment of Interstitial Cystitis/Painful Bladder Syndrome with Low-Dose Sildenafil." *Urology*, vol. 84, no. 1, 2014, pp. 51-56. doi:10.1016/j.urology.2014.02.050

Corbin, J D. "Mechanisms of Action of PDE5 inhibition in Erectile Dysfunction." *International Journal of Impotence Research*, vol. 16, no. S1, 2004, p. S4. Gale Academic Onefile, doi:10.1038/sj.ijir.3901205

Dmitrovic, R., A.R. Kunselman, and R. S. Legro. "Sildenafil Citrate in the Treatment of Pain in Primary Dysmenorrhea: A Randomized Controlled Trial." *Human Reproduction*, vol. 28, no. 11, Nov. 2013, pp. 2958–2965, doi:10.1093/humrep/det324

Iacovides, Stella, Ingrid Avidon, and Fiona C. Baker. "What We Know About Primary Dysmenorrhea Today: A Critical Review." *Human Reproduction Update*, vol. 21, no. 6, Nov./Dec. 2015, pp. 762–778, doi: 10.1093/humupd/dmv039

Paulus, Wolfgang E., et al. "Benefit of Vaginal Sildenafil Citrate in Assisted Reproduction Therapy." *Fertility and Sterility*, vol. 77, no. 4, 2002, pp. 846-847. doi.org/10.1016/S0015-0282(01)03272-1

Tramadol

CATEGORY: Addiciton Risk; Opioid
ALSO KNOWN AS: ConZip; Ultram
ANATOMY OR SYSTEM AFFECTED: Nervous system

History of Use

Tramadol was first synthesized in 1962 by the German pharmaceutical company Grünenthal. Tramadol has been in clinical use in Germany since 1977. Originally marketed as a safe painkiller with a low risk of misuse, tramadol became the most prescribed opioid on the European market. It was introduced to the prescription drug market in the United States in 1995 as Ultram, a nontraditional, centrally acting analgesic. Tramadol has a nonscheduled status, meaning it has a low potential for misuse.

Tramadol produces pleasurable sensations and relaxation without increased drowsiness, enabling people to remain productive while managing pain. It is an easily available opiate and can be habit forming because of its morphine-like properties. Because of reports of increased tramadol misuse, it has been labeled a drug of concern by the US Food and Drug Administration and thus requires additional label warnings. Some US states have classified tramadol as a controlled substance.

Effects and Potential Risks

Tramadol is a nontraditional, centrally acting opioid analgesic with morphine-like pain-relieving activity. It has a dual mechanism of pain relief because it includes a mixture of enantiomers.

Studies suggest that tramadol activity is mediated through both opioid and non-opioid or monoaminergic mechanisms. It exhibits opioid activity by binding to specific opioid receptors in the brain that decrease pain perception. Monoaminergic activity is displayed by inhibiting the reuptake of norepinephrine and serotonin, neurotransmitters responsible for altering pain response in the brain.

The short-term effects of tramadol include feelings of euphoria, mood elevation, and relaxation. Tramadol is usually well tolerated but can be associated with negative short-term effects, including nausea, vomiting, constipation, drowsiness, dizziness, vertigo, weakness, and headache.

Long-term use of tramadol can be associated with drug dependence and possible addiction. Abruptly stopping tramadol may generate opiate-like withdrawal symptoms such as anxiety, agitation, sweating, abdominal upset, and hallucinations.

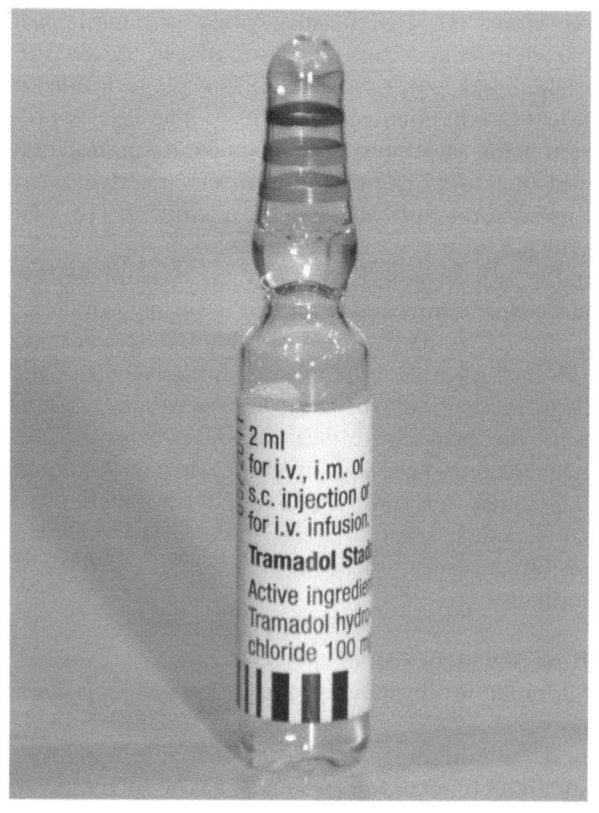

A sample of Tramadol Hydrochloride for injection, 100 mg/ml. (LhcheM via Wikimedia Commons)

—*Rose Ciulla-Bohling, PhD*

References

Hassamal, Sameer, et al. "Tramadol: Understanding the Risk of Serotonin Syndrome and Seizures." *The American Journal of Medicine*, vol. 131, no. 11, 2018, doi:10.1016/j.amjmed.2018.04.025.

Jeurgens, Jeffrey, and Theresa Parisi. "Tramadol Addiction and Abuse." *AddictionCenter*, 16 July 2019, www.addictioncenter.com/opiates/tramadol/.

Mayo Clinic. "Historically 'Safer' Tramadol More Likely than Other Opioids to Result in Prolonged Use." *ScienceDaily*, 14 May 2019, www.sciencedaily.com/releases/2019/05/190514090953.htm.

Shmerling, Robert H. "Is Tramadol a Risky Pain Medication?" *Harvard Health Blog*, Harvard Medical School, 16 Aug. 2019, www.health.harvard.edu/blog/is-tramadol-a-risky-pain-medication-2019061416844.

Subedi, Muna, et al. "An Overview of Tramadol and Its Usage in Pain Management and Future Perspective." *Biomedicine & Pharmacotherapy*, vol. 111, 2019, pp. 443–451., doi:10.1016/j.biopha.2018.12.085.

Thiels, Cornelius A, et al. "Chronic Use of Tramadol after Acute Pain Episode: Cohort Study." *Bmj*, 14 May 2019, doi:10.1136/bmj.l1849.

"Tramadol." *MedlinePlus*, U.S. National Library of Medicine, 15 Jan. 2019, medlineplus.gov/druginfo/meds/a695011.html.

■ Valium

CATEGORY: Addiction Risk; Anxiolytic; Muscle Relaxant; Sedative

ALSO KNOWN AS: Diazepam, 7-Chloro-1,3-dihydro-1-methyl-5-phenyl-2H-1,4-benzodiazepine-2-one and by other various brand names internationally.

ANATOMY OR SYSTEM AFFECTED: Musculoskeletal system; Nervous system

History of Use

Valium, a brand name of diazepam, was synthesized by chemist Leo Sternbach in 1963 while working at Hoffman-La Roche. It was the second benzodiazepine marketed by the company, the first being Librium (chlordiazepoxide) in 1960. Valium's name is based on the Latin "valere" (meaning "be strong"). Valium is indicated to treat anxiety (including preoperative anxiety), seizures, agitation, tremor and impending acute delirium tremens in acute alcohol withdrawal, and skeletal muscle spasm or spasticity caused by various disorders, including cerebral palsy, paraplegia, and stiff-man syndrome.

Valium, along with Librium and other benzodiazepines that were developed, became a popular alternative to the drugs used at the time to treat nervous and mental disorders, including chloral hydrate, reserpine, barbiturates, and meprobamate, as such drugs had serious side effects and were habit-forming. Conversely, Valium, along with Librium, was less toxic and initially appeared to cause less dependence and side effects.

As a result of these desirable drug properties, enthusiasm in the medical community and marketing campaigns, benzodiazepines became the most frequently prescribed drugs. Consequently, Americans consumed 2.3 billion tablets of Valium in 1978. Valium's prevalence in society was so great that the Rolling Stones wrote a song called "Mother's Little Helper" in 1966, which related to housewives' use of Valium to get through their busy and stressful day. The title of the song became a nickname for Valium and other similar benzodiazepine drugs. Valium was referred to in best-selling books of the time, including Jacqueline Susann's "Valley of the Dolls."

During this period of popularity, reports of misuse and dependence were published. These misuse/dependence concerns subsequently increased, especially when Valium was combined with other drugs, leading to various recommendations limiting the use of Valium. Even though newer generations of drugs have been developed to treat anxiety, Valium is still prescribed today to effectively manage the various conditions described above.

Effects and Potential Risks

Valium exerts its effects by binding to a specific portion of a protein called a receptor that the neurotransmitter gamma-aminobutyric acid (GABA) binds to. Neurotransmitters are chemical messengers which allow communication between nerve cells. Neurotransmitters regulate the majority of systems in the human body, including breathing, brain activity, movement, and heart rate. Neurotransmitters typically exert their influence by binding to receptor proteins at the end of nerve cells, which, in turn, cause one or more various cellular events to occur. GABA is an inhibitory neurotransmitter whose effects are increased upon Valium binding to the GABA receptor.

Some common side effects of Valium, which typically disappear after prolonged use, include fatigue, drowsiness, muscle weakness, and ataxia. Other adverse reactions include leucopenia, jaundice, hypersensitivity, irritability, aggression, restlessness, delusion, nightmares, hallucinations, psychoses, anterograde amnesia and physical dependence. Many of these side effects are more likely to occur in children and the elderly, so extra care is recommended in such cases.

—*Lenela Glass-Godwin, MS*
—*Jason J. Schwartz, PhD, Esq*

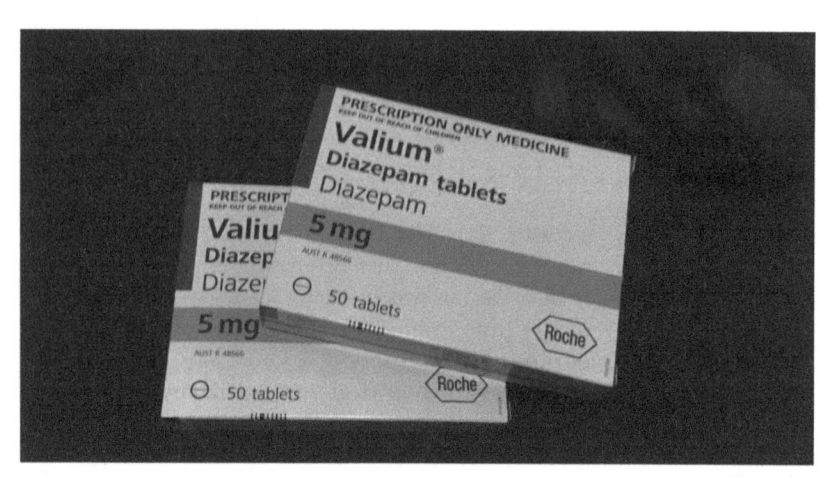

5mg of Diazepam. (National Library of Medicine)

References

Calcaterra, Nicholas E., and James C. Barrow. "Classics in Chemical Neuroscience: Diazepam (Valium)." *ACS Chemical Neuroscience*, vol. 5, no. 4, 2014, pp. 253–260., doi:10.1021/cn5000056.

Cheng, Tianze, et al. "Valium without Dependence? Individual GABAA Receptor Subtype Contribution toward Benzodiazepine Addiction, Tolerance, and Therapeutic Effects." *Neuropsychiatric Disease and Treatment*, vol. 14, 2018, pp. 1351–1361., doi:10.2147/ndt.s164307.

"Diazepam." *MedlinePlus*, U.S. National Library of Medicine, 15 July 2019, medlineplus.gov/druginfo/meds/a682047.html.

Pringle, A, et al. "Cognitive Mechanisms of Diazepam Administration: a Healthy Volunteer Model of Emotional Processing." *Psychopharmacology*, vol. 233, no. 12, 6 May 2016, pp. 2221–2228., doi:10.1007/s00213-016-4269-y.

"Valium: Side Effects, Addiction, Symptoms & Treatment: What Is Valium?" *American Addiction Centers*, 14 Nov. 2019, americanaddictioncenters.org/valium-treatment.

■ Vicodin and Norco

CATEGORY: Addiction Risk; Opioid

ALSO KNOWN AS: Hydrocodone bitartrate/acetaminophen (known in Europe as paracetamol); Lortab; Vedrocet; Xodol; Hycet; Zamicet

ANATOMY OR SYSTEM AFFECTED: Musculoskeletal system; Nervous system

History of Use

The combination of hydrocodone and acetaminophen known as *Vicodin* was approved by the U.S. Food and Drug Administration (FDA) for use as a brand-name oral prescription painkiller, marketed by Abbott in 1983. Originally, Vicodin tablets contained 500 mg of acetaminophen. However, consuming more than 4 grams of acetaminophen per day can cause liver damage. Because acetaminophen is found in so many different medications, and so widely used for pain relief, overdosing on acetaminophen is relatively easy to do. Taking more than eight Vicodin tablets in one day was enough to cause significant liver damage. Every year about 400 people died and 42,000 were hospitalized as a result of acetaminophen poisoning.

To mitigate this problem, on June 30, 2009, a FDA advisory panel recommended the removal of Vicodin and another acetaminophen/opioid combination medication called *Percocet* (oxycodone/acetaminophen) from the market because of the high incidence of acetaminophen-induced liver damage associated with these drugs. On January 13, 2011, the FDA directed drug manufacturers to limit the quantity of acetaminophen in prescription drug products to no more than 325 mg per dosage unit. Limiting the amount of acetaminophen per dosage unit in prescription products reduced the risk of severe liver injury from overdosing. Vicodin, therefore, was reformulated to only contain 300 mg of acetaminophen. The FDA had already approved a new hydrocodone/acetaminophen combination medication called *Norco* in February 1997 that contained 325 mg of acetaminophen. While the original formulation of Vicodin was discontinued, the new formulation, containing less acetaminophen and still called Vicodin, is made in the U.S. However, because of the high cost of the reformulated version of Vicodin, Norco, which is much less expensive, is the much more commonly prescribed drug. Other formulations of hydrocodone and acetaminophen are also available in solid and liquid forms. The different formulations of Vicodin and Norco are shown in the table below.

Product	Composition
Vicodin Pre-2012	
Vicodin	5 mg hydrocodone / 500 mg acetaminophen
Vicodin ES	7.5 mg hydrocodone / 750 mg acetaminophen
Vicodin HP	10 mg hydrocodone / 660 mg acetaminophen
Vicodin Post-2012	
Vicodin	5 mg hydrocodone / 300 mg acetaminophen
Vicodin ES	7.5 mg hydrocodone / 300 mg acetaminophen
Vicodin HP	10 mg hydrocodone / 300 mg acetaminophen
Norco	
Norco 5/325	5 mg hydrocodone / 325 mg acetaminophen
Norco 7.5/325	7.5 mg hydrocodone / 325 mg acetaminophen
Norco 10/325	10 mg hydrocodone / 325 mg acetaminophen

Nonmedical use of *Vicodin*, *Norco*, and other hydrocodone/acetaminophen combinations is of great concern to the medical, public health, drug misuse prevention, and law enforcement fields. Some people unintentionally become addicted to the drug after they receive a prescription for the drug to address specific pain.

Users without prescriptions buy painkillers illegally on the street; steal from pharmacies, doctors, or dentists; or steal from family or friends who may be taking the drug as prescribed. According to the 2014 National Survey on Drug Use and Health, more than 22 million persons ages twelve years and older had ever taken a prescription painkiller for a nonmedical reason. Over the past 15 years, there has been a significant decline in the misuse of prescription opioids among teens. Vicodin misuse among high school seniors dropped from 10.5 percent in 2003 to 2 percent in 2017. Teens have also reported decreased availability to prescription painkillers in 2017, with only 35.8 percent of high school seniors saying they were easy to acquire compared to 54 percent in 2010.

Effects and Potential Risks

In addition to providing temporary pain relief, Vicodin has the potential to produce many adverse reactions. It may prompt drowsiness, mood changes, and impairment of mental and physical abilities, itchiness, light-headedness, dizziness, sedation, nausea, vomiting, anxiety, and fear. Vicodin may be habit-forming and can lead to misuse, addiction, physical dependence, and tolerance. At high doses, Vicodin can affect the respiratory, dermatological, and gastrointestinal systems.

Vicodin should not be taken concomitantly with alcohol and other central nervous system (CNS) depressants, such as antihistamines, antipsychotics, or antianxiety agents. The combination may produce an additive CNS depression.

Vicodin overdose is defined as ≥90 mg of hydrocodone or ≥4 grams of acetaminophen. Hydrocodone overdose causes respiratory depression, extreme sleepiness that progresses to stupor or coma, flaccidity of skeletal muscles, cold and clammy skin, and sometimes low heart rate and abnormally low blood pressure. Respiratory and circulatory collapse, cardiac arrest, and death may occur. Acetaminophen overdose leads to potentially fatal hepatic necrosis. Other potential consequences of acetaminophen overdose include kidney failure, low blood sugar, and coma. Opioid overdose is treated with nasal naloxone (Narcan), and activated charcoal can be used to prevent absorption of ingested pills. Respiratory support and cardiovascular support are required for overdose patients. Injected N-acetylcysteine (Acetadote) is the antidote for acetaminophen intoxication.

The safety and effectiveness of Vicodin in children has yet to be determined. Pregnant women should not take Vicodin unless the potential benefit justifies the potential risk to the fetus. Regular use of opioids by pregnant women could cause the fetus to be born physically dependent on the drug. For mothers who are breastfeeding, acetaminophen is excreted in small amounts in breast milk, although it is unknown if hydrocodone is secreted also. Use of Vicodin should be avoided in these cases because of the potential for serious adverse reactions in infants, although in deciding, one should consider the importance of the drug to the mother. Dosing of Vicodin in geriatric patients should be moderated as well.

—*Patrice La Vigne*
—*Michael A. Buratovich, PhD*

References

American College of Emergency Physicians. "Street 'Norco' Looks like the Real Thing but Really, Really Isn't." *ScienceDaily*, 28 July 2016, www.sciencedaily.com/releases/2016/07/160728110433.htm.

Centers of Disease Control and Prevention. "Counterfeit Norco Poses New Danger." *JAMA Network*, vol. 315, no. 22, 14 June 2016, p. 2390., doi:10.1001/jama.2016.6975.

Holland, Kimberly, and Alyson Lozicki. "Vicodin vs. Percocet for Pain Reduction." *Healthline*, 30 Nov. 2017, www.healthline.com/health/pain-relief/vicodin-vs-percocet.

"Hydrocodone Combination Products." *MedlinePlus*, U.S. National Library of Medicine, 15 Oct. 2019, medlineplus.gov/druginfo/meds/a601006.html.

Moore, Paul A., et al. "Why Do We Prescribe Vicodin?" *The Journal of the American Dental Association*, vol. 147, no. 7, 2016, pp. 530–533., doi:10.1016/j.adaj.2016.05.005.

Non-Pharmacological Treatments

■ Arthroplasty

CATEGORY: Procedure
ANATOMY OR SYSTEM AFFECTED: Musculoskeletal system; joints of shoulder, elbow, wrist, hands, hips, knees, ankles.
SPECIALTIES AND RELATED FIELDS: Anesthesiology, general surgery, geriatrics and gerontology, orthopedics, rheumatology, sports medicine, occupational and physical therapy.

KEY TERMS
- *acetabulum*: the portion of the pelvic bone joining the femoral head to create the hip joint
- *cartilage*: flexible connective tissue between bones
- *epidural*: the injection of an anesthetic into the fluid around the spine or into the epidural space in the back
- *femur*: the leg bone extending from the knee to the hip
- *orthopedics*: a medical specialty emphasizing the prevention and correction of skeletal deformities
- *patella*: the flat, triangular bone in the front of the knee; also called the kneecap
- *tibia*: the shin bone
- *rheumatoid arthritis*: a long-term autoimmune disorder that primarily affects joints resulting in warm, swollen, and painful joints
- *viscosupplementation injections*: injections to add lubrication into the joint to make joint movement less painful

Indications and Procedures

Cartilage within a joint covers the ends of the bones, preventing bone from pressing on bone and allowing smooth, pain-free movement. Joints can become painful when cartilage on the end of each adjoining bone deteriorates, a process called osteoarthritis. A fracture, trauma, or another medical condition such as rheumatoid arthritis can also cause joint pain and disability, any of which may lead an individual to consider arthroplasty. Should initial nonsurgical treatments such as medications, physical therapy, and joint injections prove to be unsuccessful, arthroplasty, a surgery undertaken to replace deteriorating joints, becomes an option, particularly among the elderly.

Arthroplasty may be performed on the fingers, wrists, shoulders, elbows, and ankles but the most common sites of the surgery are the hips and knees. Most patients requiring hip or knee replacements are over the age of fifty, but arthroplasty may be indicated for younger people who have suffered advanced joint deterioration or trauma. Specialists in sports medicine who are typically orthopedic surgeons also frequently prescribe arthroplasty.

The hip is a ball-and-socket joint comprising the top of the femur (ball) inserted into the acetabulum (socket). During walking, the top of the femur slides within the acetabulum. Cartilage of the hip joint normally covers both bones where they join permitting smooth, painless contact between the surfaces. When the cartilage deteriorates, bones rub against each other, causing pain and restriction in movement that is eventually best relieved by hip replacement surgery.

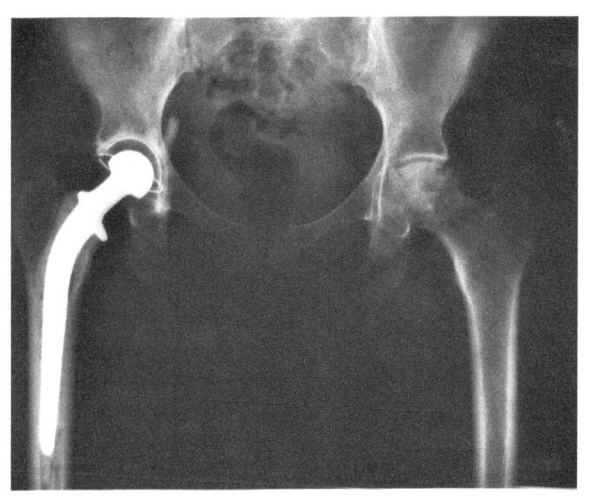

An A-P X-ray of a pelvis showing a total hip joint replacement. (National Institutes of Health)

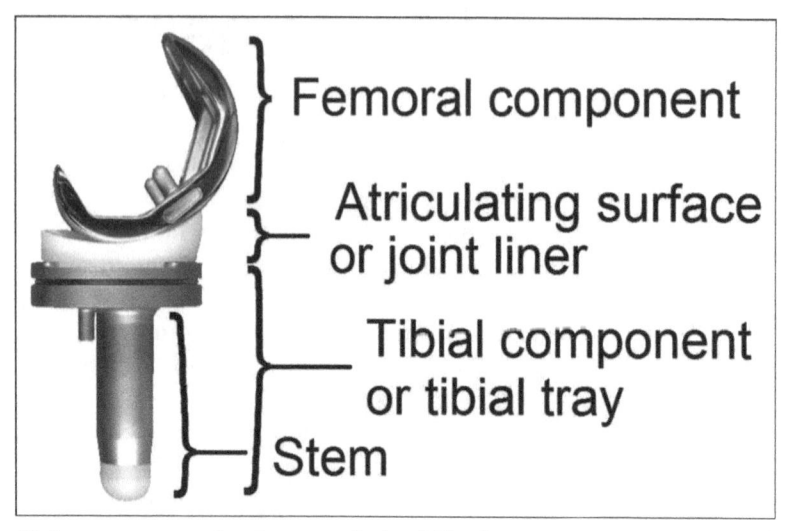

Main components of a knee prosthesis. (Mikael Häggström via Wikimedia Commons)

In hip surgery, an incision, varying in length from 2 to 12 inches, is made over the back of the hip (and more recently, the front of the hip, referred to as an anterior approach). Tissue and muscles are cut or pushed aside to expose the hip joint. The femur and acetabulum are separated. A cavity made in the acetabulum accommodates the replacement cup and allows for the insertion of a plastic-lined metal shell. The ball on the femur end of the joint is removed and replaced with a metal ball attached to a metal stem, usually made of titanium that is inserted into the femoral canal. The two parts are then cemented into place, making them adhere to the bone. Damaged muscles and tendons are repaired before the incision is closed with staples or sutures.

A similar situation can afflict the knee. In some instances, an orthopedist makes a small incision in the knee using a surgical instrument called an arthroscope or endoscope. The device inserts a narrow, illuminated tube with a camera attached into the affected site for a visual examination viewed on a monitor. If this examination, as well as previous x-rays, reveal worn bone and cartilage, a knee replacement is potentially indicated.

Knee arthroplasty consists of the worn knee joint being replaced with metal and plastic components. In knee arthroplasty, a long incision is made in the front of the knee and the patella is removed to make the joint accessible. Holes are drilled into the lower femur to affix the metal replacement. Holes are also drilled in the upper tibia to anchor a plastic plate. The back part of the patella is excised to create a flat surface into which holes are drilled to receive a plastic button. In most cases, the prosthesis is secured with cement, and the incision closed, usually with sutures or staples. Because polymethylmethacrylate cement is usually used in both the hip and knee procedures, the individual, under the guidance of a physical therapist, can gradually place weight on the surgical limb and progress as tolerated. Knee and hip arthroplasties are performed without cement and use implants with a textured or coated surface that the new bone actually grows into. Such implants may also use screws or pegs to stabilize the implant until the completion of bone ingrowth. Since cementless implants depend on new bone growth for stability, they require a longer healing time than cemented replacements. Typically, hip and knee replacements are performed on patients under general anesthesia, although a local anesthetic, either spinal or epidural, is sometimes used. In most cases, general anesthesia is preferred because patients must remain completely still during this surgery and general anesthesia causes temporary paralysis.

Uses and Complications

Arthroplasty is used to relieve pain and restore mobility in patients who have been disabled by their conditions and are reasonable surgical risks. Because many such patients are elderly, extensive preoperative evaluation is necessary. Arthroplasty may be used when medical treatments no longer effectively relieve joint pain and disability. Some medical treatments for osteoarthritis tried before arthroplasty include physical therapy, cortisone joint injections, anti-inflammatory medicines, viscosupplementation injections, and pain medicines.

Conditions such as diabetes mellitus, hypertension, heart or lung disease, and anemia increase the surgical risk. Open lesions increase the risk of infection. Nerve damage can result from cutting muscles and tendons during surgery. Blood clots can form in the lungs or legs of patients undergoing arthroplasty, and this risk may continue for two months following surgery. Blood thinners are usually administered postoperatively. Infection and loosening of prosthetic parts are additional surgical risks and complications.

Physical therapy, essential following arthroplasty of any joint, usually begins two or three days after the surgery and continues for eight weeks. Most patients are completely ambulatory within six weeks postoperatively of hip or knee arthroplasty.

Perspective and Prospects

Joint replacement is becoming more common and more than 1 million Americans have a hip or knee replaced each year. Research has shown that despite increases in age, joint replacement can help overall mobility and general wellbeing. As life expectancy increases, incidence of joint problems is increasing exponentially. In the early twentieth century, many people who lived beyond their sixties were immobilized by chronic arthritis, osteoporosis, and painful joints. When an elderly person suffered a broken hip, it often marked the beginning of a physical decline with a fatal outcome. Medical advances made during World War II had a profound effect on treating many physical problems that, although experienced in combat by relatively young people, required treatment that was soon used in dealing with the joint problems of the elderly. Hip and knee surgery were once more disabling than they currently are. Hip surgery now requires incisions as small as one inch long, although four-inch incisions are more common and ten-inch incisions are used by some surgeons.

Although arthroplasty usually involves a hospital stay of two days depending on the complexity of each individual case, some low-risk individuals without post-op complications become outpatient procedures. The use of titanium in prostheses has extended the effectiveness of such surgery, with these devices currently expected to last for over two decades. People who have arthroplasty generally have substantial improvement in their joint pain, ability to perform activities, and quality of life.

—*R. Baird Shuman, PhD*

References

"Arthroplasty." *Johns Hopkins Medicine*, 2019, www.hopkinsmedicine.org/health/treatment-tests-and-therapies/arthroplasty.

Feng, James, et al. "Total Knee Arthroplasty: Improving Outcomes with a Multidisciplinary Approach." *Journal of Multidisciplinary Healthcare*, vol. 11, 2018, pp. 63–73., doi:10.2147/jmdh.s140550.

Gogineni, Hrishikesh C., et al. "Transition to Outpatient Total Hip and Knee Arthroplasty: Experience at an Academic Tertiary Care Center." *Arthroplasty Today*, vol. 5, no. 1, Mar. 2019, pp. 100–105., doi:10.1016/j.artd.2018.10.008.

Karachalios, Theofilos, et al. "Total Hip Arthroplasty." *EFORT Open Reviews*, vol. 3, no. 5, 2018, pp. 232–239., doi:10.1302/2058-5241.3.170068.

Lee, Yong Seuk. "Comprehensive Analysis of Pain Management after Total Knee Arthroplasty." *Knee Surgery & Related Research*, vol. 29, no. 2, 1 June 2017, pp. 80–86., doi:10.5792/ksrr.16.024.

Warwick, Hunter, et al. "Immediate Physical Therapy Following Total Joint Arthroplasty: Barriers and Impact on Short-Term Outcomes." *Advances in Orthopedics*, vol. 2019, 8 Apr. 2019, pp. 1–7., doi:10.1155/2019/6051476.

Weber, Markus, et al. "Predicting Outcome after Total Hip Arthroplasty: The Role of Preoperative Patient-Reported Measures." *BioMed Research International*, vol. 2019, 29 Jan. 2019, pp. 1–9., doi:10.1155/2019/4909561.

■ Astym® therapy

CATEGORY: Therapy or Technique; Physiotherapy
ANATOMY OR SYSTEM AFFECTED: Soft tissues of the body; muscles; tendons; ligaments; musculoskeletal systems and neural pathways
SPECIALTIES AND RELATED FIELDS: Rehabilitation, Physical Therapy, Occupational Therapy, Athletic Training, Athletic Enhancement

Indications and Procedures

Astym® treatment is regenerative soft tissue therapy that rebuilds and heals the soft tissues of the body, non-invasively and without pharmaceuticals. Astym® treatment safely and effectively stimulates internal scar tissue to be resorbed by the body and regenerates damaged soft tissues. This non-invasive therapeutic approach utilizes handheld instrumentation, applied topically, to locate underlying dysfunctional soft tissue and then transfer specific pressures and shear forces via that instrumentation to the dysfunctional tissue through specific protocols and application patterns developed from scientific and clinical study. The particular pressures and shear forces are aimed at inducing a cellular response, whereby cellular mediators and growth factors assist in activating scar tissue resorption, stimulating tissue turnover and regenerating soft tissues.

Astym® therapy is typically provided in a physical or occupational therapy setting. However, elite athletes are frequently treated as part of their team care to optimize performance and treatment may occur at the site of competitions. In addition, large employers and the military routinely have Astym® therapy provided in their facilities or in the field in order to minimize interruption by resolving injuries effectively and efficiently.

Developed methodically from theory through basic science investigation to clinical study and practice, Astym® therapy engages the regenerative mechanisms of the body. It has been shown to be consistently safe and effective in the treatment of internal scar tissue that is causing pain or movement restriction, chronic tendonitis, traumatic soft tissue injury, post-surgical pain/restrictions and other soft tissue dysfunctions.

Tendinopathies and tendonitis are a widespread problem and often present a challenge to healthcare professionals, in many cases remaining unresolved. Astym® treatment is highly effective in the treatment of tendinopathy and clinical trials have demonstrated Astym® therapy to reduce pain, and increase motion and functional ability in this population. Effective both as a first-line treatment, and as a last resort when other treatments have failed, Astym® therapy is an attractive treatment option. It has a relatively short treatment course of four to six weeks (8-10 visits), and during treatment, there are usually no restrictions on activity, which is a welcome change from other more restrictive treatment options. Randomized clinical trials have shown Astym® therapy to be more effective than the standard-of-care treatments for lateral elbow tendinopathy (tennis elbow), patellar (knee) tendinopathy and Achilles tendinopathy.

Astym® therapy has also been found to reduce pain and increase function in cases where internal scar tissue is interfering with movement or causing pain. Internal scar tissue may result from a number of factors, including overuse, problematic biomechanics, trauma or surgery. Although Astym® therapy routinely demonstrates considerable success in the treatment of conditions where scar tissue is present, extraordinary improvement has been shown when Astym® therapy is used post-surgically.

There is also evidence that Astym® therapy can improve the brain-to-body connection by stimulating neuroplastic changes in damaged nervous systems. This is critically important, since Astym® therapy may alter the natural progression or prognosis for such disorders as cerebral palsy and brain injury, which has not yet been possible. The positive neural effects of Astym® therapy were demonstrated in a large, three-arm randomized controlled trial, which revealed that Astym® therapy immediately and significantly improves muscle performance after injury. These results are supported by other clinical studies indicating improvement in neural conditions such as carpal tunnel syndrome, restricted movement due to cerebral palsy and brain injury.

Uses and Complications

Astym® therapy is generally well-tolerated by patients. The treating therapist/clinician should adjust the topical pressures and forces to be within the tolerance of each patient. General contraindications include: compromised skin integrity; open wound(s); active infection; skin ulcerations; acute deep venous thrombosis (DVT); treatment involving the area of a pacemaker or internal defibrillator; active primary or metastatic tumor site; clotting disorders; and any medical condition or disorder that may be exacerbated by the application of topical pressures on the skin or underlying structures.

In order to receive proper treatment, it is important to confirm that the clinician is officially certified in Astym® therapy. Certification training educates clinicians in the scientifically developed protocols and specific treatment parameters that have been studied in the randomized controlled trials. Astym® therapy has consistently demonstrated safety and effectiveness in clinical study and is also well tolerated by patients. Astym® therapy is distinctly different from instrument-assisted soft tissue mobilization (IASTM) interventions, and it is important to recognize that IASTM interventions show neither the effectiveness nor the safety of Astym® therapy. Although the IASTM methods use tools to treat tissue, the methods and results are quite different from those of Astym® therapy, and

Diagnoses that show strong clinical results from Astym® therapy

Specific Conditions	General Conditions
• Achilles Tendinopathy	• Patellar Tendinopathy
• Anterior and Posterior Tibialis Tendinopathy	• Plantar Fasciopathy
• Arthrofibrosis	• Post-Mastectomy Scarring
• Carpal Tunnel Syndrome	• Post-Surgical Scarring/Fibrosis
• Chronic Ankle Pain and Stiffness	• Rotator Cuff Tendinopathy
• Chronic Wrist Pain and Stiffness	• Scar Tissue/Fibrosis
• DeQuervain's Tenosynovitis	• Tennis Elbow
• Golfer's Elbow	• Trochanteric Bursitis
• Hamstring Strain	• Chronic tendinopathy
• IT Band Syndrome	• Joint and muscle stiffness
• Jumper's Knee Lateral Epicondylopathy	• Sprains and strains
• Low Back Pain (nonradicular)	• Conditions resulting from dysfunctional scar tissue or fibrosis (e.g. post-traumatic, post-surgical)
• Medial Epicondylopathy	

IASTM methods are often not well tolerated by patients. IASTM methods use tooled cross-friction massage to, it is argued, break apart the tissue, whereas Astym® therapy engages the regenerative mechanisms of the body aiming to repair damaged tissue and stimulate the resorption of scar tissue. A recent systematic review evaluated the research on IASTM and concluded the research does not support the efficacy of IASTM for treating musculoskeletal pathologies.

Perspective and Prospects

Historically, treatment for soft tissue disorders centered upon treating inflammation. However, with the discovery that tendinopathies and some other soft tissue conditions are primarily degenerative in nature, scholars emphasize that treatment should now be focused on regeneration and restoration. Astym® therapy was the first conservative treatment scientifically developed to engage the regenerative mechanisms of the body and has been proven to be effective in treating a variety of soft tissue disorders. Although many available treatments today still focus on reducing inflammation, they often have little to no scientific evidence supporting their effectiveness.

—*Thomas L. Sevier, MD and Gipson Schabel*

References

Cheatham SW, Lee M, Cain M, Baker R. "The Efficacy of Instrument Assisted Soft Tissue Mobilization: A Systematic Review." *Journal of the Canadian Chiropractic Association* 60, no. 3. Sept. 2016, pp. 200-211.

Chughtai, Morad, et al. "Astym® Therapy: a Systematic Review." *Annals of Translational Medicine*, vol. 7, no. 4, Feb. 2019, p. 70., doi:10.21037/atm.2018.11.49.

Davies, Claire, et al. "Astym Therapy Improves Function and Range of Motion Following Mastectomy." *Breast Cancer: Targets and Therapy*, vol. 8, 8 Mar. 2016, pp. 39–45., doi:10.2147/bctt.s102598.

Harris, Leah S., et al. "Astym® Therapy Improves FOTO® Outcomes for Patients with Musculoskeletal Disorders: an Observational Study." *Annals of Translational Medicine*, vol. 7, no. S7, 2019, doi:10.21037/atm.2019.04.09.

Kim, Jooyoung, et al. "Therapeutic Effectiveness of Instrument-Assisted Soft Tissue Mobilization for Soft Tissue Injury: Mechanisms and Practical Application." *Journal of Exercise Rehabilitation*, vol. 13, no. 1, 28 Feb. 2017, pp. 12–22., doi:10.12965/jer.1732824.412.

Kivlan, Benjamin R., et al. "The Effect of Astym® Therapy on Muscle Strength: a Blinded,

Randomized, Clinically Controlled Trial." *BMC Musculoskeletal Disorders*, vol. 16, 29 Oct. 2015, doi:10.1186/s12891-015-0778-9.

Rodriguez-Merchan, E. Carlos, et al. "The Current Role of Astym Therapy in the Treatment of Musculoskeletal Disorders." *Postgraduate Medicine*, 28 Aug. 2019, pp. 1–6., doi:10.1080/00325481.2019.1654836.

Scheer, Nicole A., et al. "Astym Therapy Improves Bilateral Hamstring Flexibility and Achilles Tendinopathy in a Child with Cerebral Palsy: A Retrospective Case Report." *Clinical Medicine Insights: Case Reports*, vol. 9, Oct. 2016, pp. 95–98., doi:10.4137/ccrep.s40623.

Sevier, Thomas L., and Caroline W. Stegink-Jansen. "Astym Treatmentvs.eccentric Exercise for Lateral Elbow Tendinopathy: a Randomized Controlled Clinical Trial." *PeerJ*, vol. 3, May 2015, doi:10.7717/peerj.967.

■ Cervical epidural injection

CATEGORY: Procedure
SYSTEM OR ANATOMY AFFECTED: Nervous system, Spinal cord

Definition
The cervical spine is the part of the spine located in your neck. The spinal cord sits inside a tunnel created by the vertebrae (bones making up the spine). It is also protected by a soft layer of tissue called the dura. The epidural space is the area between the bony canal and the dura layer of the spinal cord.

An epidural injection is a procedure to deliver medication into this epidural space. The medication may include an anesthetic that will numb the pain and a steroid that can decrease swelling and irritation.

Reasons for Procedure
An epidural injection may be done if you have pain in your neck and upper limb that is not responding to conservative treatment, such as oral medications and physical therapy.

Damage to local joints or discs of the spine can irritate the nerves exiting the spinal cord. This can cause inflammation around the nerves, which leads to pain. The pain may be in the neck or may travel down to the shoulders and arms, and even to the hands and fingers.

The injection may provide relief for a few weeks or even a couple months depending on the exact cause of pain.

This procedure may help manage the pain until the injury that caused the nerve irritation has time to heal.

Possible Complications
Problems from the procedure are rare, but all procedures have some risk. Your doctor will review potential problems, like:

- Increase in pain
- Bleeding or fluid leakage in spinal canal
- Infection
- Spinal headaches
- Nerve damage
- Allergic reaction to the medication used, such as hives, lightheadedness, low blood pressure, or wheezing

If you smoke, talk to your doctor about ways to quit. Smoking can weaken your immune system and slow healing.

Your doctor may not want to do this injection if you have:

- Had success with conservative treatment
- Not tried other conservative treatment
- Allergies to the local anesthetic, x-ray contrast, or medications being used
- Local skin or other infection
- Bleeding disorder or take blood-thinning medication
- Cancer
- Uncontrolled high blood pressure or diabetes
- Unstable angina or heart failure

What to Expect
Prior to Procedure

Your doctor may begin with conservative treatment, such as rest, medication, physical therapy, and exercise.

Before the procedure you may need:

- A physical exam
- Imaging tests to evaluate the spinal structures with x-rays or an MRI scan

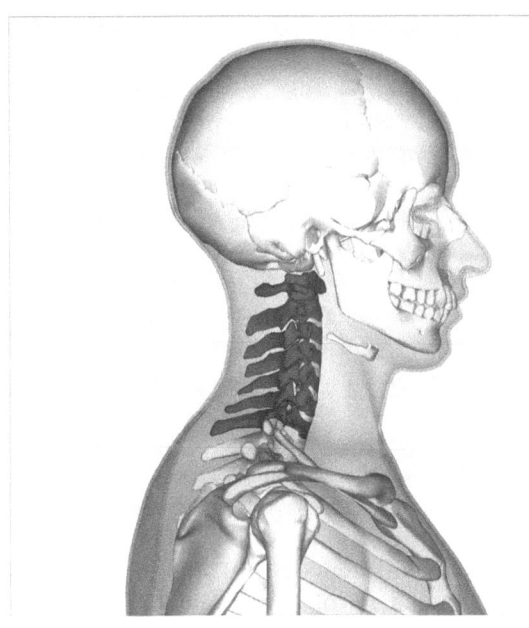

Position of human cervical vertebrae (shown in red). It consists of 7 bones, from top to bottom, C1, C2, C3, C4, C5, C6, and C7. (Anatomography via Wikimedia Commons)

- To discuss allergies that you may have to the anesthetic, pain medication, or latex

In addition, talk to your doctor about your medications. You may have to stop taking some medications up to one week or more before the procedure.

Additional considerations include:

- Your doctor may ask you to avoid food or drink a few hours before the procedure.
- You will need someone to drive you home after the procedure.

Anesthesia

You will be awake during this procedure. A local anesthetic will be used to numb the skin before the injection. Your doctor may also give you medication to help you relax.

Description of Procedure

You may have devices attached to help monitor your blood pressure, heart, and oxygen levels. You will be asked to lie on your stomach or side on an x-ray table or sit in a chair. The skin around the injection site will be cleansed. A local anesthetic will be given to numb the area.

The doctor will inject a contrast dye. This dye will help highlight the area to guide the needle. This is done using a type of x-ray called fluoroscopy. Next, when the doctor has reached the epidural space, the steroid will be delivered.

Immediately After Procedure

A small bandage will be placed over the injection site. You may be able to go home after being observed.

How Long Will It Take?

The injection only takes a few minutes. The entire procedure may be 30-60 minutes.

How Much Will It Hurt?

There is local discomfort as the numbing medication first goes in. But the rest of the procedure should not be painful. Once the injected anesthetic wears off, you may have some discomfort.

Post-procedure Care

At the Care Center

Your doctor will assess your level of pain relief.

At Home

You will have to reduce your activity level for the first day or so. You can apply ice to the affected area to relieve swelling and discomfort. Pain can be managed with medications. Proper care of the insertion site can help prevent infection. You can slowly increase your activity as tolerated or by your doctor's instructions, but injected steroids may take time to work. If you have diabetes, monitor your blood sugar levels more carefully a few weeks after an injection. The medication that was injected may cause elevated blood sugar levels.

Call Your Doctor

Call your doctor if any of these occur:

- Severe pain or headache
- Fever or chills
- Increased arm weakness or numbness
- Problems swallowing
- Redness, swelling, increasing pain, bleeding, or discharge from the injection site

If you think you have an emergency, call for emergency medical services right away.

—*Michael Woods, MD, FAAP*
EBSCO Medical Review Board

Resources

American Chronic Pain Association
https://www.theacpa.org

Ortho Info—American Academy of Orthopaedic Surgeons
https://www.orthoinfo.org

Canadian Resources

Arthritis Society
http://www.arthritis.ca

Health Canada
https://www.canada.ca

References

"Cervical Epidural." *Department of Radiology*, University of Wisconsin School of Medicine and Public Health , 18 Dec. 2017, www.radiology.wisc.edu/documents/cervical-epidural/.

"Cervical Radicular Pain and Radiculopathy." Edited by Brian C. Callaghan et al., *DynaMed*, EBSCO Information Services, 18 Nov. 2018, www.dynamed.com/condition/cervical-radicular-pain-and-radiculopathy.

"Epidural Injections." *RadiologyInfo.org*, Radiological Society of North America, Inc, 20 Mar. 2019, www.radiologyinfo.org/en/info.cfm?pg=epidural.

Rae-Grant, Alexander C. "Epidural Steroid Injection." *DynaMed*, EBSCO Information Services, 5 Sept. 2016, www.dynamed.com/topics/dmp~AN~T901362/Epidural-steroid-injection.

Simotas, Alexander C. "Cervical Radiculopathy: Nonsurgical Treatment Options." *Hospital for Special Surgery*, 1 May 2009, www.hss.edu/conditions_cervical-radiculopathy-nonoperative-treatments-epidural.asp#.VJMhbtLF-So.

■ Chiropractic

CATEGORY: Therapy or Technique; Physiotherapy
ALSO KNOWN AS: Spinal manipulation
ANATOMY OR SYSTEM AFFECTED: Musculoskeletal system

KEY TERMS

- *activator*: a small handheld spring-loaded instrument which delivers a controlled and reproducible impulse to the spine
- *high-velocity, low-amplitude*: short, quick thrust over restricted joints with the goal of restoring normal range of motion in the joint
- *low-velocity, high-amplitude*: slow, long thrusts to carry a dysfunctional joint through its full range of motion, with the therapeutic goal of increasing range of motion
- *sciatica*: pain affecting the back, hip, and outer side of the leg, caused by compression of a spinal nerve root in the lower back
- *subluxations*: a slight misalignment of the vertebrae, regarded in chiropractic theory as the cause of many health problems

Overview

Chiropractic is one of the most widely used health services. It has gained increasing acceptance as a treatment for back and neck pain, and it is covered by many health insurance plans. Millions of people would report that chiropractic spinal manipulation has brought them relief. Nonetheless, the research record for its effectiveness is inconclusive.

Daniel David Palmer founded chiropractic in 1895, after an experience in which he apparently believed he cured a man's deafness by manipulating his back. Palmer then opened the Palmer School of Chiropractic and began teaching spinal manipulation. This college still exists and has a fully accredited program.

One of Palmer's first students was his son, Bartlett Joshua (B. J.) Palmer. It was B. J. Palmer who truly popularized the technique. Later Willard Carver, an Oklahoma City lawyer, opened a competing school. He believed that chiropractic physicians needed to offer other methods of treatment in addition to spinal manipulation. This opened a schism in the chiropractic world that still exists. Followers of Palmer and his methods focus only on spinal adjustments, an approach called "straight" chiropractic. Those who, like Carver, use various approaches to healing are called "mixers." Mixers may use vitamins, herbs, and any other treatment methods they find useful (and are allowed to practice by law).

Medical treatments in the nineteenth and early twentieth centuries were not based on scientific evidence of effectiveness, and chiropractic treatment was no exception. It became a widespread technique long before there was any real evidence that it worked. Chiropractic schools utilized their profits and resources to further develop programs for

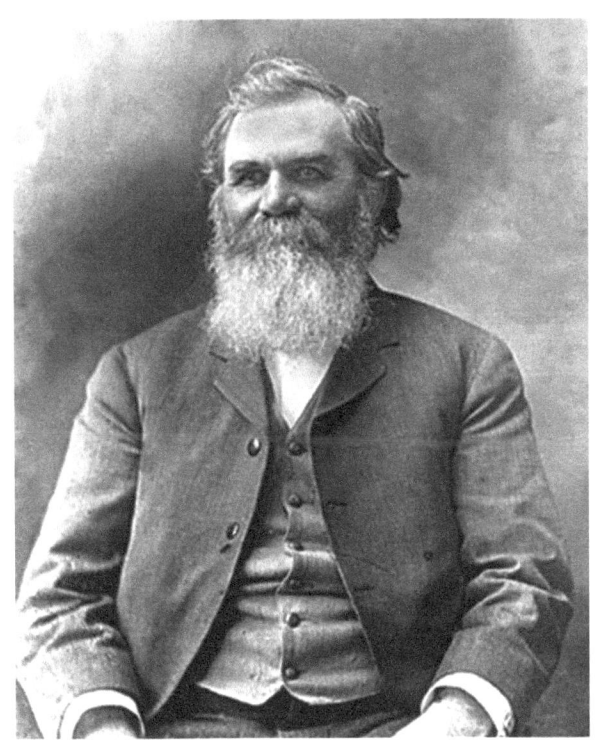

Daniel David Palmer, inventor of chiropractic. (via Wikimedia Commons)

training people in chiropractic techniques, not for verifying the theory and practice of chiropractic. However, in the 1970s, proper scientific research into chiropractic began to draw interest. In 1977, the Foundation for Chiropractic Education and Research established a program to train chiropractic researchers. Since then, efforts have been made to fund scientific trials testing the effectiveness of chiropractic techniques and to establish a scientific foundation for the practice.

There are many different chiropractic techniques, some with proprietary names such as the Gonstead and Maitland techniques. In general, most involve rapid (high-velocity) short (low-amplitude) thrusts. Manipulation may be purely manual or mechanically assisted. For example, some chiropractors use what is called an "activator," a small metal tool that applies a force directly to one vertebra.

In addition, some chiropractors use a related therapy called spinal mobilization. This method involves gentle, extended movements (low-velocity, high-amplitude) rather than the "back cracking" of classic chiropractic spinal manipulation.

Mechanism of Action

Since its origin, chiropractic theory has based itself on subluxations, or vertebrae that have shifted position in the spine. These subluxations are said to impede nerve outflow and cause disease in various organs. A chiropractic treatment is supposed to "put back in" these "popped out" vertebrae; for this reason, it is called an "adjustment."

However, no real evidence has ever been presented showing that a given chiropractic treatment alters the position of any vertebrae. In addition, there is as yet no real evidence that impairment of nerve outflow is a major contributor to common illnesses, or that spinal manipulation changes nerve outflow in such a way as to affect organ function.

Later theories suggest that chiropractic manipulation may relieve pain by "loosening" vertebrae that have become relatively immobile rather than by changing their position. In addition, the movements associated with manipulation may alter the response patterns of nerves in the central nervous system, including both the spine and the brain, leading to pain relief.

Uses and Applications

Chiropractic spinal manipulation is widely used for the treatment of back pain, neck pain, and headaches, whether acute or chronic. It is also frequently tried for pain in other areas, such as the shoulders, knees, and jaw, and for breech birth positioning of a fetus, infantile colic, frequent colds, and many other conditions.

Some chiropractic physicians promote comprehensive chiropractic care as a means of staying healthy. This approach may include diet, exercise, and supplements, along with regular chiropractic manipulation.

Scientific Evidence

Chiropractic spinal manipulation has been evaluated scientifically to determine its efficacy and its costs compared to other forms of health care. However, the evidence is not compelling in either case.

Efficacy. Although there is some evidence that chiropractic spinal manipulation may be helpful for various medical purposes, in general the evidence is not strong. There are several reasons for this, but one is fundamental: Even with the best of intentions, it is difficult to properly ascertain the effectiveness of a hands-on therapy like chiropractic.

Only one form of study can truly prove that a treatment is effective: the double-blind, placebo-controlled trial. However, it is difficult to fit chiropractic into a study design of this type. Because of this, all studies of chiropractic manipulation fall short of optimum design. Many have compared chiropractic treatment with no treatment. However, studies of this type cannot provide reliable evidence about the efficacy of a treatment. If a benefit is seen, there is no way to determine whether it was caused by chiropractic manipulation specifically or by attention generally. (Attention alone will almost always produce some reported benefit.)

More meaningful trials used some sort of unrelated fake treatment for the control group, such as phony laser acupuncture. However, it is less than ideal to use a placebo treatment that is so very different in form from the treatment under study. Better studies compare real chiropractic manipulation with sham forms of manipulation, such as light touch. Studies of this type are a definite step forward. However, it is quite likely that the practitioners unconsciously conveyed more enthusiasm and optimism when performing the real therapy than the fake therapy; this, too, could affect the outcome. It has been suggested that the only way to get around this problem would be to compare the effectiveness of trained practitioners to that of actors trained only enough to provide simulated treatment; however, such studies have not been reported.

Still other studies have simply involved treating people with chiropractic spinal manipulation and seeing whether they improve. These trials are particularly meaningless; it has been proven that both participants and examining physicians will think that they observe improvement in people given a treatment, regardless of whether the treatment does anything on its own.

Finally, other trials have compared chiropractic manipulation to competing therapies, such as massage therapy or conventional physical therapy. However, neither of these therapies has been proven effective. When one compares unproven therapies to each other, the results cannot possibly prove that any of the tested treatments are effective. Given these caveats, the following discussion will focus on what science knows about the effects of chiropractic.

Cost of care. Besides effectiveness, another important consideration is cost of care. There are many aspects to the cost of treatment, including number of visits to the chosen provider, cost of evaluation procedures such as X rays, insurance reimbursement versus patient out-of-pocket expense, and costs for missed work time.

However, it is difficult to develop accurate cost-comparison figures because there are many complicating factors in research on the subject. For example, one approach is to simply identify people with similar injuries who choose one treatment or another and add up the total cost. The results of such a study can be misleading. People with more or less severe back pain might tend to choose different forms of treatment; if those with more severe pain usually chose surgical treatment, this would tend to inflate the comparative costs of conventional care and make chiropractic seem less expensive.

Another potentially complicating factor is that, to a great extent, insurance companies control utilization of treatment. If they are less inclined to authorize chiropractic visits, people who choose chiropractic care might find their care cut off more rapidly than others who choose, say, physical therapy. This too would lead to artificially low costs of chiropractic treatment compared to physical therapy, skewing the results of the study.

These problems could be solved by conducting a study in which researchers randomly assign participants to certain treatments, with the length of treatment determined entirely by the treating physician. Studies of this type have not been conducted.

Back pain. Chiropractic spinal manipulation is one of the most popular treatments for acute and chronic back pain in the United States, and it may provide modest benefit. However, research evidence has failed to find chiropractic manipulation convincingly more effective than standard medical care.

Chiropractic does seem to be more effective than placebo, if not by a great deal. For example, a single-blind controlled study of eighty-four people with low back pain compared manipulation to treatment with a diathermy machine (a physical therapy machine that uses microwaves to create heat beneath the skin) that was not actually functioning. The researchers asked the participants to assess their own pain levels within fifteen minutes of the first treatment then three and seven days after treatment. The only statistically significant difference between the two groups was found with fifteen minutes of the manipulation. (Chiropractic had better results at that point.)

In another single-blind, placebo-controlled study, researchers assigned 209 participants to one of three groups: a high-velocity, low-amplitude (HVLA) spinal manipulation, a sham manipulation, or a back-education program. Although this has been reported as a positive study, most of the differences seen among the groups were not statistically significant. In addition, because almost one-half of the participants dropped out of the study before the end, the results cannot be regarded as meaningful.

Unimpressive results were also seen in a well-designed study of 321 people with back pain comparing chiropractic manipulation, a special form of physical therapy (the Mackenzie method), and the provision of an educational booklet in treating low back pain. All groups improved to about the same extent.

Several studies evaluated the effectiveness of chiropractic manipulation combined with a different kind of treatment called mobilization, but they too found little to no benefit. On a positive note, one study of one hundred people with back pain and sciatica symptoms (pain down the leg caused by disc protrusion) found that chiropractic manipulation was significantly more effective at relieving symptoms than was sham chiropractic manipulation.

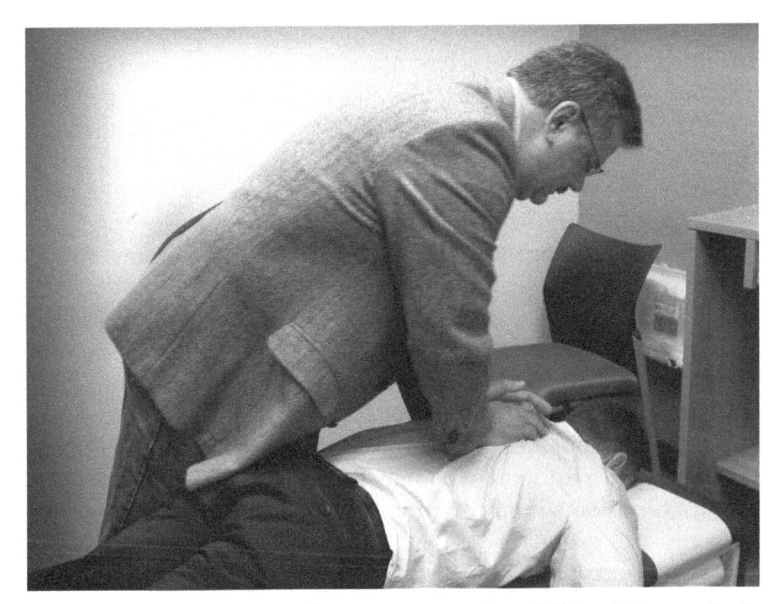

A chiropractor performs an adjustment on a patient. (Michael Dorausch via Wikimedia Commons)

Several studies have found that chiropractic is at least as helpful as other commonly used therapies for low back pain, such as muscle relaxants, anti-inflammatory medication, soft-tissue massage, conventional medical care, and physical therapy. For example, a large well-designed study found chiropractic manipulation more effective than general medical care and exercise therapy.

Physical therapy, the main conventional therapy for back pain, also lacks consistent supporting evidence. For example, in one large study of people with back pain, a single session of advice proved just as effective as a full course of physical therapy for back pain.

Neck pain. As with back pain, there is no reliable evidence that spinal manipulation works for neck pain. Of the limited number of studies performed, most have failed to find manipulation (with or without mobilization or massage) convincingly more effective than placebo or no treatment. One large study (almost two hundred participants) found that a special exercise program (MedX) was more effective than manipulation. However, a study reported in 2006 found that a single HVLA manipulation of the neck was more effective than a single mobilization procedure in improving range of motion and pain in people with neck pain.

Upper extremity pain. Persons often seek chiropractic care for painful conditions affecting their upper extremities (such as the shoulder, elbow, forearm, wrist, and hand). A recent search and analysis of all published studies examining the effectiveness of chiropractic for these conditions revealed mostly case studies, an unreliable source of evidence. The few uncovered controlled trials were of insufficient quality to draw any reliable conclusions about the effectiveness of chiropractic for painful conditions of the upper extremity.

Tension and cervicogenic headaches. Many people experience headaches caused by muscle tension, neck problems, or a combination of the two. Because these tension headaches and cervicogenic headaches (those caused by neck problems) overlap, they are discussed together here. Chiropractic spinal manipulation has shown some promise for these conditions, but the evidence remains incomplete and somewhat contradictory. In a controlled trial of 150 people, investigators compared spinal manipulation to the drug amitriptyline for the treatment of chronic tension-type headaches. By the end of the six-week treatment period, participants in both groups had improved similarly. However, four weeks after treatment was stopped, people who had received spinal manipulation showed greater reduction in headache intensity and frequency and over-the-counter medication usage than those who used the medication. The difference in the amount of improvement between the groups was statistically significant.

In another positive trial, fifty-three people with cervicogenic headaches received chiropractic spinal manipulation or laser acupuncture plus massage. Chiropractic manipulation was more effective. However, a similar study of seventy-five people with recurrent tension headaches found no difference between the two groups. Other, smaller studies of spinal manipulation have been reported too, with mixed results.

Finally, in a controlled trial, two hundred people with cervicogenic headaches were randomly assigned to receive one of four therapies: manipulation, a special exercise technique, exercise plus manipulation, or no therapy. Each participant received a minimum of eight to twelve treatments for six weeks. All three treatment approaches produced better results than no treatment, and each had approximately the same effect as the others. However, these results prove little because any treatment whatsoever will generally produce better results than no treatment.

Migraine headaches. There is some evidence that chiropractic manipulation may provide both long-term and short-term benefits for migraine headaches. In a double-blind, placebo-controlled study, 123 participants with migraine headaches were treated for two months with chiropractic manipulations or fake electrical therapy (in which electrodes were placed on the body without electrical current sent between them) as placebo. The study lasted six months: two months pre-treatment, two months of treatment, and two months post-treatment. After two months of treatment, those receiving chiropractic manipulation showed statistically significant improvement in headache severity and frequency compared with the control group. Furthermore, these benefits persisted to a two-month follow-up evaluation.

Chiropractic manipulation also produced relatively prolonged benefits in another trial. In this study, 218 people with migraine headaches were divided into three groups: manipulation, medication (amitriptyline), or manipulation plus medication. During the four weeks of treatment, all three groups experienced comparable benefits. During the follow-up four-week period, however, people who had received manipulation alone experienced more benefit than those who had been in the other two groups.

A study of eighty-five people with migraines compared spinal manipulation with two other treatments: mobilization and manipulation performed by someone other than a chiropractor. The results showed no difference among groups.

Chiropractic has been evaluated for many other conditions, including the following, but the results show little evidence of benefit.

Infantile colic. Infantile colic is a common and frustrating problem. Although chiropractic manipulation has been promoted as a treatment for this condition, there is little evidence that it offers specific benefits.

In a single-blind, placebo-controlled trial, eighty-six infants either received three chiropractic treatments or were held for ten minutes by a nurse. While a high percentage of infants improved, there was no significant difference between the two groups. Another trial compared spinal manipulation to the drug dimethicone. While chiropractic proved more effective than the medication, dimethicone itself has never been proven effective for infantile colic, and the study did not use a placebo group. For this reason, the results of this study indicate little about the effectiveness of chiropractic treatment for infantile colic.

Premenstrual syndrome. A small crossover trial of chiropractic for premenstrual symptoms found equivocal results.

Phobias. A small trial compared real and sham activator-style chiropractic treatment in people with phobias and found some evidence of benefit.

Asthma. In two controlled studies comparing spinal manipulation to sham manipulation for the treatment of people with asthma, the results showed equal improvement for participants in the two groups. These results suggest that the benefits were most likely caused by the attention given by the chiropractor and not by the spinal manipulation itself. However, one of these studies has been sharply criticized for using as a sham treatment a chiropractic method perfectly capable of producing a therapeutic effect. This could hide real benefits of the tested form of chiropractic. (If the "placebo" treatment used in a study is actually better than placebo, and the tested treatment does no better than this "placebo," the results would appear to indicate that the tested treatment is no better than placebo and, hence, is ineffective.)

Dysmenorrhea. A single-blind, placebo-controlled study of 138 women complaining of dysmenorrhea (menstrual pain) compared spinal manipulation with sham manipulation for four menstrual cycles and found no differences between the two groups.

High blood pressure. In a study of 148 people with mild high blood pressure, the use of chiropractic spinal manipulation plus dietary changes failed to prove more effective for reducing blood pressure than dietary changes alone.

Bed-wetting. A single-blind, placebo-controlled trial compared real and sham chiropractic (activator technique) in forty-six children with bed-wetting problems but failed to find a statistically significant difference between the groups.

Scoliosis. Weak evidence hints that chiropractic could be somewhat helpful for adolescent idiopathic scoliosis (curvature of the spine that occurs for no clear reason in adolescents).

What to Expect During Treatment
Depending on the condition, chiropractic treatment is usually conducted two or three times per week for one month or more. Chiropractic is also sometimes used on an as-needed basis or in a once or twice a month maintenance form. For many chiropractors, X rays are essential at the first visit and at some follow-up visits.

Each session involves hands-on manipulation following the methods of whatever manipulation technique the practitioner chooses to use. Sometimes other modalities may be used too, such as massage or hot or cold packs. Chiropractic physicians may also provide general wellness counseling and prescribe or recommend herbs or supplements.

Safety Issues
Chiropractic manipulation appears to be generally safe and rarely causes serious side effects. However, a temporary increase of symptoms may occur relatively frequently. Other side effects include temporary headache, tiredness, and discomfort radiating from the site of the adjustment.

More serious complications may occur on rare occasions. These are primarily associated with manipulation of the neck. Articles have been published that document almost two hundred cases of more serious complications associated with neck manipulation, including stroke, vertebral fracture, disc herniation, severely increased sensation of nerve pinching, and rupture of the windpipe. More than one-half of these reports involve some form of stroke, often caused by a tear in a major blood vessel at the base of the neck (the vertebral artery).

Although attempts have been made to determine in advance who will experience strokes following chiropractic, these attempts have not been successful. Thus, stroke must be considered an unpredictable, though rare, side effect of chiropractic manipulation of the neck.

To put this in perspective, however, the rate of complications from chiropractic is extremely low. According to one estimate, only one complication per million individual sessions occurs. Among people receiving a course of treatment involving manipulation of the neck, the rate of stroke is perhaps 1 per 100,000 people; the rate of death is 1 per 400,000. By comparison, serious medical complications involving common drugs in the ibuprofen family (nonsteroidal anti-inflammatory drugs, or NSAIDs) are far more common. Among people using them for arthritis, NSAIDs result in hospitalizations at a rate of about 4 in 1,000 people and death at a rate of 4 in 10,000 people. To put it another way, the rate of complications with these common over-the-counter drugs is perhaps one hundred to four hundred times greater than with chiropractic.

Certain health conditions preclude spinal manipulation. These conditions include nerve impingement causing severe nerve damage and significant disease of the spinal bones.

—*EBSCO CAM Review Board*

References
Beliveau, Peter J. H., et al. "The Chiropractic Profession: a Scoping Review of Utilization Rates, Reasons for Seeking Care, Patient Profiles, and Care Provided." *Chiropractic & Manual Therapies*, vol. 25, no. 1, 22 Nov. 2017, doi:10.1186/s12998-017-0165-8.

Blanchette, Marc-André, et al. "Effectiveness and Economic Evaluation of Chiropractic Care for the Treatment of Low Back Pain: A Systematic Review of Pragmatic Studies." *Plos One*, vol. 11, no. 8, 3 Aug. 2016, doi:10.1371/journal.pone.0160037.

"Chiropractic Care for Pain Relief." *Harvard Health*, Harvard Medical School, 6 June 2016, www.health.harvard.edu/pain/chiropractic-care-for-pain-relief.

"Chiropractic." *MedlinePlus*, U.S. National Library of Medicine, 28 Jan. 2019, medlineplus.gov/chiropractic.html.

LeFebvre, Ron, et al. "Evidence-Based Practice and Chiropractic Care." *Journal of Evidence-Based Complementary & Alternative Medicine*, vol. 18, no. 1, 28 Dec. 2012, pp. 75–79., doi:10.1177/2156587212458435.

Salehi, Alireza, et al. "Chiropractic: Is It Efficient in Treatment of Diseases? Review of Systematic Reviews." *International Journal of Community Based Nursing and Midwifery*, vol. 3, Oct. 2015, pp. 244–254.

Thiele, Rainer. *Chiropractic Treatment for Headache and Lower Back Pain Systematic Review of Randomised Controlled Trials*. Springer Fachmedien Wiesbaden GmbH, 2019.

Walker, Bruce F. "The New Chiropractic." *Chiropractic & Manual Therapies*, vol. 24, no. 1, 30 June 2016, doi:10.1186/s12998-016-0108-9.

Weber, Jim M. *Bringing It All Together: The Chiropractic Perspective for Better Structural and Functional Health*. Babypie, 2019.

■ Deep brain stimulation

CATEGORY: Therapy or Technique
ANATOMY OR SYSTEM AFFECTED: Brain, central nervous system, skull
SPECIALTIES AND RELATED FIELDS: Neurology, Neuroscience, Neurosurgery, Psychiatry, Psychology

KEY TERMS

- *dystonia*: a muscle contraction that causes repetitive movements and/or postures
- *essential tremor*: a neurological disorder that causes involuntary and rhythmic shaking. Although it can affect several different parts of the body, the trembling occurs most often in the hands
- *Parkinson's disease*: a motor system disorder that is correlated with a loss of dopamine in the brain and is characterized by tremors, muscular rigidity, and involuntary movements

Clinical Applications

Deep brain stimulation (DBS) is a surgical procedure that has received Food and Drug Administration (FDA) approval within the U.S. for alleviating symptoms associated with Parkinson's disease and essential tremor. In addition, DBS has been approved by the FDA under the Humanitarian Device Exemption for the treatment of dystonia and obsessive compulsive disorder. It is also being used as an experimental form of treatment for several other conditions and disorders such as: depression, Alzheimer's disease, Tourette's syndrome, minimally conscious state, obesity, anorexia, neuropathic pain, substance addiction, tinnitus and Huntington's disease, among others. DBS is not recommended as a first option treatment. The procedure is most commonly recommended for late stages in movement disorders after a patient has been treated with medications. Once a patient's quality of life has deteriorated due to impaired motor symptoms, and mood along with cognitive functioning are still in normal ranges, DBS becomes a viable treatment option. After DBS, these medication-refractory patients have been found to gain approximately eighty percent improvement in reduced tremor. In addition, improvements in both bradykinesia (slowness of movement) and rigidity are reported.

DBS Surgery and Risks

The primary technical goal of DBS surgery involves the accurate placement of electrodes—usually in both cerebral hemispheres—in a target with about one millimeter precision. This level of precision can occur using several different techniques. One of the more common techniques is to use a stereotactic frame that is affixed to the head while a MRI scan is obtained. Using the frame coordinates, the target location is computed using 3-dimentional x, y and z values that determine the trajectories for the electrode placement. Furthermore, to ensure that the electrodes have found their targets, clinical empirical evidence is obtained with the patient awake during the procedure. To assess neurological benefit, the surgeon will stimulate the target site using the embedded electrode and look for behavioral changes that indicate a good clinical outcome. If these tests are successful, the electrode leads are

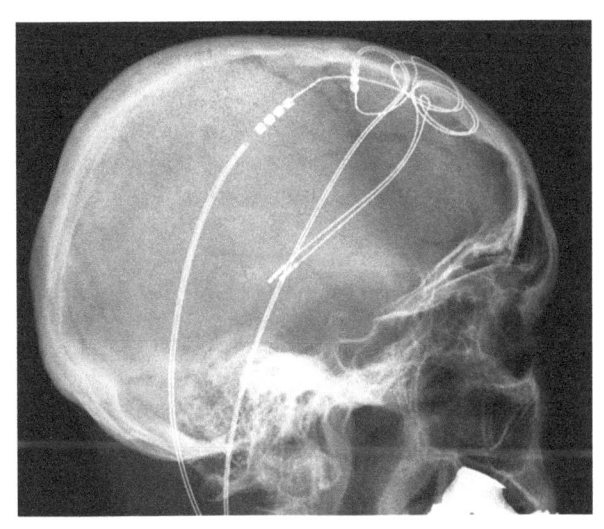

Deep brain stimulation probes shown in an X-ray of the skull. (Hellerhoff via Wikimedia Commons)

locked in place. If the tests are not optimal, the electrode can be repositioned until it attains a good result. Keeping the patient awake during the procedure is possible since the brain does not contain any pain receptors. Some patient discomfort may occur due to penetration of the dura mater covering that contains pain receptors.

The electrodes are connected to hardware that controls the frequency of the electrical pulses which are delivered to the target sites. In addition, a power supply using batteries is needed to generate the pulses. Most centers will implant the battery approximately one week later. A wire will attach to the electrode just under the scalp. This wire is then routed down the neck towards the upper chest area where the battery will be placed. Battery replacement is needed every three to five years depending on the settings used. DBS surgery includes some risks. Some of the risks can be life-threatening, such as hemorrhage; however, these are rare. Other risks include infection, seizure, electrode breakage, and electrode misplacement.

—*Bryan C. Auday, PhD, Youngeun (Grace) Park*

References

Anderson, William. *Deep Brain Stimulation Techniques and Practices*. Thieme Medical Publishers, 2019.

"Deep Brain Stimulation." *American Association of Neurological Surgeons*, 2019, www.aans.org/en/Patients/Neurosurgical-Conditions-and-Treatments/Deep-Brain-Stimulation.

Falowski, Steven M. "Deep Brain Stimulation for Chronic Pain." *Current Pain and Headache Reports*, vol. 19, no. 7, July 2015, doi:10.1007/s11916-015-0504-1.

Farrell, Sarah, et al. "The Current State of Deep Brain Stimulation for Chronic Pain and Its Context in Other Forms of Neuromodulation." *Brain Sciences*, vol. 8, no. 8, 20 Aug. 2018, p. 158., doi:10.3390/brainsci8080158.

Frank, Lone. *The Pleasure Shock: the Rise of Deep Brain Stimulation and Its Forgotten Inventor*. Dutton, 2018.

Frizon, Leonardo A, et al. "Deep Brain Stimulation for Pain in the Modern Era: A Systematic Review." *Neurosurgery*, 25 Feb. 2019, doi:10.1093/neuros/nyy552.

Jermakowicz, Walter J., et al. "Deep Brain Stimulation Improves the Symptoms and Sensory Signs of Persistent Central Neuropathic Pain from Spinal Cord Injury: A Case Report." *Frontiers in Human Neuroscience*, vol. 11, 6 Apr. 2017, doi:10.3389/fnhum.2017.00177.

Lozano, Andres M., et al. "Deep Brain Stimulation: Current Challenges and Future Directions." *Nature Reviews Neurology*, vol. 15, no. 3, Mar. 2019, pp. 148–160., doi:10.1038/s41582-018-0128-2.

Shirvalkar, Prasad, et al. "Closed-Loop Deep Brain Stimulation for Refractory Chronic Pain." *Frontiers in Computational Neuroscience*, vol. 12, 26 Mar. 2018, p. 18., doi:10.3389/fncom.2018.00018.

■ Disk removal

CATEGORY: Procedure

ANATOMY OR SYSTEM AFFECTED: Back, bones, nervous system, spine

SPECIALTIES AND RELATED FIELDS: General surgery, neurology, orthopedics, physical therapy

KEY TERMS

- *cervical vertebrae*: the first seven bones of the spinal column, located in the neck
- *disk prolapse*: the protrusion (herniation) of intervertebral disk material, which may press on spinal nerves
- *intervertebral disks*: flattened disks of fibrocartilage that separate the vertebrae and allow cushioned flexibility of the spinal column

When a disk's jellylike center bulges out through a weakened area of the firmer outer core, the disk is said to be herniated or prolapsed. This may compress the spinal cord or the nerve roots and yield such symptoms as interference with muscle strength or pain and numbness of the lower back and leg.

More than 90 percent of disk prolapses occur in the lumbar region of the back, but they may also occur in the cervical vertebrae. Occasionally, disk herniation is caused by improper lifting of heavy objects, sudden twisting of the spinal column, or trauma to the back or neck. More typically, however, a prolapsed disk develops gradually as the patient ages and the intervertebral disks degenerate.

To diagnose a prolapsed disk, a physician will likely want to visualize the vertebrae and spinal cord using X rays, computed tomography (CT) scans, or magnetic resonance imaging (MRI). Once diagnosed, most cases can be treated with analgesics, muscle relaxants (such as cyclobenzaprine and methocarbamol), and physical therapy. If the symptoms recur, however, it may be necessary to have the protruding portion of the disk or the whole disk surgically removed. This procedure usually requires that the patient have general anesthesia and remain hospitalized for several days.

For a lumbar procedure, the patient is anesthetized and placed on the operating room table in a modified kneeling position, with the abdomen suspended and the legs placed over the end of the table. The lower back is then prepared for a sterile procedure, and the surgeon makes an incision in the middle of the back along the spine. The surrounding tissues are retracted, and the vertebrae are exposed. At this time, the surgeon must make a careful dissection of the tissues in order to identify the affected nerves and intervertebral disk. Once the prolapsed disk is found, the physician will cut away the fragment of the disk impinging on the nerve. It is important that all free fragments be removed, as these could cause symptoms at a later time. Often, the surgeon must remove some of the vertebrae to gain access to the disk. This is known as a laminectomy.

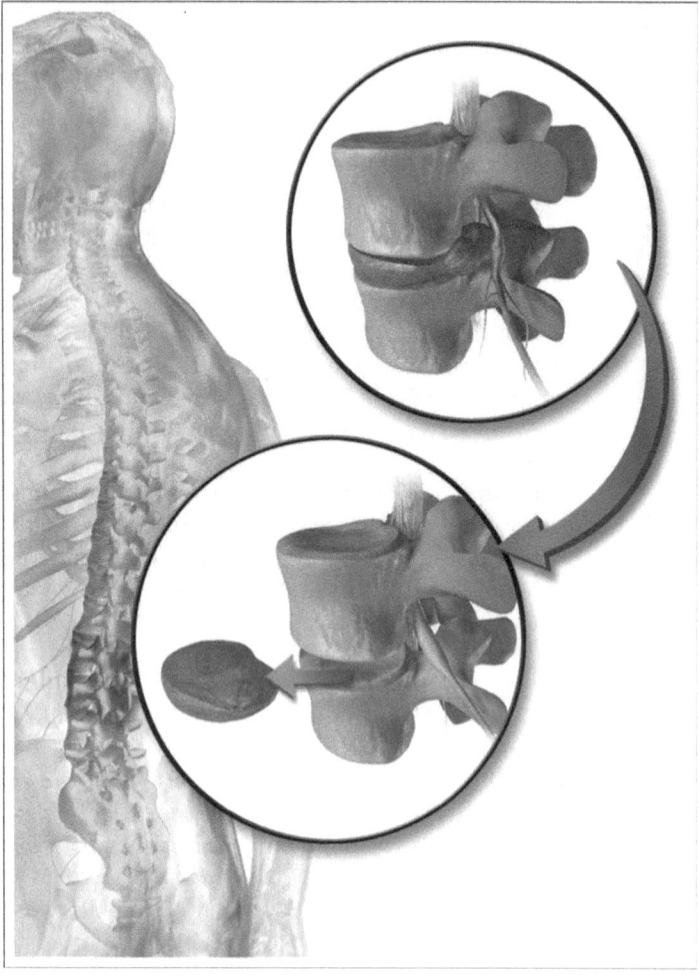

Illustration depicting a surgical discectomy. (BruceBlaus via Wikimedia Commons)

- *lumbar vertebrae*: the five bones of the spinal column in the lower back, which experience the greatest stress in the spine
- *spinal cord*: a column of nervous tissue housed in the vertebral column that carries messages to and from the brain

Indications and Procedures

A relatively common disorder that causes lower back and sometimes leg pain is the herniation or prolapse of an intervertebral disk in the lower back. These disks are made of cartilage and serve to separate the bones that make up the vertebral column. The spinal cord is located within the bony structure of the vertebrae and has nerves which enter and exit between these bones. These sensory and motor nerves must pass alongside the intervertebral disks.

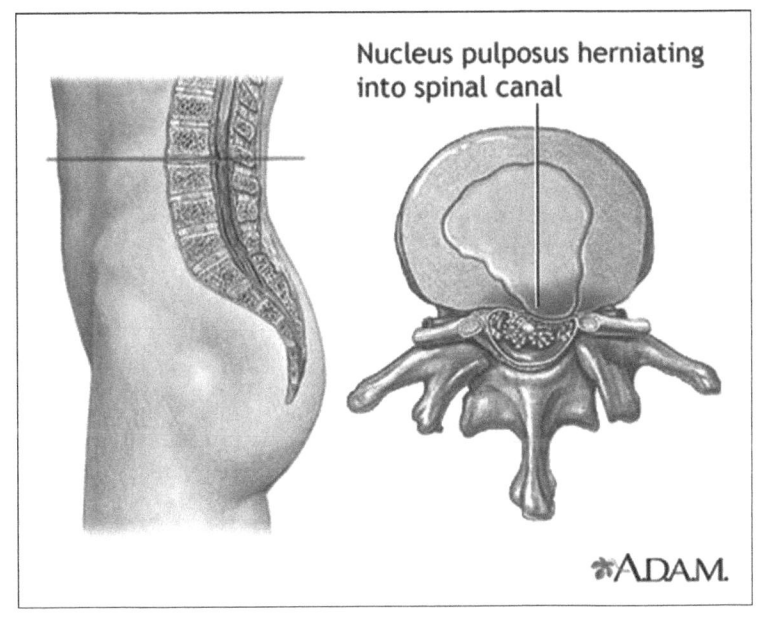

Herniated nucleus pulposus is a condition in which part or all of the soft, gelatinous central portion of an intervertebral disk is forced through a weakened part of the disk, resulting in back pain and nerve root irritation. (National Institutes of HEalth)

Uses and Complications

Because the vertebral column houses the spinal cord, any surgical manipulation of this area must be approached with extreme caution. Very large arteries (the aorta) and veins (the vena cava) lie adjacent to the spinal column, and accidental cuts can lead to rapid blood loss. The spinal cord is surrounded by a covering called the meninges, which helps to protect the cord and which contains the cerebral spinal fluid. Trauma to the meninges may cause the fluid to leak out or lead to meningitis (inflammation of the meninges). One surgical approach to reduce the adverse affects of a lesion on the meninges is to use some of the patient's fat to pack the leak and help prevent scarring. Patients with operative trauma to the meninges may complain of headache, which usually decreases in severity as the lesion heals.

Other complications that may arise include infections in approximately 3 percent of patients, thromboembolism in less than 1 percent, and death in about one patient per 1,000. Unfortunately, one of the major long-term complications reported in the study involved a worsening of symptoms after surgery.

Perspective and Prospects

Even with some potential complications, disk removal typically has a favorable outcome, although this varies somewhat depending on the patient, the treatment method, and what the patient and physician consider to be a good result. Typically, favorable outcomes range from 50 to 95 percent. The number of patients who need a second operation ranges from 4 to 25 percent.

Health care professionals are beginning to emphasize the importance of prevention of back pain. Educating patients on proper lifting techniques, such as bending the legs rather than the back and avoiding twisting, will reduce the potential for damage to the intervertebral disks. Individuals who are overweight are also at risk for developing lower back pain because of the added stress to the lumbar spine, as well as because of their relatively weak abdominal muscles. The abdominal muscles are important in stabilizing and supporting the lower back. Exercises that help strengthen these muscles are recommended for a weight-reducing exercise and diet program. Patients who must sit for long periods of time are also at risk for lower back pain. These people should take several quick breaks to stand and stretch, which reduces the constant stress on the lumbar spine.

—*Matthew Berria, Ph.D., Douglas Reinhart, M.D.*

References

Bajwa, Sukhminder Jitsingh, and Rudrashish Haldar. "Pain Management Following Spinal Surgeries: An Appraisal of the Available Options." *Journal of Craniovertebral Junction and Spine*, vol. 6, no. 3, 2015, p. 105., doi:10.4103/0974-8237.161589.

Court, C., et al. "Thoracic Disc Herniation: Surgical Treatment." *Orthopaedics & Traumatology: Surgery & Research*, vol. 104, no. 1, 2018, doi:10.1016/j.otsr.2017.04.022.

Du, Jerry, et al. "Microdiscectomy for the Treatment of Lumbar Disc Herniation: An Evaluation of Reoperations and Long-Term Outcomes."

Evidence-Based Spine-Care Journal, vol. 05, no. 02, Oct.2014,pp.77–86.,doi:10.1055/s-0034-1386750.

Gugliotta, Marinella, et al. "Surgical versus Conservative Treatment for Lumbar Disc Herniation: a Prospective Cohort Study." *BMJ Open*, vol. 6, no. 12, 2016, doi:10.1136/bmjopen-2016-012938.

Phd, Nebojsa Nick Knezevic Md, et al. "Treatment of Chronic Low Back Pain – New Approaches on the Horizon." *Journal of Pain Research*, vol. 10, 2017, pp. 1111–1123., doi:10.2147/jpr.s132769.

Shepard, Nicholas, and Woojin Cho. "Recurrent Lumbar Disc Herniation: A Review." *Global Spine Journal*, vol. 9, no. 2, 18 Dec. 2017, pp. 202–209., doi:10.1177/2192568217745063.

■ Epidural anesthesia in childbirth

CATEGORY: Procedure

DEFINITION: Epidural anesthesia is a medicine placed into the space around the spinal cord. It will block sensation in the belly and legs.

Reasons for Procedure

An epidural is used to decrease pain during labor. It blocks pain but does not put you to sleep. This allows you to interact with the care team.

After an epidural, you should no longer be able to feel:

- Intense pain with your labor contractions
- Lower back pain
- Episiotomy (if needed) or vaginal tears from labor
- Incision in your abdomen, if cesarean section (C-section) is needed

Epidural is not appropriate for everyone. You cannot have epidural anesthesia if the following occurs:

- Low platelet counts
- Blood is too thin because of blood thinners
- Bleeding (hemorrhaging) or you are in shock
- Serious infection in your back or blood
- Labor is moving too fast and there is no time to place the catheter to administer the drug

Possible Complications

Epidural can make it hard to feel contractions or the urge to push. This may lead to a longer labor. The medicine may need to be decreased. Other medicine may help to increase sensation.

An epidural can lower the mother's blood pressure. This can affect the amount of oxygen that reaches you and your baby. The baby's heart rate will be watched closely. Breathing problems can also happen if the medicine affects nerves linked to breathing.

Epidurals can cause headaches after treatment. This can be treated.

What to Expect

Prior to Procedure

Your blood pressure, heart rate, and breathing rate will be monitored. Your baby's heart rate will be checked. IV fluids will be started.

Description of the Procedure

You will be asked to lay on your side or sit. You will be asked to arch your back and remain very still. The area around your waistline on your middle

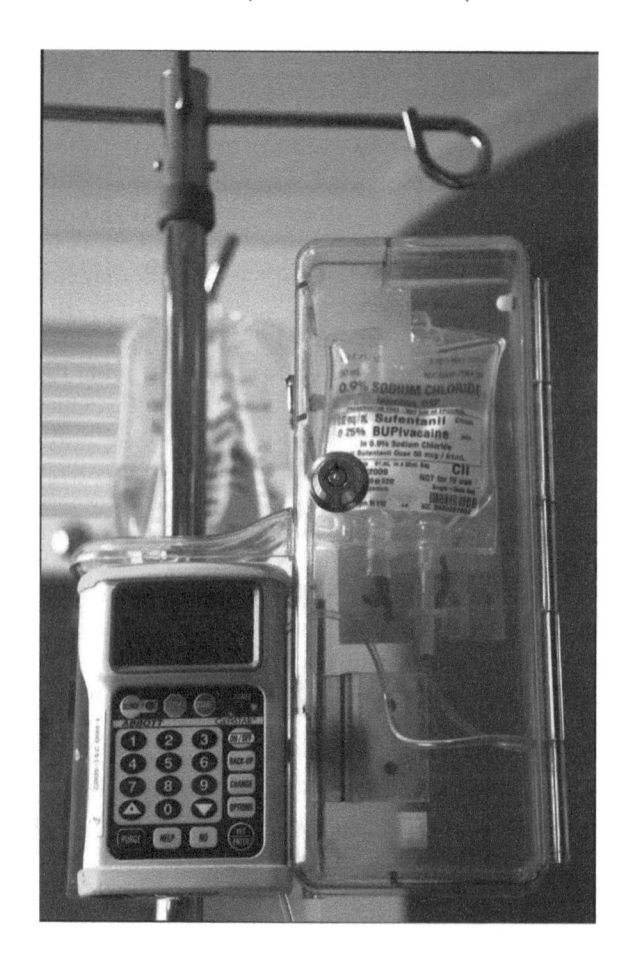

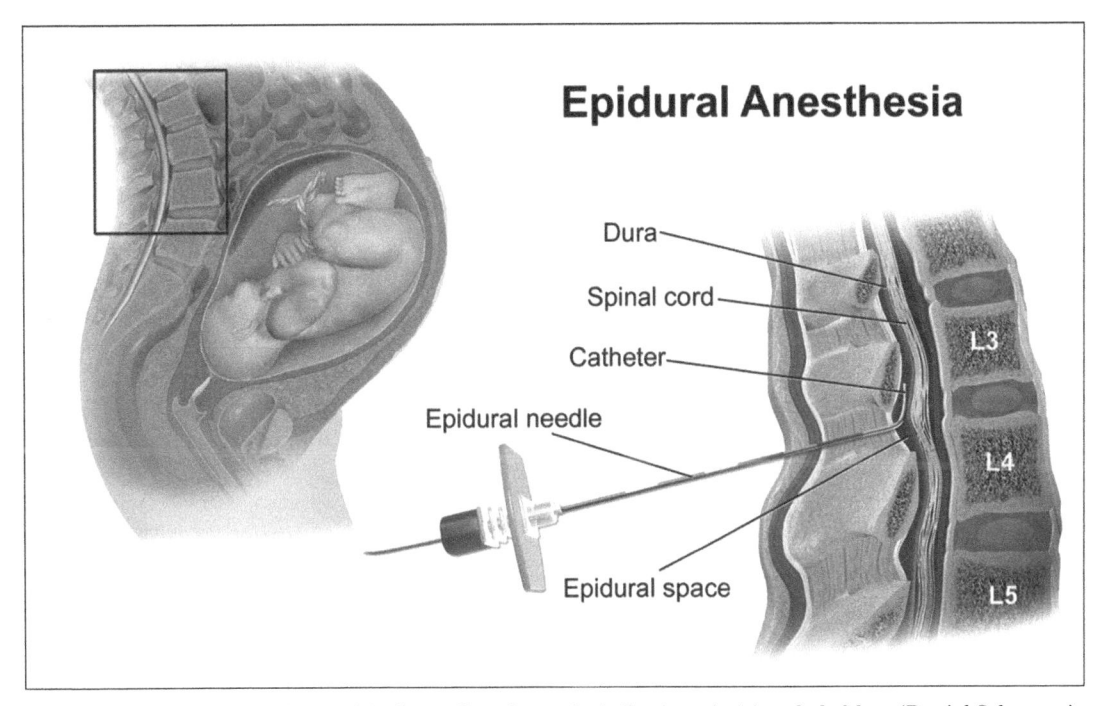

Epidural infusion pump with opioid (sufentanil) and anesthetic (bupivacaine) in a locked box. (Daniel Schwen via Wikimedia Commons)

back will be wiped. It is an antiseptic that can to reduce the chance of infection. An anesthesia medicine will be injected into the area. It will make it numb.

A needle will then be inserted into your lower back. A small tube will be threaded through the needle. It will be passed into the space around your spinal cord. The needle will be removed and the catheter taped to your back. The medicine will be given through the catheter. More medicine may be given through the tube so that the numbness lasts until the baby is born.

Immediately After Procedure

After the tube is placed you will be asked to move from side to side. You may have the following side effects:

- Shivering
- Ringing in your ears
- Backache
- Soreness where the needle is inserted
- Nausea
- Difficulty urinating

How Long Will It Take?

It will only take a few minutes to place the tube. You should feel some pain relief within a few minutes. The full effect should happen within 20 minutes.

How Much Will It Hurt?

You may feel some pressure as the needle is being inserted.

Post-procedure Care

At the Care Center

You and the baby will be closely watched for changes. Other care for delivery will continue.

A tingling feeling may be felt as the anesthesia is wearing off. You may need help to walk until the anesthesia wears off completely.

Call Your Doctor

The epidural will have worn off before you go home. Call your doctor if you have:

- Lingering or worsening back pain
- Severe headache
- Signs of infection such as redness or swelling

—Andrea Chisholm, MD

Resources

Family Doctor—American Academy of Family Physicians
https://familydoctor.org

The American Congress of Obstetricians and Gynecologists
http://www.acog.org

Canadian Resources

The Society of Obstetricians and Gynaecologists of Canada
https://sogc.org

Women's Health Matters
http://www.womenshealthmatters.ca

References

Anim-Somuah, Millicent, et al. "Epidural versus Non-Epidural or No Analgesia for Pain Management in Labour." *Cochrane Database of Systematic Reviews*, 21 May 2018, doi:10.1002/14651858.cd000331.pub4.

"Comfort Measures (Pharmacologic) During Labor." Edited by Allen Shaughnessy and Alan Ehrlich, *DynaMed*, EBSCO Information Services, 13 Aug. 2018, www.dynamed.com/topics/dmp~AN~T116857/Comfort-measures-pharmacologic-during-labor.

Herrera-Gómez, Antonio, et al. "Risk Assessments of Epidural Analgesia During Labor and Delivery." *Clinical Nursing Research*, vol. 27, no. 7, 28 July 2017, pp. 841–852., doi:10.1177/1054773817722689.

Ricciotti, Hope. "Contrary to Popular Belief, Epidurals Don't Prolong Labor. Phew." *Harvard Health Blog*, Harvard Medical School, 25 Oct. 2017, www.health.harvard.edu/blog/epidurals-dont-prolong-labor-phew-2017102512612.

Thomson, Gill, et al. "Women's Experiences of Pharmacological and Non-Pharmacological Pain Relief Methods for Labour and Childbirth: a Qualitative Systematic Review." *Reproductive Health*, vol. 16, no. 1, 30 May 2019, doi:10.1186/s12978-019-0735-4.

Van Den Bosch, A. A. S., et al. "Maternal Quality of Life in Routine Labor Epidural Analgesia versus Labor Analgesia on Request: Results of a Randomized Trial." *Quality of Life Research*, vol. 27, no. 8, 30 Mar. 2018, pp. 2027–2033., doi:10.1007/s11136-018-1838-z.

Whitley, Nancy. *A Manual of Clinical Obstetrics*. Lippincott, 1985.

■ Exercise

CATEGORY: Therapy or Technique; Physiotherapy; Prevention

ANATOMY OR SYSTEM AFFECTED: All

KEY TERMS

- *aerobic exercise*: brisk exercise that promotes the circulation of oxygen through the blood and is associated with an increased rate of breathing
- *hormone replacement therapy*: treatment with estrogens with the aim of alleviating menopausal symptoms or osteoporosis
- *resistance exercise*: exercise that causes the muscles to contract against an external resistance with the expectation of increases in strength, tone, mass, and/or endurance
- *weight training*: a system of conditioning involving lifting weights especially for strength and endurance

Overview

One of the most obvious differences between modern life and life in the past for humans can be found in the level of physical exercise. For the majority of people living in developed countries today, heavy physical exercise does not occur as a part of ordinary daily life but must be deliberately sought out. Compare this to most of human history, in which heavy daily exercise was a requirement for survival. Even among the upper classes in nineteenth-century Europe, going for a ten- to twenty-mile walk by way of recreation was not unusual.

The human body was designed to use its physical capacities. However, modern life has become a sedentary affair, in which "exercise" involves moving from couch to car to office cubicle. While decreasing strenuous exercise does have some benefits, such as reducing injuries, it also presents major drawbacks. Inadequate exercise is a major contributor to the current epidemic of obesity, which in turn leads to diabetes, heart disease, and osteoarthritis.

Conversely, increasing one's level of exercise provides a wide variety of benefits. Besides enhancing strength and endurance and improving physical attractiveness, exercise is thought to enhance overall health and to reduce symptoms in a number of specific ailments. However, while the many benefits of exercise appear self-evident, they can be quite difficult to prove in a scientific sense. The primary problem is that it is difficult, if not impossible, to design a double-blind study of exercise.

In a double-blind, placebo-controlled study, neither participants nor researchers know who is receiving a real treatment and who is receiving a placebo. Consider the following scenario: A study (technically, an observational or epidemiological study) may note that people in a given population who exercise more develop heart disease at a lower rate than those who exercise less. From this, it is tempting to conclude causality: that exercise reduces heart disease risk. However, such a conclusion might not be correct.

Observational studies show only association, not cause and effect. Studies of this type had long shown that women who used hormone replacement therapy (HRT) were less likely to develop heart disease. Furthermore, the use of HRT was known to improve one's cholesterol profile. It seemed like an obvious case. However, to researchers' surprise, when a giant double-blind study compared hormone replacement therapy with placebo, the results showed that the use of HRT actually increased heart disease risk.

It is now hypothesized that this apparent contradiction may be due to the fact that women who use HRT are generally of higher socioeconomic status than women who do not use HRT, and that it is this socioeconomic status, and not the HRT, that was responsible for the apparent benefits seen. Whatever the reason, it is now clear that HRT does not prevent heart disease, and that the conclusions drawn from observational studies were exactly backwards. Based on this, one must at least consider the possibility that people who engage in more exercise have other qualities that protect them from heart disease, and that it is these qualities, and not the exercise, that protects them. The problem here is that while it is possible to give a placebo that convincingly resembles HRT, it is difficult to conceive of a placebo form of exercise that participants and researchers would not immediately identify as different from real exercise.

Besides observational studies, other forms of scientific research involving exercise remain similarly inadequate. For example, numerous studies have attempted to prove that exercise is helpful for depression. In these studies, people who are made to exercise improve to a greater extent than those who are not interfered with. However, this finding does not prove that exercise per se aids depression. It might be, for example, that simply being enrolled in a study, and being motivated to do anything at all, might aid depression. (This suspicion is given further weight by findings that improvement in depression is not related to the intensity of the exercise done; if it were the exercise itself, one would think that more intense exercise would provide greater benefits.)

Double-blind, placebo-controlled studies eliminate all of these potential confounding factors and many others. However, it is not feasible to design a double-blind study in which people are unaware ("blind" to the fact) that they are exercising. Therefore, all results regarding the potential benefits of exercise must be taken with caution.

Scientific Evidence

The benefits of exercise with the most solid scientific foundation include the following: preventing falls in the elderly, slightly reducing blood pressure, mildly improving cholesterol profile, enhancing survival in people with heart disease, and improving metabolic syndrome. Regarding blood pressure, aerobic exercise has the best supporting evidence, but resistance exercise (weight training) has also shown promise. One study found that four ten-minute "snacks" of aerobic exercise per day were as effective at lowering blood pressure as forty minutes of continuous exercise. Aerobic exercise can also raise levels of HDL (good) cholesterol and reduce levels of triglycerides.

Other conditions for which exercise has some meaningful supporting evidence of benefit include asthma, depression, type 2 diabetes (improving blood sugar control, even in the absence of weight loss), fibromyalgia, and, osteoarthritis. Regarding osteoporosis, the general scientific consensus is that exercise does help, but the supporting evidence is surprisingly weak.

Inconsistent or otherwise weak evidence suggests potential benefit for back pain, chronic fatigue syndrome, cognitive impairment (mild dementia), colon cancer prevention, insomnia in the elderly, stroke prevention, and weight loss. It is widely believed that exercise improves immune function, but there is no meaningful supporting evidence for this belief. High- intensity exercise (such as marathon running) is known to temporarily weaken the immune system, increasing the likelihood of respiratory infection.

Evidence conflicts on whether exercise is helpful for reducing menopausal symptoms. However, it is known that heavy exercise causes increased calcium loss through sweat, and the body does not compensate for this by reducing calcium loss in the urine. The result can be a net calcium loss great enough to present health concerns for menopausal women. One study found that the use of an inexpensive calcium supplement (calcium carbonate), taken at a dose of 400 milligrams twice daily, is sufficient to offset this loss.

—*EBSCO CAM Review Board*

References

Ambrose, Kirsten R., and Yvonne M. Golightly. "Physical Exercise as Non-Pharmacological Treatment of Chronic Pain: Why and When." *Best Practice & Research Clinical Rheumatology*, vol. 29, no. 1, 2015, pp. 120–130., doi:10.1016/j.berh.2015.04.022.

Brittain, Danielle R., et al. "Moving Forward with Physical Activity: Self-Management of Chronic Pain among Women." *Women's Health Issues*, vol. 28, no. 2, 2018, pp. 113–116., doi:10.1016/j.whi.2017.12.006.

Geneen, Louise J, et al. "Physical Activity and Exercise for Chronic Pain in Adults: an Overview of Cochrane Reviews." *Cochrane Database of Systematic Reviews*, 24 Apr. 2017, doi:10.1002/14651858.cd011279.pub3.

King, Kristi Mcclary, and Olivia Estill. "Exercise as a Treatment for Chronic Pain." *ACSM s Health & Fitness Journal*, vol. 23, no. 2, 2019, pp. 36–40., doi:10.1249/fit.0000000000000461.

"The Secret to Joint Pain Relief - Exercise." *Harvard Health*, Harvard Medical School, www.health.harvard.edu/healthbeat/the-secret-to-joint-pain-relief-exercise.

Smith, Benjamin E, et al. "Musculoskeletal Pain and Exercise—Challenging Existing Paradigms and Introducing New." *British Journal of Sports Medicine*, vol. 53, no. 14, 20 June 2018, pp. 907–912., doi:10.1136/bjsports-2017-098983.

■ Exercise-based therapies

CATEGORY: Therapy or Technique; Physiotherapy; Prevention

ANATOMY OR SYSTEM AFFECTED: All

KEY TERMS

- *Alexander technique*: a process that teaches how to properly coordinate body and mind to release harmful tension and to improve posture, coordination and general health
- *Feldenkrais method*: a system of gentle movements that promote flexibility, coordination, and self-awareness
- *Pilates*: system of physical conditioning involving low-impact exercises and stretches designed to strengthen muscles of the torso and often performed with specialized equipment
- *qigong*: a Chinese system of breathing exercises, body postures and movements, and mental concentration, intended to maintain good health and control the flow of vital energy
- *Tai Chi*: a Chinese martial art and form of stylized, meditative exercise, characterized by methodically slow circular and stretching movements and positions of bodily balance
- *Trager approach*: a combination of hands-on tissue mobilization, relaxation, and movement reeducation called Mentastics
- *yoga*: comes from a Sanskrit word meaning "union;" yoga combines physical exercises, mental meditation, and breathing techniques to strengthen the muscles and relieve stress

Overview

According to a 2008 Centers for Disease Control and Prevention (CDC) health study, 7 percent of those surveyed engaged in what is considered

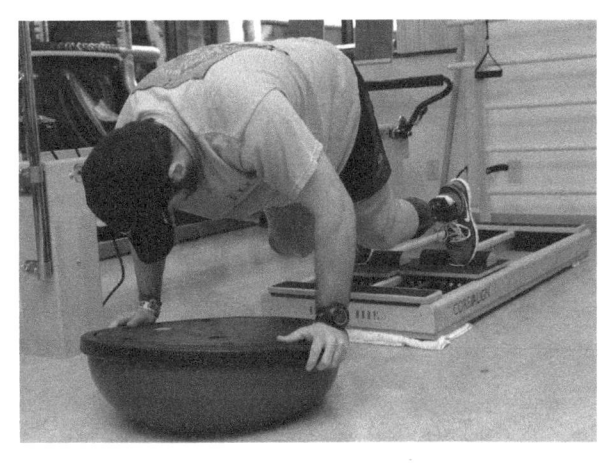

A Sailor mountain climbs using the core align pilates machine during a physical therapy appointment in the Comprehensive Combat and Complex Casualty Care facility at Naval Medical Center San Diego. (U.S. Navy photo by Mass Communication Specialist 1st Class Anastasia Puscian)

exercise-based complementary and alternative medicine (CAM) activities. These activities are considered outside the scope of conventional exercise practices. Although pain relief was the most common reason for its use, exercise-based CAM is used throughout the spectrum of medical conditions. A survey of the medical literature revealed seven exercise-based CAM activities, namely yoga, Tai Chi, qigong, pilates, the Alexander technique, the Feldenkrais method, and the Trager approach.

With an estimated sixteen million participants in the United States, yoga is the most popular exercise-based CAM activity. A five-thousand-year-old practice that originated in India, yoga seeks to integrate the mind, body, and spirit through physical poses, breathing exercises, meditation, and spiritual philosophy. Pilates is another popular exercise system in the West. This one-hundred-year-old form of exercise is designed to strengthen core muscles while focusing on posture and proper breathing. Often, props and apparatus are used.

Tai Chi, originally conceived as a martial art in China five hundred years ago, is now practiced primarily for general physical fitness. Although many forms exist, in the West, Tai Chi uses a series of slow, graceful movements to enhance strength, stamina, and balance. Tai Chi is part of a larger, five-thousand-year-old system of traditional Chinese mental, spiritual, and physical training called qigong. Other components of qigong include physical poses, meditation, and breathing exercises.

The Feldenkrais method, the Alexander technique, and the Trager approach are lesser known exercise-based CAM activities. These are movement therapies in which practitioners are guided in their posture and physical actions to improve balance, reduce pain, and increase emotional well-being.

Mechanisms of Action

Four of the seven forms of exercise-based CAM can be considered forms of general physical exercise. Yoga, Pilates, Tai Chi, and qigong involve various degrees of cardiovascular, strength, and flexibility training. Thus they promote stamina, bone health, healthy weight, muscle tone, balance, and strength. Yoga, Tai Chi, and qigong also involve meditation. Although scientific research is ongoing, it appears that meditation decreases heart rate, increases blood flow to the organs, and improves mood regulation because of changes in the nervous system. No clinical data are available to determine the exact mechanism of action of the Alexander technique, the Feldenkrais method, or the Trager approach.

Uses and Applications

Exercise-based CAM is most commonly used to improve and maintain overall fitness. Other common therapeutic uses are to reduce stress, relieve pain, and improve flexibility. Exercise-based CAM experts claim, however, that these exercise systems are helpful in treating a variety of conditions, such as asthma, osteoporosis, menstrual pain, depression, cancer, high blood pressure, diabetes, arthritis, insomnia, neuromuscular disorders, fatigue, attention deficit disorder, gastrointestinal disorders, infertility, sinusitis, and heart disease.

Scientific Evidence

Determining whether exercise-based CAM is effective in the management and prevention of illness is challenging. A limited number of well-designed clinical trials are available. The wide variety of practices within these different styles makes obtaining a consensus difficult.

In 2010, several large, well-designed studies showed that Tai Chi and qigong were beneficial in preventing osteoporosis in postmenopausal women

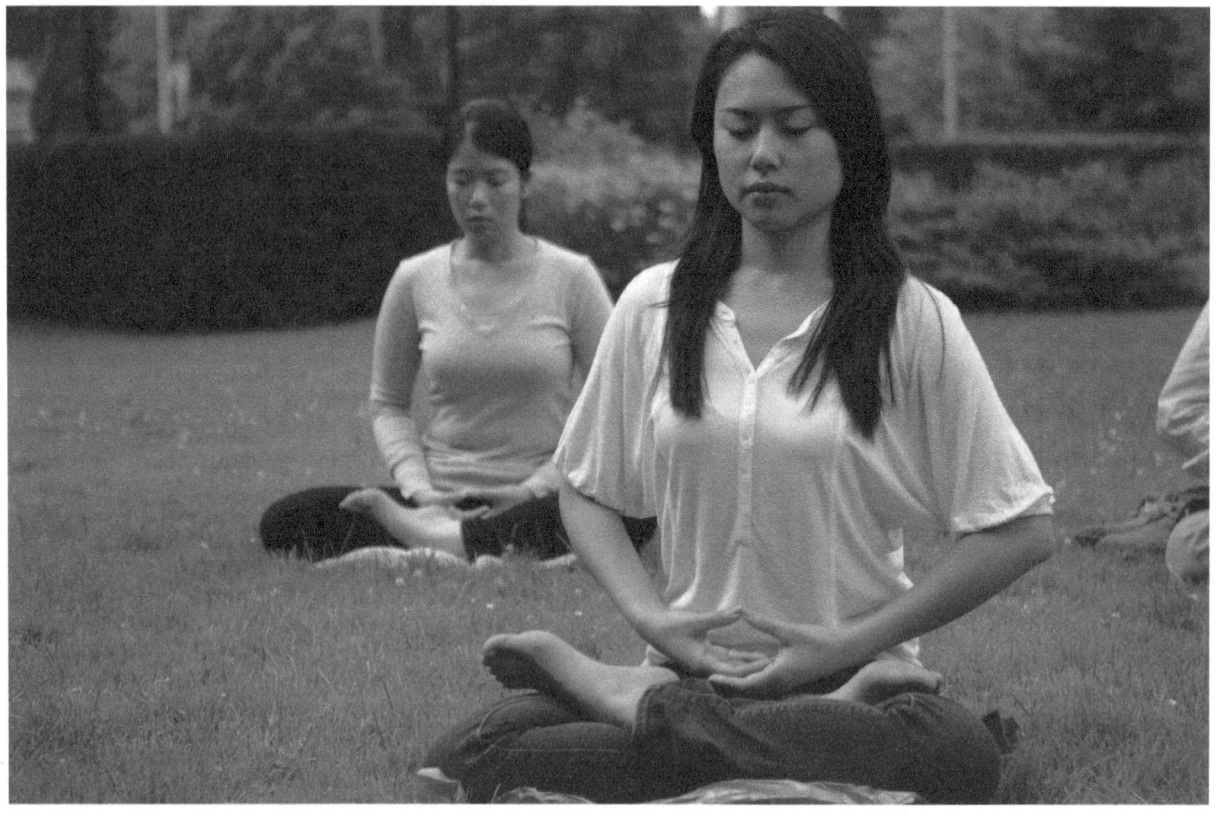

Falun Gong practitioners hold their hands in the "jeiyin" position while doing the fifth exercise (a sitting meditation) of Falun Gong in Toronto. (Joffers951 via Wikimedia Commons)

and in treating hypertension and heart disease. Additionally, these studies suggest that Tai Chi may be effective in enhancing the immune system of the elderly.

A review of the medical literature reveals promising evidence that yoga may help treat a variety of medical conditions, including mood disorders, hypertension, insomnia, back pain, and osteoporosis, and may improve overall physical conditioning. In a 2008 randomized clinical trial in the journal *Menopause*, yoga reduced hot flashes in women by 30 percent. Furthermore, numerous studies have demonstrated that yoga diminishes sex performance anxiety and enhances female sexual desire. Many health practitioners use yoga in conjunction with conventional medicine in the treatment of cancer to reduce anxiety, pain, and insomnia, although scientists continue to debate the exact mechanisms of action involved.

A gap in the literature exists regarding the use of Pilates in treating medical conditions. Experts do agree that Pilates is effective in improving strength, flexibility, and balance. Although experts in the Feldenkrais method, the Alexander technique, and the Trager approach claim that their movement exercises reduce pain, prevent injury, and improve balance, no well-designed clinical trials have been conducted to determine their efficacy.

With regard to other medical claims about exercise-based CAM, no well-designed randomized controlled trials are available; a review of the medical literature did not support the claims.

Choosing a Practitioner

Hundreds of exercise-based CAM instructor-training programs have been established in the United States. None, however, include provider licensing requirements. Standards of certification for yoga instruction are largely based on the style of yoga studied and practiced. One program, the Yoga Alliance, is a nonprofit organization in the United States that maintains standards for yoga teacher-training programs. Teacher certification with this program requires a minimum of two hundred hours of training.

Several Tai Chi and qigong organizations provide teacher certification in the United States. Various levels of certification are offered based on hours of training and desired goals. Hundreds of Pilates training programs have been established in the United States too. Although licensing is not required, the Pilates Method Alliance offers a national teacher's certification program through written examination. Instructors of the Feldenkrais method, the Alexander technique, and the Trager approach are required to complete two-to-four-year training programs that encompass four hundred to sixteen hundred hours of class and fieldwork for certification.

Safety Issues

Exercise-based CAM is generally considered safe for those without serious health conditions or injuries. Persons with spine or joint disease, uncontrolled blood pressure, or severe balance abnormalities should avoid some exercise-based CAM activities. Although uncommon, spine and joint injuries have occurred during CAM exercise activities. To avoid such injuries, participants should adhere to the directions of a certified instructor. Pregnant women, who should exercise caution when considering CAM, typically require modification of certain practices. All potential participants, especially if pregnant, looking into exercised-based CAM as a form of therapy should consult with their health care providers before joining any exercise-based program. It is advisable to choose a certified provider. Typically, a national association that confers the certification will have a list of qualified providers.

—Marie President, M.D.

References

Abbott, Ryan, and Helen Lavretsky. "Tai Chi and Qigong for the Treatment and Prevention of Mental Disorders." *Psychiatric Clinics of North America*, vol. 36, no. 1, 2013, pp. 109–119., doi:10.1016/j.psc.2013.01.011.

Brämberg, Elisabeth Björk, et al. "Effects of Yoga, Strength Training and Advice on Back Pain: a Randomized Controlled Trial." *BMC Musculoskeletal Disorders*, vol. 18, no. 1, 29 Mar. 2017, doi:10.1186/s12891-017-1497-1.

Hillier, Susan, and Anthea Worley. "The Effectiveness of the Feldenkrais Method: A Systematic Review of the Evidence." *Evidence-Based Complementary and Alternative Medicine*, 8 Apr. 2015, pp. 1–12., doi:10.1155/2015/752160.

Klein, Penelope, et al. "Meditative Movement, Energetic, and Physical Analyses of Three Qigong Exercises: Unification of Eastern and Western Mechanistic Exercise Theory." *Medicines*, vol. 4, no. 4, 23 Sept. 2017, p. 69., doi:10.3390/medicines4040069.

Nichols, Hannah. "The Research-Backed Benefits of Yoga." *Medical News Today*, MediLexicon International, 23 Sept. 2019, www.medicalnewstoday.com/articles/326414.php.

Selhub, Eva. "The Alexander Technique Can Help You (Literally) Unwind." *Harvard Health*, Harvard Medical School, 19 Nov. 2015, www.health.harvard.edu/blog/the-alexander-technique-can-help-you-literally-unwind-201511238652.

Solloway, Michele R., et al. "An Evidence Map of the Effect of Tai Chi on Health Outcomes." *Systematic Reviews*, vol. 5, no. 1, 27 July 2016, doi:10.1186/s13643-016-0300-y.

Teut, Michael, et al. "Qigong or Yoga Versus No Intervention in Older Adults With Chronic Low Back Pain—A Randomized Controlled Trial." *The Journal of Pain*, vol. 17, no. 7, 2016, pp. 796–805., doi:10.1016/j.jpain.2016.03.003.

Wells, Cherie, et al. "The Effectiveness of Pilates Exercise in People with Chronic Low Back Pain: A Systematic Review." *PLoS ONE*, vol. 9, no. 7, 1 July 2014, doi:10.1371/journal.pone.0100402.

■ Heat and cold therapy

CATEGORY: Therapy or Technique
ALSO KNOWN AS: Thermotherapy
ANATOMY OR SYSTEM AFFECTED: Musculoskeletal system

KEY TERMS
- *cryotherapy*: the therapeutic use of cold
- *thermotherapy*: treatment of disease by heat (as by hot air, hot baths, or diathermy)

Introduction

Pain control within in a society plagued by opioid dependence should be approached with utmost sensitivity and caution. Minimizing the risk of harm while providing safe and effective pain relief should be the ultimate goal of any health care provider. Utilizing heat and cold therapies is the easiest, least expensive, and the most effective non-pharmaceutical interventions available for the management of acute and chronic pain.

How Heat Therapy Works

Superficial heat application to the human body causes blood vessel to dilate, thus bringing more blood flow and oxygen delivery to the affected area and increasing tissue pliability. Heat can be applied in the form of bags filled with dried rice or bean, a heat cushion, topical heating creams (containing the ingredient capsaicin which causes the warming sensation), rubber hot water bottles or heat lamps. These items should be of warm temperature, and never hot. Heat can be reapplied after an hour if applicable. Heat therapy has a greater effect when it is used in conjunction with moderate exercises or range of motion movements . When utilized for menstrual cramps, heat therapy can inhibit the production of prostaglandins, which are short-lived hormone-like molecules produced by the uterine lining after ovulation that stimulate the contraction of smooth uterine muscle and cause menstrual cramps. Arthritis, a chronic and painful inflammation of the joints, typically reacts well to warmer temperatures. Heat increases local circulation, thus delivering more blood and nutrients to the painful area, and it also soothes and relaxes stiff muscles and joints.

How Cold Therapy Works

Cold application or cryotherapy is indicated during the acute phase of tissue injury such as immediately after surgery, exercise, or trauma to the body. The metabolic rate of tissues decreases upon the presence of cold temperatures, thereby decelerating cellular metabolism, enzymatic responses, and release histamine, all of which deter tissue damage. In addition, cold induces vasoconstriction, which decreases blood flow, membrane absorptivity, inflammation, and edema. If an open wound is present, the treated area should be protected with a plastic bag, and the ice pack should be placed over the plastic bag. Inspect the skin color after 5 minutes of cold therapy and withdraw the ice if the skin is bright pink or red. Otherwise, replace the ice for 5-15 minutes, and then reapply after an hour if still indicated.

Risks

The risks of using heat and cold therapy for pain management are low and of less severity than those applied to pharmaceutical interventions. Although the risk of injury is low, health providers and patients needed to be aware of specific injury potentials including burns and frostbite during thermotherapy interventions. Placing a cloth between a heat source and the skin for protection can minimize the risk of burns. Ice can cause frostbite if the skin is not protected or it is left on too long. Ice that is left on for an extensive amount of time can slow the healing process. The skin over which the therapy is applied must be checked at regular intervals to prevent such undesirable outcomes.

Contraindications to Using Heat and Cold Therapy

Heat or cold therapy should not be used in patients with diabetes or active infections. It should also not be used in those areas with poor circulation or poor sensation. Heat or cold therapy should also not be used around the front or side of neck, or on the left shoulder of patients with a heart condition, and it should be foregone if the patient cannot follow directions.

—*Liza Davis, RN*

References

"Pain Relief Tools for Patients & Self-Care." *American Holistic Nurses Association*, 2017, www.ahna.org/Home/Resources/Holistic-Pain-Tools.

Corti, Lisa. "Nonpharmaceutical Approaches to Pain Management." *Topics in Companion Animal Medicine*, vol. 29, no 1, 2014, pp. 24–28. doi:10.1053/j.tcam.2014.04.001

D'Arcy, Yvonne M.. Compact Clinical Guide to Women's Pain Management : An Evidence-Based Approach for Nurses. Springer Publishing Company, 2014.

Dineen, Cari W. "Heat or Ice?" *Health*, vol. 30, no. 10, 2016, pp. 65–71.

Weeks, John. "Holistic Nurse-Led Integrative Medicaid Pain Pilot 'Off the Charts' in Savings ... Plus More." Integrative Medicine: *A Clinician's Journal*, vol. 16, no. 3, 2017, pp. 18–21.

■ Hydrotherapy

CATEGORY: Therapy or Technique; Physiotherapy
ANATOMY OR SYSTEM AFFECTED: All
SPECIALTIES AND RELATED FIELDS: Alternative medicine, physical therapy, rheumatology, sports medicine

Indications and Procedures

Hydrotherapy, or water treatment, is one of the oldest therapies still in use. A procedure with origins in ancient Greece has today found a place in alternative medicine.

One use of hydrotherapy is as an alternative method of exercising for patients with chronic heart failure, since the buoyancy effect reduces loading. Exercises to improve mobility, strength, and cardiovascular fitness can be provided easily in water. Immersion in warm water has been used in bathing resorts in Europe since the beginning of the twentieth century to reduce heart failure symptoms as well as to enhance heart function.

Systemic diseases such as diabetes mellitus, peripheral heart disease, neuropathy, steroid dependence, and venous stasis are major contributing factors to forming chronic wounds. The consequence is a non-healing wound with hypoxia, infection, edema, and metabolic abnormalities. Patients with such wounds, in need of extensive debridement, have traditionally been advised to be immersed in a full-body whirlpool. The reason behind whirlpool therapy is that whirling and agitation of the water, with injected air, removes contaminants and toxic debris and dilutes bacterial contents. The common therapeutic protocol is a five- to twenty-minute session, once daily. Typically, this regimen is continued for a brief period. Other debridement techniques have been gaining in popularity in recent years due to concerns about whirlpool therapy including high water pressure, oversaturation of the skin, and cross-contamination.

Physical therapists have always recommended hydrotherapy to relieve extreme pain. Therefore, it is not surprising that it has found a place in providing relief for patients with fibromyalgia.

Another area where hydrotherapy has found popularity is in labor and childbirth. Studies indicate using hydrotherapy for relief of rapid pain and anxiety in labor. Subjective maternal responses to bathing in labor have been favorable. No maternal or infant infections have been attributed to bathing with intact or ruptured membranes. Maternal bathing in labor does not appear to affect Apgar scores at five minutes or stress hormones at birth.

A 2003 case study indicated that hydrotherapy may be beneficial in treating Rett syndrome. An eleven-year-old girl with stage III Rett syndrome was treated with hydrotherapy in a swimming pool twice a week for eight weeks. After the application of hydrotherapy, stereotypical hand movements had decreased and purposeful hand functions and feeding skills had increased. Research into the effectiveness of hydrotherapy in treating this and other neuromuscular conditions is ongoing.

Perspective and Prospects

Ancient Greek literature contains a considerably large volume of published articles concerning different types of baths and hydrotherapy. These topics were addressed for preventive, hygienic, or therapeutic purposes. These Greek baths were classified in two categories: cold water baths and hot water baths. Cold water baths were said to slow blood circulation; decrease the amount of sweat produced; increase muscular strength, the ability to work, and a sense of well-being; and improve physical, mental, and moral balance. The hot water baths were reported to be relaxing, antispasmodic, and beneficial for treating nervous disturbances.

—*Giri Sulur, Ph.D.*

References

Carere, Amy, and Robin Orr. "The Impact of Hydrotherapy on a Patient's Perceived Well-Being: a Critical Review of the Literature." *Physical Therapy Reviews*, vol. 21, no. 2, 16 Sept. 2016, pp. 91–101., doi:10.1080/10833196.2016.1228510.

Castro-Sánchez, Adelaida María, et al. "Hydrotherapy for the Treatment of Pain in People with Multiple Sclerosis: A Randomized Controlled Trial." *Evidence-Based Complementary and Alternative Medicine*, 2012, pp. 1–8., doi:10.1155/2012/473963.

Dail, Clarence W., and Charles Thomas. *Hydrotherapy: Simple Treatments for Common Ailments*. Teach Services, Inc., 2013.

Ingraham, Paul. "Hydrotherapy: Water Powered Rehab." *PainScience.com*, 1 Aug. 2016, www.painscience.com/articles/hydrotherapy.php.

Vanderlaan, Jennifer. "Retrospective Cohort Study of Hydrotherapy in Labor." *Journal of Obstetric, Gynecologic & Neonatal Nursing*, vol. 46, no. 3, 2017, pp. 403–410., doi:10.1016/j.jogn.2016.11.018.

Zamunér, Antonio Roberto, et al. "Impact of Water Therapy on Pain Management in Patients with Fibromyalgia: Current Perspectives." *Journal of Pain Research*, vol. 12, 2019, pp. 1971–2007., doi:10.2147/jpr.s161494.

Massage therapy

CATEGORY: Therapy or Technique; Physiotherapy
ANATOMY OR SYSTEM AFFECTED: All

KEY TERMS
- *deep-tissue massage:* a massage technique that's mainly used to treat musculoskeletal issues, such as strains and sports injuries; it involves applying sustained pressure using slow, deep strokes to target the inner layers of muscles and connective tissues
- *effleurage:* a series of massage strokes used in Swedish massage to warm up the muscle before deep tissue work
- *neuromuscular massage:* targets the neurological system and the muscles related to it, addressing trigger points on the body that affect mood and neurological function
- *reflexology:* a system of massage used to relieve tension and treat illness, based on the theory that there are reflex points on the feet, hands, and head linked to every part of the body
- *shiatsu:* a form of therapy of Japanese origin based on the same principles as acupuncture, in which pressure is applied to certain points on the body using the hands
- *structural integration:* a type of bodywork that focuses on the connective tissue, or fascia, of the body; fascia surrounds muscles, groups of muscles, blood vessels, organs, and nerves, binding some structures together while permitting others to slide smoothly over each other
- *Swedish massage:* the most popular type of massage in the United States, it involves the use of hands, forearms or elbows to manipulate the superficial layers of the muscles to improve mental and physical health
- *touch-based therapy:* based on the belief that vital energy flows through the human body and can be balanced or made stronger by practitioners who pass their hands over, or gently touch, a patient's body

Overview

Along with herbal treatment, touch-based therapy is one of the most ancient forms of medical care. Humans stroke and rub areas of the body that hurt; massage therapy develops this human impulse into a professional treatment. There is no doubt that massage relieves pain and induces relaxation temporarily. Whether it offers any lasting benefits, however, remains unclear.

Forms of massage. There are many schools of massage. In most cases, massage therapists combine several techniques, although there are also purists who use one method only. The most common technique is Swedish massage, which combines long strokes and gentle kneading movements that primarily affect surface muscle tissues. Deep-tissue massage utilizes greater pressure to reach deeper levels of muscles. This may be called the "hurts-good-and-feels-great-after" approach. Shiatsu or acupressure massage also uses deep pressure but does so according to the principles of acupuncture theory. Neuromuscular massage (such as the St. John method of neuromuscular therapy) applies strong pressure to tender spots, technically known as trigger points.

Several other techniques are best described as relatives of massage. Rolfing structural integration aims to affect not muscles, but the connective tissue (fascia) surrounding muscles and everything else in the body. This highly organized technique aims to permanently improve the body's structure. Reflexology is a form of foot massage based on the theory that the whole body is reflected in the foot.

Mechanism of Action

There are many theories about how massage might work, but none have been proved true. Little doubt exists that massage temporarily increases blood circulation in the massaged area, but it is not clear that this makes any lasting difference. Some massage therapists and massage therapy schools promote the notion that massage breaks up calcium deposits in the muscle, but there is no objective substantiation for this claim. A completely different explanation is that massage promotes healing in a more general way, by reducing stress and inducing relaxation. Massage also satisfies the basic human need to be touched.

Some forms of massage (such as Rolfing, acupressure, and reflexology) have elaborate theories behind them. However, there is little to no scientific evidence for these theories; moreover, there is some evidence that the theory behind reflexology is incorrect.

Uses and Applications

Massage is most commonly used to relieve muscular tension and to promote relaxation. Massage is also said to be helpful as an aid to the treatment of various conditions, including attention deficit disorder (ADD), asthma, autism, bedsores, bulimia, cystic fibrosis, diabetes, eczema, fibromyalgia, human immunodeficiency virus infection, iliotibial band pain, juvenile rheumatoid arthritis, low back pain, lymphedema, neck pain, premenstrual syndrome (PMS), pregnancy, severe burns, and spinal cord injury.

Scientific Evidence

Although there is some evidence that massage may be helpful for various medical purposes, in general the evidence is not strong. There are several reasons for this, but one is most fundamental: Even with the best of intentions, it is difficult to properly ascertain the effectiveness of a hands-on therapy like massage.

Only one form of study can truly prove that a treatment is effective: the double-blind, placebo-controlled trial. However, it is not possible to fit massage into a study design of this type. What could researchers use for placebo massage, and how could they make sure that both participants and practitioners did not know who was receiving real massage and who was receiving fake massage?

Because of these problems, all studies of massage fall short of optimum design. Many have compared massage to no treatment. However, studies of this type cannot provide reliable evidence about the efficacy of a treatment. If a benefit is seen, there is no way to determine whether it was caused by massage specifically, or just by attention generally. (Attention alone will almost always produce some reported benefit.)

More meaningful trials used some sort of fake treatment for the control group, such as phony laser acupuncture. However, using a placebo treatment that is very different in form from the treatment under study is less than ideal. One study compared real reflexology with fake reflexology. However, it is quite likely that the reflexologists unconsciously conveyed more enthusiasm and optimism when performing the real therapy than when performing the fake therapy; this, too, could affect the outcome. It has been suggested that the only way to avoid this last problem would be to compare the effectiveness of trained practitioners with actors trained only enough to provide a simulation of treatment; however, such studies have not been reported.

Still other studies have simply involved giving people massages and seeing whether they improved. These trials are particularly meaningless; it has been long since proven that both participants and examining physicians will, at minimum, think that they observe improvement in people given a treatment, whether or not the treatment does anything on its own.

Finally, other trials have compared massage to competing therapies, such as acupuncture or relaxation therapy. When one compares unproven therapies to each other, the results cannot possibly prove that any of the tested treatments are effective. Given these caveats, the following is a summary of what science knows about the effects of massage.

Low back pain. Although the evidence is far from complete, it does appear that massage may offer benefits for low back pain. However, these benefits may last for only a short time. One study compared massage with fake laser therapy in 107 people with low back pain. The results indicate that massage is more effective than fake laser therapy for relieving low back pain, and that massage therapy with exercise and posture training is even more effective.

Another study compared acupuncture, massage, and self-care education in 262 people with persistent back pain. By the end of the ten-week treatment period, massage had shown itself more effective than self-care (or acupuncture). However, at a one-year follow-up, no difference was seen in symptoms between the massage group and the self-care group. In another study, acupressure-style massage was more effective than Swedish massage for the treatment of low back pain.

In a review of thirteen randomized trials, researchers concluded that massage may be effective for nonspecific low back pain, and that the beneficial effects can last for up to one year in persons with chronic pain. Researchers also noted that exercise and education appear to enhance the effectiveness of massage.

Cancer. Massage therapy has been studied for its benefits in managing the symptoms associated with cancer and its treatment. In a randomized study investigating the effects of massage on 348 persons with advanced cancer who had moderate

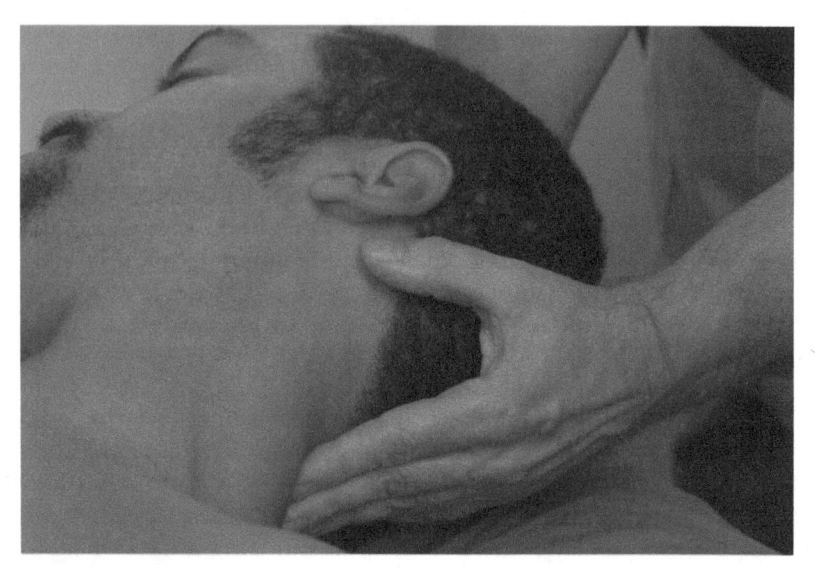

Massage therapist manipulating the head and neck during a massage session. (National Institutes of Health)

to severe pain, the researchers found that, compared with simple touch, massage was significantly more effective at reducing pain and improving mood immediately following treatment; the effect, however, was not sustained. The authors of a review of ten massage therapy studies could not draw firm conclusions about its benefits for a wide range of symptoms in persons undergoing treatment for cancer.

Massage without aromatherapy has shown promise for reducing nausea caused by chemotherapy. However, a small randomized trial found that effleurage massage, a common massage technique, had no significant effect on anxiety, depression, or quality of life among twenty-two women undergoing radiation therapy for breast cancer.

Other conditions. Preliminary controlled trials of varying quality suggest that massage may provide benefit in a number of conditions, including the following: ADD, anorexia nervosa, asthma in children, autism, bulimia, cystic fibrosis, anxiety, diabetes, eczema, fibromyalgia, iliotibial band pain (a form of tendonitis that can cause knee or hip pain), juvenile rheumatoid arthritis, migraine headaches, pregnancy and childbirth, quitting smoking, burn recovery, and spinal cord injury. One study found that massaging premature infants three times daily for ten days at acupressure locations resulted in greater weight compared with similar infants receiving routine care.

One study commonly cited as evidence that ordinary massage therapy is helpful for PMS was flawed by the absence of a control group. However, a better-designed trial compared reflexology with fake reflexology in thirty-eight women with PMS symptoms and found evidence that real reflexology was more effective.

Several studies indicate that massage with aromatherapy may be helpful for relieving anxiety. One study evaluated this combination therapy for treating anxiety or depression (or both) in people undergoing treatment for cancer. The treatment did appear to provide some short-term benefits. A 2008 review could find no convincing evidence for the effectiveness of massage therapy against depression in general.

Study results are mixed on whether massage can improve measures of immune function in people with human immunodeficiency virus infection. For chronic neck pain, one study found that massage is less effective than acupuncture. In fact, in this trial, massage was no more effective than fake acupuncture. Finally, a review of the literature published in 1997 suggests that massage is not helpful for preventing pressure sores (bedsores).

Choosing a Practitioner

As with all medical therapies, it is best to choose a licensed practitioner. Where licensure is not available, persons should seek a referral from a qualified and knowledgeable medical practitioner. However, most states in the United States license massage therapists.

Note that massage, like other hands-on therapies, involves personal talents that go beyond specific training, certification, or licensure: Some people are simply gifted with their hands. Furthermore, what works for one person may not work for another. For these reasons, some trial and error is often necessary to find the best massage therapist.

Safety Issues

Massage is generally safe. However, it can sometimes exacerbate pain temporarily, even when properly performed. In addition, massage that is performed too forcefully on fragile people could cause bone fractures and other internal injuries. However, licensed massage therapists have been trained in ways to avoid causing these problems. Finally, machines designed to perform elements of massage may be less safe than standard massage.

—*EBSCO CAM Review Board*

References

Allen, Laura. "Case Study: The Use of Massage Therapy to Relieve Chronic Low-Back Pain." International Journal of Therapeutic Massage & Bodywork: Research, Education, & Practice, vol. 9, no. 3, Sept. 2016, doi:10.3822/ijtmb.v9i3.267.

Bervoets, Diederik C, et al. "Massage Therapy Has Short-Term Benefits for People with Common Musculoskeletal Disorders Compared to No Treatment: a Systematic Review." Journal of Physiotherapy, vol. 61, no. 3, 2015, pp. 106–116., doi:10.1016/j.jphys.2015.05.018.

Hou, Wen-Hsuan, et al. "Treatment Effects of Massage Therapy in Depressed People." The Journal of Clinical Psychiatry, vol. 71, no. 07, 2010, pp. 894–901., doi:10.4088/jcp.09r05009blu.

Ingraham, Paul. "Massage Therapy: Does It Work?" PainScience.com, 18 July 2018, www.painscience.com/articles/does-massage-work.php.

Nelson, Nicole L., and James R. Churilla. "Massage Therapy for Pain and Function in Patients With Arthritis." American Journal of Physical Medicine & Rehabilitation, vol. 96, no. 9, 2017, pp. 665–672., doi:10.1097/phm.0000000000000712.

Sherman, Karen J., et al. "Effectiveness of Therapeutic Massage for Generalized Anxiety Disorder: a Randomized Controlled Trial." Depression and Anxiety, vol. 27, no. 5, 2010, pp. 441–450., doi:10.1002/da.20671.

"Therapeutic Massage for Pain Relief." Harvard Health, Harvard Medical School, July 2016, www.health.harvard.edu/alternative-and-complementary-medicine/therapeutic-massage-for-pain-relief.

Woolston, Chris. "Massage for Pain Relief." Consumer HealthDay, 1 Jan. 2019, consumer.healthday.com/encyclopedia/holistic-medicine-25/mis-alternative-medicine-news-19/massage-for-pain-relief-645793.html.

■ Neurosurgery

CATEGORY: Procedure
ANATOMY OR SYSTEM AFFECTED: Bones, brain, glands, head, nerves, nervous system, psychic-emotional system, spine
SPECIALTIES AND RELATED FIELDS: General surgery, neurology, psychiatry

KEY TERMS

- *aneurysm*: the swelling of a blood vessel, which occurs with the stretching of a weak place in the vessel wall
- *cannula*: a tube or hypodermic needle implanted in the body to introduce or extract substances
- *commissurotomy*: the severing of the corpus callosum, the fiber tract joining the two cerebral hemispheres
- *hematoma*: a localized collection of clotted blood in an organ or tissue as a result of internal bleeding
- *lesion*: a wound or tumor of the brain or spinal cord
- *lobectomy*: the removal of a lobe of the brain, or a major part of a lobe
- *lobotomy*: the separation of either an entire lobe or a major part of a lobe from the rest of the brain
- *trephination*: the opening of a hole in the skull with an instrument called a trephine

Indications and Procedures

Neurosurgery refers to any surgery performed on a part of the nervous system. Brain surgery may be used to remove a tumor or foreign body, relieve the pressure caused by an intracranial hemorrhage, excise an abscess, treat parkinsonism, or relieve pain. In cases of severe mental depression or untreatable epilepsy, psychosurgery (such as lobotomy) may alleviate the worst symptoms, although these procedures are now rare. Surgery may be performed on the spine to correct a defect, remove a tumor, repair a ruptured intervertebral disk, or relieve pain. Surgery may be performed on nerves to remove a tumor, relieve pain, or reconnect a severed nerve.

Most brain operations share some common procedures. Bleeding from the numerous tiny blood vessels in the brain is controlled by use of an electric needle, a finely pointed instrument that shoots a minute electric current into the vessel and seals it. (This same instrument can be used as an electric knife for bloodless cutting.) Brain tissue is kept moist by continued washing with a dilute salt solution. The brain tissue itself is handled with damp cotton pads attached to the end of forceps.

If the brain is swollen, it may be treated by intravenous injections of urea. The resulting increase in the salt concentration of the blood draws the water away from the brain. In addition to drawing off excess water, the brain's size is temporarily reduced, giving the surgeon extra room to maneuver. To help reduce bleeding within the brain, the patient's blood pressure can be lowered by half temporarily through an injection of a drug into the blood. The patient's temperature is also reduced, which lowers the brain's need for oxygen and ensures that the reduced blood flow will not be deleterious.

An operation in which a hole is cut into the skull is called a craniotomy. If only a small hole is required, the procedure is called trepanation (or trephination) and uses an instrument called a trephine, resembling a corkscrew with a short, nail-like tip and a threaded cutting disk. The size of the opening that is made ranges from 1.5 centimeters (0.6 inches) to 3.8 centimeters (1.5 inches) in diameter and, if necessary, may be enlarged with an instrument called a rongeur. This type of surgery is performed to insert needles or cannulas and to remove subdural hematomas. If too much of the bony skull has to be removed (or is fractured by accidental means), a substitute for the bone is inserted. The substitute is usually made of plastic, such as acrylic.

Brain surgery for advanced Parkinson's disease will not cure the disease but may help alleviate some of its symptoms. The major symptoms are tremor, stiffness, weakness, and slowed movements. For patients who do not respond well to medication, a form of neurosurgery called deep brain stimulation (DBS) can be used to reduce or stop the shaking, by implanting a small device called a brain pacemaker that emits electrical impulses to block abnormal activity in affected regions of the brain.

When pain becomes unbearable, such as the pain associated with cancer, the nerves carrying these pain messages can be interrupted anywhere between the brain and the cancerous region. The nerve to the affected organ can be severed, the nerve roots of the spinal cord can be cut, or the cut can be made within the spinal cord.

Hypophysectomy is the surgical removal of the pituitary gland. It is usually performed to slow the growth and spread of endocrine-dependent malignant tumors of the breast, ovary, or prostate gland. It may also be used to stop the deterioration of the retina that may come with diabetes mellitus or to remove a pituitary tumor. Hypophysectomy is considered only as a last resort when cryosurgery or radioactive implants fail to destroy the pituitary tissue. There are two ways to reach a diseased pituitary gland by surgery. One way is to go through the nose. The skull is entered through the sphenoid sinus, and the floor of the bony saddle of the middle of the skull is cut to reach the gland. The second means is by craniotomy. The skull is opened through an incision in the hairline above the forehead. A flap of bone, hinged at eyebrow level, is brought forward so that the surgeon can see the entire affected area clearly. The gland is completely excised.

Psychosurgery is now considered only as a last resort, when nothing else can possibly work. It is rarely undertaken because of the availability of so many drugs to control mental illnesses. In the cases when a lobotomy is performed, it can be done under local anesthesia through tiny holes drilled in the roof of the eyes' orbits. An instrument is then inserted to separate the lobes of the brain.

A laminectomy is performed to relieve compression of the spinal cord caused by injury (the displacement of a bone) or by the degeneration of a disk; it may also be used to find and remove a displaced intervertebral disk. A laminectomy is performed under general anesthesia. The surgeon makes an incision in the back, vertically over the tips of the vertebral bones. The large, thick muscles that lie on either side are peeled back from the surface of the bones. The lamina itself is the part of a vertebral bone that forms the back wall of the spinal canal. When the laminae are cut away, the spinal canal is opened so that the spinal cord covering can be cut. Once the cord is exposed, a particular condition can be treated. It may then be necessary to fuse the vertebrae. The removal of the laminae causes little interference with support or motion of the spine, although recovery from the surgery requires that the patient remain prone for several days to keep the spine in alignment.

Fusion of the vertebrae is the surgical joining of two or more spinal vertebrae to stabilize a segment of the spinal column following severe trauma, a herniated (ruptured) disk, or a degenerative disease. The surgery is performed under general anesthesia. The cartilage pads are removed from between the posterior portions of the affected vertebrae. Bone chips are cut from the vertebral ridges and inserted as a replacement for the removed cartilage. Postoperative motion must be limited until the articulating bones heal.

Severe pain that cannot be controlled by analgesics (painkillers) may be treated by surgery. One procedure, a cordotomy, removes a section of the spinal cord so that most of the nerve fibers that transmit pain messages to the brain are destroyed. At first, the patient does experience less pain, but after a few months, the pain can recur and become worse than before. The recurrence of pain is likely attributable to the reconstruction of some axons that carry ascending messages. Other painful conditions can be treated with surgery. Trigeminal neuralgia (or tic douloureux) is one such condition. These severe attacks of stabbing pain in the face may last a minute or more. The trigeminal nerve can be injected with a concentrated alcohol solution, which will prevent it from working for a year or two. This condition is usually treated surgically by drilling a burr hole in the temple and cutting across the lower two-thirds of the nerve trunk at the site.

Asympathectomy surgically interrupts a part of the sympathetic nerve pathways. It is used to relieve the pain of vascular disease. The surgery involves removing the sheath from around an artery. This sheath carries the sympathetic nerve fibers that control vasoconstriction. Once the sheath is removed, the vessel relaxes and expands so that more blood travels through it.

Uses and Complications
While neurosurgery offers the hope of recovery to people suffering with tumors, aneurysms, and brain injuries, it may result in complications that can bring disability, coma, or even death. Therefore, three issues must be taken into account before neurosurgery is performed. First, these surgeries involve higher risk than most other procedures. Second, diseases that necessitate neurosurgical treatment may render patients wholly or partially incompetent to understand the implications of their surgery. Third, sometimes matching the appropriate surgery to the patient's condition is an uncertain process. Even standard neurosurgical procedures have not been proven in every event.

Because the diagnosis of a brain tumor is often seen as fatal, many believe that surgery has little value as therapy, especially for malignant tumors. Others suggest, however, that the more radical the surgery, the greater the chance of survival for the patient. The problem arises when a tumor is found within the center area of the brain, where the primary sensory and motor cortices are situated. Surgical methods of the past tended to exacerbate the problems of the patient. The use of lasers and microscopy, however, may increase the chance of successful treatment. Using these tools, incisions of no longer than 2 centimeters can be made. Using the microscope, the surgeon can guide the laser to the tumor, which is gently melted and vaporized-all without disturbing the brain. This method is especially useful for reaching deep-seated tumors.

Stereotactic surgery is a means by which monitoring devices are inserted into the brain cortex. These devices can detect lesions, stimulate or record areas within the cortex, or in some other way study the brain. The two things necessary to perform this surgery are a stereotactic atlas (or map) of the brain and the instrumentation for the procedure. The atlas is a series of individual maps, each representing a slice of the brain. The stereotactic instrument consists of two parts: a head holder, which maintains the patient's head in a particular position and orientation, and an electrode holder, which holds the device that is to be inserted.

The purpose of the lesion method of stereotactic surgery is to remove, damage, or destroy a part of the brain in such a way that the behavior of the patient can be monitored to determine the functions of the affected area. Surgery to produce lesions is an extremely precise, and therefore dangerous, surgery. Structures within the brain are tiny, convoluted, and tightly packed, and any surgery performed on an area may therefore damage adjacent areas. There are four different methods of producing lesions.

Aspiration lesions are performed when the target site is in a more accessible area of the brain, where the surgeon can see it clearly and can use the proper instruments. The cortical tissue is aspirated by a handheld pipette, and then the tougher white matter layers are peeled away. Deeper lesions are created with high-frequency (radiofrequency) currents passed through carefully placed electrodes. The heat of the current destroys the tissue. The amount of tissue to be removed is regulated

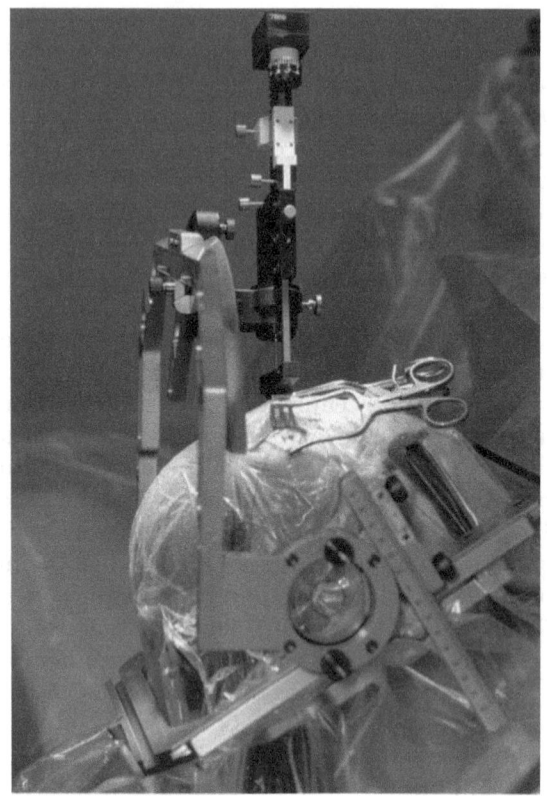

Insertion of an electrode during deep brain stimulation for Parkinson's disease. (via Wikimedia Commons)

through control of the current's duration and intensity. In the third method, a nerve or tract to be removed can be cut with a scalpel. A tiny incision severing the nerve does not have to do damage to surrounding tissues, so the lesion is small.

The fourth method is cryogenic blockade. In this method, a coolant is pumped through the tip of an implanted cryoprobe to cool the area. When the tissue is cooled, the neurons do not fire. The temperature must remain above freezing, however, to prevent destruction of the tissue. Although the result is not a true lesion, since function returns, this cooled area acts as a lesion because the behavior that it governs is interrupted. Consequently, cryogenic blockade is said to produce a reversible lesion.

A commissurotomy, or severing the connection between the two cerebral hemispheres, may be performed in cases of severe epilepsy if no other treatment is successful. After the two halves are separated (the brain stem is left intact), each hemisphere maintains all the centers that mediate its functions, except that each cortex sees only half the world. For example, visual messages are crossed so that the opposite hemisphere is stimulated by only one eye's input. If both eyes and both hemispheres are working, however, vision should be unaffected. In fact, no real deficits should occur in these patients' behavior. They retain the same verbal intelligence, reasoning, perception, motor coordination, and personality, because of the brain's extraordinary ability to preserve unity, or oneness.

Commissurotomies were first performed in the hope of reducing the severity of convulsions and seizures associated with epilepsy. The rationale was that the severity of the convulsions would be reduced if discharges could be limited to the hemisphere from which they originated. The benefits far surpassed expectations; many patients never experience another convulsion.

Perspective and Prospects

Archaeological evidence shows that people living in the Stone Age performed trepanation. This operation was likely performed to release evil spirits or demons: There is little evidence of fractures of the skulls that have been found, and the pieces of skulls that were excised were preserved and worn as talismans. Today, surgeons in some tribal cultures perform the same surgery; in some cases, some are done for ritual purposes, while others are performed for head injuries as well as headache, dizziness, and epilepsy. Trepanation laid the groundwork for brain surgery as it is still practiced.

Perhaps the most intriguing possibility for future research is transplanting brains or brain tissue. Brain transplants have come a long way from their portrayal in science fiction. In 1971, the first real evidence that transplanted tissue could survive was found. These successful attempts were made in rats. Further studies have shown that transplants have a higher survival rate in tissue richly vascularized with sufficient room to grow. It is hoped that neurotransplant surgery can be used to treat brain damage. One approach would be to develop procedures of implantation that would stimulate the regeneration of the patient's own tissue. A second approach would be to replace damaged tissue with healthy tissue of the same type.

The major question that will have to be answered before successful regeneration is accomplished is why neurons of the peripheral nervous system (PNS) regenerate but the neurons of the central nervous system (CNS) do not. One hypothesis would be that they are too structurally different. This theory is disputed by studies that show CNS neuron regeneration in the peripheral nervous system, while PNS neurons do not regenerate in the central nervous system. Other evidence to refute the hypothesis is that peripheral sensory neurons regenerate until they reach the spinal cord, then regeneration ceases. Therefore, perhaps there is an environmental factor within the central nervous system that prohibits regeneration, such as scar tissue that forms only in the area of CNS damage. Experiments to prove or disprove this theory are inconclusive. The other possibility is that the insulating cells wrapped around CNS neurons are different enough from the Schwann cells of PNS neurons that regeneration is discouraged.

Attempts to replace damaged tissue with healthy tissue have been most useful in treating Parkinson's disease (with its rigidity, tremors, and lack of spontaneous movement). One type of tissue used for replacement is fetal neural tissue. It not only survives but also innervates adjacent tissue, releases neurotransmitters (in this case dopamine), and alleviates the symptoms of parkinsonism. A possible substitute for neural tissue is autotransplantation with some of the patient's own adrenal medulla. This tissue could be used because it too releases dopamine. Investigations thus far have been controversial, but the operation is being performed worldwide.

—*Iona C. Baldridge*

References

Burchiel, Kim J., and Ahmed M. Raslan. "Contemporary Concepts of Pain Surgery." *Journal of Neurosurgery*, vol. 130, no. 4, 2019, pp. 1039–1049., doi:10.3171/2019.1.jns181620.

Follett, Kenneth A. *Neurosurgical Pain Management*. W.B. Saunders, 2004.

Giller, Cole A. "The Neurosurgical Treatment of Pain." *Archives of Neurology*, vol. 60, no. 11, Nov. 2003, pp. 1537–1540., doi:10.1001/archneur.60.11.1537.

Parks, Troy. "Neurosurgery Makes Pain Management Curricular Breakthroughs." *American Medical Association*, 2 Aug. 2016, www.ama-assn.org/delivering-care/opioids/neurosurgery-makes-pain-management-curricular-breakthroughs.

——. "Using Neurosurgical Solutions to Manage Chronic Back Pain." *American Medical Association*, 23 Aug. 2016, www.ama-assn.org/delivering-care/opioids/using-neurosurgical-solutions-manage-chronic-back-pain.

Shamji, Mohammed F., et al. "The Advancing Role of Neuromodulation for the Management of Chronic Treatment-Refractory Pain." *Neurosurgery*, vol. 80, no. 3S, 21 Feb. 2017, doi:10.1093/neuros/nyw047.

Vadivelu, Nalini, et al. "Options for Perioperative Pain Management in Neurosurgery." *Journal of Pain Research*, vol. 9, 2016, p. 37., doi:10.2147/jpr.s85782.

■ Pain management during gestation

CATEGORY: Therapy or Technique
ANATOMY OR SYSTEM AFFECTED: Low back; Pelvis; Reproductive system

About 22-72 percent of all pregnant women will experience pregnancy related pain not related to labor. Some women develop acute non-obstetrical complaints during pregnancy while others have exacerbations of chronic conditions during pregnancy. Many women choose to withhold treatment for the fear they will harm the fetus. However, leaving pain untreated or not treating it properly could be as harmful for the fetus as treating the pain. Chronic and severe pain that is left untreated is associated with hypertension and depression which can increase complications with the pregnancy.

Common non-obstetrical complaints during pregnancy include low back pain and pelvic pain in nearly 70 percent of all pregnancies. Low back pain during pregnancy increases in prevalence in Caucasian and African American women and in women who had back pain prior to pregnancy. Treatment of pain during pregnancy should include a combination of pharmacologic and non-pharmacologic treatments to promote the best outcomes.

Non-Pharmacologic Treatments

When a pregnant women presents with pain, especially low back pain, conservative non-pharmacologic therapy should be offered. It is important to initially provide postural training. These women should be taught correct posture when sitting and standing. They should also be taught how to walk and bend to prevent further injury. If instruction is not enough, there are postural support devices to enforce the training they have received. Another modality to prevent or improve back pain is to schedule rest throughout the day. If a woman's back pain persists despite the training, she should participate in physical therapy focused on posture, stretches, and back strengthening. Physical therapy in combination with education has been shown to improve back pain during pregnancy but also decrease disability and provide higher quality of life. Physical therapy is the most widely accepted non-pharmacologic treatment because it is safe during all stages of the pregnancy. Some alternative non-pharmacologic treatments that have been identified as potentially beneficial in pain during pregnancy include acupuncture, yoga, water therapy, and support belts.

Pharmacologic Treatments

Tylenol is currently the medication of choice when treating pain during pregnancy. If a pregnant woman is in severe pain and/or conservative treatments do not work, Tylenol is an acceptable medication during all stages of pregnancy. Tylenol is a non-salicylate medication with analgesic potential and little risk of increasing congenital defects.

NSAIDs, or non-steroidal anti-inflammatory drugs, may be efficacious in providing relief in pain during pregnancy but are generally avoided throughout pregnancy. This medication class commonly includes ibuprofen, naproxen, and ketorolac. NSAIDs inhibit prostaglandin production which is required to keep the ductus arteriosus patent. NSAID use in late pregnancy can lead to premature closure of the ductus which could be very harmful to the fetus.

Opioids may be utilized during pregnancy if pain cannot be adequately controlled with non-pharmacologic treatment, Tylenol, or a short course of NSAIDs. The use of opioids during pregnancy has been increasing worldwide. One study revealed 6 percent of all pregnant women in Norway filled at least one opioid prescription during their pregnancy and the number in the United States is expected to be even higher. While there is limited evidence about opioids causing harm to fetal development, there are potential adverse effects immediately after the child is born. If a fetus was repeatedly exposed to opioids in utero, they may require observation in the neonatal intensive care unit to monitor withdrawals immediately after birth. In general, the use of opioids during pregnancy is cautioned and the risk to the fetus must always be discussed with the patient.

—*Christine Gamble, MD*

References

Babb, Malaika, et al. "Treating Pain during Pregnancy." *Canadian Family Physician*, vol. 56, no. 1, Jan. 2010, pp. 25–27.

Desai, Rishi, et al. "Prescription Opioids in Pregnancy and Birth Outcomes: A Review of the Literature." *Journal of Pediatric Genetics*, vol. 4, no. 2, 2015, pp. 56–70., doi:10.1055/s-0035-1556740.

Interrante, Julia D., et al. "Risk Comparison for Prenatal Use of Analgesics and Selected Birth Defects, National Birth Defects Prevention Study 1997–2011." *Annals of Epidemiology*, vol. 27, no. 10, 2017, pp. 645–653., doi:10.1016/j.annepidem.2017.09.003.

Ray-Griffith, Shona, et al. "Chronic Pain during Pregnancy: a Review of the Literature." *International Journal of Women's Health*, vol. 10, 2018, pp. 153–164., doi:10.2147/ijwh.s151845.

Shah, Shalini, et al. "Pain Management in Pregnancy: Multimodal Approaches." *Pain Research and Treatment*, 2015, pp. 1–15., doi:10.1155/2015/987483.

Progressive muscle relaxation

CATEGORY: Therapy or Technique; Physiotherapy
ANATOMY OR SYSTEM AFFECTED: Musculoskeletal system; Nervous system

KEY TERMS

- *autonomic nervous system*: the part of the nervous system responsible for control of the bodily functions not consciously directed, such as breathing, the heartbeat, and digestive processes
- *behavioral medicine*: an interdisciplinary field of research and practice that focuses on how people's thoughts and behavior affect their health
- *vasodilation*: the dilatation of blood vessels, which decreases blood pressure

Overview

The positive effects of relaxation and the contributory influences of prolonged stress and tension on illness have long been recognized. Progressive muscle relaxation (PMR) is a technique aimed at reducing the somatic (bodily)

> **Relaxation Techniques**
>
> Relaxation techniques include a number of practices, such as progressive muscle relaxation, guided imagery, biofeedback, self-hypnosis, and deep breathing exercises. The goal is similar in all: to consciously produce the body's natural relaxation response, characterized by slower breathing, lower blood pressure, and a feeling of calm and well-being.
>
> Relaxation is more than a state of mind; it physically changes the way the body functions. Being able to produce the relaxation response using relaxation techniques may counteract the effects of long-term stress, which may contribute to or worsen a range of health problems including depression, digestive disorders, headaches, high blood pressure, and insomnia.
>
> When a person is under stress, the body releases hormones that produce the fight-or-flight response: Heart rate and breathing rate go up, and blood vessels narrow (restricting the flow of blood). This response allows energy to flow to parts of the body, such as the muscles and the heart, that need to take action. However useful this response may be in the short term, evidence shows that when the body remains in a stress state for a long time, emotional or physical damage can occur. Long-term or chronic stress (lasting months or years) may reduce the body's ability to fight illness and can lead to or worsen certain health conditions. Chronic stress may lead to high blood pressure, headaches, stomachache, and other symptoms. Stress may worsen certain conditions, such as asthma. Stress also has been linked to depression, anxiety, and other mental illnesses.
>
> In contrast to the stress response, the relaxation response slows the heart rate, lowers blood pressure, and decreases oxygen consumption and levels of stress hormones. Because relaxation is the opposite of stress, the theory is that voluntarily creating the relaxation response through regular use of relaxation techniques could counteract the negative effects of stress.

consequences of stress, such as muscle tension, by lowering physiologic arousal and, thereby, inducing relaxation.

Commonly used models of progressive relaxation are based on the principles identified by American psychiatrist Edmund Jacobson in the 1930s. The basic technique developed by Jacobson involves alternately tensing and relaxing major muscle groups of the body, while concurrently focusing on sensations associated with the tensing and relaxing.

Regardless of the reasons for its application, current PMR methods begin with a rationale for its use. The fundamental premise is that muscle tension, even when it is not overtly perceived, causes anxiety (and often pain, discomfort, and agitation) and that significant a reduction in associated symptoms will result if tense muscles are relaxed.

Participants learning PMR are requested to loosen tight clothing and to sit in a comfortable chair in a quiet setting relatively free from distraction. A trained therapist then instructs and demonstrates how to isolate, tense, and relax muscles, and then systematically guides the person through the different muscle groups in a fixed order.

During the "tensing" phase of the procedure, the person is directed to construct the identified muscle as tightly as possible while keeping other muscle groups loose and relaxed. Attention is directed to the sensations associated with tensing, such as tightness and discomfort. The tensing phase lasts approximately ten seconds and is followed by the "relaxing" or "releasing" phase, wherein muscles tension is "let go" and muscles are allowed to become limp. The participant then focuses on the feeling of tension and discomfort draining from the muscle and takes notice of the contrast between the warmth and comfort of relaxed muscles and the discomfort of tensed muscles.

After about ten to fifteen seconds of relaxing, the sequence is repeated with another muscle group. A typical sequence of muscle groups addressed in the technique is the following: hands, biceps and triceps, shoulders, chest, neck, mouth and lips, eyes, forehead and scalp, back, stomach, thighs, calves, feet, and toes. After completing the sequence of tensing and releasing phases, participants take an "inventory" of their muscle groups and relax those with remaining tension. The procedure takes about twenty to thirty minutes to complete.

During the procedure, participants are encouraged to avoid blocking thoughts that might intrude upon their consciousness, and either to allow these thoughts to flow through their mind or to shift their focus toward their breathing if they find themselves distracted. For a period of time following the exercise, participants may engage in slow, steady, and even breathing as a means of enhancing the relaxation response. They may also repeat a calming word or phrase such as "relax," "release," or "let go" each time they exhale so that the word or phrase becomes a cue for promoting relaxation, a practice known as cue-controlled relaxation.

Typically, two or three guided relaxation sessions are conducted to develop basic proficiency with the exercise. Nonguided practice sessions are encouraged to further enhance skills, with the goal of the person being able to achieve a highly relaxed state without guidance. Common variations to the procedure include abbreviated protocols such as "release only" methods, whereby the tensing phase is eliminated or emphasis is directed at specific muscle groups that are identified as particularly key in inducing overall relaxation. Audiotapes of the relaxation procedure may also be used to develop relaxation skills.

Mechanism of Action
PMR has been found to affect the autonomic nervous system, which, among other functions, regulates how the body reacts to changes in the environment. These effects include decreases in heart rate, blood pressure, and muscle tension, and general arousal. Vasodilation of blood vessels also occurs, causing increased blood flow throughout the body, most noticeably in the extremities. These responses are the opposite of those produced by anxiety and lead to subjective feelings of warmth, comfort, and calmness.

Uses and Applications
PMR has a long history of use in psychiatry, psychology, and behavioral medicine. The procedure has been employed as a stand-alone therapy and as a component of multifaceted protocols treating psychiatric and medical illnesses. In nonmedical settings, the procedure is commonly used to promote overall wellness and healthy adaptation to life stressors.

Scientific Evidence
A large body of research has demonstrated that PMR is effective in reducing symptoms stemming from a variety of medical and psychiatric conditions. A double-blind, placebo-controlled study in 2005 examined the technique as applied in a medical setting. The study showed that asthmatic female adolescents' lung function, heart rate, and blood pressure improved after learning and employing PMR. Another double-blind, placebo-controlled study, in 2009, examined the technique's psychiatric application. The study found that PMR improved anxiety symptoms in hospitalized adults with schizophrenia.

Choosing a Practitioner
Trained and licensed mental health or medical professionals should be consulted for persons seeking PMR treatment for psychiatric, psychological, or medical conditions. For nonmedical applications, trained nonprofessionals and audiotapes are usually appropriate.

Safety Issues
Before participating in PMR, interested persons should consult a physician or other health care provider.

—*Paul F. Bell, Ph.D.*

References
Corbett, Christina, et al. "A Randomised Comparison of Two 'Stress Control' Programmes: Progressive Muscle Relaxation versus Mindfulness Body Scan." *Mental Health & Prevention*, vol. 15, 2019, p. 200163., doi:10.1016/j.mph.2019.200163.

Cuncic, Arlin. "Chill Out: How to Use Progressive Muscle Relaxation to Quell Anxiety." *Verywell Mind*, 13 July 2019, www.verywellmind.com/how-do-i-practice-progressive-muscle-relaxation-3024400.

Dunford, Emma, and Miles Thompson. "Relaxation and Mindfulness in Pain: A Review." *Reviews in Pain*, vol. 4, no. 1, 2010, pp. 18–22., doi:10.1177/204946371000400105.

Pangotra, Aditi, et al. "Effectiveness of Progressive Muscle Relaxation, Biofeedback and L-Theanine in Patients Suffering from Anxiety Disorder." *Journal Of Psychosocial Research*, vol. 13, no. 1, 2018, pp. 219–228., doi:10.32381/jpr.2018.13.01.21.

Selva, Joaquin. "Progressive Muscle Relaxation (PMR): A Positive Psychology Guide." *PositivePsychology.com*, 4 July 2019, positivepsychology.com/progressive-muscle-relaxation-pmr/.

Smith, Karen E., and Greg J. Norman. "Brief Relaxation Training Is Not Sufficient to Alter Tolerance to Experimental Pain in Novices." *Plos One*, vol. 12, no. 5, 11 Mar. 2017, doi:10.1371/journal.pone.0177228.

Stone removal

CATEGORY: Procedure
ANATOMY OR SYSTEM AFFECTED: Abdomen, bladder, gallbladder, kidneys, urinary system
SPECIALTIES AND RELATED FIELDS: Gastroenterology, general surgery, nephrology, urology

KEY TERMS
- *calculus*: an abnormal crystalline formation of a mineral salt; also called a stone
- *cholecystectomy*: the removal of a diseased gallbladder or one that contains many gallstones
- *cholelithiasis*: the formation of gallstones in the gallbladder or the ducts that connect the gallbladder to the liver or small intestine
- *ureterolithotomy*: the surgical removal of a stone in the ureter
- *ureters*: the two muscular tubes that connect the kidneys to the urinary bladder and that serve as conduits for urine
- *urolithiasis*: the formation of stones in the urinary tract

Indications and Procedures

Urinary tract stones can occur in the kidneys, ureters, or urinary bladder. These stones, or calculi, are caused by substances that precipitated in the urine. The most common substance that solidifies in the urine is calcium oxalate. Stones referred to as infective, however, are present in about 20 percent of patients with urinary tract stones. These stones typically occur in patients with chronic urinary tract infections. Bacteria in the urinary tract produce ammonia, which combines with calcium or magnesium. Infective stones have the potential to block large areas of the urinary tract.

Patients with urinary tract calculi may experience a variety of symptoms depending on where the stones are located. If a stone is in the ureter, then a sharp pain that extends from the middle of the back to the groin is felt; this pain is called renal colic. Bladder stones are usually not as painful, but they may obstruct the flow of urine from the urinary bladder.

The patient's physician will have the urine examined for the presence of blood (hematuria) and

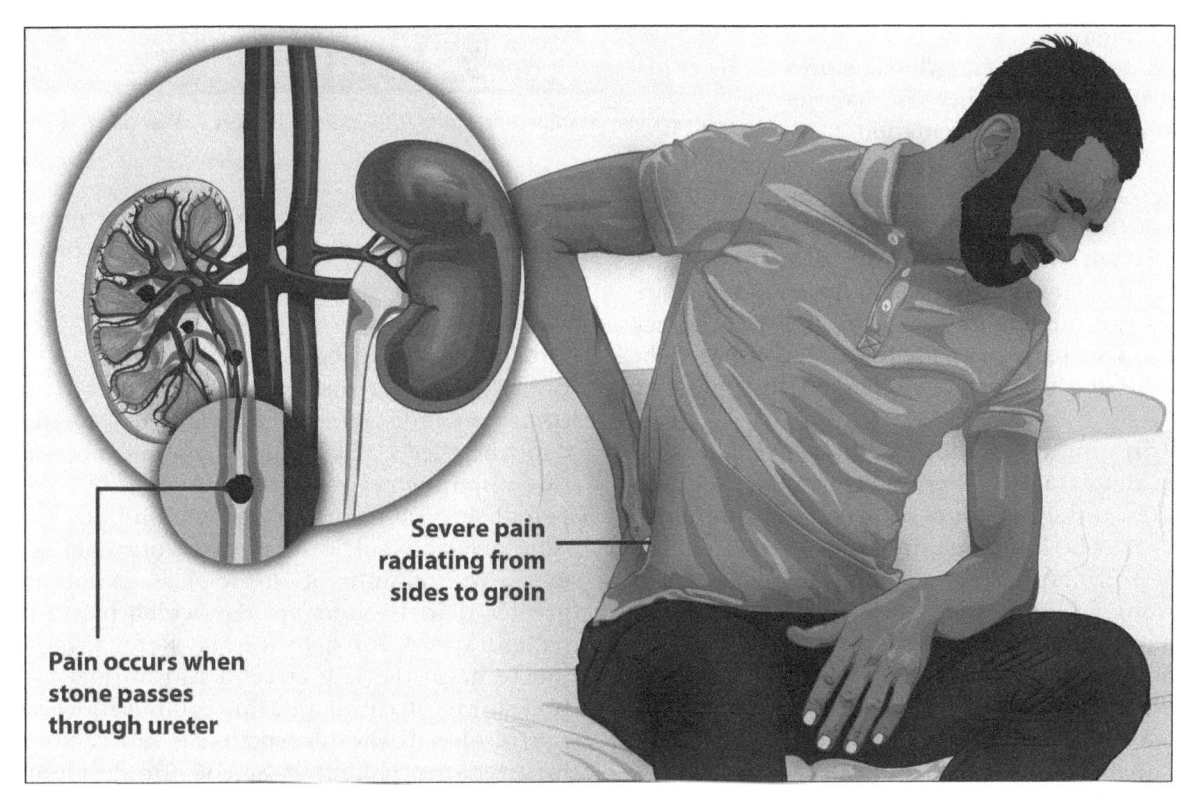

A man with kidney stones suffering from the typical symptom - pain in the sides that radiates down to the groin. Stones in the kidney have also been shown. (Myupchar via Wikimedia Commons)

crystals. X rays and/or ultrasound will show the location of the stone. Blood tests may or may not be ordered depending on whether a metabolic disorder is suspected. Hypercalcemia and hyperparathyroidism can be detected by a blood test; both indicate a problem of excess calcium.

If the urinary tract stone is relatively small, the renal colic is treated with bed rest and an analgesic, along with adequate fluid intake to promote passing of the stone. Larger stones, infective stones, or severe obstruction of urinary flow requires surgery to remove the stone. The patient is usually under general anesthesia and has a small surgical scope (a cystoscope for the bladder or a ureterorenoscope for the ureter) passed up the urethra. These scopes give the surgeon the ability to visualize and crush the stones with attachments on the instruments.

The gallbladder, which stores and concentrates bile, also has the potential for stone formation. Gallstones are usually composed of cholesterol and may be found in the ducts that connect the gallbladder to the small intestine or liver. If a stone has obstructed one of these ducts, the resulting symptoms can include intense pain known as biliary colic. This pain is usually felt in the upper right side of the abdomen or between the shoulder blades.

Ultrasound scanning of the upper abdomen can almost always detect the presence of gallstones. If the gallstones do not cause symptoms, they may be left alone, or drugs such as chenodiol and ursodeoxycholic acid may be tried to dissolve them. When symptoms are severe, removal of the gallbladder (cholecystectomy) is indicated. This surgery involves an incision under the ribcage on the right side. A laparoscope may be used or a larger incision made for an open procedure. In either case, the liver is gently lifted to expose the gallbladder, and the blood vessels and cystic duct are tied off so that

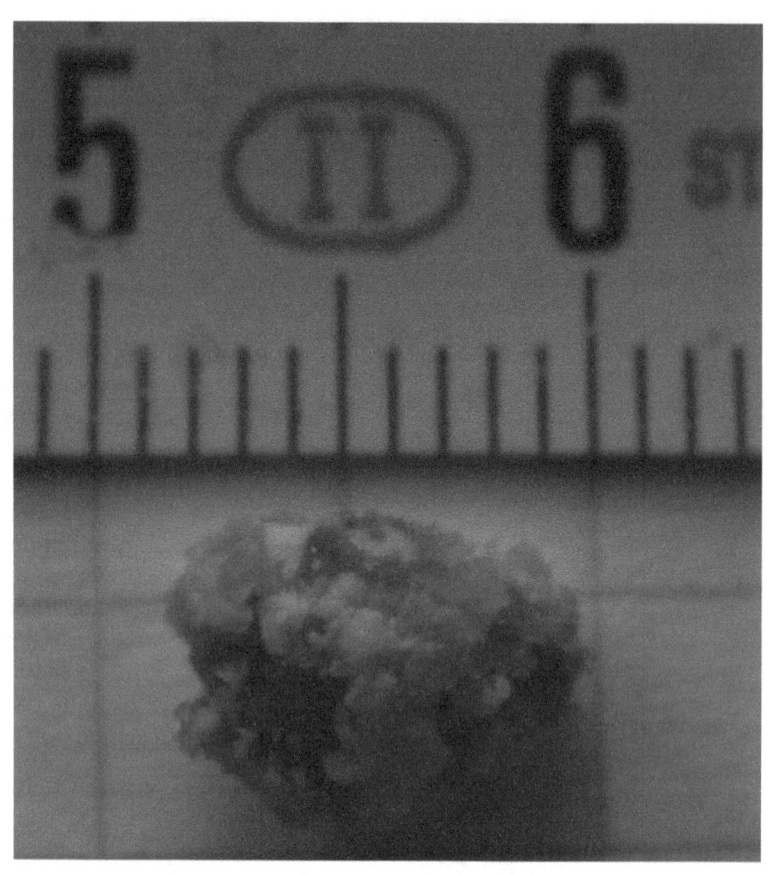

A kidney stone, 8 millimeters (0.3 in) in diameter. (Robert R. Wal via Wikimedia Commons)

blood and bile do not leak from the excised organ. The wound is then closed, and the patient may return home within a week.

Uses and Complications

Complications from removing urinary tract stones include infections, scarring, bleeding, and anesthesia risks. These complications are rare when the operation is performed by a competent surgical team. An uncommon but significant adverse result from obstruction relief is an excessive amount of urine loss, sometimes greater than 10 liters per day, which places the patient at risk for dehydration. Reducing fluid intake helps the kidney return to normal function slowly. Occasionally, this complication does not resolve. If the obstruction is not removed, however, the patient is at risk for developing chronic urinary tract infections and even renal failure.

The major risk in performing cholecystectomy is damage to the bile duct that leads to the small intestine. If scarring or inflammation occurs in this duct, it may lead to obstruction of the flow of bile from the liver. This in turn may lead to obstructive jaundice, in which pigments normally released into the intestines accumulate in the liver and blood. The patient may have a yellowish tinge to the skin and eyes until the obstruction is corrected.

If there are no complications during the cholecystectomy, then the outcome of the surgery is usually good. Approximately 90 percent of the patients have no further symptoms and recover completely in about three weeks.

Perspective and Prospects

Advances in medical technology have aided physicians in the removal of stones. Kidney and urethral stones now can be broken up using a technique called lithotripsy. An ultrasonic lithotripsy probe can break the stones using externally applied sound waves that penetrate the skin and other soft tissues. For some patients, a noninvasive technique takes advantage of sound waves transmitted through the abdominal cavity and directed at the stones. This procedure is known as extracorporeal shock-wave lithotripsy. The latter technique is also used to treat some patients with gallstones.

—*Matthew Berria, Ph.D., Douglas Reinhart, M.D.*

References

Çakici, Özer Ural, et al. "Open Stone Surgery: Still-in-Use Approach for Complex Stone Burden." *Central European Journal of Urology*, vol. 70, no. 2, 2017, doi:10.5173/ceju.2017.1205.

Kuroda, Shinnosuke, et al. "A New Prediction Model for Operative Time of Flexible Ureteroscopy with Lithotripsy for the Treatment of Renal Stones." *Plos One*, vol. 13, no. 2, 13 Feb. 2018, doi:10.1371/journal.pone.0192597.

Mayo Clinic Staff. "Bladder Stones." *Mayo Clinic*, Mayo Foundation for Medical Education and Research, 16 Aug. 2019, www.mayoclinic.org/diseases-conditions/bladder-stones/diagnosis-treatment/drc-20354345.

Mayo Clinic Staff. "Gallstones." *Mayo Clinic*, Mayo Foundation for Medical Education and Research, 8 Aug. 2019, www.mayoclinic.org/diseases-conditions/gallstones/diagnosis-treatment/drc-20354220.

Mayo Clinic Staff. "Kidney Stones." *Mayo Clinic*, Mayo Foundation for Medical Education and Research, 8 Feb. 2019, www.mayoclinic.org/diseases-conditions/kidney-stones/diagnosis-treatment/drc-20355759.

Sharbaugh, Adam, et al. "Contemporary Best Practice in the Management of Staghorn Calculi." *Therapeutic Advances in Urology*, vol. 11, 2019, p. 175628721984709., doi:10.1177/1756287219847099.

Zisman, Anna L. "Effectiveness of Treatment Modalities on Kidney Stone Recurrence." *Clinical Journal of the American Society of Nephrology*, vol. 12, no. 10, 22 Oct. 2017, pp. 1699–1708., doi:10.2215/cjn.11201016.

■ TENS machines

CATEGORY: Therapy or Technique; Physiotherapy
ANATOMY OR SYSTEM AFFECTED: Musculoskeletal system

Transcutaneous electrical nerve stimulation or TENS utilizes a machine that sends small electrical signals from a source to electrodes connected to an area on the body. TENS devices may be used to help reduce pain using electrical signals. TENS devices have been noted to aid in relief of pain associated with arthritis, muscle spasms, joint pain, pain associated with menstruation, pelvic pain caused by endometriosis, and sports injuries. A variety of different medical specialties including orthopedics, neurology, physical therapy, chiropractic, and palliative medicine have developed treatment plans using TENS devices.

TENS devices or devices with similar mechanisms have been utilized for centuries. The earliest form of TENS device dates back to approximately 60 A.D. when a Roman physician used electric eels for symptomatic relief. Today's concept of TENS units were researched and adapted by Dr. C. Norman Shealy and played an important role in therapy for migraines, back pain, and gout.

Mechanism of Action

A TENS machine transmits mild electric current to activate nerves in order to relieve pain. TENS is a non-pharmacologic and non-invasive treatment for pain relief. TENS is believed to stimulate nerves both centrally and peripherally in order to reduce pain.

TENS is believed to provide pain relief by stimulating peripheral opioid receptors. Studies revealed that peripheral nerves responded more to low frequency TENS and thus had more analgesic effect than high frequency TENS. It is proposed that TENS units may also utilize central mechanisms to reduce pain via the spinal cord. When TENS units are used there may be stimulation of opioid receptors which helps to decrease pain propagation at the spinal level. Repeated use of TENS may lead to tolerance at spinal opioid receptors thus creating a decreased analgesic effect. In order to prevent tolerance from developing quickly it is recommended to alternate low and high frequency TENS treatments. The alternation of frequencies may more than double the amount of consecutive days TENS treatments can provide analgesic relief.

Effects

TENS devices provide a non-pharmacologic and non-invasive option to provide short term pain relief. TENS is usually used in conjunction with other treatments and is almost never the only modality used for pain relief. It is more effective if used in conjunction with pharmacotherapy and possibly physical therapy. TENS is a rapid onset and efficacious short term option for pain relief. TENS is not a cure for the underlying pathology causing pain and is often not useful in the setting of chronic pain conditions.

When using a TENS device someone may feel a tingling during treatment. The treatment may be painful or uncomfortable but decreasing the frequency of stimulation should resolve the pain caused by the treatment. TENS sessions are usually well tolerated with minimal to no side effects.

Risks

There are a few situations where TENS treatment may not be appropriate. It is not recommended to use a TENS device if someone has pacemaker, a metal implant, electrical implants, epilepsy, heart problems, or are early in pregnancy. Electrodes should not be used on people who have broken or irritated skin, varicose veins, or tumors overlying treatment area. Electrodes should never be placed over front sides of the neck, the temples, in the mouth, over the eyes, or sandwich of chest and back at same time.

One common complication mentioned includes contact dermatitis or allergic reaction to the adhesive on the electrode pads. Hypoallergenic pads can be purchased to prevent this complication. Another complication discussed is the possible risk associated with driving and operating heavy machinery while using a TENS device. If the device causes pain or a muscular contraction it could cause an unintended movement and result in an accident.

Clinical Trials

There is still some debate about the using TENS as a medical treatment due to unclear efficacy of TENS in reducing pain. Due to the limited adverse effects and the potential for pain relief and positive effects TENS is a generally accepted treatment. Most studies have found TENS devices do provide pain relief; however, it is usually short term. The treatment is thought to be rapid in onset and offset and thus is usually valuable to trial TENS for pain relief. Clinical trials and research regarding the efficacy and exact mechanisms of action are ongoing to help clarify if TENS should be regularly used as a pain relief device.

—*Christine Gamble MD*

References

Desantana, Josimari M., et al. "Effectiveness of Transcutaneous Electrical Nerve Stimulation for Treatment of Hyperalgesia and Pain." *Current Rheumatology Reports*, vol. 10, no. 6, 2008, pp. 492–499., doi:10.1007/s11926-008-0080-z.

Gibson, William, et al. "Transcutaneous Electrical Nerve Stimulation (TENS) for Chronic Pain an Overview of Cochrane Reviews." *Cochrane Database of Systematic Reviews*, vol. 4, Apr. 2019, doi:10.1002/14651858.CD011890.pub3.

Grover, Casey, et al. "Transcutaneous Electrical Nerve Stimulation (TENS) in the ED for Pain Relief: A Preliminary Study of Feasibility and Efficacy." *Western Journal of Emergency Medicine*, vol. 19, no. 5, 9 Aug. 2018, pp. 872–876., doi:10.5811/westjem.2018.7.38447.

Murina, Filippo, and Stefania Di Francesco. "Transcutaneous Electrical Nerve Stimulation." *Electrical Stimulation for Pelvic Floor Disorders*, by Jacopo

Martellucci, Springer International Publishing, 2015, pp. 105–117.

Vance, Carol Gt, et al. "Using TENS for Pain Control: the State of the Evidence." *Pain Management*, vol. 4, no. 3, 2014, pp. 197–209., doi:10.2217/pmt.14.13.

■ Tooth extraction

CATEGORY: Procedure
ANATOMY OR SYSTEM AFFECTED: Gums, mouth, teeth
SPECIALTIES AND RELATED FIELDS: Dentistry, orthodontics

Indications and Procedures

A tooth may have to be extracted for one of several reasons. Impaction is a condition in which a developing tooth is forced into an adjacent tooth, blocking its progress; the impacted tooth can threaten the health and proper alignment of nearby teeth if it is not extracted. The occurrence of crooked or misaligned teeth may also require surgical removal. In tooth decay, dental tissue weakens in a gradual process and can eventually be destroyed. Decay usually begins in the outer layer of the tooth, penetrates to the underlying dentin, and kills the innermost tissue (pulp) of the tooth. Tooth extraction is necessary if this process of decay cannot be halted.

The extraction of teeth is one of the most common procedures in dentistry. Dentists usually perform simple extractions, but they often refer patients needing more complicated procedures to oral surgeons.

In simple extractions, the dentist first applies a local anesthetic to deaden the area surrounding the tooth that is to be pulled. Then, the dentist uses forceps and short levers to loosen the tooth in its socket. The tooth is removed in one piece by breaking the ligaments that hold the tooth in place. Once the tooth has been extracted, the dentist cleans the empty socket and ensures that the blood flowing from the socket is clotting properly. The socket is dressed to protect it and help it heal.

The oral surgeon may use a general anesthetic with a patient needing a complex extraction. The surgeon may need to cut through gum and bone to gain access to the tooth requiring extraction. The tooth may be cut into small pieces before it can be removed. Sutures may be required to close the wound.

The pain caused by extraction usually peaks a few hours after the procedure. Patients are given analgesics (painkillers) and are encouraged to keep the head elevated and to use an ice pack.

—*Russell Williams, M.S.W.*

References

Cohen, N., and J. Cohen-Lévy. "Healing Processes Following Tooth Extraction in Orthodontic Cases." *Journal of Dentofacial Anomalies and Orthodontics*, vol. 17, no. 3, 2014, p. 304., doi:10.1051/odfen/2014006.

Fukuda, Ken-Ichi. "Diagnosis and Treatment of Abnormal Dental Pain." *Journal of Dental Anesthesia and Pain Medicine*, vol. 16, no. 1, 2016, p. 1., doi:10.17245/jdapm.2016.16.1.1.

Gotter, Ana, and Christine Frank. "What to Expect During a Tooth Extraction." *Healthline*, 9 Feb. 2018, www.healthline.com/health/tooth-extraction.

Hong, Bosun, et al. "Minimally Invasive Vertical versus Conventional Tooth Extraction." *The Journal of the American Dental Association*, vol. 149, no. 8, 2018, pp. 688–695., doi:10.1016/j.adaj.2018.03.022.

Kumarswamy, A. "Multimodal Management of Dental Pain with Focus on Alternative Medicine: A Novel Herbal Dental Gel." *Contemporary Clinical Dentistry*, vol. 7, no. 2, 2016, p. 131., doi:10.4103/0976-237x.183066.

Peck, Sheldon. "Extractions, Retention and Stability: the Search for Orthodontic Truth." *European Journal of Orthodontics*, vol. 39, no. 2, 23 Feb. 2017, pp. 109–115., doi:10.1093/ejo/cjx004.

Wu, Song, et al. "Effect of Low-Level Laser Therapy on Tooth-Related Pain and Somatosensory Function Evoked by Orthodontic Treatment." *International Journal of Oral Science*, vol. 10, no. 3, 2 July 2018, doi:10.1038/s41368-018-0023-0.

Alternative Treatments

■ Acupressure

CATEGORY: Therapy or Technique
ANATOMY OR SYSTEM AFFECTED: All

KEY TERMS
- *meridians*: each of a set of pathways in the body along which vital energy is said to flow; there are twelve such pathways associated with specific organs
- *moxibustion*: a type of heat therapy in which an herb is burned on or above the skin to warm and stimulate an acupuncture point or affected area
- *pressure points*: a point on the surface of the body sensitive to pressure
- *qi*: the circulating life energy that in Chinese philosophy is thought to be inherent in all things; in traditional Chinese medicine the balance of negative and positive forms in the body is believed to be essential for good health

Overview

Acupressure is sometimes thought of as acupuncture without needles. Because acupressure and acupuncture support the body's natural healing powers, many conditions can be improved, corrected, or even eliminated. Like other touch therapies, acupressure conveys the care and empathy that are necessary ingredients in healing. As such, holistic therapies like acupressure are especially appropriate for problems best suited to a biopsychosocial approach.

Acupressure is part of the healing system of traditional Chinese medicine (TCM), a unique and comprehensive system for diagnosing and treating disease, preventing illness, and promoting wellness. TCM encompasses many diverse health-enhancing and energy-balancing therapies, including acupuncture, herbal medicine, Tai Chi Chuan, qigong, *Gua Sha*, cupping, moxibustion, and *tui na* acupressure. All of these techniques, and many others, manipulate qi, the essential energy of life. Originating in China thousands of years ago, TCM continues to be practiced throughout the world.

To understand acupressure, one should study some basic principles of TCM, and one theory in particular necessitates elaboration: the notion that human beings are governed by opposing but complementing forces, yin and yang, a notion at the heart of Daoism, which forms the basis of TCM. According to Daoism, this balance of forces infiltrates and influences the entire universe, including those within. One of the basic aims of TCM is to correct imbalances of yin and yang to prevent sickness and restore health. Fully comprehending the principles behind yin and yang (and many other concepts) permits Chinese medical practitioners to diagnose accurately and treat effectively.

In short, TCM offers alternative explanations for how health problems develop in the first place, and it provides many approaches for treating these problems. Depending on a person's specific clinical presentation, acupressure and other modalities, used alone or with allopathic methods, can prove quite beneficial for many health conditions.

Mechanism of Action

Acupressure relies on touch rather than needles to manipulate the flow of qi in the body. Specifically, qi is thought to move through the body by means of a complex system of meridians, or energy channels. These meridians are known by the names of body organs (the bladder channel or liver channel) and refer to energetic patterns with particular characteristics based on TCM principles and practice.

Specific areas on the skin where the meridians pass and allow the manipulation of qi are referred to as acupoints or acupressure points. During a typical acupressure session, these points are pressed, rubbed, tapped, or otherwise touched as a way of influencing qi to bring about desired results. The effects of acupressure are reinforced through a healthy diet, herbal formulas, exercise, fresh air, meditation, and spirituality.

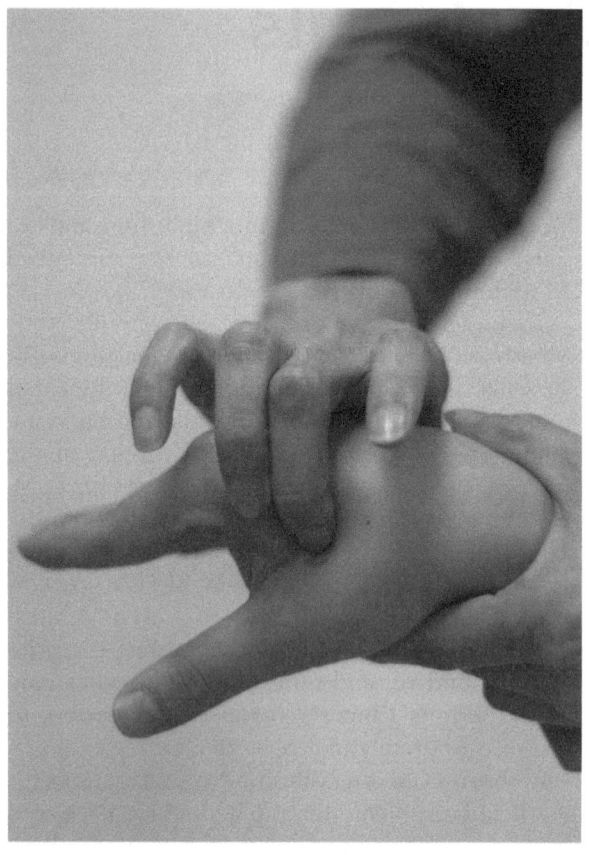

Acupuncture point LI-4 (Hegu) (Mk2010 via Wikimedia Commons)

Uses and Applications

According to data published by the World Health Organization, TCM is helpful for ophthalmological, respiratory, gastrointestinal, neurological, and musculoskeletal disorders, and disorders of the ear, nose, and throat. In the United States, acupressure (and acupuncture) are used mostly to treat painful conditions such as headaches, arthritis, bursitis, injuries, and postsurgical pain.

The effectiveness of TCM in general extends beyond controlling pain. More recently, acupressure is being used to treat chronic fatigue, anxiety, stress, insomnia, depression, addictions, smoking, eating disorders, irritable bowel syndrome, hypertension, sexual dysfunctions, premenstrual and menopausal symptoms, and many other conditions. Also, acupressure appears to improve circulation, boost immune functioning, help eliminate metabolic waste products, promote relaxation, enhance self-esteem, and create a general sense of well-being.

In its most crucial role, however, TCM presents a theoretical and practical framework for engaging in a holistic understanding of health and illness.

Scientific Evidence

Controlled double-blind studies into the efficacy of acupressure per se have not been conducted. However, many smaller studies exist that affirm the positive role of acupressure in such conditions as pain, stroke, heart disease, cancer, smoking, obesity, insomnia, allergies, and menstrual disorders. Furthermore, scientific evidence supporting the efficacy of TCM in general–and acupuncture in particular–continues to grow. This is in addition to millennia of observational information gathered throughout China, Japan, Korea, and other Asian countries.

Choosing a Practitioner

TCM is certainly more complex than the beginner or casual observer might think. This ancient discipline specifically emphasizes concepts of wellness, illness, and recovery. It further emphasizes the best of medical ideas and methodologies from the past and the present–from the wisdom of everyday people to the advanced knowledge of the best-trained TCM physicians and other healing arts practitioners. For these reasons and more, actual treatment with TCM, including acupressure, requires the expertise of a trained and licensed clinician. Simple, everyday ailments, however, respond well to acupressure performed as self-therapy.

In the United States, licensed physicians, acupuncturists, and massage therapists practice acupressure. Practitioners can be found by contacting state licensing boards and such national groups as the American Academy of Medical Acupuncture, the American Association of Acupuncture and Oriental Medicine, and the American Massage Therapy Association.

Safety Issues

Acupressure is an exceptionally safe modality because of its noninvasive nature. Contraindications (that is, conditions for which acupressure is not recommended) typically include acute illness (such as hypertensive urgency and tachycardia), serious illness (such as cancer), pregnancy, bleeding (such as with open wounds), and skin diseases and lesions (such as infections and ulcers).

—*George D. Zgourides, M.D., Psy.D.*

References

Adams, Angela, et al. "Acupressure for Chronic Low Back Pain: a Single System Study." *Journal of Physical Therapy Science*, vol. 29, no. 8, 2017, pp. 1416–1420., doi:10.1589/jpts.29.1416.

Bleecker, Deborah. *Acupuncture Points Handbook: a Patient's Guide to the Locations and Functions of Over 400 Acupuncture Points.* Draycott Design Books, 2017.

Mafetoni, Reginaldo Roque, and Antonieta Keiko Kakuda Shimo. "The Effects of Acupressure on Labor Pains during Child Birth: Randomized Clinical Trial." *Revista Latino-Americana De Enfermagem*, vol. 24, 8 Aug. 2016, doi:10.1590/1518-8345.0739.2738.

Mehta, Piyush, et al. "Contemporary Acupressure Therapy: Adroit Cure for Painless Recovery of Therapeutic Ailments." *Journal of Traditional and Complementary Medicine*, vol. 7, no. 2, 2017, pp. 251–263., doi:10.1016/j.jtcme.2016.06.004.

Noll, Eric, et al. "Randomized Trial of Acupressure to Improve Patient Satisfaction and Quality of Recovery in Hospitalized Patients: Study Protocol for a Randomized Controlled Trial." *Trials*, vol. 18, no. 1, 7 Mar. 2017, doi:10.1186/s13063-017-1839-1.

Ogal, Hans P., and Wolfram Stor. *Pictorial Atlas of Acupuncture: an Illustrated Manual of Acupuncture Points.* H.F. Ullman Publishing, 2012.

■ Acupuncture

CATEGORY: Therapy or Technique
ANATOMY OR SYSTEM AFFECTED: All

KEY TERMS

- *electroacupuncture:* a procedure in which pulses of weak electrical current are sent through acupuncture needles into acupuncture points in the skin
- *low level laser therapy:* form of medicine that applies low-level (low-power) lasers or light-emitting diodes (LEDs) to the surface of the body
- *placebo effect:* phenomenon in which a placebo (a fake treatment, an inactive substance like sugar, distilled water, saline solution, etc.) can sometimes improve a patient's condition simply because the person has the expectation that it will be helpful
- *yin and yang:* a concept of dualism in ancient Chinese philosophy, describing how seemingly opposite or contrary forces may actually be complementary, interconnected, and interdependent in the natural world, and how they may give rise to each other as they interrelate to one another

Overview

Acupuncture has been part of the medical mainstream in countries such as China and Japan for centuries. It is also one of the most widely utilized forms of alternative therapy in the United States. More than ten million acupuncture treatments are administered annually in the United States alone. In addition, third-party insurance reimbursement and managed care coverage for acupuncture are increasing.

Because of acupuncture's popularity, scientific investigation of the method has grown dramatically, with many new studies reported every week. However, the results have been mixed at best.

What Is Acupuncture?

Simply defined, acupuncture is a treatment method aimed at eliciting a response (such as pain relief) through the insertion of very fine needles in the body surface at sites called acupuncture points. A related technique called acupressure (or shiatsu) uses pressure on these points, and a related therapy known as electroacupuncture applies electricity to the points.

A variety of treatment methods, approaches, techniques, styles, and theoretical frameworks exist within the broad scope of acupuncture. Differences in forms of acupuncture are often cultural. The system of acupuncture practiced in Japan, for example, is quite different from that found in China. Many acupuncturists practice a more or less traditional style called traditional Chinese medicine (TCM). Others have adopted modern styles that have little or no reliance on traditional principles.

Acupuncture needles are most often inserted at specific locations on the skin called acupuncture points. These points are located on specific lines outlined by tradition, referred to as meridians or channels. According to Chinese medical theory,

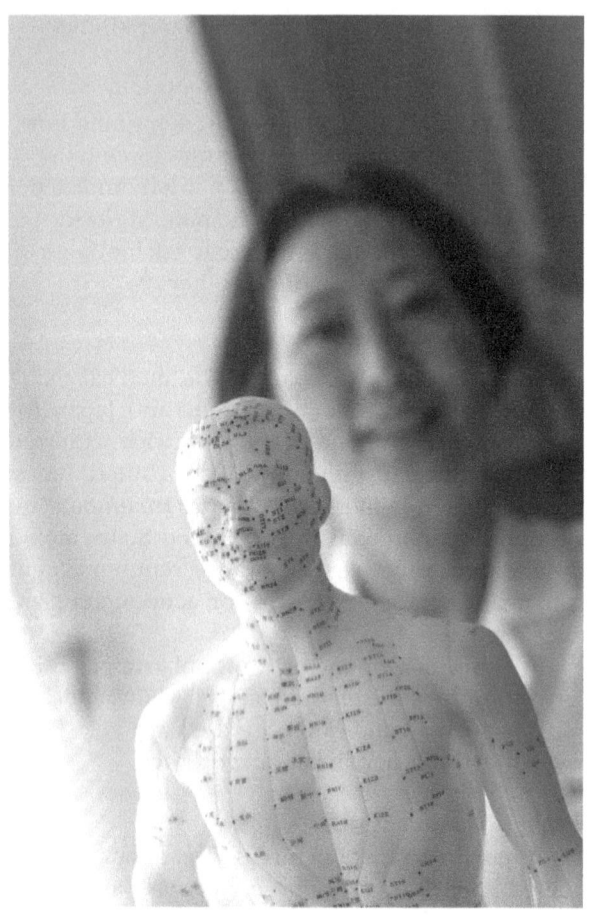

Doctor displays a model of acupuncture points on the body. (National Institutes of Health)

fourteen major meridians form an invisible network connecting the body surface with the internal organs. Meridians are to conduct qi, the energy or vital force of the body. Pain or illness is said to result from imbalances or blockages in the flow of qi through the meridians. Acupuncture is traditionally thought to remove such blockages, restore the normal circulation of qi, and improve overall health by promoting the balance of energy in the system. However, there is no scientific evidence for the existence of the meridians or qi itself. (Meridians are not visible under a microscope and, contrary to popular belief, they do not match major nerve pathways.)

In addition to meridians and qi, the concept of yin and yang is central to acupuncture theory, as it is to all of traditional Chinese philosophy. The terms "yin" and "yang" do not represent forces or substances; rather, they are, as one, a way to look at the world in terms of the interaction of polar opposites. According to this viewpoint, all movement, growth, and change in the world is a manifestation of the push and pull of these forces. Although seemingly in opposition, these forces are thought to complement and support each other. For example, without rest one cannot exert energy; without becoming tired by exerting energy, it is difficult to sleep. This is just one illustration of the harmony and interaction of yin and yang.

Yang is traditionally associated with heat, power, daylight, summer, and many other active or energetic aspects of life; yin is cold, quiet, and dark. Many illnesses are characterized in terms of an excess or deficiency of either yin or yang, or of both at the same time. For example, when the body is feverish, it is too yang as a whole. There is also a yin and yang balance in each individual organ and part of the body; these can become excessive or deficient too.

Thus, in TCM, illnesses are described as complex patterns of imbalances and blockages. Treatment is based not on medical diagnosis, but on identifying these problems in the body's energy and seeking to correct them. Does this traditional analysis contain truths about human health or is it just archaic thinking? The answer remains unknown.

History of Acupuncture

Primitive acupuncture needles dating to circa 1000 B.C.E. have been discovered in archeological finds of the Shan Dynasty in China. The theoretical framework underlying the practice of acupuncture was first set forth in the *Inner Classic of Medicine*, or *Nei Jing*, first published in 206 B.C.E. during the Han Dynasty.

As an active and growing tradition, the theory and practice of TCM evolved over the centuries, at times undergoing rapid changes. Acupuncture reached perhaps its golden age under the Ming Dynasty in the late sixteenth and early seventeenth centuries. Subsequently, it took second place to an ascending practice of herbal medicine. By the time acupuncture came back in vogue in twentieth-century China, it had undergone a major transformation, sometimes called the herbalization of acupuncture. Today's acupuncture methods given the name traditional Chinese medicine are derived to a great extent from this relatively modern revision of the theory. Present-day

Japanese acupuncture, however, dates to earlier versions of acupuncture.

Another major change occurred after the Communist Revolution in China in 1949. The new leadership, while wanting to carry through a process of modernization, decided to support and preserve traditional medicine. During the Cultural Revolution, the famous "barefoot doctors" were trained in both modern and traditional medicine and sent out to the rural areas to provide medical care for the people. Today, in the largest and most modern Chinese hospitals, Western medicine and TCM, including acupuncture and herbal treatments, are practiced side by side.

Acupuncture entered France through its colonial rule of Vietnam. It was there that, in 1957, the French physician Paul Nogier conceived the notion of auricular (ear) acupuncture. According to his theory, the entire body is "mapped" onto the ear in the form of an inverted fetus. Using this system of correspondence, one can, according to Nogier, treat any part of the body by treating the corresponding part of the ear. This approach was subsequently taken up in China, even though it had been invented in the West and had no real foundation in traditional practice. (Classic acupuncture includes only a few points on the ear and does not refer to any representation of the entire body.) Nogier claimed to have scientifically tested his theory, but the methods he used to accomplish this fall far short of anything recognizable as modern science. There are no properly designed studies to support the "little man on the ear" hypothesis, and the one well-designed study on the subject failed to find any correlation between pain in the body and tenderness in corresponding parts of the ear as predicted by Nogier's theory.

Acupuncture was virtually unheard of and unavailable in the United States until 1972, the year U.S. president Richard Nixon made his historic visit to China. Among the accompanying press was the well-known journalist James Reston, who was hospitalized while in China and received acupuncture anesthesia. Upon returning to the United States, Reston published an article about his experience, stimulating new interest in acupuncture among the public and within the medical community. Although it was later discovered that the drugs used with acupuncture anesthesia probably played a major role, the perception of acupuncture as a powerful treatment caused it to gain respect in the United States. Acupuncture schools began to open in the late 1970s and 1980s. With training available in the United States, the number of acupuncturists began to grow rapidly; there are now many thousands of certified and licensed acupuncturists.

Mechanism of Action

The exact mechanisms by which acupuncture might produce effects on the body remain unknown. Weak preliminary evidence from the 1970s hints that acupuncture encourages the release of endorphins (morphine-like compounds that function as the body's internal pain-regulating substances). Support for this theory comes from a study in which the use of the drug naloxone, which opposes the effects of endorphins, was found to block pain relief from acupuncture. However, the body releases endorphins in response to any sort of pain, and it may be that needle insertion per se, and not acupuncture, is responsible for the rise in endorphins. Furthermore, there is some evidence that the placebo effect itself works by means of endorphins; in one study, naloxone blocked the ability of a placebo treatment to reduce pain.

It has also been proposed that acupuncture may influence other chemicals in the body that control various physiologic activities. Preliminary studies have shown possible effects of acupuncture on norepinephrine, acetylcholine, and cyclic AMP, all of which are "chemical messengers" that regulate key systems in the body. However, none of this evidence is strong.

Scientific Evidence

Although there have been numerous controlled studies of acupuncture, there is no condition for which acupuncture's supporting evidence is strong. There are several reasons for this, but one is fundamental: Even with the best of intentions, it is difficult to properly ascertain the effectiveness of a hands-on therapy such as acupuncture.

Only one form of study can truly prove that a treatment is effective: the double-blind, placebo-controlled trial. However, it is not easy to fit acupuncture into a study design of this type. One problem is designing a form of placebo acupuncture, and an even more challenging problem is to ensure that participants and practitioners do not know who is receiving real acupuncture and who is receiving fake. Without such blinding, the results of the study can be skewed by numerous factors.

In an attempt to approximate double-blind studies of acupuncture, researchers have resorted to a number of clever techniques. Perhaps the most common involves sham acupuncture. In such studies, a fake version of acupuncture is used. However, because the acupuncturist knows that this is a fake treatment, he or she may subtly convey a lack of confidence in the outcome. Such studies are called single-blind and are not fully trustworthy. (The only exceptions are studies in which the patient is anesthetized before the acupuncture and is, presumably, incapable of interpreting the possibly biased actions of the acupuncturist.)

To get around this problem and produce a truly double-blind study, some studies may employ trained technicians, and not real acupuncturists, to insert needles. Such technicians might be given a list of real acupuncture points or phony acupuncture points, without being told which is which. However, it is not reasonable to suppose that an essentially untrained technician can give an acupuncture treatment as effective as that of a real acupuncturist. Furthermore, using a fixed set of points to treat a problem is not true to traditional acupuncture, which always individualizes treatment to the person seeking care.

Another approach is to use real acupuncturists to deliver treatment, but to have a separate person evaluate the effects of that treatment. Such studies may be described as partially double-blind (or observer blind); they prevent researchers from biasing their own observations, but they still do not eliminate the problem that the acupuncturist might communicate confidence (or lack of it) to the participants. The placebo effect in acupuncture is very sensitive to expectation; in one study, persons who believed they were getting real acupuncture experienced benefits and those who believed they were getting fake acupuncture failed to experience benefits. Whether or not they were actually receiving real or fake acupuncture proved to be irrelevant; it was the belief that mattered. One doubts whether acupuncturists are sufficiently adept at hiding their true feelings from their patients. Osteopathic physician Kerry Kamer suggested a whimsical approach to testing acupuncture: For the placebo group, use actors trained to convey confidence while performing fake acupuncture. However, such studies have not been reported.

Despite their limitations, most of the best studies available are single-blind or partially double-blind designs. Although imperfect, they can give some idea whether true acupuncture might be effective.

There is another problem to consider. Acupuncture causes a very strong placebo effect, whether it is real or fake. This phenomenon tends to diminish the difference in results between the treatment group and the placebo group and can potentially hide a true benefit by making it too small to reach statistical significance. As an example, consider a study in which sixty-seven people with hip arthritis received either random needle placement or actual acupuncture. The results showed improvement in both groups, but to the same extent. Does this mean that traditional acupuncture is actually no better than random acupuncture? Not necessarily. The study could simply have been too small to identify benefits that did occur. In studies that show a strong placebo effect, it may be necessary to enroll hundreds of participants to show benefit above statistical "background noise." A small study can fail to find benefit, but it cannot actually prove lack of benefit.

Some studies have compared acupuncture to other therapies, such as physical therapy or massage. Trials of this kind are good for determining relative cost effectiveness, but they cannot be taken as proof of efficacy for one simple reason: These other therapies have never been proven effective themselves.

There is one additional problem in evaluating the evidence for acupuncture: Many of the studies were performed in China, and there is evidence of systematic bias in the Chinese medical literature. In 1998, researchers evaluating the acupuncture studies from China discovered that each study found acupuncture effective. This led researchers to look further into other Chinese medical research. Review of controlled trials involving other therapies, including standard drugs, showed that Chinese trials reported positive results 99 percent of the time. Although some bias exists in all medical publications, this finding suggests a particularly high rate of bias in the Chinese research record. A subsequent analysis in 2007 continued to find grossly inadequate standards of rigor in Chinese studies of Chinese medicine.

Given these caveats, the following sections address the science regarding acupuncture. They begin with conditions in which acupuncture research has been mostly positive, continue with those for which the record is mixed, and conclude with those in which the tested form of acupuncture has not proved effective. Studies of acupressure and electroacupuncture also are discussed.

Evidence-Based Uses

Nausea and vomiting. Numerous studies have evaluated treatment on a single acupuncture point (P6), which is traditionally thought to be effective for relief of various forms of nausea and vomiting. This point is located on the inside of the forearm, about two inches above the wrist crease. Most studies have investigated the effects of pressure on this point (acupressure) rather than needling. The most common methods involve a wristband with a pearl-sized bead in it situated over P6. The band exerts pressure on the bead while it is worn, and the user can press on the bead for extra stimulation.

Although the research record is mixed, on balance it appears that P6 stimulation offers at least modest benefits for nausea. This approach has been studied in anesthesia-induced nausea, the nausea and vomiting of pregnancy, and other forms of nausea.

Anesthesia-induced nausea. General anesthetics and other medications used for surgery frequently cause nausea. A minimum of ten controlled studies enrolling about one thousand women undergoing gynecologic surgery found that P6 stimulation of various types reduced such postsurgical nausea compared with placebo.

On the negative side, a double-blind, placebo-controlled study of 410 women undergoing gynecologic surgery failed to find P6 acupressure more effective than fake acupressure (both were more effective than no treatment). A small trial of acupuncture in gynecologic surgery also failed to find benefit, as did three studies of acupressure for women undergoing cesarean section. Studies of acupuncture or acupressure in other forms of surgery have produced about as many negative results as positive ones.

A 2004 review of the entire literature regarding P6 stimulation for postoperative nausea found twenty-six studies. All of these studies suffered from significant flaws; however, on balance, the reviewers found that stimulation of P6 does reduce postoperative nausea compared with placebo. Similarly, a 2008 review of six placebo-controlled trials investigating the effectiveness of P6 stimulation on nausea and vomiting both during and after cesarean section found some benefit, though the authors concluded that the results were largely inconsistent.

One aspect of studies of acupressure for postsurgical nausea is that here a single-blind study is probably as good as a double-blind study. If the acupressure wrist band is not put on until after anesthesia has begun, no amount of confidence or lack of it by the practitioner is likely to alter the placebo effect experienced by the unconscious patient. Thus, studies of acupressure/acupuncture for this condition have a higher potential validity than studies for any of the other conditions listed here. The fact that benefits have been seen strongly suggests that stimulation of P6 does affect nausea. That there is no clear physiological reason why this should be so makes this an intriguing finding, even if the benefit is too slight to make much real difference in postoperative care.

Nausea and vomiting during pregnancy. Several controlled studies have evaluated the benefits of acupressure or acupuncture in the nausea and vomiting of pregnancy, commonly called morning sickness. The results for acupressure, though not for acupuncture, have generally been positive.

For example, a double-blind, placebo-controlled study of ninety-seven women found evidence that wristband acupressure may work. Participants wore either a real wristband or a phony one that appeared identical. Both real and fake acupressure caused noticeable improvement in more than one-half of the participants. However, women using the real wristband showed better results in terms of the duration of nausea. Intensity of the nausea symptoms was not significantly different between groups.

These results are consistent with other studies of acupressure for morning sickness, though two studies failed to find benefit for severe morning sickness. However, one large trial of acupuncture instead of acupressure failed to find benefit. This single-blind, placebo-controlled study of 593 pregnant women with morning sickness compared the effects of traditional acupuncture, acupuncture at P6 only, acupuncture at "wrong" points (sham acupuncture), and no treatment. As noted, the placebo effect of acupuncture is very strong. Women in all three treatment groups (including the fake acupuncture group) showed significant improvements in nausea and dry retching compared with the no-treatment group. However, neither form of real acupuncture proved markedly more effective than fake acupuncture.

Other forms of nausea. A single-blind, placebo-controlled study found acupressure helpful for motion sickness, though another, similar study did not. A single-blind, placebo-controlled trial of 104 people undergoing high-dose chemotherapy for breast cancer found that electrical stimulation on P6 significantly reduced episodes of vomiting. A small study in children receiving chemotherapy for a variety of cancers suggested that acupuncture may reduce the need for antinausea medication. Similar improvements were seen in four other studies of acupuncture or acupressure in persons undergoing chemotherapy or radiation. In a small sham-controlled study, acupressure wristbands showed promise, although the benefit seen just missed the conventional cutoff for statistical significance. However, equivocal or absent effectiveness was seen in three other studies of wristbands, and one study failed to find more benefit with real acupuncture than with fake acupuncture.

Tendonitis. Several small controlled studies have found acupuncture helpful for tendonitis. For example, a single-blind, placebo-controlled trial of fifty-two people with rotator cuff (shoulder) tendonitis found evidence that acupuncture is more effective than placebo. Benefits were also seen in four other studies of people with shoulder or elbow tendonitis. However, another study failed to find benefit.

In a sizable randomized trial, 425 persons receiving physical therapy for their persistent shoulder pain were divided into two groups: One group received single-point acupuncture while the other group received a sham treatment (mock transcutaneous electrical nerve stimulation) for three weeks. The acupuncture group showed significant improvement over the control group one week after treatment.

In a study of eighty-two people with elbow tendonitis, deep acupuncture was more effective than shallow acupuncture placebo in the short term, but by three months there was no difference between the groups. A comparative trial of twenty people found weak evidence that electroacupuncture may be more effective than ordinary acupuncture for elbow tendonitis. Two other trials failed to find laser acupuncture effective compared with either sham or other, similar treatments. Eight sessions of true acupuncture were no better than sham acupuncture in 123 persons treated for persistent arm pain caused by repetitive use.

A 2004 systematic review found five positive controlled studies on acupuncture for tennis elbow and concluded that "strong evidence" supports the use of acupuncture for this condition. However, this characterization of the evidence as "strong" would seem to be premature. For the reasons described in the beginning of this section, virtually all studies of acupuncture are single-blind, and such studies (except when performed on anesthetized patients) cannot exclude the possible effect of confidence conveyed by practitioners performing valid treatment, compared with lack of confidence conveyed by those delivering sham treatment.

Pregnancy support. As noted, acupuncture has shown some promise for reducing symptoms of morning sickness. This treatment has additionally been studied for aiding other aspects of pregnancy. However, the record is marred by poorly designed studies.

A well-controlled study of 210 women giving birth found that real acupuncture was more effective than sham acupuncture at reducing labor pain. Benefits were also seen in another well-controlled study. Two other studies of poorer quality also reported benefit. In one study, however, sterile water injections were found to be more effective than acupuncture for lower back pain and relaxation during labor. It is unclear whether or not the persons in the study knew what treatment they were receiving at the time. In one placebo-controlled trial and one review of ten mostly low quality trials, real acupuncture was no better than sham acupuncture in relieving pelvic pain during pregnancy before labor.

A study of forty-five pregnant women found that the use of acupuncture on the expected birth due date significantly sped up the actual date of delivery. However, this trial used a no-treatment control group instead of sham acupuncture. Another study that failed to use sham treatment found minimal evidence that the use of acupuncture may help

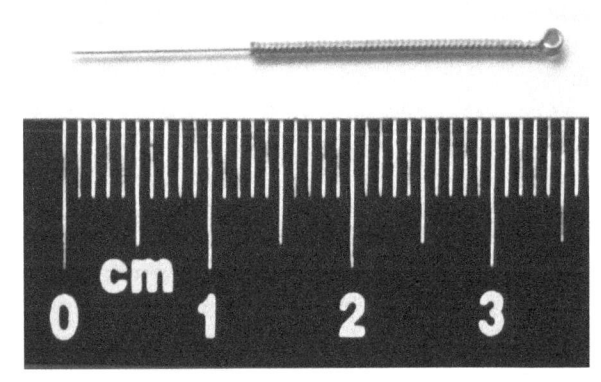

One type of acupuncture needle. (Xhienne via Wikimedia Commons)

stimulate normal term labor. A study of 106 women evaluated whether acupuncture can speed up delivery after prelabor rupture of membranes ("water breaking" too early) and failed to find benefit. However, again, no adequate control group was used; this is equally a problem for negative and for positive studies. Finally, in a placebo-controlled trial, real acupuncture administered for two days before a planned induction of labor (artificial stimulation of labor) was no better than sham acupuncture at preventing the need for induction or shortening the time of labor.

Acupuncture has also been studied for converting breech presentation of the unborn infant to normal positioning. In a study of 240 women at thirty-three to thirty-five weeks gestation, acupuncture combined with moxibustion caused the breech presentation to convert in 54 percent of women, while only 37 percent of women in the no-treatment control converted. Again, placebo acupuncture would have been better than no treatment. A much smaller study also found benefits with acupressure. In 2008, researchers published a review of six randomized-controlled trials that investigated acupuncture-like therapies (moxibustion, acupuncture, or electroacupuncture) applied to a specific point (BL67). They concluded that these therapies were effective at decreasing the incidence of breech presentations at the time of delivery. Again, however, not all of these studies employed a sham acupuncture group for comparison.

Osteoarthritis. Acupuncture has shown inconsistent benefit as a treatment for osteoarthritis. While the results of numerous smaller studies suggest that acupuncture is an effective treatment for osteoarthritis (of the knee, in particular), larger studies have generally found it be no more effective than sham acupuncture.

A 2006 meta-analysis (systematic statistical review) of studies on acupuncture for osteoarthritis found eight trials that were similar enough to be considered together. A total of 2,362 people were enrolled in these studies. The authors of the meta-analysis concluded that acupuncture should be regarded as an effective treatment for osteoarthritis.

However, one study comprised almost one-half of all the people considered in this meta-analysis, and it failed to find real acupuncture more effective than sham acupuncture. In this study, published in 2006, 1,007 people with knee osteoarthritis were given either real acupuncture, fake acupuncture, or standard therapy for six weeks. Though both real acupuncture and fake acupuncture were more effective than no acupuncture, there was no significant difference in benefits between the two acupuncture groups. In general, larger studies are more reliable than small ones. For this reason, it is always somewhat questionable when meta-analysis combines one very large negative study and a number of smaller positive ones to come up with a positive outcome.

Another review, published in 2007, concluded differently. It concluded that real acupuncture produces distinct benefits in osteoarthritis compared with no treatment, but that fake acupuncture is very effective for osteoarthritis too. When real acupuncture is compared with fake acupuncture, the difference in outcome, while it might possibly be statistically significant, is so trivial as to make no difference in real life. In other words, virtually all of the benefit of acupuncture for osteoarthritis is a placebo effect.

The apparent slight statistical difference between real and fake acupuncture could easily have been caused by problems of single-blind studies. Acupuncturists who know they are performing real acupuncture may subconsciously convey more confidence to their patients than those who know they are performing fake acupuncture. The history of medical studies makes it clear that such unconscious communications can greatly affect results; because the evidence shows only a minute difference between the results of real and fake acupuncture, it is quite possible that this transmission of confidence (or lack of it) is the entire cause of the difference, and that the specific techniques and theories of acupuncture themselves play no role.

Headache. Acupuncture has shown some promise for various types of headaches, including migraines and tension headaches; however, the research record remains mixed, and the best-designed studies have generally failed to find benefit. In a 2008 analysis of five randomized-controlled trials that were considered highest in quality, researchers determined that real acupuncture has limited benefit over sham acupuncture for tension headache. Subsequently, in a large randomized trial involving 3,182 headache patients, the group that received fifteen acupuncture sessions in three months experienced significantly fewer headache days and less pain compared with the group receiving usual care. However, there was no placebo group. While it is clear that many headache patients benefit from acupuncture, it remains unclear whether or not this presents more than a placebo effect.

Neck pain. A 2006 review of the literature found ten controlled studies of acupuncture for chronic neck pain. The pooled results suggest that acupuncture may be more effective than fake acupuncture, in the short term. However, overall the study quality was fairly low.

In a study of 177 people with chronic neck pain, fake acupuncture proved more effective than massage. In a pilot study, ten weeks of acupuncture combined with physical therapy appeared to be more effective than either acupuncture or physical therapy alone for chronic neck pain, in the short term. There has been some study of acupuncture for acute neck pain; however, in one of the best of these studies, the use of laser acupuncture failed to provide benefit for whiplash injuries.

Dental procedures. The evidence regarding acupuncture treatment of dental pain is mixed. A literature review published in 1998 identified four meaningful studies on acupuncture for reducing pain during dental procedures. Three of the studies found positive results, but the largest (with 110 participants) found no benefit. It was largely on the basis of this review that acupuncture was discussed in the media as a "proven" treatment for dental pain. However, these mixed results do not constitute proof. More recent studies have also shown mixed results. At present, therefore, the available evidence does not provide a reliable basis for concluding that acupuncture is effective for dental pain.

Chemical dependency. Although some animal studies suggest that ear acupuncture or electroacupuncture may have some benefits for chemical dependency, study results in humans have been mixed at best, with the largest studies reporting no benefits. For example, while benefits were seen in a much smaller single-blind trial, a single-blind, placebo-controlled trial that evaluated 620 cocaine-dependent adults found acupuncture no more effective than sham acupuncture or relaxation training. Similarly, a single-blind, placebo-controlled study enrolling 236 residential clients found no benefit for cocaine addiction from ear acupuncture. Finally, in a placebo-controlled trial involving 83 people addicted to drugs attending a methadone detoxification clinic, the addition of ear acupuncture did not improve withdrawal symptoms or cravings. Methadone, a relatively weak narcotic, is commonly used to treat narcotic addition over the long-term.

The situation is much the same for alcohol addiction. A single-blind, placebo-controlled study of 503 alcoholics failed to find evidence of benefit with three weeks of ear acupuncture. In addition, a ten-week, single-blind, placebo-controlled study of 72 alcoholics found no difference in drinking patterns or cravings between sham acupuncture and real acupuncture groups. There are two other small trials that also failed to find significant benefits. However, one single-blind trial of 54 people did find some evidence of improvement.

A single-blind, controlled trial of one hundred people with heroin addiction evaluated the potential benefits of ear acupuncture. However, a high dropout rate makes the results difficult to interpret.

In a meta-analysis of 12 placebo-controlled trials, acupuncture was not found more effective than sham acupuncture for smoking cessation. A more recent observer-blind, sham-controlled study of 330 adolescent smokers also found no benefit. While most addiction studies involve ear acupuncture, a randomized trial compared real versus sham acupuncture on body points. The study found no difference in quit rates, depression, or anxiety. One study found that acupuncture may not be effective on its own but may (in some unknown manner) increase the effectiveness of stop-smoking education. In this sham-controlled study of 141 adults, acupuncture plus education was twice as effective as sham acupuncture plus education and four times as effective as acupuncture alone. However, these benefits were seen only in the short term; at long-term follow-ups, the relative advantage of acupuncture disappeared.

Back pain. Research has not produced convincing evidence that acupuncture is effective for back pain. Many studies widely cited as providing such evidence were actually invalid because of a lack of a proper control group. People with back pain given acupuncture report benefits, but the problem is that people given fake acupuncture also experience benefits, often to a similar degree. In a review of twenty-three randomized trials involving more than six thousand persons with chronic low back pain, researchers concluded that acupuncture is more effective than no treatment for short-term pain relief, but there was no significant difference between the effects of true and sham acupuncture. Researchers also found that acupuncture can be a useful addition to conventional therapies.

A six-month patient-blind and observer-blind trial of 1,162 people with back pain compared real acupuncture, fake acupuncture, and conventional therapy. Both real and fake acupuncture proved to be twice as effective as conventional therapy according to the measures used. However, there was only a minimal difference between real and fake acupuncture. These results do not indicate that acupuncture is effective per se; rather, they show the significant power of acupuncture as placebo.

Similarly, in a single-blind, controlled study (using sham acupuncture and no treatment) of 298 people with chronic back pain, the use of real acupuncture failed to prove significantly more effective than sham acupuncture. Also, in a fairly large randomized trial involving 638 adults with chronic back pain, there was no difference in pain at one year in persons receiving real acupuncture compared with fake acupuncture (with neither group improving significantly over standard care). Both real and sham acupuncture were, however, associated with improved function at one year. Other studies enrolling more than three hundred people also failed to find benefit.

A trial compared the effects of acupuncture, massage, and education (such as videotapes on back care) in 262 people with chronic back pain in a ten-week period. The exact type of acupuncture and massage was left to practitioners, but only ten visits were permitted. At the ten-week point, evaluations showed benefit with massage but not with acupuncture. One year later, massage and education were nearly equivalent, and both were superior to acupuncture.

One small study found chiropractic spinal manipulation more effective than anti-inflammatory medication or acupuncture for low back pain. In another trial, acupressure-style massage was found to be more effective for back pain than Swedish massage. However, Swedish massage has not been proven effective for back pain, so this does not prove that acupressure-style massage is effective. Two single-blind, placebo-controlled trials, one with thirty participants and another with sixty, also failed to find evidence of benefit.

Two studies did find possible slight benefits with electrical acupuncture for chronic low back pain. An additional study found acupressure more effective than physical therapy for low back pain, and another found some potential benefit with electric acupuncture.

Low level laser therapy (LLLT) is a technique similar to electroacupuncture that uses precision laser energy instead of electricity conducted through a needle. In a detailed review of seven randomized trials, researchers were unable to draw any conclusions regarding the effectiveness of LLLT for nonspecific low back pain.

Several other studies have compared acupuncture with other treatments for back pain. Treatments such as transcutaneous electrical nerve stimulation (TENS), physical therapy, and chiropractic care were found equally effective. However, because TENS, physical therapy, and chiropractic care have not themselves been proven effective for back pain, studies of this type cannot be taken as evidence that acupuncture is effective. One study did find acupressure massage more effective than standard physical therapy; however, it was performed in a Chinese population that may have had more faith in this traditional approach than in physical therapy.

Stroke. Acupuncture is widely used in China for treatment of acute stroke. A few controlled studies have been published, but the best-designed and largest studies failed to find benefit.

For example, a single-blind, placebo-controlled trial of 104 people who had just experienced a stroke failed to find any benefit with ten weeks of twice-weekly acupuncture. Similarly, a single-blind, controlled study of 150 people recovering from stroke compared acupuncture (including electroacupuncture), high-intensity muscle stimulation, and sham treatment. All participants received twenty treatments for ten weeks. Neither acupuncture nor muscle stimulation produced any benefits. A ten-week study of 106 people that provided thirty-five traditional acupuncture sessions also failed to find benefit. Also, 92 persons who received either twelve acupuncture treatments or a comparable sham treatment demonstrated the same level of improvement up to one year later.

A few studies did find benefit, but they were very small, and some did not use a placebo group. One trial of sixty-two persons found that a three-week program of TENS of acupuncture points (beginning about nine days after stroke) improved muscle tone and strength in the affected leg. A large review including fifty-six mostly poor quality trials reported that acupuncture may benefit post-stroke rehabilitation (based on an analysis of thirty-eight trials), and another review of nine trials found limited evidence in support of moxibustion for stroke rehabilitation.

Surgery support. Acupuncture has been explored as a means of reducing pain after surgery with encouraging but not unequivocal results. A double-blind, placebo-controlled study of forty-two people undergoing arthroscopic knee surgery found that the use of acupuncture during surgery did not reduce pain levels during the subsequent twenty-four hours. Another double-blind, placebo-controlled trial of fifty women undergoing hysterectomy found no benefit with electroacupuncture, and a double-blind study of seventy-one people undergoing abdominal surgery failed to find acupressure helpful.

However, some benefits of acupressure were reported in a single-blind trial of forty persons undergoing arthroscopic knee surgery. In addition, a special form of needle insertion called intradermal acupuncture reduced postsurgical pain in 107 people undergoing abdominal surgery. Ear acupuncture has also shown promise. In a 2008 review of fifteen randomized-controlled trials, researchers determined that acupuncture is capable of reducing pain and the need for opioid medications (morphine and related agents) immediately following surgery compared with sham acupuncture.

Other studied uses. Bee venom acupuncture (BVA), which involves the injection of diluted bee venom directly into acupoints, has been used for the treatment of pain. An analysis of four well-designed, randomized trials, comparing bee venom plus classic acupuncture with saline injection plus classic acupuncture, found that the BVA-classic acupuncture combination was significantly more effective for musculoskeletal pain.

Acupressure and acupuncture have been tried for insomnia with mixed results. A single-blind, placebo-controlled study involving eighty-four residents of a nursing home found that real acupressure was superior to sham acupressure for improving sleep quality. Treated participants fell asleep faster and slept more soundly. In a similar study, researchers found that performing acupressure on a single point on both wrists for five weeks improved sleep quality among residents of long-term care facilities compared with lightly touching the same point. Another single-blind, controlled study reported benefits with acupuncture but failed to include a proper statistical analysis of the results. For this reason, no conclusions can be drawn from the report. In another trial, ninety-eight people with severe kidney disease were divided into three groups: no extra treatment, twelve sessions of fake acupressure (not using actual acupuncture points), and twelve sessions of real acupressure. Participants receiving real acupressure experienced significantly improved sleep compared with those receiving no extra treatment. However, fake acupressure was just as effective as real acupressure.

In a fourth randomized trial involving twenty-eight women, six weeks of auricular (outer ear) acupuncture was more effective than sham acupuncture. In one study, magnetic pearls used to stimulate acupuncture points in the ear seemed to show some benefit compared with nonmagnetic stimulation of ear points. A small, single-blind, placebo-controlled study of sixty adults with primary insomnia found that three weeks of electroacupuncture improved sleep efficiency and decreased wake time after sleep onset.

One small, double-blind, placebo-controlled study found real acupuncture more effective than sham acupuncture for menstrual pain. (This study used nonacupuncturists who were given real or fake acupuncture protocols to apply, but they did not know which they were applying.) In addition, a controlled study of sixty-one women evaluated the effects of a special garment designed to stimulate acupuncture points related to menstrual pain. In this latter study, researchers chose to compare treatment to no treatment, rather than to sham treatment. For this reason, the results (which were positive) mean little. In another trial, a seed-pressure method of auricular acupressure appeared to improve menstrual pain compared with sham auricular acupressure in seventy-four women. The potentially inadequate blinding of participants in this study, however, may have limited these results. Indeed, in a review of thirty controlled trials on menstrual pain, researchers were unable to draw conclusions about the effectiveness of acupuncture and similar treatments for menstrual pain because of widespread study design problems. Also, a review of twenty-seven trials with 2,960 persons concluded that acupuncture might be more effective than medications or herbs for relieving menstrual pain, but the studies were of limited quality.

Although anesthesia apparently performed entirely with acupuncture first raised Western interest in acupuncture, the original demonstrations of acupuncture anesthesia have been discredited. It now appears that if acupuncture has any anesthetic effect, that effect is extremely modest. At most, acupuncture may be capable of slightly decreasing the required dose of general anesthetic necessary to induce anesthesia (but even this has not been consistently seen in studies).

A six-month, single-blind, controlled study of sixty-seven women with frequent bladder infections found that acupuncture therapy reduced the frequency of infection. Another study found that acupuncture may be helpful for hyperactive bladder (the frequent need to urinate but without the presence of an infection to cause the need).

A study of fifty-two people with allergic rhinitis (hay fever) found that acupuncture plus traditional Chinese herbal treatment was slightly more effective than fake acupuncture plus fake Chinese herbal treatment. However, another study failed to find acupuncture alone beneficial for allergic rhinitis. Moreover, a carefully conducted review of seven placebo-controlled trials failed to find convincing evidence for acupuncture's effectiveness against allergic rhinitis.

A Chinese study found that acupuncture plus moxibustion was more effective for Bell's palsy than was drug treatment. In a review of six studies involving 537 persons with Bell's palsy, researchers could draw no conclusions about the beneficial effects of acupuncture because of poor study quality.

Five small, controlled studies reported that acupuncture can improve menopausal symptoms, but most of these studies had significant problems in design or statistical analysis. Two additional trials failed to find acupuncture beneficial for hot flashes. One trial of 175 perimenopausal and postmenopausal women concluded that adding acupuncture to usual care reduced hot flash frequency compared with usual care alone in the first four weeks after treatment. However, another fairly large randomized trial involving 267 postmenopausal women found that while the addition of acupuncture to self-care advice significantly reduced the frequency and intensity of hot flashes in the first twelve weeks, the benefits were lost six months later. A 2009 review of six trials found that true acupuncture was no more effective than sham acupuncture for this indication. Finally, one small study found no benefit for the psychological distress associated with menopause.

Another small, placebo-controlled study in women with breast cancer who also had hot flashes caused by their treatments suggested some benefit for acupuncture, though the results were inconclusive for similar reasons. However, another study did not find acupuncture effective in these women, and a 2008 review of all existing studies on the subject concluded that the evidence does not support a beneficial effect for acupuncture in women with breast cancer who have hot flashes.

Acupuncture has been studied for use in cancer treatment support. In a small randomized trial of forty-three women with breast cancer, six weeks of acupuncture twice-weekly reduced joint pain attributed to aromatase-inhibitor therapy. Another small randomized trial of seventy persons found that acupuncture may decrease xerostomia and pain after neck dissection for cancer treatment.

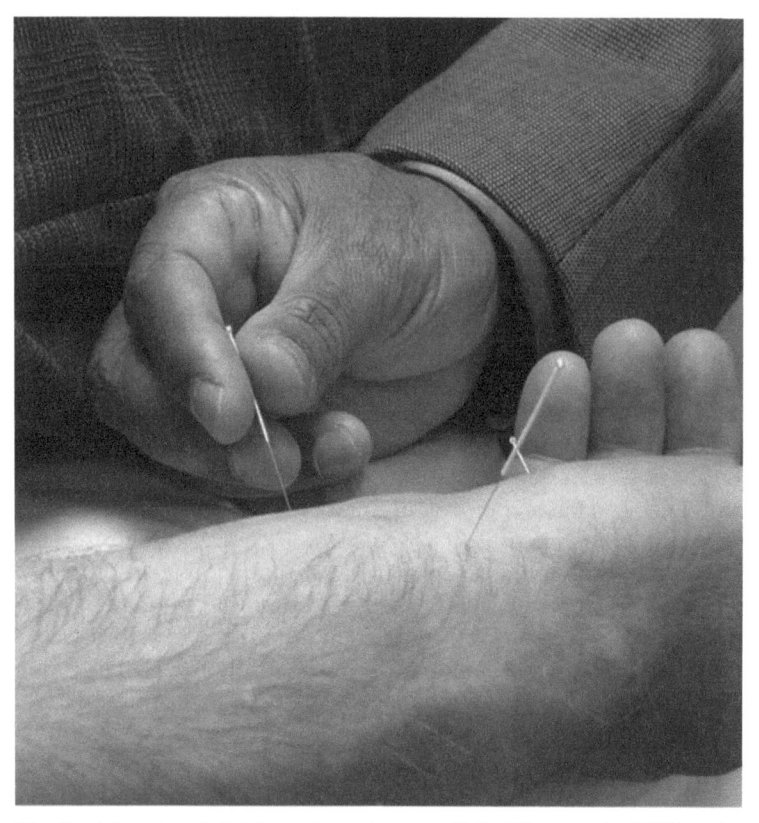

Needles being inserted into a person's arm. (Kyle Hunter via Wikimedia Commons)

A 2006 review of acupuncture for treatment of fibromyalgia found five controlled studies, none of which were of high quality. The authors of another review of seven trials could not determine the effectiveness of acupuncture for fibromyalgia because of the unreliability of the studies. Overall, the results do not provide reliable evidence that acupuncture is helpful.

Evidence for acupuncture's effectiveness for depression has been mixed. In a study of 151 depressed persons, twelve sessions of acupuncture failed to prove more effective than fake acupuncture. However, another sham-acupuncture controlled trial evaluated 43 people with depression and 13 people with generalized anxiety disorder. The results suggest that ten (but not five) acupuncture sessions can significantly improve symptoms.

One study of eight persons with major depressive disorder found that adding acupuncture to a lower dose of antidepressant (fluoxetine) improved anxiety and had an overall therapeutic effect similar to sham acupuncture with a higher dose of antidepressant. In a mathematical review of the results of eight randomized trials, the impact of acupuncture on depression was unconvincing. However, in another review of twenty trials involving two thousand persons with major depression, real acupuncture's effectiveness was comparable to that of antidepressants but no greater than that of sham acupuncture for this population.

Another trial compared real and sham ear acupuncture in healthy people and found some evidence that real acupuncture can relieve normal daily stress. A 2010 review of nine mostly poor quality trials determined that there is insufficient evidence to conclude that acupuncture is effective for premenstrual syndrome.

Although open trials appeared to show benefit, a minimum of three controlled studies failed to find acupuncture helpful for improving the success rate of in vitro fertilization (IVF). A 2008 analysis of seven randomized trials found that, on balance, acupuncture may significantly improve the odds of pregnancy in women undergoing IVF. However, because not all of these studies used sham acupuncture as a control, the reliability of this conclusion is questionable. Moreover, a second analysis in the same year of thirteen randomized-controlled trials investigating the effectiveness of acupuncture in 2,500 women undergoing a specialized IVF procedure, in which sperm is injected directly into the egg, found no evidence of any benefit. However, the story does not end here. In a subsequent review of thirteen trials, a different group of researchers concluded that acupuncture may improve the success rate of IVF, but only if it is used on the day of embryo transfer (when the fertilized egg is placed into the womb). According to this study, acupuncture is not effective when used up to three days after embryo transfer or when eggs are being retrieved from the ovaries.

Acupuncture may be more effective than sham acupuncture and as effective as standard treatments for temporomandibular joint (TMJ) pain. One study of 110 people with pain found acupuncture at least as effective as standard occlusal splint therapy. Another small study involving forty persons with TMJ pain, however, found no difference between placebo and low-level laser therapy (LLLT) directed at painful points; both groups benefitted equally. However, in a double-blind, randomized trial comparing real LLLT with sham LLLT, the real therapy was more effective for TMJ pain after eight sessions. Instead of needles, LLLT involves the use of laser energy directed on or off acupuncture points.

A single-blind trial tested acupuncture on a group of thirty-six healthy young men and found some evidence of improvement in sports performance. However, a single-blind, controlled study of forty-eight people found that the use of acupuncture did not reduce muscle soreness caused by exercise.

One study purportedly found that acupressure reduced fatigue in people with severe kidney disease. In fact, it found that both sham acupuncture and real acupuncture reduced fatigue compared with no treatment, but that real acupuncture was not more effective than fake acupuncture.

One study found minimal benefits for Parkinson's disease. Another study failed to find any benefits. In two comprehensive reviews of multiple clinical trials, independent sets of researchers concluded that there was no well-established evidence for acupuncture's effectiveness in this condition.

People with cancer often experience fatigue. Acupuncture has shown a bit of promise for improving this symptom. A Chinese study reported that acupuncture is helpful for vocal cord dysfunction.

A study that reported acupuncture's benefits for chronic prostatitis failed to use a control group and is, therefore, meaningless. However, another study found that real acupuncture was more effective than sham acupuncture at reducing the symptoms of chronic prostatitis both during treatment and for six months after treatment. Another study suggested that electroacupuncture may improve symptoms in men with chronic prostatitis (or a related condition called chronic pelvic pain syndrome), but this study was very small.

After an acute attack of shingles, pain may linger for months or years, causing what is known as postherpetic neuralgia. A single-blind, placebo-controlled study of sixty-two people with pain of this type failed to find any benefit with acupuncture. Two separate groups of researchers conducting detailed reviews of eight randomized controlled trials found some beneficial effects of acupuncture for rheumatoid arthritis, but they were unconvinced that it was more beneficial than sham acupuncture or other standard treatments. There have been numerous reports about acupuncture treatment for asthma, but most published studies are of low quality, with results being contradictory at best. One study failed to find acupuncture helpful for shortness of breath associated with advanced cancer.

Peripheral neuropathy (nerve pain in the extremities) is a common complaint for those with human immunodeficiency virus (HIV) infection. A placebo-controlled trial of 239 people with HIV found acupuncture no more effective than placebo in peripheral neuropathy. The study also tested drug therapy for peripheral neuropathy and also found it ineffective.

A substantial study (192 participants) failed to find acupuncture more helpful than fake acupuncture for high blood pressure. However, another study, this one enrolling 160 people, did report benefit. A much smaller study also reported benefits, but there were problems in its statistical analysis. In a review of eleven randomized-controlled trials on the subject, researchers determined that acupuncture's ability to lower blood pressure remains inconclusive.

Acupuncture is probably not effective for epilepsy. A single-blind, controlled trial of individualized acupuncture for thirty-four people with severe epilepsy found no benefit, and subsequently, a comprehensive review of eleven studies found no reliable evidence of its effectiveness.

One controlled study failed to find electroacupuncture effective for reducing discomfort during colonoscopy. A controlled study purportedly found acupuncture helpful for speeding recovery in people with spinal cord injuries, but it failed to use a sham-acupuncture control group. Several controlled and open trials of acupuncture for tinnitus (ringing in the ear) found no benefit.

A well-designed, single-blind, placebo-controlled study of sixty people with irritable bowel syndrome (IBS) compared traditional acupuncture to sham acupuncture. In the thirteen-week study period, both groups improved to the same extent. A larger trial of 230 adults with IBS found that acupuncture (six treatments in three weeks) was not associated with improved symptoms or severity compared with sham acupuncture. Two smaller studies have also failed to find acupuncture more effective than placebo acupuncture.

In a placebo-controlled trial, sixty nursing women received needle acupuncture, fifty-six women received laser acupuncture, and sixty women received placebo acupuncture. The results showed no differences in milk production. In one small study, light needling at one acupuncture point on both hands was more effective than no needling among forty infants with colic.

What to Expect During Treatment
Acupuncture therapy has its own style and atmosphere, both like and unlike an ordinary medical encounter. The first session will begin with a thorough analysis of the condition and the patient's health history. If the acupuncturist practices according to the principles of TCM, the patient will be asked a number of questions about his or her specific complaint and general health, including how well he or she sleeps, digests food, eliminates, and breathes, and about the level of his or her energy. All of these factors are considered relevant. The acupuncturist may ask questions that seem to have little bearing on the patient's condition, questions such as whether or not the patient feels cold or hot most of the time. TCM looks for overall patterns in both physical and emotional well-being, which guide the acupuncturist in developing a treatment plan that is specific not only for the patient's symptoms but also for the patient's overall health pattern.

Depending on the specific complaint and on the patient's individual symptom pattern, the acupuncturist may use only a few needles or as many as twenty or more. Acupuncture needle sizes are typically 32- to 36-gauge, which means they are about one-quarter millimeter in diameter, much smaller than a hypodermic needle. Unlike hollow hypodermic needles, acupuncture needles are solid, which allows them to penetrate the skin easily and relatively painlessly. Acupuncture needles may produce a mild pricking sensation when inserted, but sometimes nothing is felt at insertion. The needles are generally inserted to a depth ranging from a few millimeters to one-half inch. Insertion depth is greater at the more fleshy areas of the body, such as the thighs and buttocks.

Acupuncture needles are typically inserted through a plastic tube that guides the needle into the skin. This is a fairly modern needle insertion technique. Traditional freehand insertion is also used; most acupuncturists are trained in this method. Virtually all acupuncturists in the United States now use sterilized, one-time-use disposable needles, which eliminate any risk of cross-infection.

The acupuncturist may twirl the inserted needles and ask the patient to indicate when he or she feels a mild, achy, heavy sensation or when the area may feel slightly numb or tingly. These sensations, described in TCM as the arrival of qi, are regarded as a positive response that will enhance the effectiveness of the treatment.

Whatever the sensation, it should be mild, should not be overly unpleasant, and should subside within a few minutes. If any needles are genuinely painful, one should inform the practitioner so he or she can adjust the depth or remove the needle altogether. The needles are generally left in place for twenty to thirty minutes. During this time, the patient should feel comfortable and relaxed and may fall asleep.

Acupuncturists may also employ a technique known as electroacupuncture, in which electrodes are attached to the needles and a mild current is applied. This is intended to increase the stimulation of the needle and is generally used for more painful conditions. Electroacupuncture produces a tingly, pulsating sensation. The acupuncturist can control the intensity and adjust it to a level that is comfortable.

Traditionally trained acupuncturists often use needles and heat to stimulate acupuncture points with a procedure called moxibustion, which involves a mixture of herbs rolled into a cigar-like shape. The roll is lit, and the burning end is held over the skin, allowing the heat to penetrate the area around the acupressure point. The moxa roll never touches the skin, so the patient will not be burned. The acupuncturist will ask the patient to inform him or her know before the moxa gets too hot. Moxibustion is generally quite pleasant. It is regarded as a "tonifying" treatment, which means it is intended to strengthen function.

Choosing a Practitioner

Acupuncture is a licensed health profession in the United States in thirty-nine states and the District of Columbia. Most states require at least three years of training at an accredited school of acupuncture and passage of a national board certification examination administered by the National Certification Commission for Acupuncture and Oriental Medicine. Most states grant the title licensed acupuncturist, certified acupuncturist, registered acupuncturist, or simply acupuncturist upon certification. A few states allow acupuncturists who have a doctorate from an approved or accredited college to use the title doctor of Oriental medicine (D.O.M.) or Oriental medical doctor (O.M.D.).

In most states, medical doctors can practice acupuncture with no training; in many states, chiropractors may practice acupuncture with one hundred or fewer hours of training. Approximately one-third of the states that license acupuncturists require their clients to have a referral from a Western medical practitioner (a medical doctor, osteopath, chiropractor, or dentist) before or in conjunction with acupuncture treatment. In the remaining states, acupuncturists may accept persons for treatment without prior referral.

Training programs have become fairly standardized, so an acupuncturist with qualifications in one state has essentially the same training as those certified in other states. If a prospective patient is in a state that does not license acupuncturists, he or she should ask to see evidence that the acupuncturist has completed a minimum of three years of training at an accredited institution. One can check with the state's medical board for the exact licensure title and requirements.

Safety Issues

Serious adverse effects associated with the use of acupuncture are rare. The most commonly reported problems include short-term pain from needle insertion, tiredness, and minor bleeding. There is one report of infection caused by acupuncture given to a person with diabetes.

Some acupuncture points lie over the lungs, so insertion to an excessive depth could conceivably cause a pneumothorax (punctured lung). Because acupuncturists are trained to avoid this complication, it is a rare occurrence.

A report from China contained an example of another complication caused by excessively deep needling. A forty-four-year-old man was needled on the back of the neck at a commonly used acupuncture point just below the bony protuberance at the base of the skull. However, the acupuncturist inserted the needle too deeply and punctured a blood vessel in the skull. The client developed a severe headache with nausea and vomiting; a scan showed bleeding in the brain, and a spinal tap found a small amount of blood in the cerebrospinal fluid. The severe headache, along with neck stiffness, continued for twenty-eight days. The man was treated with standard pain medication, and the condition resolved itself without any permanent effects. Also, infection caused by the use of unclean needles has been reported, but the modern practice of using disposable sterile needles appears to have eliminated this risk.

—*EBSCO CAM Review Board*

References

Chen, Yan-Jiao, et al. "What Is the Appropriate Acupuncture Treatment Schedule for Chronic Pain? Review and Analysis of Randomized Controlled Trials." *Evidence-Based Complementary and Alternative Medicine,* 18 June 2019, pp. 1–10., doi:10.1155/2019/5281039.

Devitt, Michael. "Research Finds Acupuncture Effective for Chronic Pain." *American Academy of Family Physicians,* 21 May 2018, www.aafp.org/news/health-of-the-public/20180521acupuncture.html.

Filshie, Jacqueline, et al. *Medical Acupuncture: a Western Scientific Approach.* 2nd ed., Elsevier, 2016.

Ning, Zhipeng, and Lixing Lao. "Acupuncture for Pain Management in Evidence-Based Medicine." *Journal of Acupuncture and Meridian Studies,* vol. 8, no. 5, 2015, pp. 270–273., doi:10.1016/j.jams.2015.07.012.

Swanberg, Sarah. *A Patient's Guide to Acupuncture: Everything You Need to Know.* Althea Press, 2019.

Xiang, Anfeng, et al. "The Immediate Analgesic Effect of Acupuncture for Pain: A Systematic Review and Meta-Analysis." *Evidence-Based Complementary and Alternative Medicine,* 25 Oct. 2017, pp. 1–13., doi:10.1155/2017/3837194.

Yang, Ziyi, et al. "The Effectiveness of Acupuncture for Chronic Pain with Depression." *Medicine,* vol. 96, no. 47, 27 Nov. 2017, doi:10.1097/md.0000000000008800.

Biofeedback

CATEGORY: Therapy or Technique
ANATOMY OR SYSTEM AFFECTED: All
SPECIALTIES AND RELATED FIELDS: Alternative medicine, cardiology, exercise physiology, family medicine, internal medicine, neurology, occupational health, physical therapy, preventive medicine, psychology, sports medicine, vascular medicine

KEY TERMS

- *biodisplay*: audio or visual information about the physiological activity within an organism displayed by various instruments and processes
- *biofeedback*: the provision of information about the biological or physiological processes of an individual to him or her, with the objective of empowering the individual to make conscious changes in the processes being monitored; it can be instrumental (using devices that monitor physiological or biological processes) or noninstrumental (using bodily sensations)
- *biofeedback instrument*: a device (usually electronic) that is capable of measuring and displaying information about a physiologic process in a way that allows an individual to monitor the physiologic activity through his or her own senses
- *electrodermal response (EDR) biofeedback*: the monitoring and displaying of information about the conductivity of the skin; used for anxiety reduction, asthma treatment, and the treatment of sleep disorders
- *electroencephalographic (EEG) biofeedback*: the monitoring and displaying of brain wave activity; used for the treatment of substance abuse disorders, epilepsy, attention-deficit disorders, and insomnia
- *electromyograph* (EMG): an instrument that is capable of monitoring and displaying information about electro-chemical activity in a group of muscle fibers
- *neuromuscular rehabilitation*: the process of employing electromyographic biofeedback to correct physiological disorders that have both muscular and neurological components, such as the effects of strokes and fibromyalgia; also called myoneural rehabilitation
- *physiological autoregulation*: the process by which an individual utilizes information about a physiological activity to effect changes in that activity in a direction that contributes to normal (or desirable) functioning

Indications and Procedures

Biofeedback has been utilized in both research and clinical applications. The term itself denotes the provision of information (feedback) about a biological process. It has been found that individuals (laboratory animals included), when given feedback that is reinforcing, are able to change physiological processes in a desired direction; homeostatic processes being what they are, these changes are in a positive direction. In the case of humans, the feedback is provided about a physiological function of which the individual would not otherwise be aware were it not for the provision via a biodisplay-of information about that process.

Human maladies range from the purely structural to the purely functional, with various gradations. An example of a structural disorder is a broken bone, while an example of a functional disorder might be a person who manifests symptoms of blindness for which there is no known or identifiable organic cause. Looking at the spectrum of human maladies, one can consider the continuum as "structural," "psychophysiological," "mental-emotional," "hysterical," and "feigned." The category of psychophysiological lies midway between structural and mental-emotional. A psychophysiological disorder has elements of both mind and body interactions; it is a physiological disorder brought about by thoughts, feelings, and emotions. There are those who take the position that all human maladies and disorders have a mental-emotional component to them, that there can be no change in the mental-emotional state without a corresponding change in the physiological state and no change in the physiological state without a corresponding change in the mental-emotional state.

It is currently the preference of many scientifically and technologically oriented practitioners to deal with the more structural disorders (or to treat the disorder as if it were mostly structural). It is also the case that many mental health practitioners prefer to deal with disorders that fall more into the mental-emotional category. A growing number of practitioners, however, have an interest in and training for dealing with psychophysiological disorders. This emerging field is referred to as behavioral medicine, and a large percentage of the practitioners in this field employ biofeedback as a modality.

A classic example of biofeedback being used to correct a physiological problem would be the employing of electromyograph (EMG) biofeedback for the correction of a simple tension (or psychophysiologic) headache. The headache is caused by inappropriately high muscle tension in the neck, head, or shoulders. In surface electromyographic biofeedback, the biofeedback practitioner attaches electronic sensors to the muscles of the forehead, neck, or shoulders of the patient. The electronic sensors pick up signals from electrochemical activity at the surface of the skin in the area of the involved muscle groups. The behavior of the muscles being monitored is such that minute changes in the electrochemical activity in the muscles-tension and relaxation-occur naturally.

The sensitivity of the biofeedback instrument (the magnification of the signal may be as high as one thousand times) and the display of the signal make the individual aware of these changes via sound or visual signals (biodisplays). When the biofeedback signal indicates that the muscle activity is in the direction of relaxation, the individual makes an association between that muscle behavior and the corresponding change in the strength of the signal. The individual can then increase the duration, strength, and frequency of the relaxation process. Having learned to relax the involved muscles, the individual is able to prevent or abort headache activity.

It is axiomatic that any physiological process (behavior) that is capable of being quantified, measured, and displayed is appropriate for biofeedback applications. The following are some of the more commonly used biofeedback instruments.

An electromyograph is an instrument that is capable of monitoring and displaying information about electrochemical activity in a group of muscle fibers. Common applications of surface electromyography (in which sensors are placed on the surface of the skin, as opposed to the insertion of needles into the muscle itself) include stroke rehabilitation. Surface electromyography is also used in the treatment of tension headaches and fibromyalgia.

An galvanic skin or electrodermal response (EDR) biofeedback instrument is capable of monitoring and displaying information about the conductivity of the skin. An increase in the conductivity of the skin is a function of moisture accumulating in the space recently occupied by blood. The rate of blood flow depends on the amount of autonomic nervous system arousal present within the organism at the time of measurement. The higher the level of autonomic nervous system arousal, the greater the amount of skin conductivity. Common applications of EDR biofeedback are the reduction of anxiety caused by phobic reactions, the control of asthma (especially in young children), and the treatment of sleep disorders. For example, many insomniacs are unable to drop off to sleep because of higher-than-appropriate autonomic nervous system activity.

An instrument that is capable of monitoring and displaying the surface temperature of the skin, as correlated with an increase in vascular (blood flow) activity in the area of the skin in question, can also be used for biofeedback. Such an instrument is helpful in treatment for high blood pressure and migraine headaches.

Electroencephalographic (EEG) biofeedback involves the monitoring and displaying of brain wave activity as a correlate of autonomic nervous system activity. Different brain waves are associated with different levels of autonomic nervous system arousal. Common applications of EEG biofeedback are in the treatment of substance abuse disorders, epilepsy, attention-deficit disorders, and insomnia.

Heart rate variability (HRV) biofeedback monitors and displays the changing intervals between heart beats. Studies have indicated that HRV biofeedback may be beneficial in treating cardiovascular, respiratory, and emotional conditions.

Uses and Complications

Biofeedback is gaining in popularity because of a number of factors. One of the principal reasons is a growing interest in alternatives to the lifetime use of medications to manage a disorder.

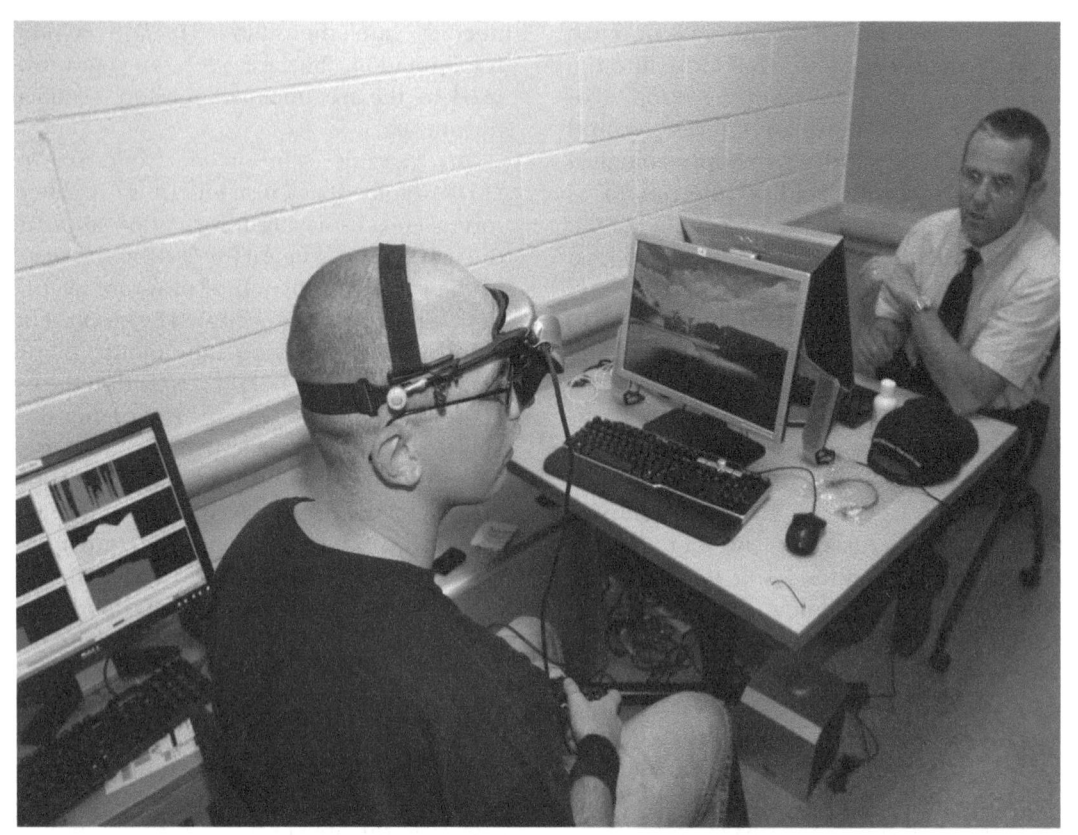

Through a DoD grant, Dr. Carmen Russoniello of East Carolina University is working toward a portable biofeedback training program that could prevent or reduce post-traumatic stress symptoms. (Photo by Dr. Carmen Russoniello)

To understand the rationale for biofeedback in a clinical setting, it is essential to discuss the types of disorders for which it is commonly employed. As pointed out in the National Institute of Mental Health's publication *Biofeedback*, the more common usages of biofeedback treatment techniques include "migraine headaches, tension headaches, and many other types of pain; disorders of the digestive system; high blood pressure and its opposite, low blood pressure; cardiac arrhythmias (abnormalities, sometimes dangerous, in the rhythm of the heartbeat); Raynaud's disease (a circulatory disorder that causes uncomfortably cold hands); epilepsy; paralysis and other movement disorders."

Thus, biofeedback can be safely and effectively employed in the alleviation of numerous disorders. One example worth noting-in terms of the magnitude of the problem-is the treatment of cardiovascular disorders. Myocardial infarctions, commonly known as heart attacks, are one of the major health problems in the industrialized world and an area of special concern to those practitioners with a psychophysiological orientation.

One of the principal causes of heart attacks is hypertension (high blood pressure). Emotions have much to do with the manifestation of high blood pressure (hypertension), which places this condition in the category of a psychophysiological disorder. Researchers have demonstrated that biofeedback is an effective methodology to correct the problem of high blood pressure. The data reveal that many individuals employing biofeedback have been able to decrease (or eliminate entirely) the use of medication to manage their hypertension. Studies also show that these individuals maintain normal blood pressure levels for as long as two years following the completion of biofeedback training.

Because of its noninvasive properties and its broad applicability in the clinical setting, biofeedback is also increasingly becoming one of the more commonly utilized modalities in many fields, such as behavioral medicine. Researchers have provided documented evidence showing that biofeedback is effective in the treatment of so-called stress-related disorders. Research has also shown that biofeedback has beneficial applications in the areas of neuromuscular rehabilitation (working with stroke victims to help them develop greater control and use of afflicted muscle groups) and myoneural rehabilitation (working with victims of fibromyalgia and chronic pain to help them obtain relief from debilitating pain).

Research in the 1960s pointed to the applicability of EEG biofeedback for seizure disorders, such as epilepsy. Advanced technology and later research findings have demonstrated EEG biofeedback to be effective in the treatment of attention-deficit disorder, hyperactivity, and alcoholism as well.

Biofeedback appears to have particular applicability for children. Apparently, there is an innate ability on the part of the young to learn self-regulation skills, such as the lowering of autonomic nervous system activity, much more quickly than older persons. Since this activity is highly correlated with respiratory distress, biofeedback is often used in the treatment of asthma in prepubescent children. Biofeedback is also being successfully used as an alternative to prescription medications (such as Ritalin) for youngsters with attention-deficit disorder.

The use of biofeedback is also found in the field of athletics and human performance. Sports psychologists and athletic coaches have long recognized that there is an inverted U pattern of performance where autonomic nervous system activity and performance are concerned. In the field of sports psychology, this is known as the Yerkes-Dobson law. The tenets of this law state that as the level of autonomic nervous system arousal rises, performance will improve-but only to a point. When autonomic nervous system arousal becomes too high, a corresponding deterioration in performance occurs. At some point prior to an athletic competition, it may be desirable for an athlete to experience an increase (or a decrease) in the level of autonomic nervous system activity (the production of adrenaline, for example). Should adrenaline levels become too high, however, the athlete may "choke" or become tense.

To achieve physiological autoregulation (often referred to in this athletic context as "self-regulation"), athletes have used biofeedback to assist them with establishing better control of a variety of physiologic processes. Biofeedback applications have ranged from hand-warming techniques for cross-country skiers and mountain climbers to the regulation of heartbeat for sharpshooters, such as biathletes and archers, to the lowering of adrenaline levels for ice-skaters, gymnasts, and divers.

Biofeedback, apart from empirical studies or research on both animal and human subjects, is seldom used in isolation. In most treatment protocols, it is employed in combination with such interventions as behavioral management, lifestyle counseling, exercise, posture awareness, and nutritional considerations. In most biofeedback applications, the individual is also taught a number of procedures that he or she is encouraged to use between therapy sessions. The conscientious and effective practice of these recommended procedures has been proven to be a determining factor in the success rate of biofeedback. The end aim of biofeedback is self-regulation, and self-regulation must extend to situations outside the clinical setting.

Biofeedback (when employed as a part of a behavioral medicine program) is usually offered as a component of a treatment team approach. The biofeedback practitioner commonly interfaces with members of other disciplines to design and implement a treatment protocol to correct the presenting problem (for example, fibromyalgia) for which the referral was made.

One commonly found model of biofeedback is for the patient, the biofeedback practitioner, and the primary medical care provider to constitute a team. The team concept applies even to the extent that the biofeedback practitioner (in many ways acting as a coach) will give the patient a number of procedures to follow between treatment sessions and will then evaluate, with the patient and the medical practitioner, the effectiveness of the procedure. Modifications in the modalities and in the interventions follow from these evaluations. Biofeedback interventions are dynamic and measurable so that the effectiveness of the protocol can be adjusted to meet the needs of the patient.

Perspective and Prospects

Biofeedback, as a treatment modality, is relatively new. The history of biofeedback as a research tool, however, dates back to early attempts to quantify physiological processes. From the time of Ivan

Pavlov and his research on the salivary processes in canines, both psychologists and physiologists have long been interested in the measurement of human behavior (including physiological processes).

Early in the twentieth century, the work of Walter B. Cannon, with his book *The Wisdom of the Body* (1932), helped to set the stage for the field of self-regulation. Another landmark was the 1929 publication of Edmund Jacobson's *Progressive Relaxation*. More recently, the work of such pioneers as John V. Basmajian, Neal Miller, Elmer Green, Joseph Kamiya, and many others spawned research and development efforts that by 1975 produced more than twenty-five hundred literature references utilizing biofeedback as a part of a study.

The evolution of biofeedback as a treatment modality has its historical roots in early research in the areas of learning theory, psychophysiology, behavior modification, stress reactivity, electronics technology, and biomedical engineering. The emerging awareness-and acceptance by the general public-that individuals do in fact have the potential to promote their own wellness and to facilitate the healing process gave additional impetus to the development of both the theory and the technology of biofeedback treatment. Several other factors have combined to produce the climate within which biofeedback has gained recognition and acceptance. One of these was widespread recognition that many of the disorders that afflict humankind have, as a common basis, some disruption of the natural feedback processes. Part of this recognition is attributable to the seminal work of Hans Selye on stress reactivity.

Developments in the fields of electronics, physiology, psychology, endocrinology, and learning theory produced a body of knowledge that spawned the evolution and growth of biofeedback. Further refinement and an explosion of technology have resulted in procedures and techniques that have set the stage for the use of biofeedback as an effective intervention with wide applications in the treatment of numerous disorders.

A number of devices have been designed for home biofeedback use. Some are computer-based while others are stand-alone, handheld devices. Consumers interested in such equipment should consult with their biofeedback team regarding the safety and reputability of the products under consideration.

A new version of biofeedback has promising hope for people with brain damage due to injury, paralysis, or stroke. Known as "neuroprosthetics," "nanobiotechnology," or occasionally, "brain interface chips," this technology is in the early stages of research but is enabling people to control machinery with their thoughts.

Some research and clinical trial studies have shown that quadriplegic people can learn to operate a computer, manipulate a robotic arm, or play video games through the use of an implanted electrode. Signals from the chip are sent to an analog-to-digital converter, which processes the simultaneous firings of neurons into digital data. For example, if a person thinks about turning off a computer, the analog information translates this into an actual motion, controlling the cursor on the computer screen. Other research has utilized noninvasive methods of assimilating neuronal activity. In some research studies, quadriplegic persons and persons with no neuromuscular impairment could control a cursor by controlling their EEG patterns. Participants are able to do this by learning to identify, over time, feedback from brain-wave activity.

Both electrode implants and EEG methods have their positives and negatives. EEGs are a bit cumbersome, due to the wires and electronic equipment; however, wireless EEG technology in the future may be possible. Implanted electrodes may provide more precise information, but this approach requires surgery and is expensive and potentially risky.

Neither method directly affects actual movement; that is, it does not read minds but instead enables the mind to act directly on an external object. The futuristic prospect of controlling machinery with thoughts has many psychological, medical, and ethical implications that will need to be uncovered as research progresses.

—*Ronald B. France, Ph.D.*
—*LeAnna DeAngelo, Ph.D.*

References

"Biofeedback Glossary." *Association for Applied Psychophysiology and Biofeedback*, 2011, www.aapb.org/i4a/pages/index.cfm?pageid=3462.

Del Pozo, Jessica. "Biofeedback." *Institute for Chronic Pain*, 2017, www.instituteforchronicpain.org/treating-common-pain/what-is-pain-management/biofeedback.

Giggins, Oonagh M, et al. "Biofeedback in Rehabilitation." *Journal of NeuroEngineering and Rehabilitation*, vol. 10, no. 60, 18 June 2013, doi:10.1186/1743-0003-10-60.

Lee, Courtney, et al. "Mind–Body Therapies for the Self-Management of Chronic Pain Symptoms." *Pain Medicine*, vol. 15, no. S1, Apr. 2014, pp. S21–S39., doi:10.1111/pme.12383.

Schwartz, Mark S., and Frank Andrasik. *Biofeedback: a Practitioner's Guide*. 4th ed., The Guilford Press, 2017.

Sielski, Robert, et al. "Efficacy of Biofeedback in Chronic Back Pain: a Meta-Analysis." *International Journal of Behavioral Medicine*, vol. 24, no. 1, Feb. 2017, pp. 25–41., doi:10.1007/s12529-016-9572-9.

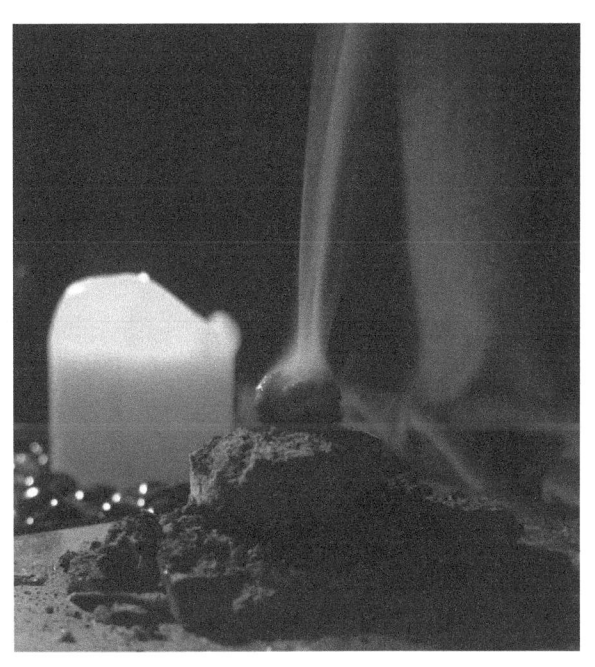

Indirect burning of frankincense on a hot coal. (Spacebirdy via Wikimedia Commons)

■ Boswellia

CATEGORY: Herbs and Supplements; Anti-Inflammatroy

ALSO KNOWN AS: Indian frankincense; Indian olibanum, Salai guggul, and Sallaki

ANATOMY OR SYSTEM AFFECTED: Gastrointestinal system; Musculoskeletal system; Respiratory system

Overview

The gummy resin of the *Boswellia* tree has a long history of use in Indian herbal medicine as a treatment for arthritis, bursitis, respiratory diseases, and diarrhea.

Therapeutic Dosages

A typical dose of *Boswellia* is 300 to 400 mg three times a day of an extract standardized to contain 37.5 percent boswellic acids. Some studies have used dosages as high as 1,200 mg three times daily.

Therapeutic Uses

Growing evidence suggests that *Boswellia* has anti-inflammatory effects. On this basis, the herb has been tried for a number of conditions in which inflammation is involved, including painful conditions such as bursitis, osteoarthritis, rheumatoid arthritis, and tendonitis. For the same reason, it has also been tried for asthma and inflammatory bowel disease (ulcerative colitis or Crohn's disease). In addition, *Boswellia* has shown promise for the relatively rare disease of the colon in which inflammation plays a role: collagenous colitis.

Furthermore, extracts of *Boswellia* have been studied as an aid to standard care for malignant glioma (a type of incurable brain tumor). Use of *Boswellia* appears to decrease symptoms, probably by decreasing inflammation in the brain (as well as through other mechanisms). However, this has not been proven, and individuals with cancer should not use *Boswellia* (or any other herb or supplement) except on a physician's advice.

Scientific Evidence

Rheumatoid arthritis. According to a review of unpublished studies, preliminary double-blind trials have found *Boswellia* effective in relieving the symptoms of rheumatoid arthritis. Two placebo-controlled studies, involving a total of eighty-one people with rheumatoid arthritis, reportedly found significant reductions in swelling and pain over the course of three months. In addition, a comparative study of sixty

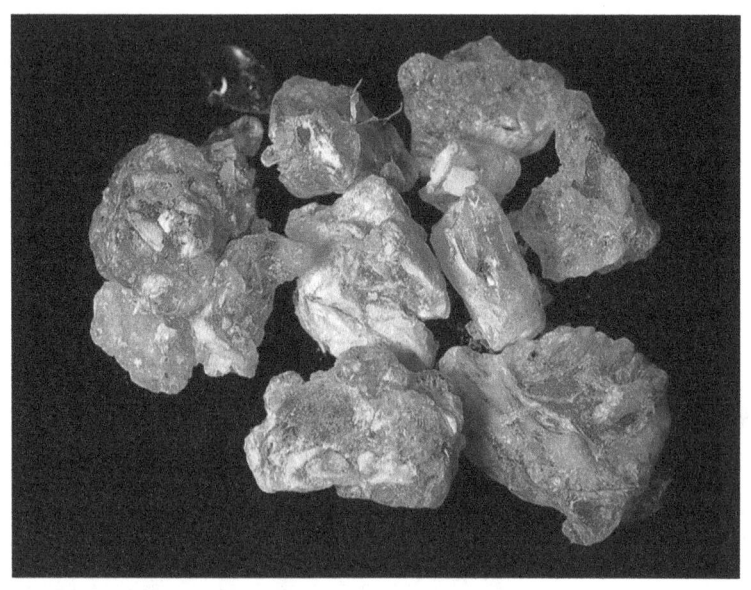

Frankincense from Yemen. (via Wikimedia Commons)

people over six months found that *Boswellia* extract produced symptomatic benefits comparable to oral gold therapy. However, this review was rather sketchy on details.

A more recent double-blind, placebo-controlled study that enrolled seventy-eight people with rheumatoid arthritis found no benefit. However, about one-half of the patients dropped out, which seriously diminishes the significance of the results.

Asthma. A six-week double-blind, placebo-controlled study of eighty people with relatively mild asthma found that treatment with *Boswellia* at a dose of 300 milligrams (mg) three times daily reduced the frequency of asthma attacks and improved objective measurements of breathing capacity.

Osteoarthritis. In a double-blind study of thirty people with osteoarthritis of the knee, researchers compared *Boswellia* against placebo. Participants received either *Boswellia* or placebo for eight weeks and were then switched over to the opposite treatment for an additional eight weeks. The results showed significantly greater improvement in knee pain, knee mobility, and walking distance with *Boswellia* compared to a placebo.

Inflammatory bowel disease. An eight-week double-blind, placebo-controlled trial of 102 people with Crohn's disease compared a standardized *Boswellia* extract against the drug mesalazine. Participants taking *Boswellia* fared at least as well as those taking mesalazine, according to a standard score of Crohn's disease severity. A small, poorly designed trial found some indications that *Boswellia* might also offer benefit in ulcerative colitis.

Safety Issues

In clinical trials of pharmaceutical grade standardized *Boswellia* extract, no serious side effects have been reported. Crude herb preparations, however, may not be as safe as the specially manufactured extract. Safety in young children, pregnant or nursing women, and individuals with severe liver or kidney disease has not been established.

—EBSCO CAM Review Board

References

Euștice, Carol. "*Boswellia* Frankincense for Osteoarthritis." *Verywell Health*, 15 May 2019, www.verywellhealth.com/*Boswellia*-for-osteoarthritis-2551981.

Iram, Farah, et al. "Phytochemistry and Potential Therapeutic Actions of Boswellic Acids: A Mini-Review." *Asian Pacific Journal of Tropical Biomedicine*, vol. 7, no. 6, 2017, pp. 513–523., doi:10.1016/j.apjtb.2017.05.001.

Lemerond, Terry. "Reduce Inflammation from Respiratory Diseases with *Boswellia*." *Chiropractic Economics*, 4 June 2018, www.chiroeco.com/breathing-easier-*Boswellia*/.

Moncivaiz, Aaron, and Debra Rose Wilson. "*Boswellia* (Indian Frankincense)." *Healthline*, 9 Nov. 2017, www.healthline.com/health/*Boswellia*.

Prabhavathi, K, et al. "A Randomized, Double Blind, Placebo Controlled, Cross over Study to Evaluate the Analgesic Activity of *Boswellia* Serrata in Healthy Volunteers Using Mechanical Pain Model." *Indian Journal of Pharmacology*, vol. 46, no. 5, 2014, p. 475., doi:10.4103/0253-7613.140570.

Shader, Richard I. "An Anecdote About Arthritis and *Boswellia* Serrata." *Clinical Therapeutics*, vol. 40, no. 5, 2018, pp. 669–671., doi:10.1016/j.clinthera.2018.04.008.

Siddiqui, Mahtab Z. "*Boswellia* Serrata, A Potential Antiinflammatory Agent: An Overview." *Indian Journal of Pharmaceutical Sciences*, vol. 73, no. 3, May 2011, pp. 255–261., doi:10.4103/0250-474X.93507.

Bromelain

CATEGORY: Herbs and Supplements; Anti-Inflammatory
Origin: Pineapple juice; Pineapple stem
ANATOMY OR SYSTEM AFFECTED: Immune system; Sinus system

Overview

Bromelain is not actually a single substance, but rather a collection of protein-digesting enzymes (also called proteolytic enzymes) found in pineapple juice and in the stem of pineapple plants. It is primarily produced in Japan, Hawaii, and Taiwan, and much of the original research was performed in the first two of those locations. Subsequently, European researchers developed an interest, and by 1995, bromelain had become the thirteenth most common individual herbal product sold in Germany.

Therapeutic Dosages

Recommended dosages of bromelain vary with the form used. Because of the wide variation, one should follow the label's instructions.

Therapeutic Uses

Bromelain (often in combination with other proteolytic enzymes) is used in Europe to aid in recovery from surgery and athletic injuries, as well as to treat sinusitis and phlebitis. Other proposed uses of bromelain include chronic venous insufficiency (closely related to varicose veins), hemorrhoids, other diseases of the veins, bruising, rheumatoid arthritis, gout, ulcerative colitis, and dysmenorrhea (menstrual pain). However, there is no real evidence that bromelain is effective for these conditions. One study failed to find bromelain effective for osteoarthritis.

Bromelain is definitely useful as a digestive enzyme. Unlike most digestive enzymes, bromelain is active in both the acid environment of the stomach and the alkaline environment of the small intestine. This may make it particularly effective as an oral digestive aid for those who do not digest food properly.

Bromelain may also increase the absorption of various drugs, particularly antibiotics such as amoxicillin and tetracycline. This could offer both risks and benefits. Bromelain is widely available in grocery stores as a meat tenderizer.

Scientific Evidence

While most large enzymes are broken down in the digestive tract, those found in bromelain appear to be absorbed whole to a certain extent. This finding makes it reasonable to suppose that bromelain can actually produce systemic (whole-body) effects. Once in the blood, bromelain appears to reduce inflammation, "thin" the blood, and affect the immune system. These influences may be responsible for some of bromelain's therapeutic effects.

Injury and surgery. The evidence for bromelain as a treatment for injuries and surgeries is mixed. A double-blind, placebo-controlled study evaluated 160 women who received episiotomies (surgical cuts in the perineum) during childbirth. Participants given 40 milligram (mg) of bromelain four times daily for three days, beginning four hours after delivery, showed a statistically significant decrease in edema, inflammation, and pain. Ninety percent of persons taking bromelain demonstrated excellent or good responses, compared with 44 percent in the placebo group. However, another double-blind study of 158 women who received episiotomies failed to find significant benefit.

In a double-blind controlled trial, ninety-five patients undergoing treatment for cataracts were given 40 mg of bromelain or a placebo (along with other treatments) four times daily for two days prior to surgery and five days post-operatively. Overall, less inflammation was noted in the bromelain-treated group compared with the placebo group.

Benefits were also seen in double-blind, placebo-controlled studies of dental, nasal, or foot surgery. However, a study of 154 people undergoing facial plastic surgery found no benefit.

A somewhat informal controlled study of 146 boxers suggested that bromelain helps bruises to heal more quickly. Another study–this one without any type of control group–found that bromelain reduced swelling, pain at rest, and tenderness among 59 patients with blunt trauma injuries, including bruising.

People who engage in intense exercise to which they are not accustomed may experience a set of symptoms called delayed onset muscle soreness (DOMS), consisting of pain, reduced flexibility, and weakness of the muscles involved. Bromelain has been proposed for this condition, but a small double-blind, placebo-controlled study failed to find it effective.

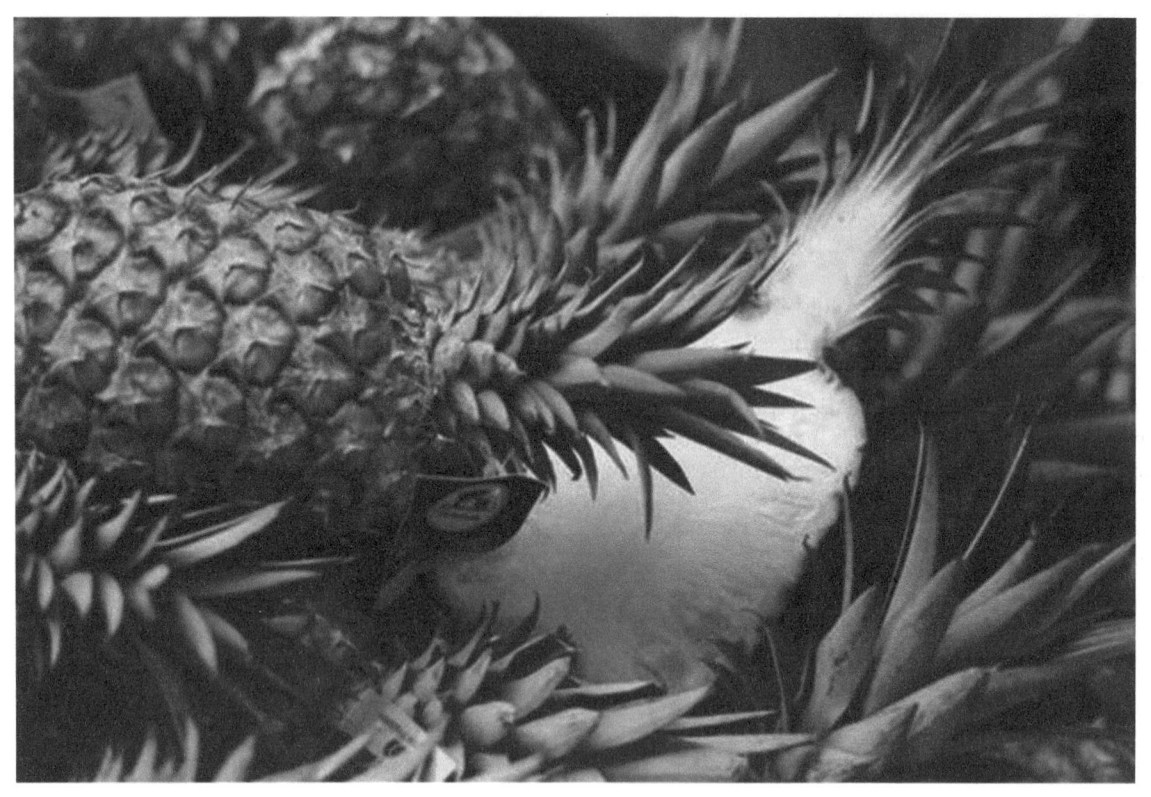

Bromelain is an enzyme extract derived from the stems of pineapples, although it exists in all parts of the fresh pineapple. (via Wikimedia Commons)

Sinusitis. In a double-blind trial, forty-eight patients with moderately severe to severe sinusitis received bromelain or a placebo for six days. All patients were placed on standard therapy for sinusitis, which included antihistamines, analgesics, and antibiotics. Upon completion of the study, inflammation was reduced in 83 percent of those taking bromelain compared with 52 percent of the placebo group. Breathing difficulty was relieved in 78 percent of the bromelain group and 68 percent of the placebo group. Overall, good to excellent results were observed in 87 percent of patients treated with bromelain compared with 68 percent on placebo. Benefits were also seen in two other studies enrolling a total of more than one hundred individuals with sinusitis.

Safety Issues

Bromelain appears to be essentially nontoxic, and it seldom causes side effects other than occasional mild gastrointestinal distress or allergic reactions. However, because bromelain "thins" the blood to some extent, it should not be combined with drugs such as warfarin (Coumadin) without a doctor's supervision.

According to one small animal study, bromelain might interact with sedative medications, increasing their effect. As noted above, it might also increase blood levels of various antibiotics, which could present risks in some cases. In addition, one trial suggests that doses of bromelain eight times higher than standard recommendations might increase heart rate (but not blood pressure). Safety in young children, pregnant or nursing women, and those with liver or kidney disease has not been established.

Important Interactions

Bromelain might amplify the effect of medications that thin the blood, such as warfarin (Coumadin) or heparin, sedative drugs such as benzodiazepines, or antibiotics.

—*EBSCO CAM Review Board*

References

Pavan, Rajendra, et al. "Properties and Therapeutic Application of Bromelain: A Review." *Biotechnology Research International*, 2012, pp. 1–6., doi:10.1155/2012/976203.

Ramli, Aizi Nor Mazila, et al. "Bromelain: from Production to Commercialisation." *Journal of the Science of Food and Agriculture*, vol. 97, no. 5, 28 Oct. 2016, pp. 1386–1395., doi:10.1002/jsfa.8122.

Rathnavelu, Vidhya, et al. "Potential Role of Bromelain in Clinical and Therapeutic Applications." *Biomedical Reports*, vol. 5, no. 3, 18 July 2016, pp. 283–288., doi:10.3892/br.2016.720.

Whelan, Corey, and Debra Rose Wilson. "Bromelain." *Healthline*, 22 Dec. 2017, www.healthline.com/health/bromelain.

◼ Capsaicin

CATEGORY: Analgesic; Anti-inflammatory
ALSO KNOWN AS: A chili pepper extract with analgesic properties
ANATOMY OR SYSTEM AFFECTED: Neurological system; Nervous system; Musculoskeletal system, Dermatological system

Overview

Capsaicin is pro-nociceptive (causes pain) and when eaten evokes pain in the mouth, cornea, skin, joints, and muscles. Found in red peppers, capsaicin is a staple spice in many cuisines around the world. Because of its pro-nociceptive properties, it is used as the primary agent in pepper spray and has been a valuable component of self-defense strategies for many years.

Therapeutic Uses

When applied topically, capsaicin causes no harm to tissues when used for pain control, unlike heat, chemical or mechanical stimuli. Low-dose capsaicin cream is available over the counter and has been for many years. Daily, repeated applications of capsaicin cream may be necessary to achieve the desired pain control effect. In 2009, the FDA approved a long-term capsaicin patch (*Qutenza*) for the treatment of postherpetic neuralgia, a common complication of shingles, in which burning pain remains long after the rash and blisters of shingles have disappeared.

Scientific Evidence

Chronic pain is estimated to affect 20.4% of the United States population and is known to be one of the most common reasons people seek medical treatment. Studies indicate capsaicin to be an effective treatment for chronic neurological pain, as in the case of post herpetic neuralgia, and osteoarthritic pain. Double-blinded, placebo-controlled studies have established that capsaicin is also an effective treatment for osteoarthritis of the hand, knee, hip and/or shoulder. Clinical trials have also shown that capsaicin is an effective treatment for other types of neuropathic pain besides post-herpetic neuralgia. Capsaicin gel, lotions, or ointments do not have a long duration of action and usually require multiple administrations. Several studies have shown that the topical capsaicin patch, *Qutenzas*, lasts an average of five months. Capsaicin injections work for at least four weeks, although limited studies have been conducted to date.

Safety Issues

Capsaicin in its pure form can be harmful if swallowed, can cause skin irritation, and can damage the eyes if it contacts them. As a precaution, capsaicin users should thoroughly wash their hands and any part of their skin that encounters the medication with soap and water, especially after handling it. Topical capsaicin should be applied to the desired site and care should be used not to contact any mucous membranes (e.g., gums, nasal cavity, vagina, rectum) until your hands have been washed thoroughly. Injectable capsaicin has not been shown to cause concerns in clinical trials. Overall studies indicate medical capsaicin poses minimal safety concerns as an analgesic and is probably a better choice for pain relief than some alternatives.

—*Cathy Shell BSN, RN*

References

Dahlhamer J, et al. "Prevalence of Chronic Pain and High-Impact Chronic Pain Among Adults—United States, 2016." *MMWR Morb Mortal Wkly Rep,*. vol. 67, no. 36, 2018, pp. 1001-1006. doi:10.15585 /mmwr.mm6736a2

Kelly, S., et al. "Increased Function of Pronociceptive TRPV1 at the Level of the Joint in a Rat Model of Osteoarthritis Pain." *Ann. Rheum. Dis.* vol. 74, 2015, pp. 252–259.

Guedes, V., et al. "Topical Capsaicin for Pain in Osteoarthritis: A Literature Review." *Rheumatologia Clinica*, vol. 14, no. 1, 2018, pp. 40–45. doi:10.1016/j.reuma.2016.07.008.

Man-Kyo Chung, & James N. Campbell. "Use of Capsaicin to Treat Pain: Mechanistic and Therapeutic Considerations." *Pharmaceuticals*, vol 9, no. 4, 2016, p. 66. doi:10.3390/ph9040066

Mou, J., et al, "Qutenza (capsaicin) 8% Patch Onset and Duration of Response and Effects of Multiple Treatments in Neuropathic Pain Patients. *Clinical Journal of Pain*, vol. 30, 2014, pp. 286–294.

National Center for Biotechnology Information. "Capsaicin." *PubChem Compound Database*, U.S. National Library of Medicine, pubchem.ncbi.nlm.nih.gov/compound/Capsaicin.

■ Comfrey

CATEGORY: Herbs and Supplements; Anti-inflammatory
ALSO KNOWN AS *Symphytum officinale*
ANATOMY OR SYSTEM AFFECTED: Musculoskeletal system

Overview

Comfrey is a high-yielding leafy green plant that has been used for centuries as a feed crop for animals and a medicine for humans. However, in 2001, it was removed as an oral dietary supplement from the American market, and soon afterwards, it was removed as a commercial animal food source. These actions were taken because comfrey contains dangerous levels of toxic pyrrolizidine alkaloids, and its use has led to severe liver injury and death.

Traditionally, oral or topical use of comfrey was said to help bones heal more rapidly, and this is the origin of its Latin name *Symphytum* ("drawing together"). It was also used orally for the treatment of digestive and lung problems. Topical comfrey creams have been used to treat minor wounds, bruises, sprains, and varicose veins.

Therapeutic Dosages

The tested form of topical comfrey contains 10 percent of a 2.5:1 juice extract made from fresh pressed plant sap; in other words, every 100 grams (g) of cream contains the equivalent of 25 g of comfrey sap.

Therapeutic Uses

Comfrey is commonly included in salves and creams that also contain such herbs as aloe, goldenseal, calendula, and vitamin E. Such preparations are marketed for treatment of minor wounds. However, for safety reasons, comfrey should not be applied to broken skin. Therefore, it should not be used for the treatment of lacerations or abrasions (cuts and scrapes). There is some evidence that topical comfrey might be useful in the treatment of various conditions involving pain in the joints or muscles where skin is unbroken. Safety, however, does remain a concern.

In a double-blind, placebo-controlled study of 142 people with acute ankle sprain, use of comfrey cream for eight days significantly enhanced rate of recovery. Comfrey proved more effective than a placebo in measurements of pain, swelling, and mobility. More modest benefits were seen in another double-blind trial, this one enrolling 203 people with ankle sprain and comparing a high-comfrey product to a low-comfrey product.

Another double-blind, placebo-controlled study, this one enrolling 215 people, found comfrey cream helpful for treatment of back pain. Finally, in a three-week double-blind study of 220 people with osteoarthritis of the knee, comfrey cream reduced symptoms significantly more than a placebo cream.

In a recent, well-designed trial, two concentrations of comfrey creams were evaluated for the treatment of fresh abrasions among 278 patients (almost one-quarter of whom were under age twenty). The higher-concentration cream (10 percent) contained ten times more comfrey than the low-concentration cream (considered the reference or placebo cream). The 10 percent comfrey cream led to significantly faster wound healing than the reference cream after two to three days of application. Although the researchers reported no adverse effects in either group, the use of comfrey has been associated with severe and even life-threatening, toxic effects when used orally, and its use over open wounds should be undertaken with extreme caution.

Additional studies, generally of lower quality, suggest possible benefit for shoulder tendonitis and knee injuries. The active ingredients in comfrey are not known but may include rosmaric acid, choline, and allantoin.

Safety Issues

As noted above, comfrey contains substances called pyrrolizidine alkaloids that are both toxic to the liver and carcinogenic. The main form of liver disease seen with comfrey is a blockage of small veins

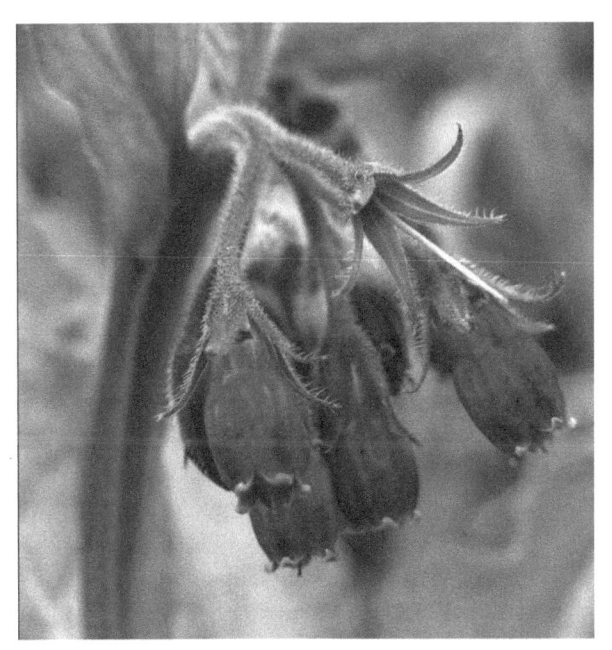

Symphytum officinale *flowers*. (Müller Tamás via Wikimedia Commons)

that can lead to liver cirrhosis and eventually liver failure (hepato-occlusive disease). Liver transplantation may be required. Oral use of comfrey for as brief a time as five to seven days in a child and nineteen to forty-five days in adults has resulted in severe liver disease and death. Long-term use of very low dosages may also cause harm.

In general, the root of the plant contains more pyrrolizidine alkaloids than the leaves. Related species of comfrey such as *S. uplandicum* and *S. asperum* contain even higher levels of these toxins and may be mistakenly sold as ordinary comfrey.

Pyrrolizidine alkaloids in comfrey can be absorbed through the skin. For this reason, it has been recommended that when using comfrey preparations, the daily amount of pyrrolizidine alkaloids should not exceed 100 micrograms (mcg). Few products are labeled to indicate their pyrrolizidine alkaloid content. Furthermore, the common analytic methods used for testing pyrrolizidine alkaloid content may fail to measure a certain chemical form of these toxins (the N-oxide form), leading to results that are too low by a factor of ten or more. For all these reasons, it may be prudent to avoid topical comfrey products entirely. If comfrey is used as a topical treatment, experts recommend that it not be applied for more than four to six weeks per year or more than ten days in a row and that it never be applied on broken skin. In addition, comfrey should not be used by children, pregnant or nursing women, or people with liver disease.

—*EBSCO CAM Review Board*

References

Goldman, Rena, and Debra Rose Wilson. "What Is Comfrey?" *Healthline*, 18 July 2016, www.healthline.com/health/what-is-comfrey.

Johannes, Laura. "A Plant to Ease Muscle and Joint Pain." *The Wall Street Journal*, Dow Jones & Company, 20 Apr. 2015, www.wsj.com/articles/a-plant-to-ease-muscle-and-joint-pain-1429568686.

Kucera, Alexander, et al. "Tolerability and Effectiveness of an Antitrauma Cream with Comfrey Herb Extract in Pediatric Use with Application on Intact and on Broken Skin." *International Journal of Pediatrics and Adolescent Medicine*, vol. 5, no. 4, 2018, pp. 135–141., doi:10.1016/j.ijpam.2018.11.002.

Lucille, Holly. *The Healing Power of Trauma Comfrey*. Take Charge Books, 2013.

Seigner, Jacqueline, et al. "A Symphytum Officinale Root Extract Exerts Anti-Inflammatory Properties by Affecting Two Distinct Steps of NF- B Signaling." *Frontiers in Pharmacology*, vol. 10, 26 Apr. 2019, doi:10.3389/fphar.2019.00289.

Staiger, Christiane. "Comfrey Root: from Tradition to Modern Clinical Trials." *Wiener Medizinische Wochenschrift*, vol. 163, no. 3-4, Feb. 2013, pp. 58–64., doi:10.1007/s10354-012-0162-4.

——. "Comfrey: A Clinical Overview." *Phytotherapy Research*, vol. 26, no. 10, 23 Feb. 2012, pp. 1441–1448., doi:10.1002/ptr.4612.

■ Devil's claw

CATEGORY: Herbs and Supplements; Anti-inflammatory

ALSO KNOWN AS: *Harpagophytum procumbens;* Grapple plant; Wood spider

ANATOMY OR SYSTEM AFFECTED: Musculoskeletal system

Overview

Devil's claw is a native herb of South Africa, so named because of its rather peculiar appearance. Its large tuberous roots are used medicinally, after being chopped up and dried in the sun for three days. Native South Africans used the herb to reduce pain and fever and to stimulate digestion. Colonists brought devil's claw home to Europe, where it became a popular treatment for arthritis.

Therapeutic Dosages

A typical dosage of devil's claw is 750 milligrams three times daily of a preparation standardized to contain 3 percent iridoid glycosides.

Therapeutic Uses

In modern Europe, devil's claw has been used to treat all types of joint pain, including osteoarthritis, rheumatoid arthritis, and gout. Devil's claw also is used for soft-tissue (muscle-related or tendon-related) pain. Like other bitter herbs, devil's claw is said to improve appetite and relieve mild stomach upset.

Scientific Evidence

The evidence for devil's claw is fairly preliminary, with the largest and most well-designed studies showing marginal benefits at best. Most studies have evaluated the herb for treatment of arthritis.

A double-blind study compared devil's claw to the European drug diacerhein. Diacerhein is a member of a drug category not recognized in the United States: the so-called slow-acting drugs for osteoarthritis (SADOAs). Unlike anti-inflammatory drugs such as ibuprofen, SADOAs do not provide immediate relief, but rather act over a period of weeks to gradually reduce arthritis pain. The supplements glucosamine and chondroitin have been proposed as natural SADOAs.

In this trial, 122 persons with osteoarthritis of the hip or knee (or both) were given either devil's claw or diacerhein for four months. The results showed that devil's claw was as effective as diacerhein, as measured by pain levels, mobility, and need for pain-relief medications (such as acetaminophen or ibuprofen). While this might seem impressive, diacerhein itself is only slightly effective, and in such cases, comparative studies must use a placebo group to achieve reliable results.

Another double-blind study followed eighty-nine persons with rheumatoid arthritis for two months. The group given devil's claw showed a significant decrease in pain intensity and improved mobility. A third double-blind study of fifty people with various types of arthritis found that ten days of treatment with devil's claw provided significant pain relief. A fourth study compared devil's claw against Vioxx, an anti-inflammatory drug no longer on the market. While it was widely reported that devil's claw was as effective as the drug, the study was too small to produce statistically meaningful results.

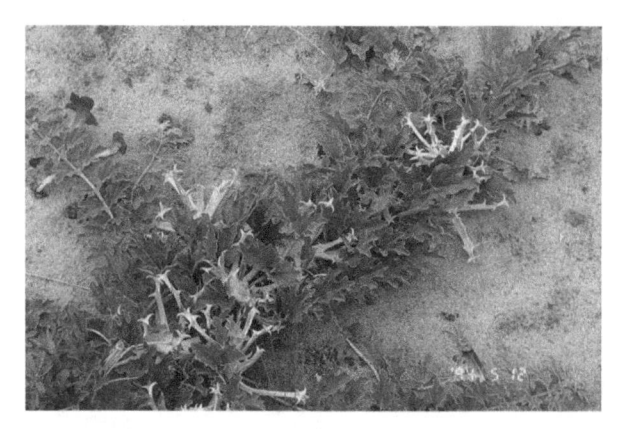

Harpagophytum procumben. (© CITES Secretariat)

Other studies have evaluated devil's claw for treatment of muscular tension and discomfort. One of these studies was a four-week, double-blind, placebo-controlled trial that evaluated sixty-three persons with muscular tension or pain in the back, shoulder, and neck. The results showed significant pain reduction in the treatment group, compared with the placebo group. However, a double-blind study of 197 persons with back pain found devil's claw marginally effective at best. Similarly unimpressive results were seen in an earlier double-blind study of 118 people with back pain.

It remains unclear how devil's claw might work. Some studies have found an anti-inflammatory effect, but others have not. Apparently, the herb does not produce the same changes in prostaglandins as standard anti-inflammatory drugs.

Safety Issues

Devil's claw appears to be safe, at least for short-term use. In one study, no evidence of toxicity emerged at doses many times higher than recommended. In a review of twenty-eight clinical trials, researchers found no instances where adverse effects were more common than those associated with a placebo. Minor adverse effects, most gastrointestinal in nature, occurred in roughly 3 percent of patients.

Devil's claw is not recommended for people with ulcers. Also, a six-month open study of 630 people with arthritis showed no side effects other than

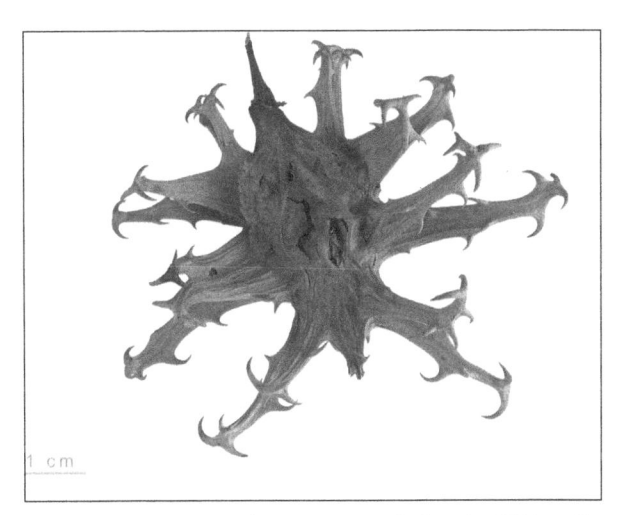

Dry fruit of H. procumbens. (Roger Culos via Wikimedia Commons)

occasional mild gastrointestinal distress. According to one case report, devil's claw might increase the potential for bleeding in persons taking warfarin (Coumadin).

Safety in young children, pregnant or nursing women, or those with severe liver or kidney disease has not been established. Persons taking blood-thinning medications such as warfarin or heparin should note that devil's claw might enhance the effect of these drugs, possibly producing a risk of bleeding.

—*EBSCO CAM Review Board*

References

Brien, Sarah. "Trial Evaluating Devil's Claw for the Treatment of Hip and Knee Osteoarthritis." *ClinicalTrials.gov*, U.S. National Library of Medicine, 12 Sept. 2011, clinicaltrials.gov/ct2/show/NCT00295490.

"Devil's Claw: MedlinePlus Supplements." *MedlinePlus*, U.S. National Library of Medicine, 22 Mar. 2018, medlineplus.gov/druginfo/natural/984.html.

Mcgregor, Gerard, et al. "Devil's Claw (Harpagophytum Procumbens): An Anti-Inflammatory Herb with Therapeutic Potential." *Phytochemistry Reviews*, vol. 4, no. 1, 2005, pp. 47–53., doi:10.1007/s11101-004-2374-8.

Mncwangi, Nontobeko, et al. "Devil's Claw—A Review of the Ethnobotany, Phytochemistry and Biological Activity of Harpagophytum Procumbens." *Journal of Ethnopharmacology*, vol. 143, no. 3, 2012, pp. 755–771., doi:10.1016/j.jep.2012.08.013.

Park, Kyoung Sik. "A Systematic Review on Anti-Inflammatory Activity of Harpagoside." *Journal of Biochemistry and Molecular Biology Research*, vol. 2, no. 3, 2016, pp. 166–169., doi:10.17554/j.issn.2313-7177.2016.02.27.

■ Eucalyptus

CATEGORY: Herbs and Supplements; Anti-bacterial; Anti-inflammatory
ALSO KNOWN AS: *Eucalyptus globulus*
ANATOMY OR SYSTEM AFFECTED: Respiratory system

Overview

The eucalyptus tree originated in Australia and Tasmania, but it has spread to all other inhabited continents. There are many different varieties of eucalyptus, with somewhat differing constituents. The most common type used medicinally is eucalyptus globules. Its essential oil contains eucalyptol (cineol or cineole).

Eucalyptus oil has a long history of use as a topical antiseptic. It also has been used as a lozenge or inhalation therapy for asthma, cough, sore throat, and other respiratory conditions.

Therapeutic Dosages

The studied dosage of cineole is 200 mg three times daily for adults. Internal use of cineole or eucalyptus oil should be avoided in children. In the gingivitis study, chewing gum containing 0.4 and 0.6 percent eucalyptus extracts were used. For use as an insect repellent, 25 to 50 milliliters (ml) of the oil is added to 500 ml of water. One should not use in children age twelve years or younger. As an inhalant, a few drops of eucalyptus oil are added to a vaporizer.

Therapeutic Uses

A standardized combination of cineol from eucalyptus, d-limonene from citrus fruit, and alpha-pinene from pine has been studied for effectiveness in a variety of respiratory conditions. These oils are all in a chemical family called monoterpenes, and for this reason the combined treatment is called essential oil monoterpenes. This combination is discussed in a separate article of that name.

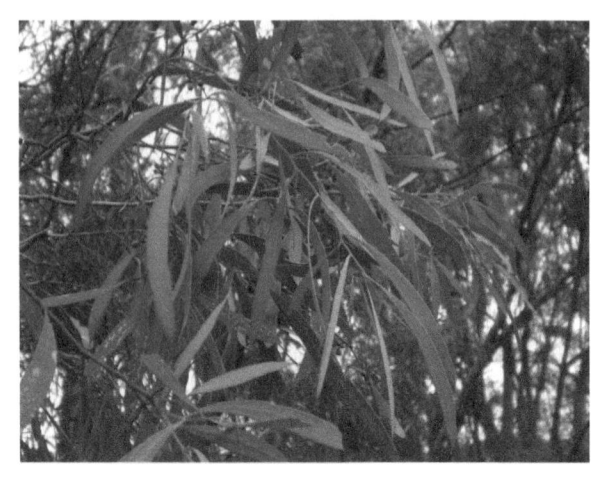

Eucalyptus polybractea *or Blue-leaf Mallee, a species yielding high quality eucalyptus oil.* (John Moss via Wikimedia Commons)

Eucalyptus oil or its constituents taken alone have undergone only limited study. It appears to be most promising as a treatment for the common cold. However, concerns about safety have limited its use.

In a double-blind, placebo-controlled study of 152 people, use of cineol at a dose of 200 milligrams (mg) three times daily markedly improved symptoms of the common cold. Benefits were seen in such symptoms as nasal congestion, headache, and overall malaise. Because the participants in this study suffered, in particular, from sinus symptoms, this study has been used to indicate that cineol may be helpful for viral sinusitis. Few significant side effects were seen in this study, but the product used was of pharmaceutical grade, and not all dietary supplements of eucalyptus oil may be equally safe. A second placebo-controlled study involving 150 subjects also demonstrated favorable results for cineol, compared with a combination of five other herbal products.

In another study, thirty-two people on steroids to control severe asthma (steroid-dependent asthma) were given either placebo or cineole (200 mg three times daily) for twelve weeks. The results showed that people using cineole were able to gradually reduce their steroid dosage to a greater extent than those taking placebo. Reduction of steroid dosage should be done only under the supervision of a physician.

Cineole or eucalyptus oil applied topically also has shown some potential value for repelling mosquitoes. In one double-blind study, chewing gum containing eucalyptus extract was more beneficial for moderate gingivitis than a placebo gum.

Safety Issues

Internal use of eucalyptus oil at appropriate doses by healthy people can cause nausea, heartburn, vomiting, diarrhea, and skin rash. Excessive dosages can be fatal, especially to children. Inhalation of the oil can exacerbate asthma in some people. Application of cineole to the entire body resulted in severe nervous system poisoning in a six-year-old child. In general, eucalyptus oil should not be used by young children, pregnant or nursing women, or people with severe liver or kidney disease.

Although no drug interactions of eucalyptus are firmly documented, there are theoretical reasons to believe it could interact with a number of medications, either raising or lowering their levels. Therefore, people taking any oral or injected medication that is critical to their health or well-being should avoid internal use of eucalyptus until more is known.

—*EBSCO CAM Review Board*

References

Ali, Babar, et al. "Essential Oils Used in Aromatherapy: A Systemic Review." *Asian Pacific Journal of Tropical Biomedicine*, vol. 5, no. 8, 2015, pp. 601–611., doi:10.1016/j.apjtb.2015.05.007.

Jun, Yang Suk, et al. "Effect of Eucalyptus Oil Inhalation on Pain and Inflammatory Responses after Total Knee Replacement: A Randomized Clinical Trial." *Evidence-Based Complementary and Alternative Medicine*, 2013, pp. 1–7., doi:10.1155/2013/502727.

Lakhan, Shaheen E., et al. "The Effectiveness of Aromatherapy in Reducing Pain: A Systematic Review and Meta-Analysis." *Pain Research and Treatment*, 2016, pp. 1–13., doi:10.1155/2016/8158693.

Silva, Jeane, et al. "Analgesic and Anti-Inflammatory Effects of Essential Oils of Eucalyptus." *Journal of Ethnopharmacology*, vol. 89, no. 2-3, 2003, pp. 277–283., doi:10.1016/j.jep.2003.09.007.

Wong, Cathy. "The Health Benefits of Eucalyptus Oil." *Verywell Health*, 24 June 2019, www.verywellhealth.com/steam-inhalation-with-eucalyptus-essential-oil-88169.

Feverfew

CATEGORY: Herbs and Supplements
ALSO KNOWN AS: *Tanacetum parthenium*
ANATOMY OF SYSTEM AFFECTED: Craniofacial

Overview
Originally native to the Balkans, feverfew, a relative of the common daisy, was spread by deliberate planting throughout Europe and the Americas. Feverfew's feathery and aromatic leaves have long been used medicinally to improve childbirth, promote menstruation, induce abortions, relieve rheumatic pain, and treat severe headaches.

Contrary to popular belief, feverfew is not used for lowering fevers. Actually, according to one source, "feverfew" is a corruption of the name "featherfoil." Featherfoil became featherfew and ultimately feverfew. In an odd historical reversal, this name then led to a widespread belief among herbalists that feverfew could lower fevers. After a while they noticed that it did not work, and they then rejected feverfew as a useless herb. Feverfew remained unpopular until a serendipitous event occurred in the late 1970s.

At that time, the wife of the chief medical officer of the National Coal Board in England had serious migraine headaches. When workers in the industry learned of this, a sympathetic miner suggested she try a folk treatment he had used. She followed his advice and chewed feverfew leaves. The results were dramatic: Her migraines disappeared almost completely.

Her husband was impressed, too. He used his high office to gain the ear of a physician who specialized in migraine headaches, E. Stewart Johnson of the London Migraine Clinic. Johnson subsequently experimented with feverfew in his practice and seemed to observe good results. This led to the studies described here.

Therapeutic Dosages
The tested liquid-carbon-dioxide feverfew extract is taken at a dose of 6.25 milligrams (mg) three times daily. To replicate the dosage of feverfew used in the two positive studies of whole leaf described above, one should take 80 to 100 mg of powdered whole feverfew leaf daily.

Therapeutic Uses
Feverfew is used primarily for the prevention of migraine headaches. For this purpose, it is taken daily. There has been no formal investigation of feverfew as a treatment for migraines that have already started, although one double-blind study evaluating feverfew as a preventive agent did find hints of possible symptom-reducing benefits.

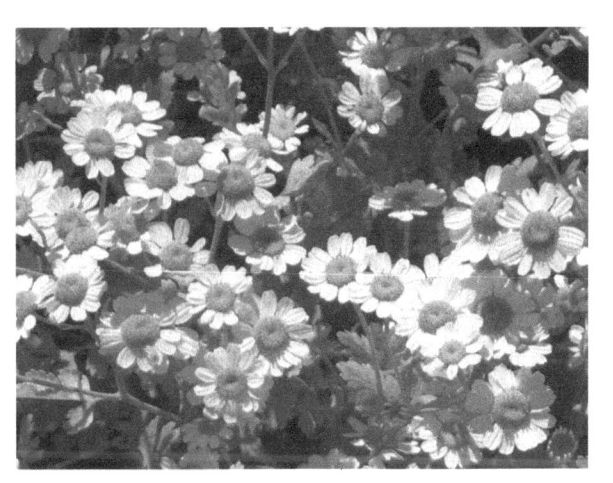

Tanacetum parthenium. (Vsion via Wikimedia Commons)

It is important to remember that serious diseases may occasionally first present themselves as migraine-type headaches. For this reason, proper medical diagnosis is essential if one suddenly starts having migraines without a previous history or if the pattern of one's migraines changes significantly. Feverfew is sometimes recommended for osteoarthritis or rheumatoid arthritis, but there is no evidence that it works.

Scientific Evidence
Five meaningful double-blind, placebo-controlled studies have been performed to evaluate feverfew's effectiveness as a preventive treatment for migraines. The best of the positive trials used a feverfew extract made by extracting the herb with liquid carbon dioxide. Two other trials that used whole feverfew leaf also found it effective; however, two studies that used feverfew extracts did not find benefit.

In a well-conducted sixteen-week, double-blind, placebo-controlled study of 170 people with migraines, use of a feverfew extract at a dose of 6.25 mg three times daily resulted in a significant decrease in headache frequency, compared with the effect of the placebo treatment. In the treatment group, headache frequency decreased by 1.9 headaches per month, compared with a reduction of 1.3 headaches per month in the placebo group. The average number of headaches per month prior to treatment was 4.76 headaches. The extract used in this study was made utilizing liquid carbon dioxide. A previous study using the same extract had failed to find benefit, but it primarily enrolled people with less frequent migraines.

Two other studies used whole feverfew leaf and found benefit. The first followed fifty-nine people for eight months. For four months, half received a daily capsule of powdered feverfew leaf; the other half took placebo. The groups were then switched and followed for an additional four months. Treatment with feverfew produced a 24 percent reduction in the number of migraines and a significant decrease in nausea and vomiting during the headaches. A subsequent double-blind study of fifty-seven people with migraines found that use of feverfew leaf could decrease the severity of migraine headaches. This trial did not report whether there was any change in the frequency of migraines; it is possible, therefore, that this study actually showed a symptom-reducing effect rather than a preventive benefit. One study using an alcohol extract failed to find benefit.

Safety Issues

Animal studies suggest that feverfew is essentially nontoxic. In one eight-month study, there were no significant differences in side effects between the treated and control groups. There also were no changes in measurements on blood tests and urinalysis.

In a survey involving three hundred people, 11.3 percent reported mouth sores from chewing feverfew leaf, occasionally accompanied by general inflammation of tissues in the mouth. A smaller percentage reported mild gastrointestinal distress. However, mouth sores do not seem to occur in people who use encapsulated feverfew leaf powder, the usual form.

In view of its use as a folk remedy to promote abortions, feverfew should probably not be taken during pregnancy. Because feverfew might slightly inhibit the activity of blood-clotting cells known as platelets, it should not be combined with strong anticoagulants, such as warfarin (Coumadin) or heparin, except on medical advice. Feverfew might also increase the risk of stomach problems if combined with anti-inflammatory drugs, such as aspirin. Safety in young children, pregnant or nursing women, and those with severe kidney or liver disease has not been established.

Important Interactions

If one is taking warfarin (Coumadin), heparin, aspirin, or other nonsteroidal anti-inflammatory drugs, one should use feverfew only on medical advice.

—*EBSCO CAM Review Board*

References

Moscano, Filomena, et al. "An Observational Study of Fixed-Dose Tanacetum Parthenium Nutraceutical Preparation for Prophylaxis of Pediatric Headache." *Italian Journal of Pediatrics*, vol. 45, no. 1, 12 Mar. 2019, doi:10.1186/s13052-019-0624-z.

Pareek, Anil, et al. "Feverfew (Tanacetum Parthenium L.): A Systematic Review." *Pharmacognosy Reviews*, vol. 5, no. 9, 2011, pp. 103–110., doi:10.4103/0973-7847.79105.

Pourianezhad, Farzaneh, et al. "Review on Feverfew, a Valuable Medicinal Plant." *Journal of Herbmed Pharmacology*, vol. 5, no. 2, 2016, pp. 45–49.

Wider, Barbara, et al. "Feverfew for Preventing Migraine." *Cochrane Database of Systematic Reviews*, 20 Apr. 2015, doi:10.1002/14651858.cd002286.pub3.

Wong, Cathy. "What Is Feverfew and What Does It Do?" *Verywell Health*, 17 July 2019, www.verywellhealth.com/the-health-benefits-of-feverfew-89562.

■ Flaxseed

CATEGORY: Herbs and Supplements; Functional Food
ALSO KNOWN AS: *Linum usitatissimum*; Linseed
ANATOMY OR SYSTEM AFFECTED: Cardiovascular system; Immune system

Overview

Flaxseed is the hard, tiny seed of *Linum usitatissimum*, the flax plant, which has been widely used for thousands of years as a source of food and clothing. There are a minimum of three flaxseed components with potential health benefits. The first is fiber, valuable in treating constipation. Flaxseed also contains alpha-linolenic acid, a type of omega-3 fatty acid similar to the omega-3 fatty acids found in fish oil but significantly different in other ways and perhaps offering some of the same benefits. Finally, substances called lignans in flaxseed have phytoestrogenic properties, making them somewhat similar to the isoflavones in soy.

The oil made from flaxseed has no appreciable amounts of lignans, but it does contain alpha-linolenic acid.

Therapeutic Dosages
According to the European Scientific Cooperative on Phytotherapy, the usual dose of flaxseed for constipation is 5 grams (g) of whole, cracked, or freshly crushed seeds soaked in water and taken with a glassful of liquid three times a day. Effects begin in eighteen to twenty-four hours. Because of this time delay, it is recommended to take flaxseed for a minimum of two to three days. Children age six to twelve years should be given one-half the adult dose, while children younger than age six years should be treated only under the guidance of a physician.

To soothe an upset stomach, one should soak 5 to 10 g of whole flaxseed in one-half cup of water, strain after twenty to thirty minutes, then drink. For painful skin inflammations, the recommended dose is 30 to 50 g of crushed or powdered seed applied externally as a warm poultice or compress.

Like other sources of fiber, flaxseed should be taken with plenty of fluids, or it may actually worsen constipation. Also, it is best to start with smaller doses and then increase.

Uses and Applications
The fiber in flaxseed binds with water, swelling to form a gel that, like other forms of fiber, helps soften the stool and move it along in the intestines. One study found that flaxseed can help with chronic constipation in irritable bowel disease. German health authorities approve of the use of flaxseed for various digestive problems, such as chronic constipation, irritable bowel syndrome, diverticulitis, and general stomach discomfort.

Flaxseed may be slightly helpful for improving cholesterol profile, according to some studies. Purified alpha linolenic acid or lignans alone have not consistently shown benefits. It may be the generic fiber and not the other specific ingredients in flaxseed that improve cholesterol levels.

Flaxseed, its lignans, and its oil have undergone a small amount of investigation for potential cancer prevention or cancer treatment possibilities. Flaxseed has shown some promise for treating kidney disease associated with lupus (lupus nephritis). Because it is believed to have soothing properties, flaxseed is sometimes used for symptomatic relief of stomach distress and is applied externally for inflammation of the skin. However, research on these potential uses is essentially nonexistent.

Although flaxseed is often advocated for the treatment of symptoms related to menopause, a sizable twelve-month study failed to find it more helpful than wheat germ placebo. Besides failing to improve immediate symptoms such as hot flashes, flaxseed did not appear to provide any protection against loss of bone density. An earlier, much smaller study by the same researchers found it equally effective for menopausal symptoms as hormone replacement therapy, but because of the absence of a placebo group and the high rate of placebo response in menopausal symptoms, these results cannot be taken as indicating much. Another study tested flaxseed without comparing it with placebo and reported a 50 percent reduction in hot flashes. The researchers went on to state that this reduction in hot flashes was "greater than what would be expected with placebo," a rather curious claim because menopausal women given placebo typically experience almost exactly a 50 percent decrease in hot flashes.

In a preliminary double-blind trial of seventy-eight older men, flaxseed extract modestly improved the urinary symptoms associated with benign prostatic hyperplasia (prostate enlargement) after four months of treatment. The use of essential fatty acids in the omega-3 family has also shown some promise for the treatment of nonalcoholic fatty liver.

Scientific Evidence
Constipation. In a double-blind study, fifty-five people with chronic constipation caused by irritable bowel syndrome received either ground flaxseed or psyllium seed (a well-known treatment for constipation) daily for three months. Those taking flaxseed had significantly fewer problems with constipation, abdominal pain, and bloating than those taking psyllium. The flaxseed group had even further improvements in constipation and bloating while continuing their treatment in the three months after the double-blind part of the study ended. The researcher concluded that flaxseed relieved constipation more effectively than psyllium.

Cholesterol and atherosclerosis. Some human studies have found that flaxseed improves cholesterol profile. However, the benefits, if they do exist, are very

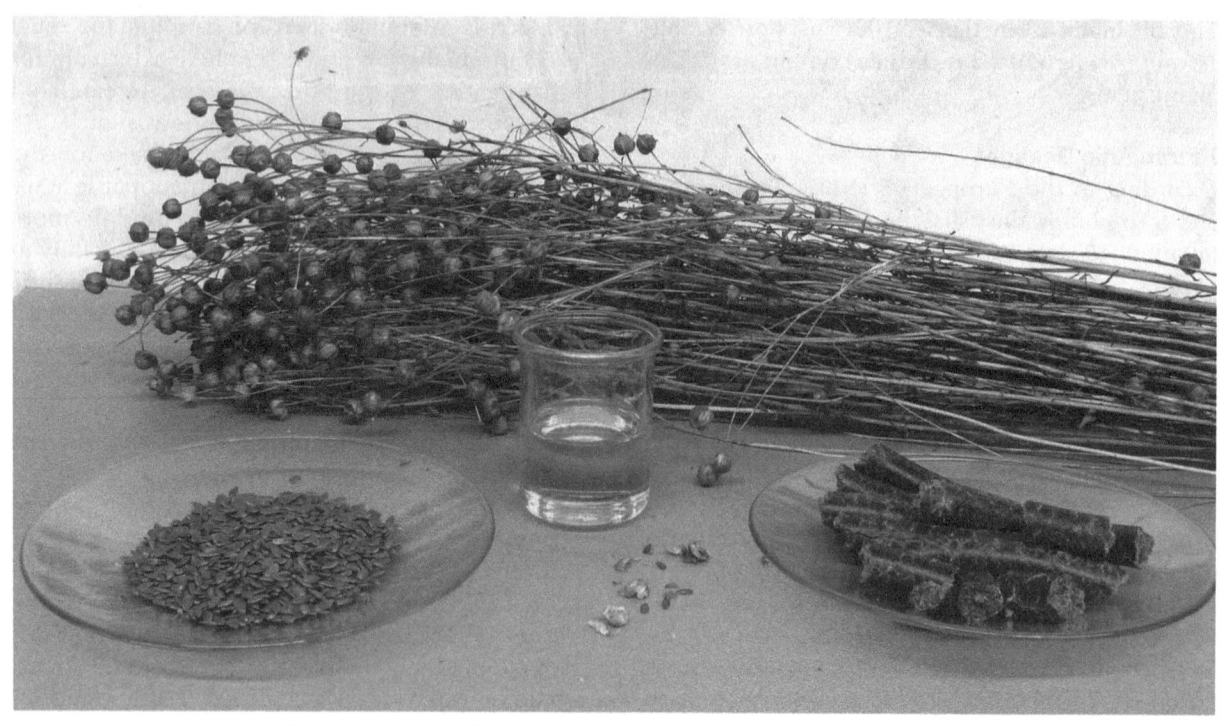

For the production of high quality linseed oil the seeds of the flax plant are cold pressed. The residue, called linseed cake (right) is a high quality and nutritious animal food. (Handwerker via Wikimedia Commons)

modest. For example, in a double-blind study of about two hundred postmenopausal women, the use of flaxseed at a dose of 40 g daily produced measurable improvements in cholesterol profile, but the improvements were so small that the researchers considered them "clinically insignificant." It has been claimed that flaxseed might also have a direct effect in helping to prevent atherosclerosis based on its lignan ingredients, but the evidence upon which these claims are based is limited to studies in rabbits.

Cancer. Some evidence hints that flaxseed or its lignan components might have cancer-preventive properties. Observational studies and other forms of preliminary evidence suggest that people who eat more lignan-containing foods have a lower incidence of breast cancer and perhaps colon cancer.

The lignans in flaxseed are phytoestrogens, plant chemicals mimicking the effects of estrogen in the body: Phytoestrogens hook onto the same spots on cells where estrogen attaches. If there is little estrogen in the body, for example after menopause, lignans may act like weak estrogen. However, when natural estrogen is abundant, lignans may reduce the hormone's effects by displacing it from cells; displacing estrogen in this manner might help prevent those cancers that depend on estrogen, such as breast cancer, from starting and developing. (This is also, in part, how soy is believed to work in breast cancer prevention, although the phytoestrogens in soy are isoflavones.)

Some preliminary research indicates that these lignans may also fight cancer in other ways, perhaps by acting as antioxidants. Animal studies using flaxseed and its lignans offer supporting evidence for a potential cancer-preventive or even cancer-treatment effect; several found that one or the other inhibited breast and colon cancer in animals and reduced metastases from melanoma (a type of skin cancer) in mice. Test-tube studies have found that flaxseed or one of its lignans inhibited the growth of human breast cancer cells, and that the lignans enterolactone and enterodiol inhibited the growth of human colon tumor cells. This preliminary research is promising, but much more is needed before any conclusions can be drawn. Although much of this anticancer work has focused on the lignans in flaxseed, one study also found that flaxseed oil, which contains no appreciable amounts of lignans, slowed the growth of malignant breast tumors in rats.

Safety Issues

Flaxseed is generally believed to be safe. However, there are some potential risks to consider. As with many substances, there have been reports of life-threatening allergic reactions to flaxseed.

Because of its potential effects on estrogen, pregnant or breast-feeding women should probably avoid flaxseed. One study found that pregnant rats who ate large amounts of flaxseed (5 or 10 percent of their diet) or one of its lignans, gave birth to offspring with altered reproductive organs and functions (in humans, eating 25 g of flaxseed per day amounts to about 5 percent of the diet). Lignans were also found to be transferred to baby rats during nursing. Additionally, a study of postmenopausal women found that the use of flaxseed reduced estrogen levels and increased levels of prolactin. This suggests hormonal effects that could be problematic in pregnancy.

Flaxseed may not be safe for women with a history of estrogen-sensitive cancer, such as breast or uterine cancer. A few test-tube studies suggest that certain cancer cells can be stimulated by lignans such as those present in flaxseed. Other studies found that lignans inhibit cancer cell growth. As with estrogen, lignans' positive or negative effects on cancer cells may depend on dose, type of cancer cell, and levels of hormones in the body. Persons with a history of cancer, particularly breast cancer, should consult a doctor before consuming large amounts of flaxseed.

Flaxseed (like other high-fiber foods) may delay glucose absorption. This may lead to better blood sugar control but it also may increase the risk of hypoglycemic reactions. Persons with diabetes should consult a doctor about appropriate use.

Finally, flaxseed contains tiny amounts of cyanide-containing substances, which can be a problem among livestock eating large amounts of flax. While normal cooking and baking of whole flaxseed or flour eliminates any detectable amounts of cyanide, it is theoretically possible that eating huge amounts of raw or unprocessed flaxseed or flaxseed meal could pose a problem. However, most authorities do not think this presents much of a risk in real life.

—*EBSCO CAM Review Board*

References

American Physiological Society. "Flaxseed Fiber Ferments in Gut to Improve Health, Reduce Obesity." *ScienceDaily*, 5 Feb. 2019, www.sciencedaily.com/releases/2019/02/190205090541.htm.

Calado, Ana, et al. "The Effect of Flaxseed in Breast Cancer: A Literature Review." *Frontiers in Nutrition*, vol. 5, 7 Feb. 2018, doi:10.3389/fnut.2018.00004.

Goyal, Ankit, et al. "Flax and Flaxseed Oil: an Ancient Medicine & Modern Functional Food." *Journal of Food Science and Technology*, vol. 51, no. 9, 10 Jan. 2014, pp. 1633–1653., doi:10.1007/s13197-013-1247-9.

Nordqvist, Joseph, and Debra Rose Wilson. "Flaxseed: Health Benefits, Nutritional Content, and Risks." *Medical News Today*, MediLexicon International, 20 Nov. 2017, www.medicalnewstoday.com/articles/263405.php.

Setayesh, Mohammad, et al. "A Topical Gel From Flax Seed Oil Compared With Hand Splint in Carpal Tunnel Syndrome: A Randomized Clinical Trial." *Journal of Evidence-Based Complementary & Alternative Medicine*, vol. 22, no. 3, 2016, pp. 462–467., doi:10.1177/2156587216677822.

Zeratsky, Katherine. "Why Buy Ground Flaxseed?" *Mayo Clinic*, Mayo Foundation for Medical Education and Research, 18 Jan. 2019, www.mayoclinic.org/healthy-lifestyle/nutrition-and-healthy-eating/expert-answers/flaxseed/faq-20058354.

■ Garlic

CATEGORY: Herbs and Supplements; Functional Food
ALSO KNOWN AS: *Allium sativum*
ANATOMY OR SYSTEM AFFECTED: Cardiovascular system

Overview

The story of garlic's role in human history could fill a book, as indeed it has, many times. Its species name, *sativum*, means "cultivated," indicating that garlic does not grow in the wild. So fond have humans been of this herb that garlic can be found almost everywhere in the world, from Polynesia to Siberia.

From Roman antiquity through World War I, garlic poultices were used to prevent wound infections. The famous microbiologist Louis Pasteur performed some of the original work showing that garlic could kill bacteria. In 1916, the British government issued a general plea for the public to supply it with garlic to meet wartime needs. Garlic was called Russian penicillin during World War II because, after running out of antibiotics, the Russian government turned to this ancient treatment for its soldiers. After World War II, Sandoz Pharmaceuticals manufactured a garlic compound for intestinal spasms, and the Van Patten Company produced another for lowering blood pressure.

Uses and Applications

Garlic is widely used as an all-around treatment for preventing or slowing the progression of atherosclerosis (the cause of most heart attacks and strokes). However, there is actually relatively little in the way of meaningful evidence that it works for this purpose. The balance of the evidence suggests that garlic is not effective for treating high cholesterol; there is only minimal evidence that it offers any benefits for people with high blood pressure. According to some studies, garlic might have blood-thinning effects, but whether this translates into any medical benefit remains unclear.

One study found preliminary evidence that the use of garlic could enhance blood sugar control in diabetes. Also, garlic has a long folkloric history as a treatment for colds and is commonly stated to strengthen the immune system. However, not until 2001 was there supporting evidence for this use. A well-designed double-blind study suggested that the regular use of garlic extract can help prevent colds.

In addition, folklore suggesting that garlic ingestion can ward off insect bites may have some truth to it, at least when garlic is taken regularly for several weeks. When applied topically, garlic can kill fungi, and there is preliminary evidence suggesting that ajoene, a compound derived from garlic, might help treat athlete's foot. Topical garlic can also kill bacteria on contact; however, if taken by mouth, garlic will not work like an antibiotic (that is, throughout the body). Furthermore, oral garlic has failed to prove effective for killing *Helicobacter pylori*, the stomach bacteria implicated as a major cause of ulcers.

Traditionally, garlic was often combined with the herb mullein in oil products designed to reduce the pain of middle ear infections (otitis media) but not of external ear infections (known commonly as swimmer's ear). Two double-blind studies support this use. While these products may reduce pain, it is very unlikely that they have any actual effect on the infection because the eardrum prevents them from reaching the site of infection.

Preliminary evidence, including one small double-blind trial, suggests that regular intake of garlic as food or as aged garlic supplements may reduce the risk of various forms of cancer. Based on extremely weak evidence, garlic has been proposed as a treatment for problems related to the yeast *Candida albicans*, problems such as vaginal yeast infection, oral yeast infection (thrush), and the purported condition discussed in some alternative medicine circles as yeast hypersensitivity syndrome.

Scientific Evidence

Atherosclerosis. Scant evidence hints that garlic might help prevent atherosclerosis, the most common cause of heart attacks and strokes. Garlic preparations have been found to slow hardening of the arteries in animal studies.

In a double-blind, placebo-controlled study that followed 152 people for four years, standardized garlic powder at a dosage of 900 milligrams (mg) daily significantly slowed the development of atherosclerosis as measured by ultrasound. However, this study had some statistical problems that make its results less than fully reliable.

An observational study of two hundred people measured the flexibility of the aorta, the main artery exiting the heart. Participants who took garlic showed more flexibility, indicating less atherosclerosis. However, because this was not a double-blind trial, its results prove little.

Heart attack prevention. In one study, 432 people who had experienced a heart attack were given either garlic oil extract or no treatment for a period of three years. The results showed a significant reduction of second heart attacks and about a 50 percent reduction in death rate among those taking garlic.

High cholesterol. A number of studies published in the 1980s and early 1990s found evidence that garlic preparations can reduce high cholesterol. However, virtually all subsequent studies have failed to find any significant benefit. One carefully designed study failed to find benefits with raw garlic, garlic powder, or aged garlic. The accumulating impact of these repeated negative results

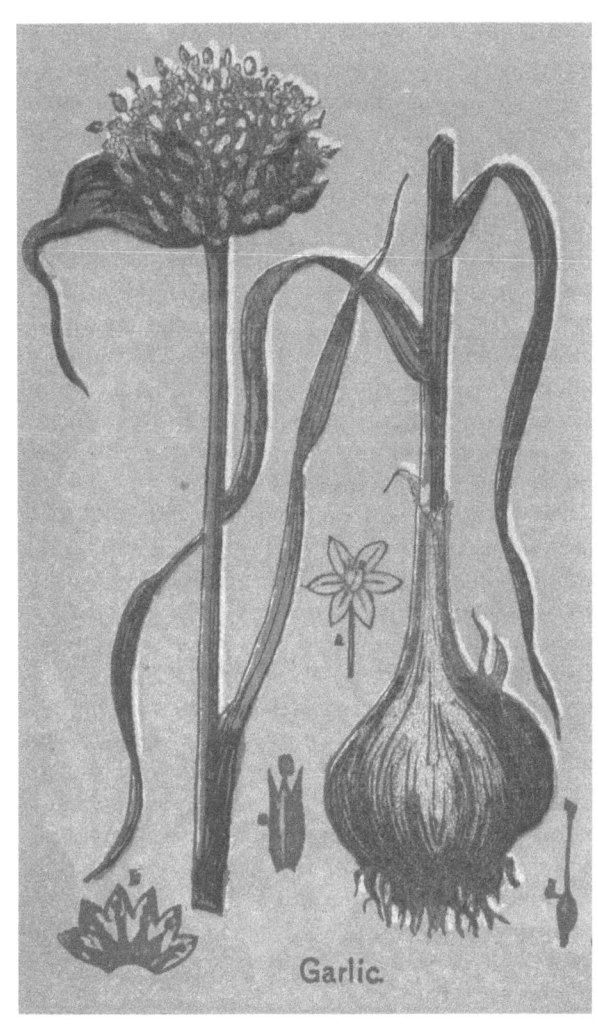

Garlic from "Plate No. 6: Medicinal Plants." part of The Book of Health. *Providence, Rhode Island: W. P. Mason, 1898.* (Henry M. Lyman via Wikimedia Commons)

indicates that garlic is not effective for improving cholesterol profile.

Hypertension. Numerous studies have found weak evidence that garlic lowers blood pressure slightly, perhaps in the neighborhood of 5 to 10 percent more than placebo. It remains unclear whether garlic supplements can help persons with high blood pressure safely eliminate or avoid antihypertensive medications.

One study followed forty-seven persons with an average starting blood pressure of 171/101. In a period of twelve weeks, one-half were treated with 600 mg of garlic powder daily standardized to 1.3 percent alliin, while the other one-half were given placebo. The results showed a statistically significant drop of 11 percent in the systolic blood pressure and 13 percent in the diastolic pressure. In comparison, blood pressure fell in the placebo group by 5 and 4 percent, respectively. However, this study had a significant problem: The average starting blood pressures of the placebo and the treated groups were quite different, making comparisons unreliable.

Prevention of colds. The herb garlic has a long history of use for treating or preventing colds. An American study reported in 2001 provides meaningful preliminary evidence that garlic might possess cold-fighting powers. In this twelve-week, double-blind, placebo-controlled trial, 146 people received either placebo or a garlic extract between the months of November and February.

The results showed that participants receiving garlic were almost two-thirds less likely to catch cold than those receiving placebo. Furthermore, participants who did catch cold recovered about one day faster in the garlic group compared with the placebo group. Thus, the regular use of garlic might help prevent colds. However, there is no evidence that taking garlic at the onset of a cold will help a person recover more quickly.

Insect repellent. A twenty-week, double-blind, placebo-controlled crossover trial followed eighty Swedish soldiers and measured the number of tick bites they received while undergoing the garlic and the placebo treatments. The results showed a modest but statistically significant reduction in tick bites when soldiers consumed 1,200 mg of garlic daily for eight to ten weeks. However, the type of garlic used in this study was not stated. Another study failed to find one-time use of garlic helpful for repelling mosquitoes.

Cancer prevention. Evidence from observational studies suggests that garlic may help prevent cancer, particularly cancer of the stomach and colon. In one of the best of these trials, the Iowa Women's Study, 41,837 women were questioned as to their lifestyle habits (beginning in 1986) and then followed in subsequent years. At the four-year follow-up, questionnaires showed that women whose diets included significant quantities of garlic were approximately 30 percent less likely to develop colon cancer.

The interpretations of studies like this one are always a bit controversial. For example, it is possible that the women who ate a lot of garlic also made other healthful lifestyle choices. While researchers

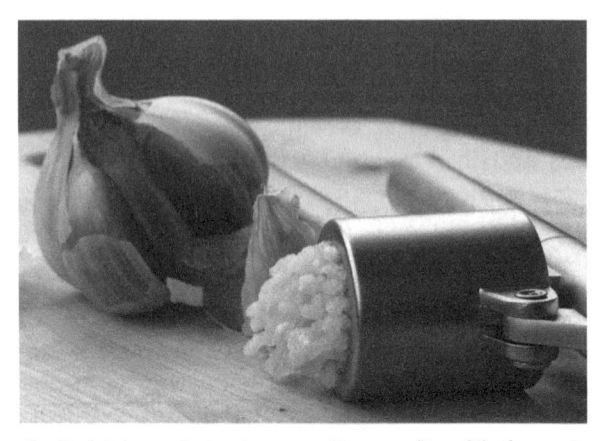

Garlic being crushed using a garlic press. (Lee Kindness via Wikimedia Commons)

looked at this possibility carefully and concluded that garlic was a common factor, it is not clear that the researchers are right. What is really needed to settle the question is an intervention trial, in which some people are given garlic and others are given placebo. However, no studies have been performed to evaluate garlic for cancer prevention.

Antimicrobial. There is no question that raw garlic can kill a wide variety of microorganisms, including fungi, bacteria, viruses, and protozoa, by direct contact. A double-blind study reported in 1999 found that a cream made from the garlic constituent ajoene was just as effective for fungal skin infections as the standard drug terbinafine. These findings may explain why garlic was traditionally applied directly to wounds to prevent infection (but it also can burn the skin). Nevertheless, there is no real evidence that taking garlic orally can kill organisms throughout the body. Thus, it is not an antibiotic in the usual sense; it is more of an antiseptic.

Oral garlic could theoretically offer benefits against organisms in the stomach or intestines because it can come into direct contact with them. However, there is only the slightest evidence that it works for any specific infection of this type. For example, despite test-tube evidence that garlic can kill *H. pylori*, studies in people have not been promising.

Dosage

A typical dosage of garlic is 900 mg daily of a garlic powder extract standardized to contain 1.3 percent alliin, providing about 12,000 micrograms of alliin daily, or 4 to 5 mg of "allicin potential." Alliin-free aged garlic is taken at a dose of 1 to 7.2 grams daily.

Alliin is a relatively odorless substance found in garlic. When garlic is crushed or cut, an enzyme called allinase is brought in contact with alliin, turning it into allicin. Allicin is responsible for much of the typical odor of garlic. It is very active chemically and probably helps the garlic bulb defend itself from attack by insects and other threats. However, allicin is unstable, and it soon breaks down into a variety of other substances. When garlic is ground up and encapsulated, the effect is similar to cutting the bulb: Alliin contacts allinase, yielding allicin, which then breaks down. Unless something is done to prevent this process, garlic powder will not have any alliin or allicin left by the time it is purchased.

Some garlic producers believe that alliin and allicin are not essential for garlic's effectiveness and do not worry about this breakdown. Aged garlic, for example, has very little of either compound, but other manufacturers believe that allicin is the primary active ingredient in garlic. Because allicin is an unstable chemical, these manufacturers are faced with a challenge.

One solution might be to chemically stabilize allicin so that it does not break down. However, allicin has a strong garlic smell, and a relatively odorless product is preferable. Many manufacturers of garlic powder products seek to stabilize the alliin in the product, and to do so in such a way that the alliin converts to allicin after it is consumed. How well their methods work remains a matter of controversy.

One should not confuse essential oil of garlic with garlic oils. The term "garlic oil" refers to garlic extracted by means of oil. Garlic essential oil is the pure oily component of the herb, and, like other essential oils, it is potentially toxic.

Safety Issues

As a commonly used food, garlic is on the GRAS (Generally Recognized As Safe) list of the U.S. Food and Drug Administration. Test rats have been fed gigantic doses of aged garlic (2,000 mg per kilogram of body weight) for six months without any signs of negative effects. Long-term treatment with standardized garlic powder at a dose equivalent to three times the usual dose, along with fish oil, produced no toxic effects in rats.

The only common side effect of garlic is unpleasant breath odor. Even "odorless garlic" produces an offensive smell in up to 50 percent of those who use it. Other side effects occur only rarely. For example, a study that followed 1,997 people who were given a normal dose of deodorized garlic daily for sixteen weeks showed a 6 percent incidence of nausea, a 1.3 percent incidence of dizziness on standing (perhaps a sign of low blood pressure), and a 1.1 percent incidence of allergic reactions. There were also a few reports of bloating, headaches, sweating, and dizziness.

When raw garlic is taken in excessive doses, it can cause numerous symptoms, such as stomach upset, heartburn, nausea, vomiting, diarrhea, flatulence, facial flushing, rapid pulse, and insomnia. Topical garlic can cause skin irritation, blistering, and even third-degree burns.

Because garlic might "thin" the blood, it is probably imprudent to take garlic pills immediately before or after surgery or labor and delivery because of the risk of excessive bleeding. Similarly, garlic should not be combined with blood-thinning drugs such as warfarin (Coumadin), heparin, aspirin, clopidogrel (Plavix), ticlopidine (Ticlid), or pentoxifylline (Trental). In addition, garlic could conceivably interact with natural products with blood-thinning properties, such as ginkgo, policosanol, or high-dose vitamin E. However, a placebo-controlled study found that actual raw garlic consumed in food at the fairly high dose of 4.2 mg once daily did not impair platelet function. In addition, volunteers who continued to consume the dietary garlic for one week did not show any changes in their normal platelet function.

Garlic may also combine poorly with certain medications for human immunodeficiency virus (HIV) infection. Two HIV-positive persons experienced severe gastrointestinal toxicity from the HIV drug ritonavir after taking garlic supplements. Garlic might also reduce the effectiveness of some drugs used for HIV infection. Garlic is presumed to be safe for pregnant women (except just before and immediately after delivery) and nursing mothers, although this has not been proven.

Important Interactions

Persons should not use garlic except on medical advice if also taking blood-thinning drugs. Taking garlic at the same time as ginkgo, policosanol, or high-dose vitamin E might conceivably cause a risk of bleeding problems. Finally, one should not use garlic if also taking medications for HIV infection.

—*EBSCO CAM Review Board*

References

Arreola, Rodrigo, et al. "Immunomodulation and Anti-Inflammatory Effects of Garlic Compounds." *Journal of Immunology Research*, 19 Apr. 2015, pp. 1–13., doi:10.1155/2015/401630.

Arrowhead Health. "Remedies for Muscle and Joint Pain." *Arrowhead Health Centers*, 7 Aug. 2015, arrowheadhealth.com/home-remedies-for-muscle-and-joint-pain/.

Bisen, Prakash S., and Mila Emerald. "Nutritional and Therapeutic Potential of Garlic and Onion (Allium Sp.)." *Current Nutrition & Food Science*, vol. 12, no. 3, 2016, pp. 190–199., doi:10.2174/1573401312666160608121954.

Courtney, Suzanne Whitney, et al. "Is Garlic Effective in Reducing Cardiovascular Risk Factors?" *Evidence-Based Practice*, 22 July 2019, doi:10.1097/EBP.0000000000000566.

Newman, Tim. "Garlic: Proven Health Benefits and Uses." *Medical News Today*, MediLexicon International, 18 Aug. 2017, www.medicalnewstoday.com/articles/265853.php.

Qidwai, Waris, and Tabinda Ashfaq. "Role of Garlic Usage in Cardiovascular Disease Prevention: An Evidence-Based Approach." *Evidence-Based Complementary and Alternative Medicine*, 2013, pp. 1–9., doi:10.1155/2013/125649.

■ Ginger

CATEGORY: Herbs and Supplements; Antiemetic; Functional Food
ALSO KNOWN AS: *Zingiber officinale*
ANATOMY OR SYSTEM AFFECTED: Gastrointestinal system

Overview

Native to southern Asia, ginger is a perennial that is two to four feet in length and produces grasslike leaves up to one foot long and almost one inch wide. Although it is called ginger root in the grocery store, the part of the herb used is actually the rhizome, the underground stem of the plant, with its outer covering (similar to bark) scraped off.

Ginger has been used as food and medicine for millennia. Arabian traders carried ginger root from China and India to be used as a food spice in ancient Greece and Rome, and tax records from the second century show that ginger was a source of revenue for the Roman treasury.

Chinese medical texts from the fourth century B.C.E. suggest that ginger is effective in treating nausea, diarrhea, stomachache, cholera, toothaches, bleeding, and rheumatism. Ginger was later used by Chinese herbalists to treat a variety of respiratory conditions, including coughs and the early stages of colds.

Ginger's modern use dates to the early 1980s, when a scientist named D. Mowrey noticed that ginger-filled capsules reduced his nausea during an episode of flu. Inspired by this, he performed the first double-blind study of ginger. Germany's Commission E subsequently approved ginger as a treatment for indigestion and motion sickness.

One of the most prevalent ingredients in fresh ginger is the pungent substance gingerol. However, when ginger is dried and stored, its gingerol rapidly converts to the substances shogaol and zingerone. It remains unknown if any of these substances has medicinal effects.

Uses and Applications
Some evidence suggests that ginger may be slightly helpful for the prevention and treatment of various forms of nausea, including motion sickness, the nausea and vomiting of pregnancy (morning sickness), and postsurgical nausea. (Women who are pregnant and persons undergoing surgery should not self-treat with ginger except under physician supervision.)

Scant preliminary evidence suggests that ginger might be helpful for osteoarthritis. One small study suggests that it may be beneficial for high cholesterol. Ginger has been suggested as a treatment for numerous other conditions, including atherosclerosis, migraine headaches, rheumatoid arthritis, ulcers, depression, and impotence. However, there is negligible evidence for these uses.

In traditional Chinese medicine, hot ginger tea taken at the first sign of a cold is believed to offer the possibility of averting the infection. However, there is no scientific evidence for this use.

Scientific Evidence
Nausea. The evidence for ginger's effectiveness in various forms of nausea remains mixed. It has been suggested that in some negative studies, poor-quality ginger powder might have been used. In general, while most antinausea drugs influence the brain and the inner ear, ginger appears to act directly on the stomach.

Motion sickness. Ginger has shown inconsistent promise for the treatment of motion sickness. A double-blind, placebo-controlled study of seventy-nine Swedish naval cadets at sea found that 1 gram (g) of ginger could decrease vomiting and cold sweating, but without significantly decreasing nausea and vertigo. Benefits were also seen in a double-blind study of thirty-six persons given ginger, dimenhydrinate, or placebo.

However, a 1984 study funded by the National Aeronautics and Space Administration using intentionally stimulated motion sickness found that ginger was not any more effective than placebo. Two other small studies have also failed to find any benefit. The reason for the discrepancy may lie in the type of ginger used or in the severity of the stimulant used to bring on motion sickness.

Nausea and vomiting during pregnancy. Four double-blind, placebo-controlled studies enrolling 246 women found ginger more effective than placebo for the treatment of morning sickness. For example, a double-blind, placebo-controlled trial of seventy pregnant women evaluated the effectiveness of ginger for morning sickness. Participants received either placebo or 250 milligrams of powdered ginger three times daily for four days. The results showed that ginger significantly reduced nausea and vomiting. No significant side effects occurred.

A minimum of three studies compared ginger to vitamin B_6, a commonly recommended treatment for morning sickness. Two studies found them to be equally beneficial, while the third found ginger to be somewhat better. However, because the effectiveness of vitamin B_6 for morning sickness is not solidly established (the evidence rests largely on one fairly old study), these findings are of questionable value. Despite its use in these studies, ginger has not been proven safe for pregnant women.

Postsurgical nausea. Although there have been some positive studies, on balance, the evidence regarding ginger for reducing nausea and vomiting following surgery is discouraging. A double-blind British study compared the effects of ginger, placebo, and metoclopramide (Reglan) in the treatment of nausea following gynecological surgery. The results in sixty women indicated that both treatments produced similar benefits compared with placebo.

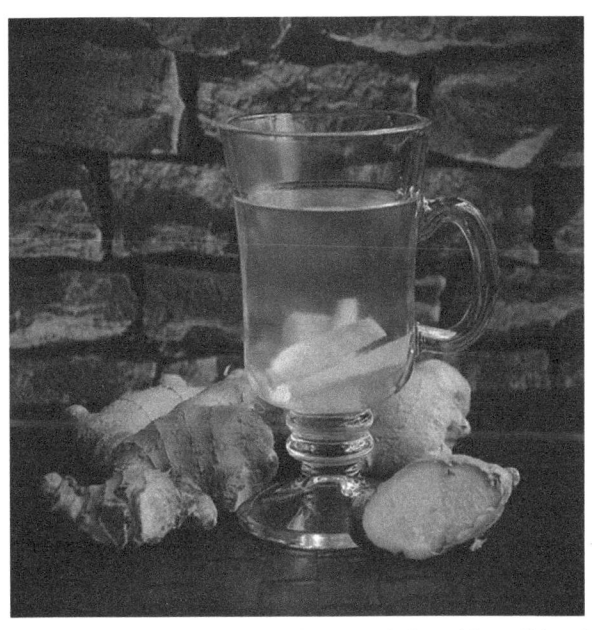

Ginger tea can be drunk by itself, or served alongside traditional accompaniments, such as milk, orange slices, or lemon. (congerdesign via Wikimedia Commons)

A similar British study followed 120 women receiving elective laparoscopic gynecological surgery. Whereas nausea and vomiting developed in 41 percent of the participants given placebo, in the groups treated with ginger or metoclopramide, these symptoms developed in only 21 and 27 percent, respectively. Benefits were also seen in a double-blind study of eighty people. A study of sixty people found marginally positive results. However, a double-blind study of 108 people undergoing similar surgery found no benefit with ginger compared with placebo. If ginger is effective for postsurgical nausea, the effect is very slight.

Other forms of nausea. One study failed to find ginger helpful for reducing nausea caused by the cancer chemotherapy drug cisplatin. In a second study, ginger did not add to the effectiveness of standard medications to treat chemotherapy-induced nausea and vomiting.

Osteoarthritis. A large double-blind study (more than 250 participants) found that a combination of ginger and another Asian spice called galanga (*Alpinia galanga*) can significantly improve arthritis symptoms. This study was widely publicized as proving that ginger is effective for osteoarthritis. However, the study design makes it impossible to draw any conclusions on the effectiveness of the ginger component of the mixture. Ginger alone has been tested only in two small double-blind studies, and they had contradictory results.

Dosage

For most purposes, the standard dosage of powdered ginger is 1 to 4 g daily, divided into two to four doses per day. To prevent motion sickness, one should begin treatment one or two days before a trip and continue it throughout the period of travel.

Safety Issues

Ginger is on the GRAS (Generally Recognized As Safe) list of the U.S. Food and Drug Administration as a food, and the treatment dosages of ginger are comparable to dietary usages. No significant side effects have been observed.

Like onions and garlic, extracts of ginger inhibit blood coagulation in test-tube experiments. European studies with actual oral ginger taken alone in normal quantities have not found any significant effect on blood coagulation, but it is still theoretically possible that a weak anticoagulant could amplify the effects of drugs that have a similar effect, such as warfarin (Coumadin), heparin, clopidogrel (Plavix), ticlopidine (Ticlid), pentoxifylline (Trental), and aspirin. One fairly solid case report appears to substantiate these theoretical concerns: The use of a ginger product markedly (and dangerously) increased the effect of an anticoagulant drug closely related to Coumadin. However, a double-blind study failed to find any interaction between ginger and Coumadin, leaving the truth regarding this potential risk unclear. Finally, the maximum safe doses of ginger for pregnant or nursing women, young children, or persons with severe liver or kidney disease has not been established.

Important Interactions

Ginger could amplify the effects of strong blood-thinning drugs such as Coumadin, heparin, clopidogrel, ticlopidine, pentoxifylline, and aspirin. Also, ginger might increase the risk of bleeding problems.

—*EBSCO CAM Review Board*

References

Ware, Megan. "Ginger: Health Benefits and Dietary Tips." *Medical News Today*, MediLexicon International, 11 Sept. 2017, www.medicalnewstoday.com/articles/265990.php.

Black, Christopher D., et al. "Ginger (Zingiber Officinale) Reduces Muscle Pain Caused by Eccentric Exercise." *The Journal of Pain*, vol. 11, no. 9, 2010, pp. 894–903., doi:10.1016/j.jpain.2009.12.013.

Lakhan, Shaheen E., et al. "Zingiberaceae Extracts for Pain: a Systematic Review and Meta-Analysis." *Nutrition Journal*, vol. 14, no. 1, 14 May 2015, doi:10.1186/s12937-015-0038-8.

Rahnama, Parvin, et al. "Effect of Zingiber Officinale R. Rhizomes (Ginger) on Pain Relief in Primary Dysmenorrhea: a Placebo Randomized Trial." *BMC Complementary and Alternative Medicine*, vol. 12, no. 1, 2012, doi:10.1186/1472-6882-12-92.

Rayati, Farshid, et al. "Comparison of Anti-Inflammatory and Analgesic Effects of Ginger Powder and Ibuprofen in Postsurgical Pain Model: A Randomized, Double-Blind, Case–Control Clinical Trial." *Dental Research Journal*, vol. 14, no. 1, 2017, p. 1., doi:10.4103/1735-3327.201135.

Terry, Rohini, et al. "The Use of Ginger (Zingiber Officinale) for the Treatment of Pain: A Systematic Review of Clinical Trials." *Pain Medicine*, vol. 12, no. 12, 2011, pp. 1808–1818., doi:10.1111/j.1526-4637.2011.01261.x.

Therkleson, Tessa. "Topical Ginger Treatment With a Compress or Patch for Osteoarthritis Symptoms." *Journal of Holistic Nursing*, vol. 32, no. 3, Sept. 2013, pp. 173–182., doi:10.1177/0898010113512182.

University of Georgia. "Daily Ginger Consumption Eases Muscle Pain by 25 Percent, Study Suggests." *ScienceDaily*, 20 May 2010, www.sciencedaily.com/releases/2010/05/100519131130.htm.

■ Herbal medicine

CATEGORY: Therapy or Technique
ANATOMY OR SYSTEM AFFECTED: All

KEY TERMS

- *herbology*: the study of herbs and their medical properties, especially when combined
- *traditional Chinese medicine*: a branch of traditional medicine that is said to be based on more than 3,500 years of Chinese medical practice that includes various forms of herbal medicine, acupuncture, cupping therapy, gua sha, massage (tui na), bonesetter (die-da), exercise (qigong), and dietary therapy
- *Western herbal medicine*: a clinical practice of healing using naturally occurring plant material or plants with little or no industrial processing

Overview

Along with massage therapy, herbal treatment is one of the most ancient forms of medicine. By the time written history began, herbal medicine was already in full swing and being used all over the world.

There are several major surviving schools of herbal medicine. Two of the most complex systems are Ayurveda (the traditional herbal medicine of India) and traditional Chinese herbal medicine (TCHM). Both Ayurveda and TCHM make use of combinations of herbs. However, the herbal tradition in the West focuses more on individual herbs, sometimes known as simples. This is the form of herbology discussed here.

History of herbal medicine. Originally, herbal medicine in Europe was primarily a women's art. The classic image of witches boiling herbs in a cauldron stems to a large extent from this period. Beginning in about the thirteenth century, however, graduates of male-only medical schools and members of barber-surgeon guilds began to displace the traditional female village herbalists. Ultimately, much of the original lore was lost. (So-called traditional herbal compendiums, such as *Culpeper's Complete Herbal*, are actually of fairly recent vintage.)

Another major change took place in the nineteenth century, when chemistry had advanced far enough to allow extraction of active ingredients from herbs. The old French word for herb, *drogue*, became the name for chemical "drugs." Subsequently, these chemical extracts displaced herbs as the standard of care. Several forces led to the predominance of chemicals over herbs, but one of the most important of these forces remains a major issue today: the problem of reproducibility.

Herbal Medicine's Greatest Problem: Reproducibility

In purchasing drugs, consumers generally know exactly what they are getting. Drugs are single chemicals that can be measured and quantified down to their molecular structure. Thus, a tablet of extra-strength Tylenol, for example, contains 500

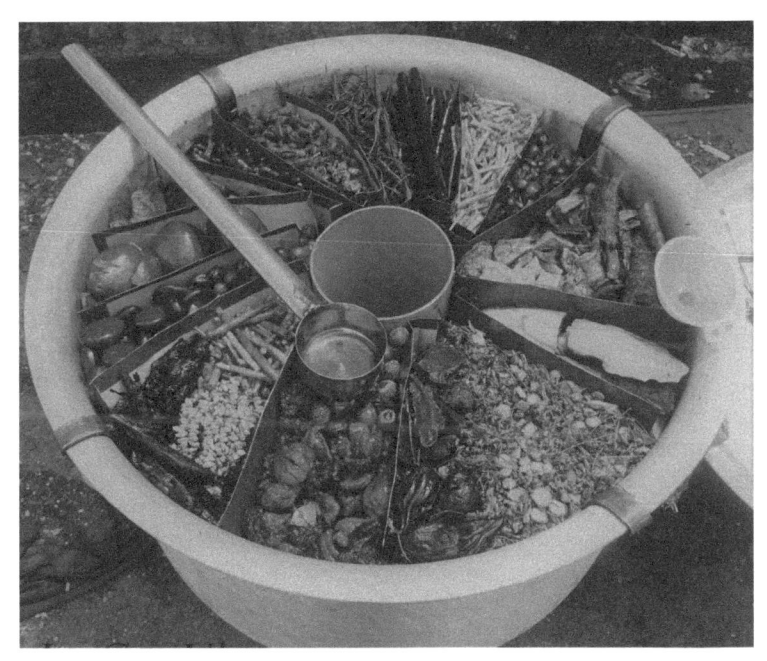

A platter of herbal medicines at Goa, India. (Joegoauk Goa via Wikimedia Commons)

milligrams of acetaminophen, regardless of where or when one buys it. Although it contains a vitamin, not a drug, the same is true of a vitamin C tablet, provided that it is correctly labeled.

Herbs, however, are living organisms comprising thousands of ingredients, and the proportions of all these ingredients may differ dramatically between two plants. Numerous influences can affect the nature of a given crop. Whether it was grown at the top or the bottom of a hill, what the weather was like, what time of year it was picked, what other plants lived nearby, and what kind of soil predominated are only a few of the factors that can affect an herb's chemical makeup.

This presents a real problem for people who wish to use herbs medicinally (as opposed to, say, for taste or fragrance). Because so much variation is possible, it is difficult to know whether one batch of an herb is equivalent in effectiveness to another.

The desire to overcome this problem provided the main initial motivation for finding the active principles of herbs and purifying them into single-chemical drugs. However, by now, most of the common herbs that possess an identifiable active ingredient have long since been turned into drugs. Today's popular herbs do not contain any known, single, active ingredients. For this reason, there is no simple way to determine the effectiveness of a given herbal batch.

This difficulty can be partially overcome by a method called herbal standardization. In this process, manufacturers make an extract of the whole herb and boil off the liquid until the concentration of some ingredient reaches a certain percentage. Contrary to popular belief, this ingredient is not usually the active ingredient; it is merely a "tag" or "handle" used for standardization purposes.

The extract is then made into tablets or capsules or bottled as a liquid, with the concentration of the tag ingredient listed on the label. This method is far from perfect, because two products with the same concentration of tag ingredients may still differ widely in other unlisted or even unidentified active constituents. Nonetheless, this form of partial standardization is better than nothing, and it allows a certain amount of reproducibility. For this reason, it is recommended that whenever possible, one should use standardized herbal extracts. Even better, one should use the very same products that were tested in double-blind studies.

Effectiveness of Herbs

There is no doubt that herbs can be effective treatments in principle, if for no other reason than that up through perhaps the 1970s, most drugs used in medicine came from herbs. Many of today's medicinal herbs have been studied in meaningful double-blind, placebo-controlled trials that provide a rational basis for believing them effective. Some of the best substantiated include *Ginkgo biloba* for Alzheimer's disease, St. John's wort for mild to moderate depression, and saw palmetto for benign prostatic hypertrophy.

However, even the best-documented herbs have less supporting evidence than the majority of drugs for one simple reason: An herb cannot be patented; therefore, no single company has the financial incentive to invest millions of dollars in research when another company can "steal" the product after it is proved to work. In addition, the problem of reproducibility always makes it difficult or impossible to know whether the batch of herbs a person is buying is as effective as the one tested in published studies.

The traditional uses of herbs are discussed here, but one should note that such uses are not reliable indicators of an herb's effectiveness. For many reasons, it simply is not possible to accurately evaluate the effectiveness of a medical treatment without performing double-blind, placebo-controlled studies, and many herbs lack these.

Safety Issues

There is a common belief that herbs are by nature safer and gentler than drugs. However, there is no rational justification for this belief. An herb is simply a plant that contains one or more drugs, and it is just as prone to side effects as any medicine, especially when taken in doses high enough to cause significant benefits.

Nonetheless, the majority of the most popular medicinal herbs are at least fairly safe. The biggest concern in practice tends to involve interactions with medications. Many herbs are known to interact with drugs, and as research into this area expands, more such interactions will be discovered.

—*EBSCO CAM Review Board*

References

Bauer, Brent A., et al. "Complementary and Alternative Medicine Therapies for Chronic Pain." *Chinese Journal of Integrative Medicine*, vol. 22, no. 6, 2016, pp. 403–411., doi:10.1007/s11655-016-2258-y.

Bhatia, ByJuhie, et al. "Herbal Remedies for Natural Pain Relief." *EverydayHealth.com*, 10 Feb. 2016, www.everydayhealth.com/pain-management/natural-pain-remedies.aspx.

Bost, Jeffreyw, et al. "Natural Anti-Inflammatory Agents for Pain Relief." *Surgical Neurology International*, vol. 1, no. 1, 2010, p. 80., doi:10.4103/2152-7806.73804.

Evans, Nicole. *Herbal Remedies: the Ultimate Guide to Herbal Remedies for Pain Relief, Stress Relief, Weight Loss, and Skin Conditions*. VDV Publishing, 2014.

Park, Kyung Moo, and Ji Hwan Kim. "Herbal Medicine for the Management of Postoperative Pain." *Medicine*, vol. 98, no. 1, 2019, doi:10.1097/md.0000000000014016.

■ Hypnotherapy

CATEGORY: Therapy or Technique
ALSO KNOWN AS: Ericksonian hypnosis, hypnosis, neurolinguistic programming, self-hypnosis
ANATOMY OR SYSTEM AFFECTED: Brain

Overview

Hypnotherapy is a poorly understood technique that has multiple definitions, descriptions, and forms. It is generally agreed that the hypnotic state is different from both sleep and ordinary wakefulness, but just exactly what it consists of remains unclear. Hypnosis is sometimes described as a form of heightened attention combined with deep relaxation, uncritical openness, and voluntarily lowered resistance to suggestion. Thus, one might say that when a person watches an engrossing film and allows himself or herself to surrender to it as if it were reality, then that person is undergoing something indistinguishable from hypnosis.

In therapeutic hypnosis, the hypnotherapist uses one of several techniques to induce a hypnotic state. The best-known (but dated) technique is the swinging watch accompanied by the suggestion to fall asleep. Such "fixed gaze" hypnosis is no longer the mainstay.

More often, hypnotists use progressive relaxation methods. Other methods include mental misdirection (as when a person is fooled during a suspenseful film) and deliberate mental confusion. The net effect is the same; the person being hypnotized is in a state of heightened willingness to accept outside suggestions.

Once the person is in this state, the hypnotherapist can make a suggestion aimed at producing therapeutic benefit. At its most straightforward, this involves direct affirmation of the desired health benefit, such as, "You are now relaxing the muscles of your neck, and you will keep them relaxed." Indirect or paradoxical suggestions may be used too, especially in schools of hypnotherapy such as Ericksonian hypnosis and neurolinguistic programming. It is also possible to learn to give oneself suggestions by inducing a state of hypnosis; this is called self-hypnosis.

Uses and Applications

Hypnotherapy is commonly used for the treatment of addictions and for reducing fear and anxiety surrounding stressful situations, such as surgery or severe illness. Other relatively common uses for hypnotherapy include insomnia, childbirth, pain control in general, and nocturnal enuresis (bedwetting). However, the evidence that hypnotherapy is effective for these uses remains incomplete at best.

Scientific Evidence

It is more difficult to ascertain the effectiveness of a therapy like hypnosis than a drug or a pill for one simple reason: It is difficult to design a proper double-blind, placebo-controlled study of this therapy. Researchers studying the herb St. John's wort, for example, can use placebo pills that are indistinguishable from the real thing. However, it is difficult to conceive of a form of placebo hypnosis that cannot be detected as such by both practitioners and participants. For this reason, all studies of hypnosis have made various compromises to the double-blind design. Some studies randomly assigned participants to receive either hypnosis or no treatment. In the best of these studies, results were rated by examiners who did not know which participants were in which group (in other words, the examiners were blinded observers). However, it is not clear whether benefits reported in such studies come from the hypnosis or less specific factors, such as mere attention.

Other studies have compared hypnosis with various psychological techniques, including relaxation therapy and cognitive psychotherapy. However, the same issues arise when trying to study these latter therapies as with hypnosis, and the results of a study that compares an unproven treatment to an unproven treatment are not meaningful.

In some studies, participants were allowed to choose whether they received hypnosis or some other therapy. Such nonrandomized studies are highly unreliable; the people who chose hypnosis, for example, might have been different in another way.

Even less meaningful studies of hypnotism simply involved giving people hypnosis and monitoring them to see whether they improved. Studies of this type have been used to support the use of hypnotherapy for hundreds of medical conditions. However, for many reasons, such open-label trials prove nothing.

In studies of most medical therapies, researchers must be sure to eliminate the possibility of a placebo effect. This concern, however, loses its relevance when hypnotism is in question. It is not a criticism of a study on hypnosis if an observed benefit turns out to be caused by the power of suggestion. After all, hypnosis consists precisely of the power of suggestion. (The placebo effect is only one of many problems with open-label studies, however.) Given these caveats, this article discusses what science knows about the medical benefits of hypnotherapy.

Possible benefits of hypnotherapy. A minimum of twenty controlled studies, enrolling more than fifteen hundred people in total, evaluated the potential benefit of hypnosis for people undergoing surgery. The combined results of the studies suggest that hypnosis may provide benefits both during and after surgery, benefits including reducing anxiety, pain, and nausea; normalizing blood pressure and heart rate; minimizing blood loss; speeding recovery; and shortening hospitalization. Many of these studies, however, were of poor quality.

Hypnosis has also shown some promise for reducing nausea, pain, and anxiety in adults and children undergoing treatment for cancer. It also may be useful in persons with breast cancer who also have hot flashes.

Numerous anecdotal reports suggest that warts can sometimes disappear in response to suggestion. In three controlled studies enrolling a total of 180 people with warts, the use of hypnosis showed superior results compared to no treatment. In one of these studies, hypnosis also was superior to salicylic acid (a standard treatment for warts). In that trial, hypnosis also was better than fake salicylic acid, hinting that the power of suggestion is greater with hypnosis than with an ordinary placebo.

Many smokers have tried hypnotherapy to break their addiction. While hypnotherapy benefits some smokers, it does not appear to be superior to other methods. In a review of nine studies, researchers found no consistent evidence that hypnotherapy was better than fourteen other interventions for nicotine addiction. Also, a later trial found that, when combined with a nicotine patch, hypnotherapy was no better than cognitive behavioral therapy.

Other conditions for which hypnosis has shown promise in controlled trials include the following: asthma, burn injury (reducing pain), fibromyalgia, hay fever, irritable bowel syndrome, labor and delivery and other gynecologic procedures, nocturnal enuresis, chest pain of unknown cause (unrelated to the heart), peptic ulcers, psoriasis, pain associated with diagnostic procedures, tension headache and other forms of headache, and vertigo and headache caused by head injury. However, the quality of many of the supporting studies was poor, and their results were frequently inconsistent.

Hypnosis is particularly popular as an aid to weight loss. However, a careful analysis of published studies shows that hypnosis is not effective for this condition; at best, the evidence points toward only a marginal benefit.

What to Expect During Treatment

Hypnotherapy sessions usually last thirty to sixty minutes. They typically involve some questions and answers, followed by the hypnosis itself. Some hypnotists teach their clients self-hypnosis so they can reinforce the formal session.

Choosing a Practitioner

As with all medical therapies, it is best to choose a licensed practitioner in states where a hypnotherapy license is available. Where licensure is not available, one should seek a referral from a qualified and knowledgeable medical provider.

Safety Issues

In the hands of a competent practitioner, hypnotherapy should present no more risks than any other form of psychotherapy. These risks might include worsening of the original problem and temporary fluctuations in mood.

Contrary to various works of fiction, hypnosis does not give the hypnotist absolute power over his or her subject. However, as with all forms of psychotherapy, the hypnotherapist does gain some power over the client through the client's trust; an unethical therapist can abuse this power.

—*EBSCO CAM Review Board*

References

Brugnoli, Maria Paola, et al. "The Role of Clinical Hypnosis and Self-Hypnosis to Relief Pain and Anxiety in Severe Chronic Diseases in Palliative Care: a 2-Year Long-Term Follow-up of Treatment in a Nonrandomized Clinical Trial." *Annals of Palliative Medicine*, vol. 7, no. 1, 2018, pp. 17–31., doi:10.21037/apm.2017.10.03.

Lee, Jin-Seong, and Young Don Pyun. "Use of Hypnosis in the Treatment of Pain." *The Korean Journal of Pain*, vol. 25, no. 2, 2012, p. 75., doi:10.3344/kjp.2012.25.2.75.

Newman, Tim. "Just How Effective Is Hypnosis at Relieving Pain?" *Medical News Today*, MediLexicon International, 28 Apr. 2019, www.medicalnewstoday.com/articles/325041.php#1.

Norton, Amy. "Could Hypnotherapy Be Alternative to Opioids for Pain?" *U.S. News & World Report*, 17 May 2019, www.usnews.com/news/health-news/articles/2019-05-17/could-hypnotherapy-be-alternative-to-opioids-for-pain.

Roberts, R Lynae, et al. "Hypnosis for Burn-Related Pain: Case Studies and a Review of the Literature." *World Journal of Anesthesiology*, vol. 6, no. 1, 2017, pp. 1–13., doi:10.5313/wja.v6.i1.1.

Williams, Sarah C.P. "Study Identifies Brain Areas Altered during Hypnotic Trances." *Stanford Medicine*, 28 July 2016, med.stanford.edu/news/all-news/2016/07/study-identifies-brain-areas-altered-during-hypnotic-trances.html.

■ Integrative medicine

CATEGORY: Therapy or Technique
ANATOMY OR SYSTEM AFFECTED: All

RELATED TERMS

Ayurveda: the traditional Hindu system of medicine, which is based on the idea of balance in bodily systems and uses diet, herbal treatment, and yogic breathing

cross-cultural medicine: the ability of providers and organizations to effectively deliver health care services that meet the social, cultural, and linguistic needs of patients

functional medicine: a personalized, systems-oriented model that empowers patients and practitioners to achieve the highest expression of health by working in collaboration to address the underlying causes of disease

homeopathy: the treatment of disease by minute doses of natural substances that in a healthy person would produce symptoms of disease

guided imagery: the use of words and music to evoke positive imaginary scenarios in a subject with a view to bringing about some beneficial effect

manual therapy: the skilled application of passive movement to a joint either within or beyond its active range of movement

mind/body therapy: techniques designed to enhance the mind's positive impact on the body

self-healing: the process of recovery (generally from psychological disturbances, trauma, etc.), motivated by and directed by the patient, guided often only by instinct

Overview

According to Andrew Weil, a prominent physician and a proponent of this system, integrative medicine (IM) works with the body's natural potential for healing. In the human body, many pathways and mechanisms serve to maintain health and promote healing. The IM perspective recognizes that treatment, often a combination of allopathic and alternative medicine, should unblock and enhance these mechanisms.

In practice, the therapeutic process addresses the whole person and relies on the main pillars of a person's well-being: mind, body, spirit, and community. This paradigm emphasizes the importance of a sound physician-patient relationship for a successful healing process. Developing rapport and empathy greatly facilitates the efficacy of lifestyle changes and the use of therapies such as pharmaceuticals, homeopathy, dietary supplements, traditional Chinese medicine, Ayurveda, manual methods, mind/body techniques, and movement therapy.

Until the 1970s, little was done to connect traditional, ancient healing modalities to biomedicine. At that time, the holistic health movement in the United States and in Western Europe started a "dynamic alliance" of therapists, including Native American healers, yoga teachers, and homeopaths. Modern medicine began taking steps to reduce the excessive use of technology and the inherent disconnect from the patient, while rediscovering more natural, less invasive avenues of healing.

The Consortium of Academic Health Centers for Integrative Medicine, founded in 2000, brings together many highly esteemed academic medical centers dedicated to promoting IM through educational opportunities, health policies, research, and collaborative initiatives. The term "integrative medicine" will most likely be used until the value of this balanced approach becomes widely recognized as simply good medicine.

Mechanism of Action

Integrative medicine combines conventional medical treatments with carefully selected alternative therapies that are proven to be safe and effective. The goal of the integrative movement is to bring back the art of healing and to address the root of the pathological process, not just the symptoms. In addition to acquiring the foundations of medical knowledge, physicians should be able to release, explore, and exploit the intrinsic healing responses of the body. Practitioners are therefore encouraged to become familiar with, and critically assess, the modalities of complementary and alternative medicine (CAM).

Core areas of education include the philosophy of science, cross-cultural medicine, principles of mind/body medicine, self-healing, and spirituality. The practitioner's ability to self-explore and maintain his or her own health balance are considered essential for the therapeutic act. The physician strives to become a partner and a mentor, who understands the important coordinates of his or her patient's life events, culture, beliefs, and relationships. By acknowledging a person's uniqueness, the processes of health maintenance and healing are tailored to best address a person's background and conditions. Matching the patient's belief system can, especially in chronic illness, lead to the activation of an internal healing response, often known as the placebo effect. Far from being a useless phenomenon based on deception, this response ultimately results in enhanced health.

Uses and Applications

Overall, IM is a combination of art and science that seeks health maintenance and disease prevention and treatment using the most natural, least invasive interventions available. Virtually all categories of disorders, and especially chronic diseases, can benefit from an integrated approach.

Cardiovascular disorders. Cardiovascular disorders such as congestive heart failure, coronary artery disease, hypertension, and peripheral vascular disease can be treated with conventional methods and with lifestyle modifications, nutrition, dietary supplements (omega-3 fatty acids, coenzyme Q_{10}, carnitine, arginine, hawthorn, and garlic), relaxation, meditation, and hydrotherapy. Primary prevention is critical in coronary artery disease and hypertension.

Cancer. Cancer can be treated with the synergistic reduction of the sequellae and by limiting the toxicity or trauma of conventional therapies and by alleviating psychological distress. Nutritional changes, dietary supplements (vitamins, immunomodulators, ginger, marijuana, and St. John's wort), acupuncture, mind/body techniques, and group support are often recommended. Preventive approaches (for breast cancer, for example) involve lifestyle changes (exercise, nutrition, limiting toxins, and breast-feeding), botanicals (seaweed, rosemary, and green tea), and mind/body methods.

Endocrine and metabolic disorders. Endocrine and metabolic disorders are also amenable to integrated therapies. Insulin resistance is often treated with metformin hydrochloride, lifestyle changes, and a low-carbohydrate diet. Supplements such as chromium, vanadium, alpha-lipoic acid, American ginseng, and fenugreek can provide benefits too. In persons with diabetes mellitus, essential care includes diet, exercise, and pharmaceuticals. Dietary supplements, such as vitamins, bilberry, and *Ginkgo biloba*, and mind/body techniques (for example, relaxation and yoga) may mitigate vascular disease and even lower glucose levels. Alternative therapies to consider in persons with hypothyroidism include dietary supplements such as vitamins, zinc, selenium, and traditional Chinese botanicals, and practices such as yoga. Pharmaceuticals are available for the treatment of osteoporosis, and vitamin D, ipriflavone, and exercise constitute useful adjuvants.

Gastrointestinal disorders. Gastroesophageal reflux, peptic ulcer disease, and irritable bowel syndrome can be treated with lifestyle changes and with botanicals (licorice, chamomile, and marshmallow root), homeopathics, and mind/body therapies (including stress management and guided imagery).

Neurological disorders. Stroke, multiple sclerosis, Alzheimer's disease, Parkinson's disease, seizures, and migraine have been linked to oxidative stress, neurotoxic factors, and inflammatory processes. Thus, they can greatly benefit from integrative methods. The complementary therapies include, but are not limited to, dietary and nutritional supplementation (omega-3 fatty acids, glutathione, coenzyme Q_{10}, alpha-lipoic acid, N-acetylcysteine, niacin, vitamins, melatonin, and magnesium), herbal supplementation (*Ginkgo biloba*, milk thistle, turmeric, vinpocetine, and skullcap), meditation, yoga, and exercise.

Asthma and allergies. Asthma and allergies respond well to alternative methods that include nutritional and environmental changes, exercise, botanicals (ginkgo, coleus, licorice, kanpo, bioflavonoids, and stinging nettle), vitamins and minerals, homeopathics, massage, inhalation, breathing techniques, and mind/body therapy.

Upper respiratory infections and sinusitis. Upper respiratory infections and sinusitis can be treated with pharmaceuticals, dietary changes, hydration, steam inhalation, supplements (vitamins, antioxidants, zinc, magnesium, garlic, and echinacea), and homeopathic remedies.

Depression and anxiety. Depression and anxiety represent a spectrum of disorders ideally suited for IM. In addition to pharmaceuticals, persons can benefit from lifestyle changes, physical activity, nutritional remedies (omega-3 fatty acids, B vitamins, folic acid, and hydroxytryptophan), botanical remedies (St. John's wort, kava kava, and ginkgo), psychotherapy, relaxation training, yoga, acupuncture, and transcranial stimulation.

Pain. Pain management represents a challenge for both the physician and the person in pain. Truly integrating allopathic and alternative medicines can offer relief and reduce frustration. Reassurance and lifestyle changes are often the first step of the therapeutic plan. A vast array of useful approaches includes pharmacotherapy, exercise, supplements (arnica and omega-3 fatty acids), homeopathy, manual methods, acupuncture, transcutaneous nerve stimulation, and mind/body therapy. Surgery is considered after conservative therapies have failed.

Pregnancy and menopause. The integrative approach to pregnancy and menopause reaches beyond the use of combined mainstream and alternative therapies. These conditions require a careful initial encounter and subsequent consideration of the mind, body, spirit, and community context. The patient-practitioner interaction is oriented toward health rather than disease, and listening to the person seeking care is essential. In pregnancy especially, the need for noninvasive, natural approaches becomes crucial. Nausea and vomiting, for example, are treated with supplements (vitamin B_6, red raspberry leaf, ginger root, and chamomile), homeopathics, acupuncture, and mind/body therapies.

Alcoholism and substance abuse. Therapeutic options for alcoholism and substance abuse include botanicals (valerian, kudzu, kava kava), acupuncture, mind/body therapies, and spirituality. The options also include twelve-step programs.

Scientific Evidence

Integrative practice is committed to the scientific method and is rooted in evidence. At the same time, the integrative practitioner aims to transcend the confines of "scientific truth" and connect with the people he or she serves on multiple levels.

A number of CAM therapies have proved effective as complements to conventional medical treatments. These CAM therapies include dietary and herbal supplements, acupuncture, manual therapy, biofeedback, relaxation training, and movement therapy. When a strong evidence base is developed for a particular complementary method, it can become part of the integrative armamentarium. After it reviewed the evidence base, for example, the Society for Integrative Oncology supported the use of acupuncture in cases in which cancer-related pain is poorly controlled.

According to the American Academy of Pediatrics, a review conducted in 2002 found more than fourteen hundred randomized-control trials of pediatric CAM; the quality of these trials was determined to be as good as those focusing on conventional therapies. It is important to note that different levels of evidence are required to prove the safety and efficacy of complementary therapies, depending on the goals of the treatment. Lower levels of evidence (that is, nonrandomized and observational studies) are acceptable for preventive or supportive goals and for noninvasive approaches. Furthermore, integrating represents more than combining; it involves holistic treatment and the synergistic application of an array of treatments. Thus, the extent of the combination or integration varies. This leads to unique challenges for the scientific validation of integrative methods. Traditional research models often appear inadequate. More studies are needed that examine the appropriateness and manner of integration for specific diseases and conditions.

Choosing a Practitioner

Approximately 70 percent of medical schools in the United States have courses in CAM. Integrative medicine centers and fellowship programs exist at many prominent universities and hospitals in the United States, including the University of Arizona, Duke University, Harvard University, the University of Michigan, and the Mayo Clinic. These centers tend to be directed by conventional physicians (doctors of medicine and doctors of osteopathy) and staffed by various practitioners.

The American Board of Integrative Holistic Medicine establishes standards for the application of IM principles and offers certification. The American Association of Integrative Medicine provides an accreditation program. Even so, qualified IM practitioners are still difficult to find, and the demand greatly exceeds the supply. Oftentimes, the collaboration between conventional physicians of various specialties and certified CAM practitioners provides the foundation and benefits of integrative care. The American Holistic Medical Association maintains a directory of integrative and holistic practitioners holding relevant degrees.

Safety Issues

When implemented by physicians and CAM practitioners who are well versed in the integrative method, IM is safe and beneficial.

—*Mihaela Avramut, M.D., Ph.D.*

References

Altug, Ziya. *Integrative Healing: Developing Wellness in the Mind and Body.* Plain Sight Publishing, An Imprint of Cedar Fort, Inc., 2018.

Chen, Lucy, and Andreas Michalsen. "Management of Chronic Pain Using Complementary and Integrative Medicine." *Bmj*, 24 Apr. 2017, doi:10.1136/bmj.j1284.

Clark, Stephanie D., et al. "Effect of Integrative Medicine Services on Pain for Hospitalized Patients at an Academic Health Center." *Explore*, vol. 15, no. 1, 2019, pp. 61–64., doi:10.1016/j.explore.2018.07.006.

Ellis, Deborah. " Holistic Approaches to Chronic Pain." *U.S. Pain Foundation*, 6 Mar. 2019, uspainfoundation.org/blog/holistic-approaches-to-chronic-pain/.

Kress, Hans-Georg, et al. "A Holistic Approach to Chronic Pain Management That Involves All Stakeholders: Change Is Needed." *Current Medical Research and Opinion*, vol. 31, no. 9, 20 Aug. 2015, pp. 1743–1754., doi:10.1185/03007995.2015.1072088.

Mao, Jun J., and Jeffery A. Dusek. "Integrative Medicine as Standard Care for Pain Management: The Need for Rigorous Research." *Pain Medicine*, vol. 17, no. 6, 26 May 2016, pp. 1181–1182., doi:10.1093/pm/pnw102.

McGregor, Jennifer. "How Holistic Methods May Help Your Chronic Pain." *Pain Connection*, 1 Sept. 2016, www.painconnection.org/blog/how-holistic-methods-may-help-your-chronic-pain/.

Saha, Felix J., et al. "Integrative Medicine for Chronic Pain." *Medicine*, vol. 95, no. 27, 2016, doi:10.1097/md.0000000000004152.

■ Kratom

CATEGORY: Addiction Risk; Herbs and Supplements
ALSO KNOWN AS: Biak-Biak; Ithang; Ketum; Kakuam; *Mitragyna speciosa*; Thom
ANATOMY OR SYSTEM AFFECTED: Nervous system; Spinal cord

Kratom is an herb derived from a tropical tree (*Mitragyna specisosa*) commonly found in Thailand, Myanmar, Papua New Guinea, and Malaysia. Kratom is currently a legal drug widely available in the United States. The U.S. Food and Drug Administration (FDA) are cautioning consumers not to use Kratom and there are currently no FDA-approved uses for Kratom. However, there are conflicting initiatives from the public pushing to have the drug approved as a substitute for other opioids due its promising therapeutic potential and relatively decreased side effect profile.

Mechanism of Action

Kratom has been known to act as both an opioid and a stimulant dependent on the dose someone ingests. Kratom binds to mu and delta-opioid receptors and causes similar effects as opioid medications without the respiratory depression expected by traditional prescription or illicit opioids. It may also bind to serotonergic and noradrenergic pathways in the spinal cord. It may act as a stimulant when someone is utilizing lower doses which may result in increased alertness, more energy, and more social behavior. When ingesting higher doses the opioid-like response will be greater and someone may experience relaxation, pain relief, sociability, and even euphoria. Kratom is commonly being used to treat musculoskeletal pain, diarrhea, opiate addiction, and opiate withdrawal. Many other consumers report using the herb as an anti-inflammatory, antipyretic, antitussive, or antihypertensive medication.

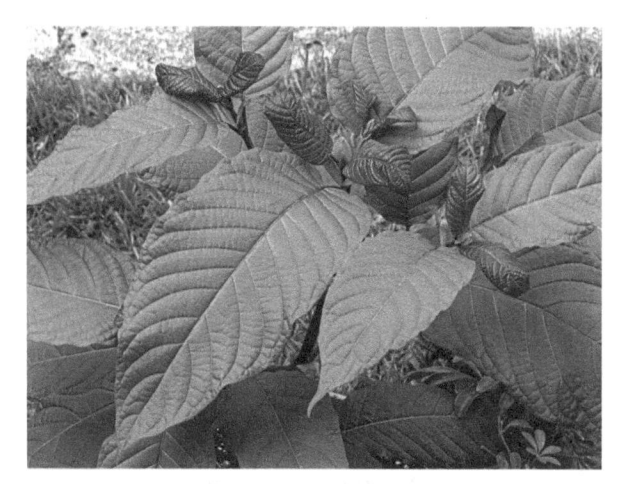

A young M. speciosa *tree.* (ThorPorre via Wikimedia Commons)

Risks

Kratom is still being researched for uses, dosing, efficacy, and safety. Some common adverse effects associated with using Kratom include nausea, itching, sedation, constipation, loss of appetite, dizziness, and confusion. There have been several reported cases of psychosis with hallucinations and delusions induced by Kratom use. Even though Kratom does not typically cause respiratory depression, there have been several reported overdoses related to Kratom use. Most, but not all, overdose cases identified had simultaneous use of other drugs which may have contributed to the adverse outcome.

Since Kratom acts on opioid receptors in the same manner as other opioid drugs there is serious concern for abuse, addiction, and detrimental health consequences. A regular user may develop a physical dependence for the drug and possibly experience withdrawal symptoms after discontinuing the herb. Regular Kratom users may experience irritability, anxiety, yawning, rhinorrhea, stomach cramps, sweating, diarrhea, and strong drug cravings when abruptly discontinuing the drug. The withdrawal from Kratom appears to be very similar to the withdrawal symptoms exhibited when withdrawing from prescription and illicit opioid medications.

There are several reports of hepatotoxicity in people who use Kratom regularly. Regular use for several weeks is associated with occasional acute liver injury. People may present with abdominal pain, nausea, fatigue, pruritus, or dark urine. There is no clear cause of liver injury but it is suspected the concurrent use of other drugs of abuse may contribute. In most cases, the discontinuation of Kratom has resulted in rapid improvement of the liver injury.

Aside from the insufficient knowledge about the drug and the potential health problems, there are several concerns associated with Kratom use at this time due to limited regulation of the herb. Kratom is often distributed as a tablet, leaf, powder, or tea which is not regulated by the FDA. Many of the labels on Kratom packaging report the content is not fit for human consumption. There have also been several reported cases of salmonella related to Kratom use. While further studies are conducted and regulation policies are created, extreme caution is recommended for people utilizing Kratom.

—*Christine Gamble MD*

References

American Chemical Society. "Kratom's Reputed Pain-Relief Benefits Could Come from One of Its Metabolites." *ScienceDaily*, 29 May 2019, www.sciencedaily.com/releases/2019/05/190529113045.htm.

Grinspoon, Peter. "Kratom: Fear-Worthy Foliage or Beneficial Botanical?" *Harvard Health Publishing*, Harvard Medical School, 26 Sept. 2019, www.health.harvard.edu/blog/kratom-fear-worthy-foliage-or-beneficial-botanical-2019080717466.

NIDA. "Kratom." *National Institute on Drug Abuse*, National Institutes of Health, Apr. 2019, www.drugabuse.gov/publications/drugfacts/kratom.

Prozialeck, Walter C., et al. "Kratom Policy: The Challenge of Balancing Therapeutic Potential with Public Safety." *International Journal of Drug Policy*, vol. 70, 2019, pp. 70–77., doi:10.1016/j.drugpo.2019.05.003.

Roth, Christine. "Study Pokes Holes in Kratom's 'Bad Rap'." *University of Rochester Medical Center*, 14 Dec. 2017, www.urmc.rochester.edu/news/story/5202/study-pokes-holes-in-kratoms-bad-rap.aspx.

Tayabali, Khadija, et al. "Kratom: a Dangerous Player in the Opioid Crisis." *Journal of Community Hospital Internal Medicine Perspectives*, vol. 8, no. 3, 4 June 2018, pp. 107–110., doi:10.1080/20009666.2018.1468693.

Veltri, Charles, and Oliver Grundmann. "Current Perspectives on the Impact of Kratom Use." *Substance Abuse and Rehabilitation*, vol. 10, 2019, pp. 23–31., doi:10.2147/sar.s164261.

■ Lavender

CATEGORY: Herbs and Supplements

ALSO KNOWN AS: English lavender, essential oil of lavender, lavender oil, *Lavandula angustifolia*, *L. officinalis*

ANATOMY OR SYSTEM AFFECTED: Nervous system

Overview

There are many plants in the lavender family, but the type most commonly used medicinally is English lavender. Traditionally, the essential oil of lavender was applied externally to treat joint pain, muscle aches, and a variety of skin conditions, including insect stings, acne, eczema, and burns. Lavender essential oil was also inhaled to relieve headaches, anxiety, and stress. Tincture of lavender was taken by mouth for joint pain, depression, migraines, indigestion, and anxiety. Lavender was additionally used as a hair rinse and as a fragrance in "dream pillows" and potpourri.

Therapeutic Dosages

When used internally, lavender tincture is taken at a dose of 2 to 4 milliliters three times a day. Lavender essential oil is used externally or by inhalation only; it should not be used internally.

Therapeutic Uses

Lavender continues to be recommended for all its traditional uses. Only a few of these uses, however, have any supporting scientific evidence whatsoever, and for none of these is the evidence strong.

A few studies suggest that lavender oil, when taken by inhalation (aromatherapy) might reduce agitation in people with severe dementia. For example, in one well-designed but small study, a hospital ward was suffused with either lavender oil or water for two hours. An investigator who was unaware of the study's design and who wore a device to block inhalation of odors entered the

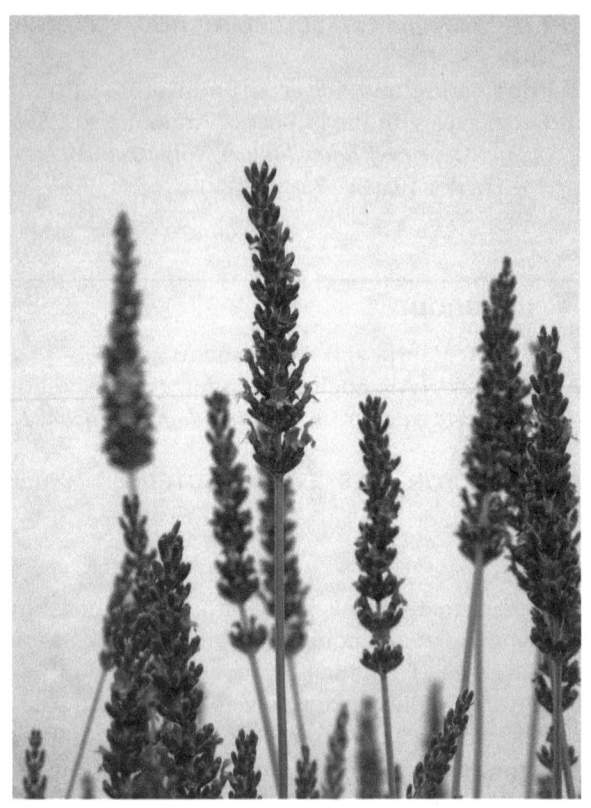

Close-up of lavender flower. (Sacamol via Wikimedia Commons)

ward and evaluated the behavior of the fifteen residents, all of whom had dementia. The results indicated that the use of lavender oil aromatherapy modestly decreased agitated behavior. A somewhat less rigorous study reported similar benefits. Rigor is essential in such studies, as it has been shown that merely creating expectations about the effects of aromas may be sufficient to cause these effects.

A preliminary controlled trial found some evidence that lavender, administered through an oxygen face mask, reduced the need for pain medications following gastric banding surgery. A small study performed in Iran reported that oral use of lavender tincture augmented the effectiveness of a pharmaceutical treatment for depression. However, this study suffered from numerous problems, both in design and reporting, and in the scientific reputation of the investigators involved.

In a controlled trial with more than six hundred participants, lavender oil in bath water failed to improve perineal pain after childbirth. One poorly designed study found weak hints that lavender might be useful for insomnia. One animal study failed to find that lavender oil enhances wound healing. Lavender is also used in combination with other essential oils.

Safety Issues

No form of lavender has undergone comprehensive safety testing. Internal use of lavender essential oil is unsafe and should be avoided. Topical use is considered much safer. Allergic reactions are relatively common, as with all essential oils. In addition, one case suggests that a combination of lavender oil and tea tree oil applied topically caused gynecomastia (male breast enlargement) in three young boys.

A controlled study found that inhalation of lavender essential oil might impair some aspects of mental function. (Presumably, this was caused by the intended sedative effects of the treatment.) Oral use of tincture of lavender has not been associated with any severe adverse effects, but comprehensive safety testing has not been performed. Finally, the maximum safe doses of any form of lavender remain unknown for pregnant or nursing women, for young children, and for people with severe liver or kidney disease.

—*EBSCO CAM Review Board*

References

Koulivand, Peir Hossein, et al. "Lavender and the Nervous System." *Evidence-Based Complementary and Alternative Medicine*, 2013, pp. 1–10., doi:10.1155/2013/681304.

Nordqvist, Joseph. "Lavender: Health Benefits and Uses." *Medical News Today*, MediLexicon International, 4 Mar. 2019, www.medicalnewstoday.com/articles/265922.php.

O'Malley, Patricia Anne. "Lavender for Sleep, Rest, and Pain." *Clinical Nurse Specialist*, vol. 31, no. 2, 2017, pp. 74–76., doi:10.1097/NUR.0000000000000273.

Peterson, Stacy M. "Why Aromatherapy Is Showing up in Hospital Surgical Units." *Mayo Clinic*, Mayo Foundation for Medical Education and Research, 27 Oct. 2017, www.mayoclinic.org/healthy-lifestyle/stress-management/in-depth/why-aromatherapy-is-showing-up-in-hospital-surgical-units/art-20342126.

Sen, Ingrid. *Lavender Essential Oil: Your Complete Guide to Lavender Essential Oil Uses, Benefits, Applications and Natural Remedies.* CreateSpace Independent Publishing Platform, 2016.

Magnesium

CATEGORY: Herbs and Supplements
ALSO KNOWN AS: Magnesium chloride, magnesium citrate, magnesium fumarate, magnesium gluconate, magnesium malate, magnesium orotate, magnesium oxide, magnesium sulfate
ANATOMY OR SYSTEM AFFECTED: All

Overview

Magnesium is an essential nutrient, meaning that the body needs it for healthy functioning. It is found in significant quantities throughout the body and used for numerous purposes, including muscle relaxation, blood clotting, and the manufacture of ATP (adenosine triphosphate, the body's main energy molecule).

Magnesium has been called nature's calcium channel blocker because of its ability to block calcium from entering muscle and heart cells. A group of prescription heart medications work in a similar way, although much more powerfully. This may be the basis for some of magnesium's effects when it is taken as a supplement in fairly high doses.

Requirements and Sources

Requirements for magnesium increase as people grow and age. The official U.S. and Canadian recommendations for daily intake are as follows: 30 milligrams (mg) for infants up to six months old, 75 mg for infants seven to twelve months old, 80 mg for children one to three years old, 130 mg for children four to eight years old, and 240 mg for persons nine to thirteen years old. For those fourteen to eighteen years old, the recommendations are 410 mg for males and 360 mg for females; for those nineteen to thirty years old, 400 mg for males and 310 for females; and for those aged thirty-one and over, 420 mg for males and 320 mg for women. The recommendations for pregnant women are 400 mg for those eighteen and younger, 350 mg for those nineteen to thirty years old, and 360 mg for those thirty-one to fifty years old; for nursing women, they are 360 mg for those aged eighteen and younger, 310 mg for those nineteen to thirty, and 320 mg for those thirty-one to fifty years old.

These recommendations refer to total intake from food plus supplements. The average diet provides a daily intake of magnesium very close to these amounts. In the United States, the average dietary intake of magnesium is lower than the recommended daily allowance; however, it is unclear whether this truly indicates deficiency, or if the recommended allowance is too high. Alcohol abuse, surgery, diabetes, zinc supplements, certain types of diuretics (thiazide and loop diuretics, but not potassium-sparing diuretics), estrogen and oral contraceptives, and the medications cisplatin and cyclosporin have been reported to reduce the body's level of magnesium or increase magnesium requirements. Those taking potassium supplements may receive greater benefit from them if they take extra magnesium as well. While it is sometimes said that calcium interferes with magnesium absorption, this effect is apparently too small to have a significant effect on overall magnesium status.

Kelp is very high in magnesium, as are wheat bran, wheat germ, almonds, and cashews. Other good sources include blackstrap molasses, brewer's yeast (not to be confused with nutritional yeast), buckwheat, nuts, and whole grains. One can also get appreciable amounts of magnesium from collard greens, dandelion greens, avocado, sweet corn, cheddar cheese, sunflower seeds, shrimp, dried fruit (figs, apricots, and prunes), and from many other common fruits and vegetables.

Therapeutic Dosages

A typical supplemental dosage of magnesium ranges from the nutritional needs described above to as high as 600 mg daily. For premenstrual syndrome (PMS) and dysmenorrhea (painful menstruation), an alternative approach is to start taking 500 to 1,000 mg daily, beginning on day fifteen of the menstrual cycle and continuing until menstruation begins. Magnesium citrate may be slightly more absorbable than other forms of magnesium.

Therapeutic Uses

Preliminary double-blind studies suggest that regular use of magnesium supplements may help prevent migraine headaches, hearing loss caused by exposure to loud noises, and kidney stones and may help treat high blood pressure, angina, dysmenorrhea (menstrual cramps), pregnancy-induced leg cramps, and premenstrual syndrome (including menstrual migraines).

People with diabetes are often deficient in magnesium, and according to some (but not all) studies, magnesium supplementation may enhance blood sugar control and insulin sensitivity in people with diabetes or prediabetic conditions. Magnesium may also help control blood pressure in people with both hypertension and diabetes.

One study found that magnesium supplements might be helpful for people with mitral valve prolapse who also have low levels of magnesium in the blood. There is some evidence that magnesium may decrease the atherosclerosis risk caused by hydrogenated oils, the margarine-like fats found in many junk foods.

Magnesium supplements do not appear to be helpful for preventing preeclampsia. (Magnesium, taken by injection rather than orally, however, is probably helpful for treating preeclampsia that already exists.)

Magnesium is sometimes said to decrease symptoms of restless legs syndrome, but the evidence that it works consists solely of open trials without a placebo group, and such studies are not trustworthy. Weak evidence hints at possible benefits for insomnia.

It is often said that magnesium supplements are essential for preventing or treating osteoporosis, but there is only minimal supporting evidence for this claim. Studies on magnesium supplements for improving sports performance have returned contradictory results.

Magnesium has also been suggested as a treatment for Alzheimer's disease, attention deficit disorder, fatigue, fibromyalgia, low high-density lipoproteins (HDL, or good cholesterol), periodontal disease, rheumatoid arthritis, and stroke. However, there is virtually no evidence that it is helpful for any of these conditions. Despite some early enthusiasm, combination therapy with vitamin B_6 and magnesium has not been found helpful in autism. One double-blind, placebo-controlled study failed to find magnesium helpful in glaucoma.

Magnesium is sometimes advocated for stabilizing the heart after a heart attack, but one study actually found that use of magnesium slightly increased risk of sudden death, repeat heart attack, or need for bypass surgery in the year following the initial heart attack. However, magnesium may be helpful in congestive heart failure. In a well-designed trial involving seventy-nine patients with severe congestive heart failure, magnesium (as magnesium orotate) significantly improved survival and clinical symptoms after one year compared with a placebo.

Alternative medical literature frequently mentions magnesium as a treatment for asthma. However, this idea seems to be based primarily on the use of intravenous magnesium as an emergency treatment for asthma. Taking something by mouth is very different from having it injected into the veins. Studies of oral magnesium for asthma have shown more negative than positive results. Inhaled, aerosolized magnesium, however, has shown some promise.

Although magnesium is sometimes mentioned as a treatment to help keep the heart beating normally, a six-month double-blind trial of 170 people did not find it effective for preventing a particular heart rhythm abnormality called atrial fibrillation. However, a small double-blind, placebo-controlled trial found that magnesium supplements reduced episodes of arrhythmia in individuals with congestive heart failure (CHF). One possible explanation: People with congestive heart failure often take drugs (loop diuretics) that deplete magnesium. The combination of magnesium deficiency with digoxin (another drug given for CHF) may cause arrhythmias. Thus, it is possible that the benefits seen here were caused by correction of that depletion.

Scientific Evidence

Migraine headaches. A double-blind study found that regular use of magnesium helps prevent migraine headaches. In this twelve-week trial, eighty-one people with recurrent migraines were given either 600 mg of magnesium daily or a placebo. By the last three weeks of the study, the treated group's migraines had been reduced by 41.6 percent, compared with a reduction of 15.8 percent in the placebo group. The only side effects observed were diarrhea (in about one-fifth of the participants) and, less often, digestive irritation.

Similar results have been seen in other, smaller double-blind studies. One study found no benefit, but it has been criticized on many significant points, including using an excessively strict definition of what constituted benefit.

Noise-related hearing loss. One double-blind, placebo-controlled study on three hundred military recruits suggests that 167 mg of magnesium daily can prevent hearing loss due to exposure to high-volume noise.

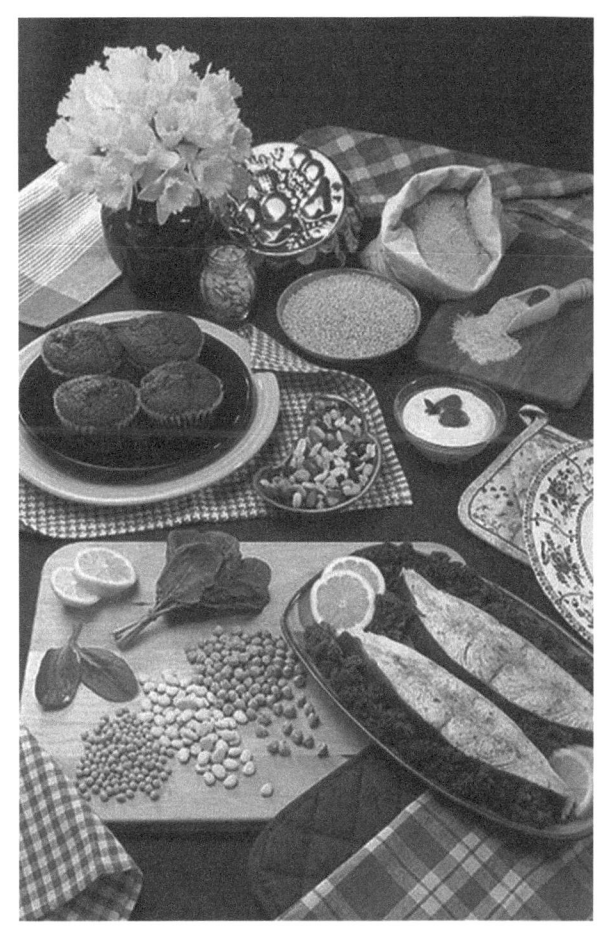

Examples of food sources of magnesium (clockwise from top left): bran muffins, pumpkin seeds, barley, buckwheat flour, low-fat vanilla yogurt, trail mix, halibut steaks, garbanzo beans, lima beans, soybeans, and spinach. (Peggy Greb via Wikimedia Commons)

Kidney stones. Magnesium inhibits the growth of calcium oxalate stones in the test tube and decreases stone formation in rats. However, human studies have had mixed results. In one two-year open study, 56 people taking magnesium hydroxide had fewer recurrences of kidney stones than 34 people not given magnesium. In contrast, a double-blind (and, hence, more reliable) study of 124 people found that magnesium hydroxide was essentially no more effective than a placebo.

Hypertension. Magnesium works with calcium and potassium to regulate blood pressure. Several studies suggest that magnesium supplements can reduce blood pressure in people with hypertension, although some studies have not shown this.

In one study, eighty-two people (ages forty to seventy-five years) with diabetes, high blood pressure, and low levels of magnesium were randomized to receive 2.5 g of magnesium chloride or a placebo for four months. Those in the treatment group had lower blood pressure readings compared with those in the control group.

Angina. In a double-blind, placebo-controlled trial of 187 people with angina, six months of treatment with magnesium at a dose of 730 mg daily improved exercise tolerance and enhanced overall quality of life. Benefits were also seen in a similar, smaller double-blind trial.

After a heart attack. In a one-year double-blind, placebo-controlled trial of 468 individuals who had just experienced a heart attack, use of a magnesium supplement at a dose of 360 mg daily failed to prevent heart-related events (defined as heart attack, sudden cardiac death, or need for cardiac bypass) and actually may have increased the risk slightly.

Dysmenorrhea. A six-month double-blind, placebo-controlled study of fifty women with menstrual pain found that treatment with magnesium significantly improved symptoms. The researchers reported evidence of reduced levels of prostaglandin F 2 alpha, a hormone-like substance involved in pain and inflammation. Similarly positive results were seen in a double-blind, placebo-controlled study of twenty-one women.

Premenstrual syndrome (PMS). A double-blind, placebo-controlled study of thirty-two women found that magnesium taken from day fifteen of the menstrual cycle to the onset of menstrual flow could significantly improve PMS symptoms, specifically mood changes.

Another small, double-blind preliminary study found that regular use of magnesium could reduce symptoms of PMS-related fluid retention. In this study, thirty-eight women were given magnesium or placebo for two months. The results showed no effect after one cycle, but by the end of two cycles, magnesium significantly reduced weight gain, swelling of extremities, breast tenderness, and abdominal bloating. In addition, one small double-blind study (twenty participants) found that magnesium supplementation can help prevent menstrual migraines. Preliminary evidence suggests that the combination of magnesium and vitamin B_6 might be more effective than either treatment alone.

Pregnancy-induced leg cramps. Pregnant women frequently experience painful leg cramping. One double-blind trial of seventy-three pregnant women found that three weeks of magnesium supplements significantly reduced leg cramps compared with a placebo.

Safety Issues

The U.S. government has set the following upper limits for use of magnesium supplements: 65 mg for children aged one to three, 110 mg for children four to eight, 350 mg for adults, and 350 mg for pregnant or nursing women. In general, magnesium appears to be quite safe when taken at or below recommended dosages. The most common complaint is loose stools. However, people with severe kidney or heart disease should not take magnesium (or any other supplement) except on the advice of a physician. Maximum safe dosages have not been established for children of all ages. There has been one case of death caused by excessive use of magnesium supplements in a developmentally and physically disabled child. Pregnant or nursing women should not exceed the nutritional dosages presented in the Requirements and Sources section.

If taken at the same time, magnesium can interfere with the absorption of antibiotics in the tetracycline family and, possibly of the drug nitrofurantoin. Also, when combined with oral diabetes drugs in the sulfonylurea family, magnesium may cause blood sugar levels to fall more than expected.

Important Interactions

Persons taking potassium supplements, manganese, loop and thiazide diuretics, oral contraceptives, estrogen replacement therapy, cisplatin, digoxin, or medications that reduce stomach acid may need extra magnesium. Persons taking antibiotics in the tetracycline family or nitrofurantoin (Macrodantin) should separate their magnesium dose from doses of these medications by at least two hours to avoid absorption problems. Those taking oral diabetes medications in the sulfonylurea family (Tolinase, Micronase, Orinase, Glucotrol, Diabinese, DiaBeta) should work closely with their physicians when taking magnesium to avoid hypoglycemia. Those taking amiloride should not take magnesium supplements except on medical advice.

—*EBSCO CAM Review Board*

References

Castro, Jessica, and Maureen F. Cooney. "Intravenous Magnesium in the Management of Postoperative Pain." *Journal of PeriAnesthesia Nursing*, vol. 32, no. 1, Feb. 2017, pp. 72–76., doi:10.1016/j.jopan.2016.11.007.

Crosby, Vincent, et al. "Magnesium." *Journal of Pain and Symptom Management*, vol. 45, no. 1, 2013, pp. 137–144., doi:10.1016/j.jpainsymman.2012.10.005.

Dean, Carolyn. *The Magnesium Miracle*. 2nd ed., Ballantine Books, 2017.

George, Renuka, et al. "'Oh Mg!' Magnesium: A Powerful Tool in the Perioperative Setting." *ASRA News*, American Society of Regional Anesthesia and Pain Medicine, Aug. 2018, www.asra.com/asra-news/article/105/oh-mg-magnesium-a-powerful-tool-in-the.

Park, Rex, et al. "Magnesium for the Management of Chronic Noncancer Pain in Adults: Protocol for a Systematic Review." *JMIR Research Protocols*, vol. 8, no. 1, 11 Jan. 2019, doi:10.2196/11654.

Teitelbaum, Jacob. "Magnesium for Pain Relief." *Psychology Today*, Sussex Publishers, 16 Sept. 2010, www.psychologytoday.com/us/blog/complementary-medicine/201009/magnesium-pain-relief.

■ Magnet therapy

CATEGORY: Therapy or Technique
ANATOMY OR SYSTEM AFFECTED: All

KEY TERMS

- *alternating pole devices*: magnets that expose the skin to both north and south magnetic fields
- *pulsed electromagnetic field therapy*: uses electromagnetic fields in an attempt to heal non-union fractures and depression
- *repetitive transcranial magnet therapy*: a form of brain stimulation therapy used to treat depression and anxiety
- *static magnets*: a magnet that retains its magnetism after being removed from a magnetic field
- *unipolar magnets*: magnets with north on one side and south on the other; the north (or negative) side is typically applied to the skin

Overview

Long popular in Japan, magnet therapy has entered public awareness in the United States, stimulated by golfers and tennis players extolling the virtues of magnets in the treatment of sports-related injuries. Magnetic knee, shoulder, and ankle pads, and insoles and mattress pads, are widely available and are thought to provide myriad healing benefits.

Despite this enthusiasm, there is little scientific evidence to support the use of magnets for any medical condition. However, some small studies suggest that various forms of magnet therapy might have a therapeutic effect in certain conditions.

History of magnet therapy. Magnet therapy has a long history in traditional folk medicine. Reliable documentation indicates that Chinese doctors have believed in the therapeutic value of magnets for two thousand years or more. In sixteenth-century Europe, Paracelsus used magnets to treat a variety of ailments. Two centuries later, Franz Mesmer became famous for treating various disorders with magnets.

In the middle decades of the twentieth century, scientists in various parts of the world began performing studies on the therapeutic use of magnets. From the 1940s on, magnets became increasingly popular in Japan. Yoshio Manaka, one of the influential Japanese acupuncturists of the twentieth century, used magnets in conjunction with acupuncture. Magnet therapy also became a commonly used technique of self-administered medicine in Japan. For example, a type of plaster containing a small magnet became popular for treating aches and pains, especially among the elderly. Magnetic mattress pads, bracelets, and necklaces also became popular, mainly among the elderly. During the 1970s, both magnets and electromagnetic machines became popular among athletes in many countries for treating sports-related injuries.

These developments led to a rapidly growing industry creating magnetic products for a variety of conditions. However, the development of this industry preceded any reliable scientific evidence that static magnets actually work for the purposes intended. In the United States, it was only in 1997 that properly designed clinical trials of magnets began to be reported. Subsequently, results of several preliminary studies suggested that both static magnets and electromagnetic therapy may indeed offer therapeutic benefits for several disorders. These findings have escalated research interest in magnet therapy.

Types of magnet therapy and their uses. The term "magnet therapy" usually refers to the use of static magnets placed directly on the body, generally over regions of pain. Static magnets are either attached to the body by tape or encapsulated in specially designed products such as belts, wraps, or mattress pads. Static magnets are also sometimes known as permanent magnets.

Static magnets come in various strengths. The units of measuring magnet strength are gauss (G) and tesla (T); 1 tesla equals 10,000 G. A refrigerator magnet, for example, is around 200 G. Therapeutic magnets measure anywhere from 200 to 10,000 G, but the most commonly used measure from 400 to 800 G.

Therapeutic magnets come in two different types of polarity arrangements: unipolar magnets and alternating-pole devices. Magnets that have north on one side and south on the other are known, rather confusingly, as unipolar magnets. Bipolar or alternating-pole magnets are made from a sheet of magnetic material with north and south magnets arranged in an alternating pattern, so that both north and south face the skin. This type of magnet exerts a weaker magnetic field because the alternating magnets tend to oppose each other. Each type of magnet has its own recommended uses and enthusiasts. (There are many heated opinions, with no supporting evidence, on this matter.)

More complex magnetic devices have also been studied, not for home use, but for use in physicians' offices and hospitals. A special form of electromagnetic therapy, repetitive transcranial magnetic stimulation (rTMS), is undergoing particularly close study. rTMS is designed specifically to treat the brain with low-frequency magnetic pulses. A large body of small studies suggest that rTMS might be beneficial for depression. It is also being studied for the treatment of amyotrophic lateral sclerosis (ALS), Parkinson's disease, epilepsy, schizophrenia, and obsessive-compulsive disorder.

Mechanism of Action

Many commercial magnets have such a weak field that it is hard to believe they could affect the body at all. Some, however, are quite powerful and could conceivably cause effects at some depth. Nonetheless, biophysicists are skeptical that static magnets

> ## Paracelsus on Magnets and Disease
>
> *Physician-botanist-alchemist Paracelsus (1493-1541), an early proponent of what is now called magnet therapy, discusses the use of magnets in treating disease in humans. Two perspectives are presented here.*
>
> Fortified by experience which is the mistress of all things, and by mature theory, based on experience, I affirm that the Magnet is a stone which not only undeniably attracts steel and iron, but has also the same power over the matter of all diseases in the whole body of man.
>
> By the attractive power of a magnet acting upon the diseased aura of the blood in an affected part, that aura may be made to return into the center from which it originated, and be absorbed therein, and thereby we may destroy the herd of the virus and cure the patient, and we need not wait idly to see what Nature will do. The magnet is therefore useful in all inflammations, in fluxes and ulcerations, in diseases of the bowels and uterus, in internal as well as in external disease.

could significantly affect the body. (The moving magnetic fields of rTMS and pulsed electromagnetic therapy, or PEMF, act differently, and there is little doubt that they can affect nerve tissue and possibly other parts of the body.)

A commonly held misconception is that magnets attract the iron in blood cells, thus moving the blood and stimulating circulation. However, the iron in the blood is not in a magnetic form. Static magnets could affect charged particles in the blood, nerves, and cell membranes or subtly alter biochemical reactions, although whether the effect is strong enough to make a difference remains to be shown. Some research results suggest that static magnets affect local blood circulation, but a rigorously designed double-blind trial found that commercially available static magnets have no effect on blood flow. Another well-designed trial also failed to find effects on blood circulation. However, there is some weak evidence that static magnets may affect muscle metabolism. Further research will be necessary to sort out these possibilities.

Scientific Evidence

Static magnets. In double-blind, placebo-controlled trials, static magnets have shown promise for a number of conditions, but in no case is the evidence strong enough to be relied upon. In a 2007 review of all studies of static magnets as a treatment for pain, researchers concluded that there is no meaningful evidence that they are effective; they further concluded that current evidence suggests that, for some pain-related conditions, static magnets are not effective (a much stronger statement than the first).

Some magnet proponents claim that it is impossible to carry out a truly double-blinded study on magnets because participants can simply use a metal pin or a similar object to discover whether they have a real magnet or not. Some researchers have gotten around this by using a weak magnet as the placebo treatment. Other researchers have designed more complicated placebo devices that participants have been found unable to identify as fake treatments.

Rheumatoid arthritis. A double-blind, controlled trial of sixty-four people with rheumatoid arthritis of the knee compared the effects of strong alternating polarity magnets with the effects of a deliberately weak unipolar magnet. Researchers used the weakened magnet as a control group so that participants would not find it easy to break the blind by testing the magnetism of their treatment.

After one week of therapy, 68 percent of the participants using the strong magnets (the treatment group) reported relief, compared with 27 percent in the control group. This difference was statistically significant. Two of four other subjective measurements of disease severity also showed statistically significant improvements. However, no significant improvements were seen in objective evaluations of the condition, such as blood tests for inflammation severity or physician's assessment of joint tenderness, swelling, or range of motion. This study suggests that magnet therapy may reduce the pain of rheumatoid arthritis without altering actual inflammation. However, the mixture of statistically significant and insignificant results indicates that a larger trial is necessary to factor out "statistical noise."

Post-polio syndrome. A double-blind, placebo-controlled study of fifty people with post-polio syndrome found evidence that magnets are effective for relieving pain. The magnets or placebo magnets were placed on previously determined trigger points (one per person) for forty-five minutes. (Trigger points are sore areas within muscle that, when pressed, cause relief in other areas of the muscle and conversely, when inflamed, cause pain in other parts of the muscle.) In the treatment group, 76 percent of the participants reported improvement, compared with 19 percent in the placebo group.

Fibromyalgia. A six-month, double-blind, placebo-controlled trial of 119 people with fibromyalgia compared two commercially available magnetic mattress pads with sham treatment and no treatment. Group 1 used a mattress pad designed to create a uniform magnetic field of negative polarity. Group 2 used a mattress pad that varied in polarity. In both groups, manufacturer's instructions were followed. Groups 3 and 4 used sham treatments designed to match in appearance the magnets used in groups 1 and 2. Group 5 received no treatment.

On average, participants in all groups showed improvement in the six months of the study. Participants in the treatment groups, especially group 1, showed a trend toward greater improvement; however, the differences between real treatment and sham or no treatment failed to reach statistical significance in most measures. This outcome suggests that magnetic mattress pads might be helpful for fibromyalgia, but a larger study would be necessary to identify benefits.

An earlier double-blind, placebo-controlled study of thirty women with fibromyalgia did find significant improvement with magnets compared with placebo. The women slept on magnetic mattress pads (or sham pads for the control group) every night for four months. Of the twenty-five women who completed the trial, participants sleeping on the experimental mattress pads experienced a significant decrease in pain and fatigue compared with the placebo group, along with significant improvement in sleep and physical functioning.

A single-blind study of somewhat convoluted design provides weak evidence that a gown made from a special "electromagnetic shielding fabric" can reduce fibromyalgia symptoms. The rationale for using this fabric is, however, somewhat scientifically implausible.

Peripheral neuropathy. A four-month, double-blind, placebo-controlled, crossover study of nineteen people with peripheral neuropathy found a significant reduction in symptoms compared with placebo. Participants wore magnetic foot insoles during the day throughout the trial period. Reduction in the symptoms of burning, numbness, and tingling were especially marked in those cases of neuropathy associated with diabetes.

Based on these results, a far larger randomized, placebo-controlled, follow-up study was performed by the same researchers. This trial enrolled 375 people with peripheral neuropathy caused by diabetes and tested the effectiveness of four months of treatment with magnetic insoles. The results indicated that the insoles produced benefits beyond that of the placebo effect, reducing such symptoms as burning pain, numbness, tingling, and exercise-induced pain.

Surgery support. A double-blind, placebo-controlled study looked at the effect of magnets on healing after plastic surgery. The study examined the use of magnets on twenty persons who had suction lipectomy (liposuction). Magnets contained in patches were placed over the operative region immediately after surgery and left in place for fourteen days. The treatment group experienced statistically significant reduction of pain and swelling on postoperative days one through four, and of discoloration on days one through three, compared with the control group. Another study of 165 people, however, failed to find that the use of static magnets over the surgical incision reduced post-surgical pain. Furthermore, the positioning of static magnets at the acupuncture/acupressure point P6 in persons undergoing ear, nose, and throat or gynecological surgeries reduced nausea and vomiting no better than placebo in a randomized trial.

Low back pain and other forms of chronic musculoskeletal pain. A double-blind, placebo-controlled, crossover trial of fifty-four people with knee or back pain compared a complex static magnet array with a sham magnet array. Participants used either the real or the sham device for twenty-four hours; then, after a seven-day rest period, they used the opposite therapy for another twenty-four hours. Evaluations showed that the use of the real magnet was associated with greater improvements than the sham treatment.

Benefits were also seen in a double-blind, placebo-controlled trial of forty-three people with chronic knee pain who used fairly high-power but otherwise ordinary static magnets continuously for two weeks. In another placebo-controlled trial, the use of a magnetic knee wrap for twelve weeks was associated with a significant increase in quadriceps (thigh muscle) strength in persons with knee osteoarthritis.

A double-blind, placebo-controlled, crossover study of twenty people who had chronic low back pain for a minimum of six months failed to find any evidence of benefit. However, the alternating-pole magnet used in this study produced a very weak magnetic field. Another study found some benefit that failed to reach statistical significance.

In a double-blind study of 101 people with chronic neck and shoulder pain, the use of a magnetic necklace failed to prove more effective than placebo treatment. Another study failed to find magnetic insoles helpful for heel pain.

Osteoarthritis. A widely publicized twelve-week study of 194 people reportedly found that the use of magnetic bracelets reduced osteoarthritis pain in the hip and knee. However, the study actually found statistically similar benefits among participants given a placebo treatment. The researchers suggest that this failure to show superior effects may have been caused, in part, by an error: The study utilized weak magnets as the placebo treatments, but thirty-four persons in the placebo group accidentally received strong magnets instead. This would tend to decrease the difference in outcome seen between the treatment and the placebo group and could therefore hide a real treatment benefit. Nonetheless, this study does not provide evidence that magnetic bracelets offer any benefit for osteoarthritis beyond that of the placebo effect.

A much smaller study also failed to find statistically significant benefit, but it was too small to be able to produce statistically meaningful results. Rather, it was designed to evaluate a special placebo magnet device. After the study, researchers polled the participants to see if they could correctly identify whether they had been given the real treatment or the placebo: They could not.

Pelvic pain. A double-blind, placebo-controlled study of 14 women with chronic pelvic pain (from endometriosis or other causes) found no significant benefit when magnets were applied to abdominal trigger points for two weeks. However, statistical analysis showed that it would have been necessary to enroll a larger number of participants to detect an effect. A larger study did find some evidence of benefit after four weeks of treatment, but a high dropout rate and other design problems compromise the meaningfulness of the results. Another small study found possible evidence of benefit in menstrual pain.

Carpal tunnel syndrome. A double-blind, placebo-controlled study of thirty people with carpal tunnel syndrome found that a single treatment with a static magnet produced dramatic and long-lasting benefits. However, identical dramatic benefits were seen in the placebo group. In two more small, randomized trials, researchers again found that there were no differences between the treatment and the placebo groups. Both groups experienced similar improvements in symptoms.

In a small study involving thirty-one people with long-standing carpal tunnel syndrome, a combination of static magnet and pulsed electromagnetic field therapy modestly improved deep pain but had no significant effect on overall pain in a two-month period.

Sports performance. People who undergo intense exercise often experience muscle soreness afterwards. One study tested magnet therapy for reducing this symptom. However, while the use of magnets did reduce muscle soreness, so did placebo treatment, and there was no significant difference between the effectiveness of magnets and placebo. Another study, of more complex design, also failed to find benefit.

Magnetic insoles have been advocated for increasing sports performance. However, a study of fourteen college athletes failed to find that magnetic insoles improved vertical jump, bench squat, forty-yard dash, or performance of a soccer-specific fitness test.

Pulsed electromagnetic field therapy. Pulsed electromagnetic field therapy (PEMF) is quite distinct from magnet therapy itself. (The term "electromagnetic field" does not, in this case, refer to magnetism in the ordinary sense.) Nonetheless, for historical reasons, PEMF is often classified with true magnetic therapies.

Bone has a remarkable capacity to heal from injury. In some cases, though, the broken ends do not join, leading to what is called nonunion fractures. PEMF therapy has been used to stimulate bone repair in nonunion and other fractures since the 1970s; this is a relatively accepted use. More controversially, PEMF has shown promise for osteoarthritis, stress incontinence, and possibly other conditions.

Osteoarthritis. Three double-blind, placebo-controlled studies enrolling more than 350 people suggest that PEMF therapy can improve symptoms of osteoarthritis. For example, a double-blind, placebo-controlled study tested PEMF in eighty-six people with osteoarthritis of the knee and eighty-one people with osteoarthritis of the cervical spine. Participants received eighteen half-hour sessions with either a PEMF machine or a sham device. The treated participants showed significantly greater improvements in disease severity than those given placebo. For both osteoarthritis conditions, benefits lasted for a minimum of one month after treatment was stopped.

A later double-blind trial evaluated low-power, extremely low-frequency PEMF for the treatment of knee osteoarthritis. A total of 176 people received eight sessions of either sham or real treatment for two weeks. The results showed significantly greater pain reduction in the treated group.

Urinary incontinence. Many women experience stress incontinence, the leakage of urine following any action that puts pressure on the bladder. Laughter, physical exercise, and coughing can all trigger this unpleasant occurrence. A recent study suggests that PEMF treatment might be helpful. In this placebo-controlled study, researchers applied high-intensity pulsating magnetic fields to sixty-two women with stress incontinence. The intention was to stimulate the nerves that control the pelvic muscles.

The results showed that one session of magnetic stimulation significantly reduced episodes of urinary leakage over the following week, compared with placebo. In the treated group, 74 percent experienced significant improvement, compared with only 32 percent in the placebo group. Presumably, the high-intensity magnetic field used in this treatment created electrical currents in the pelvic muscles and nerves. This was confirmed by objective examination of thirteen participants, which found that magnetic stimulation was increasing the strength of closure at the exit from the bladder. However, there was one serious flaw in this study: It does not appear to have been double-blind. Researchers apparently knew which participants were getting real treatment and which were not and, therefore, might have unconsciously biased their observations to conform to their expectations. Thus, the promise of electromagnetic therapy for stress incontinence still needs to be validated in properly designed trials.

Similarly, magnetic stimulation has been studied for the treatment of bed-wetting (nocturnal enuresis). In a small preliminary study, the use of PEMF day and night for two months was helpful in girls.

Multiple sclerosis. A two-month, double-blind, placebo-controlled study of thirty people with multiple sclerosis was conducted using a PEMF device. Participants were instructed to tape the device to one of three different acupuncture points on the shoulder, back, or hip. The study found statistically significant improvements in the treatment group, most notably in bladder control, hand function, and muscle spasticity. Benefits were seen in another small study too.

Erectile dysfunction. In a three-week, double-blind, placebo-controlled trial, twenty men with erectile dysfunction received PEMF therapy or placebo. The magnetic therapy was administered by means of a small box worn near the genital area and kept in place as continuously as possible during the study period; neither participants nor observers knew whether the device was activated or not. The results showed that the use of PEMF significantly improved sexual function compared with placebo.

Migraines. In a double-blind trial, forty-two people with migraine headaches were given treatment with real or placebo PEMF therapy to the inner thighs for one hour, five times per week for two weeks. The results showed benefits in headache frequency and severity. However, the study design was rather convoluted and nonstandard, so the results are difficult to interpret.

Postoperative pain. In a small, randomized trial, eighty women undergoing breast augmentation

> ### How Magnet Therapy Might Work
>
> No scientific theory or manufacturer claim about how magnet therapy might work has been proven. Although some preliminary research has been conducted in animals and in small clinical trials, the mechanisms by which magnets might affect the human body are not yet known. Scientific researchers and magnet manufacturers have proposed that magnets might work by:
> - Changing how nerve cells function and by blocking pain signals to the brain
> - Restoring the balance between cell death and growth
> - Increasing the flow of blood and the delivery of oxygen and nutrients to tissues
> - Increasing the temperature of the area of the body being treated

surgery were divided into three groups. The first group received PEMF therapy for seven days after surgery to both breasts, the second group received fake PEMF therapy to both breasts as a control, and the third group received real and fake PEMF therapy to either breast. Compared to the control, women receiving PEMF therapy reported significantly less discomfort and used less pain medications by the third postoperative day.

Electromagnetic therapy. Unlike PEMF, repetitive transcranial magnetic stimulation (rTMS) involves magnetic fields and is, therefore, more closely related to standard magnet therapy. rTMS, which involves applying low-frequency magnetic pulses to the brain, has been investigated for treating emotional illnesses and other conditions that originate in the brain. The results of preliminary studies have been generally promising.

Depression. About twenty small studies have evaluated rTMS for the treatment of depression, including severe depression that does not respond to standard treatment and the depressive phase of bipolar illness, and most found it effective. In one of these studies, seventy people with major depression were given rTMS or sham rTMS in a double-blind setting of two weeks. The results showed that participants who had received actual treatment experienced significantly greater improvement than did those receiving sham treatment. In a far larger study involving 301 depressed persons, none of whom were being treated with antidepressant medications, real rTMS was significantly more effective than fake rTMS after four to six weeks of treatment.

In another trial involving ninety-two elderly persons whose depression had been linked to poor blood flow to the brain (vascular depression), actual rTMS was significantly more effective than sham rTMS. Benefits were more notable in younger participants. In a particularly persuasive piece of evidence, researchers pooled the results of thirty double-blind trials involving 1,164 depressed persons and determined that real rTMS was significantly more effective than sham rTMS.

Two separate studies suggest that rTMS may be an effective additional treatment for the 20 to 30 percent of depressed people for whom conventional drug therapy is not successful. Another group of researchers pooled the results of twenty-four studies involving 1,092 persons and found rTMS to be more effective than sham for treatment-resistant depression. Electroconvulsive therapy (shock treatment) is often used for people in this category, but rTMS may be an equally effective alternative.

Epilepsy. In a double-blind, placebo-controlled trial, twenty-four people with epilepsy (technically, partial complex seizures or secondarily generalized seizures) not fully responsive to drug treatment were given treatment with rTMS or sham rTMS twice daily for one week. The results showed a mild reduction in seizures among the people given real rTMS. However, the benefits rapidly disappeared when treatment was stopped. Similarly short-lived effects were seen in an open trial.

Schizophrenia. A double-blind, placebo-controlled, crossover trial looked at the use of low-frequency rTMS in twelve people diagnosed with schizophrenia and manifesting frequent and treatment-resistant auditory hallucinations (hearing voices). Participants received rTMS for four days, with the length of treatment building from four minutes on the first day to sixteen minutes on the fourth day. Active stimulation significantly reduced the incidence of auditory hallucinations compared with sham stimulation. The extent of the benefit varied widely, lasting from one day in one participant to two months in another. Possible benefits were seen in other small studies. Researchers pooling the results of six controlled trials, which involved 232 persons with schizophrenia resistant to conventional treatment, found that real, low-frequency rTMS was significantly better at reducing auditory hallucinations than sham rTMS.

Parkinson's disease. In a double-blind, placebo-controlled trial of ninety-nine people with Parkinson's disease, real rTMS was more effective than sham rTMS delivered in eight weekly treatments. Similar benefits were seen in three other small studies. Even more encouraging, the combined results of ten randomized trials in persons with Parkinson's indicated significant benefit for rTMS (using higher frequencies).

Chronic pain syndromes. rTMS technology has also been applied to areas other than the brain. Myofascial pain syndrome is a condition similar to fibromyalgia but is more localized. Whereas fibromyalgia involves tender trigger points all over the body, myofascial pain syndrome involves trigger points clustered in one portion of the body only. One controlled trial found indications that a form of repetitive magnetic stimulation applied to the painful area may be effective for myofascial pain syndrome of the trapezius muscle.

In a placebo-controlled trial involving sixty-one people with long-standing diabetes, low-frequency repetitive magnetic stimulation failed to diminish the pain associated with diabetic peripheral neuropathy. However, in another study involving twenty-eight people with peripheral neuropathy, high-frequency rTMS applied to the brain was more effective at reducing pain and improving quality of life than was fake rTMS.

Tinnitus. One preliminary study found indications that rTMS may be helpful for tinnitus (ringing in the ear).

Post-traumatic stress disorder. A small, double-blind, placebo-controlled study found that the use of rTMS may be able to reduce symptoms of post-traumatic stress disorder.

Cigarette addiction. A small, double-blind, placebo-controlled study found evidence that rTMS may reduce the craving for cigarettes in people attempting to quit smoking.

Obsessive-compulsive disorder. A double-blind, placebo-controlled study of eighteen people with obsessive-compulsive disorder found no evidence of benefit with rTMS.

Amyotrophic lateral sclerosis. Amyotrophic lateral sclerosis, also called Lou Gehrig's disease, is a nerve disorder that causes progressive muscle weakness. A small pilot study hinted that rTMS may be beneficial at least temporarily.

How to Use Magnet Therapy

The following is a brief description of the use of magnet therapy. However, one should keep in mind that the ways that magnets are used have not been fully evaluated by long-term clinical testing. A full medical evaluation is advisable before using magnets. One should not treat a painful back with magnets if the underlying cause of pain is a fracture or a tumor.

Types of magnets. There are a number of theories on the best size and type of magnets to use and where to apply them, based on the type of condition being treated and other factors. Because unipolar magnets have greater depth of magnetic field penetration, some researchers consider these more effective in treating deeper tissues. Conversely, it is considered that alternating-pole magnet devices might be more effective at stimulating surface tissue. Thus, it might be appropriate to use a unipolar high-gauss magnet for low back pain that originates deep in the tissue and an alternating-pole configuration for an injury closer to the surface, such as a wrist sprain. However, there is no meaningful scientific evidence to support these distinctions.

In addition, some practitioners hold that the north side of the magnet calms and the south side excites, and that using the correct side of the magnet is crucial. However, from a scientific perspective, it is difficult to see how there could be any difference between the two poles of the magnet in terms of the effect upon body tissue.

There is general consensus that the magnet should be placed as close to the affected part of the body as possible. This can be done by taping the magnet to the skin, slipping the magnet inside a bandage over the affected area, or using a wrap device that has embedded magnets.

Taping magnets to the body might irritate the skin; in addition, some research scientists and practitioners suspect that the body may accommodate to the magnetic field over time, thus reducing the therapeutic effect. To prevent both the irritation and the accommodation, practitioners usually recommend intermittent use, such as five days on, two days off or twelve hours on, twelve hours off.

Magnetic devices available. Manufacturers make a wide range of magnetic devices. For treating large areas of the body, wraps and belts containing magnets are available. Wraps are specifically designed for the wrist, elbow, knee, ankle, neck, shoulder, and back, and are often made from thermal material to have the added effect of warming the area. These wraps are often recommended in cases of injury and arthritis, where heat feels better. Proponents of magnet therapy often recommend the use of magnetic mattress pads and mattresses for people with problems affecting several areas of the body, such as fibromyalgia or arthritis; they also recommend magnetic mattress pads for insomnia and fatigue.

Proponents of magnet therapy recommend magnetic foot insoles for people with diabetic peripheral neuropathy, leg aches and pains, circulatory problems of the lower extremities, or foot injuries and problems, and for people who stand all day. Magnetic necklaces are said to be useful for neck and shoulder pain and for generalized aches and pains, and magnetic bracelets are advocated for wrist pain and general problems.

Safety Issues

In general, magnets appear to be safe; the biggest risk appears to be skin irritation from any tape that is used to hold them in place. Magnetic resonance imaging (MRI) machines, for example, expose the body to gigantic magnetic fields, and extensive investigation has found no evidence of harm. However, during the MRI, a person is subjected to a high level of magnetism for a short period of time, whereas people who use static magnets daily or sleep on them every night are subjected to a low level of magnetism over a long period of time. It is not known whether this type of exposure has any deleterious effects. Nonetheless, one study, in which participants slept on a magnetic mattress pad every night for four months, found no side effects. In addition, a safety study of rTMS found no evidence of harm. In a large study in which rTMS was administered to numerous people with depression, totaling more than ten thousand cumulative treatment sessions, no significant adverse effects were reported. Transient headache and scalp discomfort were the most frequent problems reported. There were no seizures or changes in hearing or cognition.

It was previously thought that persons with an implantable cardioverter-defibrillator (ICD) or a pacemaker should not use magnetic devices at all, but this recommendation has been adjusted. One study found that with the exception of magnetic mattresses and mattress pads, most magnets sold for therapeutic purposes do not interfere with the magnetically activated switches present in most pacemakers. Magnetic mattress pads can deactivate and alter the function of ICDs and pacemakers, but other therapeutic magnets are safe if kept six inches or farther from these devices.

There are theoretical concerns that magnets might be risky for people with epilepsy. Similarly, until the physiological effects of magnet treatments are better understood, pregnant women should avoid them.

—*EBSCO CAM Review Board*

References

Abdulla, Fuad A., et al. "Effects of Pulsed Low-Frequency Magnetic Field Therapy on Pain Intensity in Patients with Musculoskeletal Chronic Low Back Pain: Study Protocol for a Randomised Double-Blind Placebo-Controlled Trial." *BMJ Open*, vol. 9, no. 6, 9 June 2019, doi:10.1136/bmjopen-2018-024650.

Kulish, Peter. *Conquering Pain: the Art of Healing with BioMagnetism*. 6th ed., BioMag Science, 2016.

"Magnets for Pain." *National Center for Complementary and Integrative Health*, U.S. Department of Health and Human Services, 27 Dec. 2017, nccih.nih.gov/Health/magnets-for-pain.

Palermo, Elizabeth. "Does Magnetic Therapy Work?" *LiveScience*, Future US, Inc., 12 Feb. 2015, www.livescience.com/40174-magnetic-therapy.html.

Sandoiu, Ana. "Treating Pain with Magnetic Fields." *Medical News Today*, MediLexicon International, 9 Aug. 2018, www.medicalnewstoday.com/articles/322718.php#1.

Vadalà, Maria, et al. "Mechanisms and Therapeutic Effectiveness of Pulsed Electromagnetic Field Therapy in Oncology." *Cancer Medicine*, vol. 5, no. 11, 17 Oct. 2016, pp. 3128–3139., doi:10.1002/cam4.861.

Marijuana

CATEGORY: Addiction Risk; Herbs and Supplements
ALSO KNOWN AS: Cannabis; dope; ganja; grass; hashish; hemp; mary jane; pot; smoke; weed
ANATOMY OR SYSTEM AFFECTED: Central nervous system; Circulatory system; Gastrointestinal system; Immune system; Respiratory system

KEY TERMS

- *cannabinoid*: one of a class of diverse chemical compounds that acts on cannabinoid receptors, which are part of the endocannabinoid system found in cells that alter neurotransmitter release in the brain
- *indica*: a species of Cannabis with broader leaves that is typically used for relaxation, appetite stimulation, sleep aid, and pain relief
- *sativa*: a species of Cannabis with taller plants with narrower leaves that is typically used for increased energy and its uplifting and euphoric effects

Overview

Marijuana consists of the dried, shredded leaves, stems, seeds and flowers of plants in the genus *Cannabis*. *Cannabis indica* is a strain that provides a sense of bodily relaxation when inhaled or otherwise ingested. *Cannabis sativa*, on the other hand, provides a more energetic experience. Marijuana is one of the first drugs to be used for its psychoactive qualities. It is the most commonly used illicit drug in the United States. Archeological evidence dates its cultivation to around 8,000 BCE in China, where its fibers were used to make textiles and later paper. The type of marijuana used for such purposes is more fibrous and is called hemp. It is unclear when the psychoactive effects of marijuana were discovered. The discovery of these psychoactive effects also coincides with the discovery of the medicinal uses of the drug, which has pervaded its history and is a significant feature of its contemporary status. The most common use of the drug is for its psychoactive effects. The psychoactive effects derive from a substance in the resin of the plant, called delta-9-tetraydrocannabinol (also known as THC).

History of Use

The common misconception of marijuana is that there are no other qualities of the plant besides the psychoactive effects produced when ingested. This is not the case, which is shown in both the historical and present-day usage of the plant. In India, records show that psychoactive effects of marijuana were known since at least the second millennium BCE. The Vedas state it was originally given by the god Shiva because it "releases us from anxiety." Marijuana also was an important aspect of the practice of Tantric sex. The Persians, the Scythians, and especially the Arabs, also used marijuana for its psychoactive effects, but most cultures familiar with the plant knew it only for the quality of its fibers for rope and clothing.

Throughout European history, the economic value of hemp contributed to its prevailing use, though medieval magicians, witches, and sorcerers used marijuana for its psychoactive powers. Mainstream Europeans learned of such effects only when they began to colonize Asia in the seventeenth and eighteenth centuries. By the nineteenth century, marijuana was used by leading artists and writers, especially in France and most famously at the Paris Hashish Club.

In the United States, interest in marijuana's psychoactive properties increased in the mid-nineteenth century, especially with the 1857 publication of Fitz Hugh Ludlow's *The Hasheesh Eater*. Popular magazines and books included stories of its use, and marijuana was available at local pharmacies. By the end of the century, some of the most prominent psychologists in the United States also studied the drug through personal use. Even so, by the twentieth century, marijuana was largely limited to upper-class intellectuals. Most Americans did not know anything about marijuana; their drugs of choice were opium, morphine, cocaine, and alcohol.

Racism against Chinese immigrants, combined with a desire to build commercial interests in China, contributed to the US Congress passing the Harrison Act in 1914. The Harrison Act imposed recordkeeping and taxation requirements on the sale of opium and included other previously popular narcotic drugs, such as morphine and cocaine, which were recognized as having problematic addictive properties. Marijuana was also included due to its classification as a narcotic, though it had no similar reputation for addiction. Five years later, the adoption of the Eighteenth Amendment to the US Constitution prohibited alcohol and began an era in which the federal government had authority over matters of morality, cast in the light of the

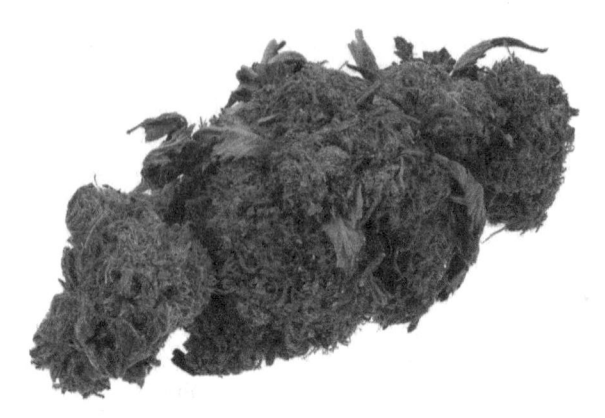

A dried flower bud of the Cannabis *plant.* (Evan-Amos via Wikimedia Commons)

intensifying class warfare as minorities and the working class fought for labor rights.

Marijuana was primarily used by Mexican immigrants in the western United States, immigrants who had been welcomed for the inexpensive labor they supplied. They were then blamed for job losses as agribusiness reduced farm workforces during the 1910s and 1920s. During those decades every western state passed laws to make marijuana illegal. Its criminalization was supported by alleged links between marijuana use and laziness, promiscuity, mental illness, and violence, all of which were based on the apparently greater incidence of such symptoms in the minority populations who tended to use marijuana.

As the Great Depression accelerated job losses during the 1930s, the rhetoric of violence-prone minorities fueled by marijuana next targeted African Americans in major cities. Led by Harry Anslinger, the director of the newly formed Federal Bureau of Narcotics, public advocacy for marijuana's criminalization as a "killer weed" convinced Congress in 1937 to prohibit its possession with the Marijuana Tax Act. Subsequent legislation in 1951 and 1956 increased penalties.

In the 1960s, marijuana use increased dramatically and became the focus of intense controversy that has continued as a national debate into the present. Marijuana, used especially by college-age youth disaffected by the dominant culture, became an expression of the youth rebellion those on both sides of a cultural divide. President Richard M. Nixon's "War on Drugs" was his attempt to curtail the rebellion. As middle-class youths became subject to arrest and incarceration, the justification for marijuana's criminalization came into question. Even as strictures against its use were increased in 1968 and 1970, presidential commissions in 1962, 1963, 1967, and 1972 concluded that the claims against marijuana were exaggerated or false.

Trends in marijuana use continued at high levels despite mandatory penalties. Statistics for twelfth graders who have used marijuana is over 60 percent in the late 1970s. But by the early 1990's usage declined to a low just under 40 percent. This no-tolerance policy began to be challenged by the middle of the 1990's as a resurgence of research into the properties of marijuana showed its medicinal benefits. This research led to several US states allowing medical cannabis use, beginning with California in 1996. A World Health Organization (WHO) survey in 2008 found that 42 percent of the US population, more than 100 million people, had used marijuana at least once, the highest rate in WHO's seventeen-country study. In 2009, the National Institute on Drug Abuse reported that 28.5 million Americans age twelve years and older had used marijuana at least once in the year prior. That same year, US attorney general Eric Holder announced that the federal government would adopt new guidelines tolerating medicinal use of marijuana according to states' regulations, though the drug remained federally illegal.

Modern Use

The last decade has seen the most dramatic shift in marijuana legislation since the 1960's. On the federal level, marijuana is still considered a Schedule 1 controlled substance, making possession of the substance a criminal offense. Despite this, several states have passed legislation that has made medicinal or recreational use of the drug legal. Currently, recreational marijuana is legal in nine states; Maine, Colorado, Washington, Alaska, Oregon, Maine, Nevada, California and Vermont. It is also legal in Washington D.C. Medical marijuana is legal in 30 states and Washington D.C. Marijuana laws vary on a state-to-state basis.

There are three principle reasons that the legalization movement has continued to build momentum. The first reason is that research has concluded that marijuana is a viable medicine that can be used to treat a wide range of symptoms. Some of the more popular applications of medical marijuana are as an alternative to opioid-based medication to manage pain, as an anti-nausea medication for patients undergoing chemotherapy treatment, and as an anti-anxiety medication for PTSD treatment. The second reason is that legalizing marijuana has been shown to have financial benefits for a state's economy government. These benefits include an economic boon from tax revenue and reducing government expenditure on the enforcement of marijuana. The final reason is that marijuana is at its height of popularity among the American public. Public support of marijuana legislation has grown significantly, with 64% of Americans in favor of legalization. Nearly 41 million Americans used marijuana in 2017, compared to around 37.5 million in 2016.

Worldwide, marijuana legalization remains controversial. In 2013 Uruguay became the first nation to legalize growing, selling, and consuming marijuana, although with strict regulations.

Effects and Potential Risks

Marijuana is a mild intoxicant, with aspects of both a stimulant and a tranquilizer. When smoked, the effects of marijuana begin in minutes and can last for hours; the maximum intensity occurs within the first hour. These effects, colloquially known as getting high, vary considerably according to the potency, the dosage, the setting, and the person's experience and attitude.

Positive short-term experiential effects include feelings of light-heartedness, well-being, euphoria, and increased sensory sensitivity. Negative effects include difficulty with concentration, poor short-term memory retention, decreased motor performance skills, increased levels of anxiety and paranoia. At high dosages, new users may experience disorientation and panic, which can account for some emergency room visits associated with marijuana use.

Longer-term experiential effects are more speculative. Users report that insights remained significant and even life-changing. Negative effects also have been proposed, including a motivational syndrome and an increased tendency to later use other, more dangerous drugs (the "gateway drug" theory). The long-term negative effects are contentious, research fails to definitively produce widely agreed upon risk factors.

Short-term physical effects include dilated blood vessels and increased heart rate. No permanently damaging effects on the body have been found from occasional use of marijuana. The tendency to combine marijuana with other drugs, most notably tobacco, poses health hazards. Several such effects have been asserted, most prominently chromosomal damage, lung damage, brain damage, and depressed immune response.

Research findings on long term effects of heavy marijuana use are highly varied. First, some studies have found a correlation with psychotic or affective mental health outcomes. Whether this correlational link implicates a causal one is hotly debated, but the possibility persists that marijuana use may exacerbate preexisting mental disorders. Second, marijuana smoke contains a number of carcinogens that can be irritants to the lungs. Third, studies on animals also indicate that the cannabinoids in marijuana may accumulate on the brain for days afterward, and it is assumed that larger and more frequent use would result in a longer period of such accumulation.

While marijuana does not cause physical dependence, it is hard not to describe long-term usage as not demonstrating some additive potential. Professionals in the field of substance use disorder have long recognized evidence of psychological dependency, at least anecdotally and empirically. Detailed, well designed research is simply lacking. Withdrawal symptoms are rare, but after prolonged heavy use, may include general unease, insomnia, lethargy, boredom, a reduced experience of pleasure, and a desire to continue use. Based on studies of acute toxicity in animals, it has been determined that a lethal dose of marijuana would be roughly five thousand times a normal dose, impossible to ingest by conventional means. No human deaths directly from marijuana use have been documented.

—*Christopher M. Aanstoos, PhD*
—*Michael Moglia*

References

DeAngelo, Steve. *The Cannabis Manifesto: a New Paradigm for Wellness.* 2nd ed., North Atlantic Books, 2015.

Donk, Tine Van De, et al. "An Experimental Randomized Study on the Analgesic Effects of Pharmaceutical-Grade Cannabis in Chronic Pain Patients with Fibromyalgia." *Pain*, vol. 160, no. 4, 2019, pp. 860–869., doi:10.1097/j.pain.0000000000001464.

Hall, Kevin P., et al. "Cannabis and Pain: A Clinical Review." *Cannabis and Cannabinoid Research*, vol. 2, no. 1, 1 May 2017, pp. 96–104., doi:10.1089/can.2017.0017.

Ivker, Rav. *Cannabis for Chronic Pain: a Proven Prescription for Using Marijuana to Relieve Your Pain and Heal Your Life.* Touchstone, 2017.

Salottolo, Kristin, et al. "The Grass Is Not Always Greener: a Multi-Institutional Pilot Study of Marijuana Use and Acute Pain Management Following Traumatic Injury." *Patient Safety in Surgery*, vol. 12, no. 16, 19 June 2018, doi:10.1186/s13037-018-0163-3.

Taylor & Francis Group. "Could Marijuana Be an Effective Pain Alternative to Prescription Medications?" *ScienceDaily*, 1 July 2019, www.sciencedaily.com/releases/2019/07/190701224523.htm.

Vu kovi , Sonja, et al. "Cannabinoids and Pain: New Insights From Old Molecules." *Frontiers in Pharmacology*, vol. 9, 13 Nov. 2018, doi:10.3389/fphar.2018.01259.

Wachter, Kerri. "Navigating Cannabis Options for Chronic Pain." *Practical Pain Management*, 24 June 2019, www.practicalpainmanagement.com/patient/treatments/marijuana-cannabis/navigating-cannabis-options-chronic-pain.

■ Medical marijuana

CATEGORY: Herbs and Supplements
ANATOMY OR SYSTEM AFFECTED: Central nervous system; Circulatory system; Gastrointestinal system; Immune system; Respiratory system
SPECIALTIES AND RELATED FIELDS: Pulmonology, cardiology, internal medicine, emergency medicine, neurology, OBGYN, pediatrics, among many others.

Medical marijuana uses the marijuana plant or chemicals in it to treat diseases or conditions. It's basically the same product as recreational marijuana, but it's taken for medical purposes. The marijuana plant contains more than 100 different chemicals called cannabinoids. Each one has a different effect on the body. Delta-9-tetrahydrocannabinol (THC) and cannabidiol (CBD) are the main chemicals used in medicine. THC also produces the "high" people feel when they smoke marijuana or eat foods containing it. Medical marijuana is any part of the marijuana plant that you use to treat health problems. People use it to get relief from their symptoms, not to try to get high.

Most marijuana that's sold legally as medicine has the same ingredients as the kind that people use for pleasure. But some medical marijuana is specially grown to have less of the chemicals that cause feelings of euphoria.

Marijuana is the most commonly used illicit drug in the United States. Its use is widespread among young people. In 2015, more than 11 million young adults ages 18 to 25 used marijuana in the past year. According to the Monitoring the Future survey, rates of marijuana use among middle and high school students have dropped or leveled off in the past few years after several years of increase. However, the number of young people who believe regular marijuana use is risky is decreasing.

Uses

Cannabinoids, the active chemicals in medical marijuana, are similar to chemicals the body makes that are involved in appetite, memory, movement, and pain. Research suggests cannabinoids might: reduce anxiety, reduce inflammation and relieve pain, control nausea and vomiting caused by cancer chemotherapy, kill cancer cells and slow tumor growth, relax tight muscles in people with multiple sclerosis, just to name a few.

How do you get medical marijuana?

To get medical marijuana, you need a written recommendation from a licensed doctor in states where that is legal. (Not every doctor is willing to recommend medical marijuana for their patients.) You must have a condition that qualifies for medical marijuana use. Each state has its own list of qualifying conditions. Your state may also require you to get a medical marijuana ID card. Once you have that card, you can buy medical marijuana at a store called a dispensary.

Administration

To take medical marijuana, you can: smoke it, inhale it through a vaporizer, eat it, apply to skin in lotion, spray, oil or cream, and place drops of liquid under the tongue. How you take it is up to you. Each method works differently in your body. If you smoke or vaporize cannabis, you feel the effects very quickly, if you eat it, it takes significantly longer.

Side Effects

Side effects that have been reported include: bloodshot eyes, depression, dizziness, fast heartbeat, hallucinations, and hypotension. The drug

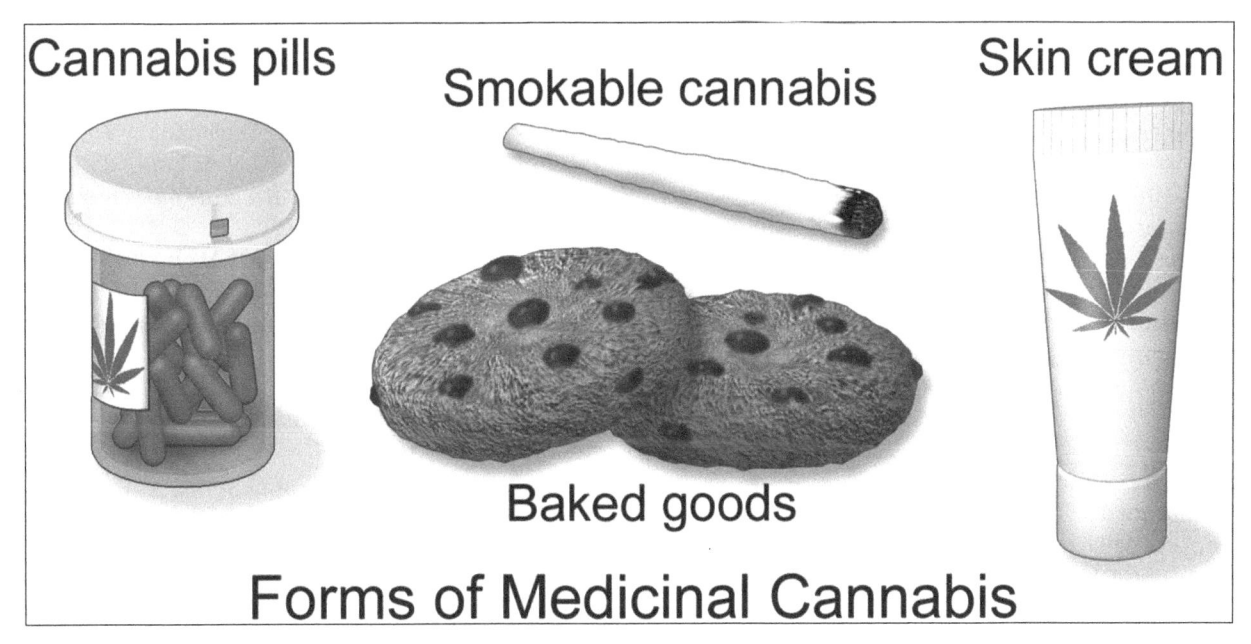

(BruceBlaus via Wikimedia Commons)

can also affect judgment and coordination, which could lead to accidents and injuries. When used during the teenage years when the brain is still developing, marijuana might affect IQ and mental function. It can also change your mood, making you feel happy, relaxed, sleepy, or anxious, disrupt your short-term memory and decision-making ability.

Large doses of medical marijuana can make some people have hallucinations, delusions, and paranoia. Research suggests that smoking marijuana can make breathing problems, like bronchitis, worse.

Long-term Side Effects
Regular smokers of medical marijuana may get respiratory problems, such as a daily cough and a higher risk of lung infections.

Studies also link routine use to mental illness, depression, anxiety, less motivation, and suicidal thoughts among young people. Marijuana use during pregnancy can raise the risk of health problems in babies. Marijuana use can result in addiction.

Problems with child development during and after pregnancy. If a pregnant woman uses marijuana, the drug may affect certain developing parts of the fetus's brain. Children exposed to marijuana in the womb have an increased risk of problems with attention, memory, and problem solving compared to unexposed children.

Intense Nausea and Vomiting. Regular, long-term marijuana use can lead to some people to develop Cannabinoid Hyperemesis Syndrome. This causes users to experience regular cycles of severe nausea, vomiting, and dehydration, sometimes requiring emergency medical attention.

Breathing problems. Marijuana smoke irritates the lungs, and people who smoke marijuana frequently can have the same breathing problems as those who smoke tobacco. These problems include daily cough and phlegm, more frequent lung illness, and a higher risk of lung infections. Researchers so far haven't found a higher risk for lung cancer in people who smoke marijuana.

Increased heart rate. Marijuana raises heart rate for up to 3 hours after smoking. This effect may increase the chance of heart attack. Older people and those with heart problems may be at higher risk.

Future Trends
Medical marijuana can still be used to alleviate many other conditions. For example, its benefit treating seizures is still being studied. In the future, medical marijuana could be used as a treatment option for many other conditions. Additionally,

more medications containing cannabinoid should be approved by the FDA.

Another issue is that the FDA doesn't oversee medical marijuana like it does prescription drugs. Although states monitor and regulate sales, they often don't have the resources to do so. That means the strength of and ingredients in medical marijuana can differ quite a bit depending on where you buy it. As a result, in the future, there should be more regulation on the manufacturing and regulation of medical marijuana sales.

—*Elizabeth Marie McGhee Nelson, PhD*
—*David Hernandez, ScB*

References

Backes, Michael. *Cannabis Pharmacy: the Practical Guide to Medical Marijuana.* Black Dog & Leventhal Publishers, 2017.

Bellnier, Terrance, et al. "Preliminary Evaluation of the Efficacy, Safety, and Costs Associated with the Treatment of Chronic Pain with Medical Cannabis." *Mental Health Clinician*, vol. 8, no. 3, 2018, pp. 110–115., doi:10.9740/mhc.2018.05.110.

Boehnke, Kevin F., et al. "Pills to Pot: Observational Analyses of Cannabis Substitution Among Medical Cannabis Users With Chronic Pain." *The Journal of Pain*, vol. 20, no. 7, 2019, pp. 830–841., doi:10.1016/j.jpain.2019.01.010.

Bridgeman, Mary Barna, and Daniel T. Abazia. "Medicinal Cannabis: History, Pharmacology, And Implications for the Acute Care Setting." *Pharmacy & Therapeutics*, vol. 42, no. 3, Mar. 2017, pp. 180–188.

C, Griffith, and La France B. "The Benefits and Effects of Using Marijuana as a Pain Agent to Treat Opioid Addiction." *Journal of Hospital & Medical Management*, vol. 04, no. 02, 2018, doi:10.4172/2471-9781.100051.

Carter, Greg T. "The Argument for Medical Marijuana for the Treatment of Chronic Pain." *Pain Medicine*, vol. 14, no. 6, 2013, pp. 800–800., doi:10.1111/pme.12137_2.

Deshpande, Amol, and Angela Mailis. "Medical Cannabis and Pain Management: How Might the Role of Cannabis Be Defined in Pain Medicine?" *The Journal of Applied Laboratory Medicine: An AACC Publication*, vol. 2, no. 4, Dec. 2017, pp. 485–488., doi:10.1373/jalm.2017.023184.

"FDA and Marijuana." *U.S. Food and Drug Administration*, 19 June 2019, www.fda.gov/news-events/public-health-focus/fda-and-marijuana.

Grinspoon, Peter. "Medical Marijuana." *Harvard Health Blog*, Harvard Medical School, 25 June 2019, www.health.harvard.edu/blog/medical-marijuana-2018011513085.

Wolf, Laurie Goldrich, and Mary Wolf. *The Medical Marijuana Dispensary: Understanding, Medicating, and Cooking with Cannabis.* Althea Press, 2016.

■ Oregano oil

CATEGORY: Herbs and Supplements; Anti-bacterial; Anti-inflammatory; Functional Food
ALSO KNOWN AS: *Origanum vulgare*
ANATOMY OR SYSTEM AFFECTED: Musculoskeletal system

Overview

The common food spice oregano grows wild in the mountains of Mediterranean countries. In ancient Greece, oregano or its essential oil was used for the treatment of wounds, snake bites, spider bites, and respiratory problems. Respiratory uses dominated the medicinal history of oregano in medieval Europe, but in the nineteenth century, physicians in the Eclectic School (a medical movement that emphasized herbal treatment) used oregano for promoting menstruation.

Therapeutic Dosages

A typical dose of oregano oil is 100 milligrams (mg) three times daily of a product standardized to contain 55 to 65 percent of the presumed active ingredient carvacrol.

Therapeutic Uses

In the 1990s, the concept of the yeast hypersensitivity syndrome (often called systemic candidiasis, or candida) became popular in alternative medicine circles. This theory states, in brief, that many people develop excessive levels of the yeast *Candida albicans* and subsequently experience symptoms of allergy to the yeast in their bodies. The symptoms of this purported syndrome include common conditions such as fatigue and headache. A succession of anticandidal treatments have been offered. Oregano oil is one of the more recent of these products.

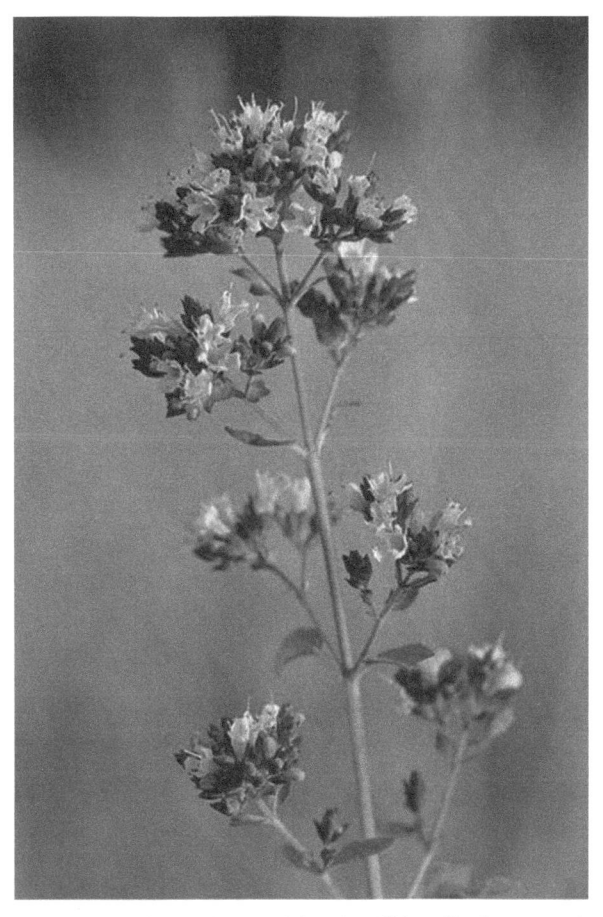

Origanum vulgare. (Ivar Leidus via Wikimedia Commons)

Scientific Evidence

It is true that oregano oil is toxic to many different types of microorganisms, including fungi and parasites. However, the same is the case with hundreds of essential oils of herbs, not to mention vinegar, alcohol, and bleach. It is a long way from killing microorganisms in a test tube or on the surface of a block of cheese to medicinal effects in the body. Only double-blind, placebo-controlled studies in humans can prove a treatment effective, and none have been performed on oregano oil. Nonetheless oregano oil is widely marketed as a treatment for candida.

There is a related theory that many people suffer from undiagnosed intestinal parasites; oregano oil is marketed for treatment of this purported problem as well. Oregano oil is also advocated for dozens of other illnesses, ranging from asthma and human immunodeficiency virus infection to rheumatoid arthritis, though without any reliable justification.

Web sites selling oregano oil additionally point out that it has antioxidant properties. While true, this does not, by itself, indicate any health benefits. Most major studies of antioxidants have failed to identify the specific benefits that were once seen as likely to result from supplementation with these substances.

Safety Issues

There are no specific safety risks known to be associated with use of oregano oil products. However, in general, essential oils of herbs can be toxic when taken even in relatively small quantities. Allergic reactions are also possible. Safety in young children, pregnant or nursing women, and people with severe liver or kidney disease has not been established.

—*EBSCO CAM Review Board*

References

De Cássia Da Silveira E Sá, Rita, et al. "Analgesic-Like Activity of Essential Oil Constituents: An Update." *International Journal of Molecular Sciences*, vol. 18, no. 12, 9 Dec. 2017, p. 2392., doi:10.3390/ijms18122392.

Cronkleton, Emily, and Debra Rose Wilson. "Oregano Oil for Cold and Flu: Does It Work?" *Healthline*, 6 Mar. 2018, www.healthline.com/health/oregano-oil-for-cold.

Han, Xuesheng, and Tory L. Parker. "Anti-Inflammatory, Tissue Remodeling, Immunomodulatory, and Anticancer Activities of Oregano (Origanum Vulgare) Essential Oil in a Human Skin Disease Model." *Biochimie Open*, vol. 4, 2017, pp. 73–77., doi:10.1016/j.biopen.2017.02.005.

Kelsey, Amber. "The Healing Properties of Oregano Oil." *Livestrong.com*, Leaf Group, 20 Jan. 2019, www.livestrong.com/article/153766-the-healing-properties-of-oregano-oil/.

Leyva-López, Nayely, et al. "Essential Oils of Oregano: Biological Activity beyond Their Antimicrobial Properties." *Molecules*, vol. 22, no. 6, 14 June 2017, p. 989., doi:10.3390/molecules22060989.

Rodriguez-Garcia, I., et al. "Oregano Essential Oil as an Antimicrobial and Antioxidant Additive in Food Products." *Critical Reviews in Food Science and Nutrition*, vol. 56, no. 10, 2015, pp. 1717–1727., doi:10.1080/10408398.2013.800832.

■ Peppermint

CATEGORY: Herbs and Supplements; Anti-inflammatory; Functional Food
ALSO KNOWN AS: *Mentha piperita*
ANATOMY OR SYSTEM AFFECTED: Gastrointestinal system; Respiratory system; Sinus system

Overview
Peppermint is a relative of numerous wild mint plants, deliberately bred in the late seventeenth century in England to become the delightful-tasting plant so well known today. It is widely used as a beverage tea and as a flavoring or scent in a wide variety of products.

Peppermint tea also has a long history of medicinal use, primarily as a digestive aid and for the symptomatic treatment of cough, colds, and fever. Peppermint oil is used for chest congestion (Vicks VapoRub), as a local anesthetic (Solarcaine, Ben-Gay), and most recently in the treatment of irritable bowel disease, also known as spastic colon.

Therapeutic Dosages
The proper dosage of peppermint oil when treating irritable bowel syndrome is 0.2 to 0.4 milliliter (ml) three times a day of an enteric-coated capsule. The capsule has to be enteric-coated to prevent stomach distress. When used in herbal combinations to treat stomach problems, peppermint oil is taken at lower doses, and it is not enteric-coated.

Therapeutic Uses
Peppermint oil has shown promise for a variety of conditions that involve spasm of the intestinal tract. Most studies have involved irritable bowel syndrome (IBS), for which peppermint oil has shown considerable promise. Peppermint oil may also be helpful for reducing the pain caused by medical examinations of the colon and stomach, as well for decreasing the intestinal gas pain that frequently follows surgery. Peppermint oil may also be helpful for dyspepsia (a condition that is similar to IBS but involves the stomach instead of the intestines). Weak evidence, far too preliminary to rely upon, hints that peppermint oil might help dissolve gallstones.

Peppermint oil is also used in another way: as aromatherapy. This means that it is inhaled, often by adding it to a humidifier. Weak evidence hints

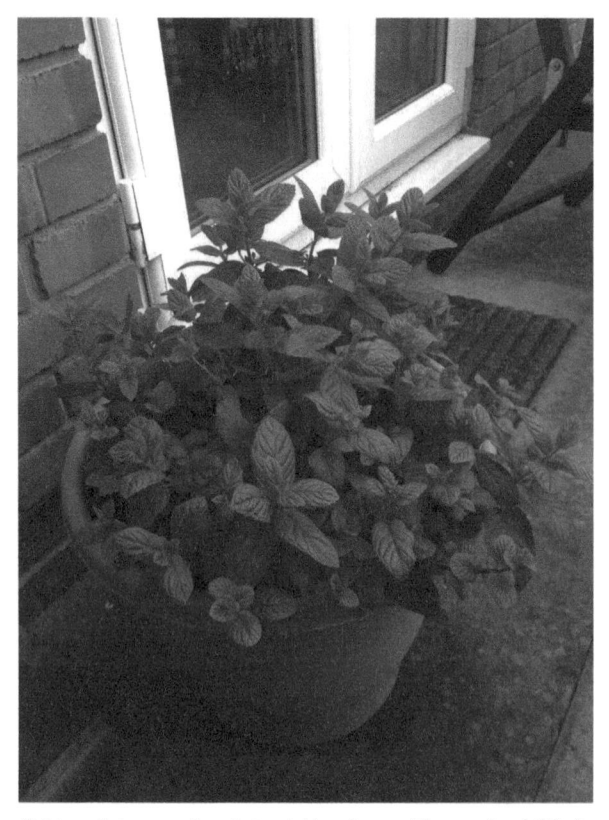

Peppermint grown in a pot outside a house. (Sunnysingh22 via Wikimedia Commons)

that inhaled peppermint oil might be helpful for relief of mucus congestion of the lungs and sinuses. Even weaker evidence hints that inhaled peppermint oil might relieve postsurgical nausea. Similarly weak evidence hints that peppermint oil, applied to the forehead, might relieve tension headaches. Finally, a study performed in Iran reported that applying peppermint water (essentially, lukewarm peppermint tea) directly to the nipples helped prevent dryness and cracking caused by breast-feeding.

Scientific Evidence
Irritable bowel syndrome (IBS). There have been numerous studies of peppermint oil for IBS. In one of the larger studies, 110 people with IBS were given either enteric-coated peppermint oil (187 milligrams, or mg) or a placebo three to four times daily, fifteen to thirty minutes before meals, for four weeks. The results showed significant improvements in abdominal pain, bloating, stool frequency, and flatulence. In a similar study, people who took

> ## Peppermint Oil for Irritable Bowel Syndrome
>
> Peppermint oil has shown promise as a treatment for irritable bowel syndrome (IBS). Peppermint contains menthol, a substance that relaxes the muscles of the small intestine. A number of studies have found that a special formulation of peppermint oil (enteric-coated, which is designed to open up only once the capsule has passed out of the stomach) can relieve symptoms. However, other studies of peppermint oil for IBS have failed to find benefit; the evidence has been sufficiently contradictory to keep the effectiveness of peppermint oil an open question.
>
> It has been suggested that the inconsistencies seen in previous studies were caused by the accidental inclusion of people who had conditions that are unrelated to IBS but cause similar symptoms. Presumably, peppermint oil may be less effective for these conditions.
>
> A study published in 2007 attempted to correct this problem by pretesting participants for the two conditions most easily mistaken for IBS: lactose intolerance and celiac disease. Fifty-seven people with IBS symptoms and evidence that they were free of the other two conditions were enrolled in the study. Over a period of four weeks, participants were given either placebo or peppermint oil.
>
> At the end of the study period, 75 percent of the participants in the peppermint oil group showed a marked improvement in IBS symptoms. ("Marked improvement" was defined as a reduction of IBS symptom scores by more than 50 percent). In comparison, only 38 percent of the participants given placebo showed an improvement of this magnitude. The difference between these outcomes was statistically significant.
>
> —*Steven Bratman, M.D.*

peppermint oil capsules for eight weeks also had less abdominal pain and discomfort compared with the placebo group.

Not all of these studies have shown that peppermint oil is beneficial, though. It has been suggested that these inconsistencies were caused by the accidental inclusion of people who had conditions unrelated to IBS that cause similar symptoms. Presumably, peppermint oil may be less effective for these problems. A study published in 2007 pretested participants for lactose intolerance and celiac disease, the two conditions most easily mistaken for IBS. A total of fifty-seven people with IBS symptoms and no evidence of the other two problems were enrolled in the study. Over a period of four weeks, participants were given either a placebo or peppermint oil. At the end of the study period, 75 percent of the patients in the peppermint oil group showed a marked reduction of IBS symptoms (defined, for this purpose, as a reduction of IBS symptom scores by more than 50 percent). In comparison, only 38 percent of the participants given a placebo showed an improvement of this magnitude, and this difference was statistically significant.

Other forms of spasm in the digestive tract. A barium enema involves introducing a solution containing the metal barium into the lower intestines. It commonly causes intestinal pain and spasm. A double-blind study of 141 individuals found that adding peppermint oil to the barium reduced the severity of intestinal spasm that occurred. Benefits were also seen in a large study conducted by different researchers. Another study found that peppermint oil reduced spasm in the stomach during a procedure called upper endoscopy. One study found that use of peppermint oil after C-section surgery reduced discomfort caused by intestinal gas.

Dyspepsia (minor indigestion). Peppermint oil is often used in combination with other essential oils to treat minor indigestion. For example, a double-blind, placebo-controlled study including thirty-nine individuals found that an enteric-coated peppermint-caraway oil combination taken three times daily for four weeks significantly reduced dyspepsia pain compared with placebo. Of the treatment group, 63.2 percent was free of pain after four weeks, compared with 25 percent of the placebo group.

Results from a double-blind, comparative study including 118 individuals suggest that the combination of peppermint and caraway oil is comparably effective to the no-longer-available drug cisapride. After four weeks, the herbal combination reduced dyspepsia pain by 69.7 percent, whereas the conventional treatment reduced pain by 70.2 percent.

A preparation of peppermint, caraway, fennel, and wormwood oils was compared with the drug

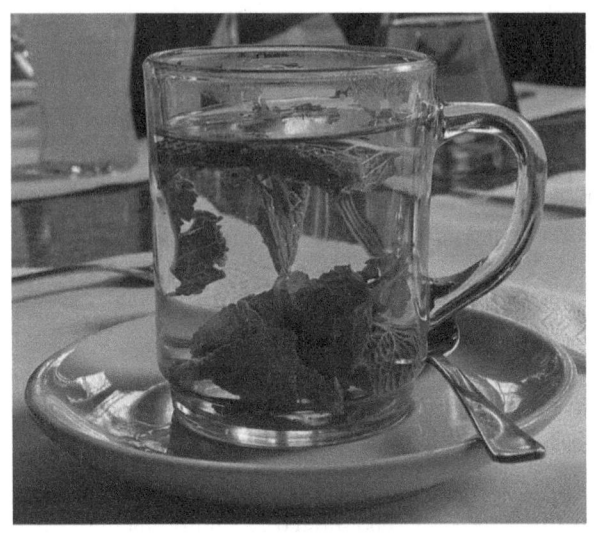

Peppermint tea with fresh leaves. (Hannes Grobe via Wikimedia Commons)

metoclopramide in another double-blind study enrolling sixty individuals. After seven days, 43.3 percent of the treatment group was pain free compared with 13.3 percent of the metoclopramide group. Metoclopramide works by reducing gastric emptying time (in other words, speeding the passage of food from the stomach into the intestines). Interestingly, some evidence suggests that peppermint oil may have the same effect.

Safety Issues

At the normal dosage, enteric-coated peppermint oil is believed to be reasonably safe in healthy adults. However, case reports and one study in rats hint that peppermint might reduce male fertility. The species *Mentha spicata* may be more problematic in this regard than the more common *M. piperita*. Excessive doses of peppermint oil can be toxic, causing kidney failure and even death. Very high intake of peppermint oil can also cause nausea, loss of appetite, heart problems, loss of balance, and other nervous system problems. Safety in young children, pregnant or nursing women, and those with severe liver or kidney disease has not been established. In particular, peppermint can cause jaundice in newborn babies, so it should not be used for colic.

Use of peppermint oil may increase levels of the drug cyclosporine in the body. Persons taking cyclosporine who wish to take peppermint oil should notify their physician in advance, so that their blood levels of cyclosporine can be monitored and their dose adjusted if necessary. Conversely, those persons already taking both peppermint oil and cyclosporine should not stop taking the peppermint without informing their physicians. Ceasing to take peppermint may cause cyclosporine levels to fall.

Important Interactions

Those taking cyclosporine should not use peppermint oil (or stop using it) except in consultation with a physician.

—*EBSCO CAM Review Board*

References

Alammar, N., et al. "The Impact of Peppermint Oil on the Irritable Bowel Syndrome: a Meta-Analysis of the Pooled Clinical Data." *BMC Complementary and Alternative Medicine*, vol. 19, no. 1, 17 Jan. 2019, doi:10.1186/s12906-018-2409-0.

Brazier, Yvette. "Peppermint: Health Benefits and Precautions." *Medical News Today*, MediLexicon International, 27 June 2017, www.medicalnewstoday.com/articles/265214.php.

Haber, Stacy L., and Shareen Y. El-Ibiary. "Peppermint Oil for Treatment of Irritable Bowel Syndrome." *American Journal of Health-System Pharmacy*, vol. 73, no. 2, 15 Jan. 2016, pp. 22–31., doi:10.2146/ajhp140801.

Johannes, Laura. "Can Mint Make Migraines Less Miserable?" *The Wall Street Journal*, Dow Jones & Company, 19 Oct. 2015, www.wsj.com/articles/can-mint-make-migraines-less-miserable-1445271218.

L, Mercy Aparna, et al. "Assessment of Sputum Quality and Its Importance in the Rapid Diagnosis of Pulmonary Tuberculosis." *Archives of Clinical Microbiology*, vol. 08, no. 04, 2017, doi:10.4172/1989-8436.100053.

"Peppermint Oil." *National Center for Complementary and Integrative Health*, U.S. Department of Health and Human Services, 1 Dec. 2016, nccih.nih.gov/health/peppermintoil.

Seladi-Schulman, Jill. "About Peppermint Oil Uses and Benefits." *Healthline*, 25 Apr. 2019, www.healthline.com/health/benefits-of-peppermint-oil.

Rosemary

CATEGORY: Herbs and Supplements; Functional Food
ALSO KNOWN AS: *Rosmarinus officinalis*
ANATOMY OR SYSTEM AFFECTED: Circulatory system; Gastrointestinal system; Musculoskeletal system

Overview
The herb rosemary has been used as a food spice and as a medicine since ancient times. Traditional medicinal uses of rosemary leaf preparations taken internally include digestive distress, headaches, and anxiety. The fragrance of rosemary leaf has been said to enhance memory. Rosemary oil has been applied to the skin to treat muscle and joint pain and taken internally to promote abortions.

Therapeutic Dosages
A typical dosage of rosemary leaf is 4 to 6 grams daily. Rosemary essential oil should not be used internally.

Therapeutic Uses
Germany's Commission E has approved rosemary leaf for treatment of dyspepsia (nonspecific digestive distress) and rosemary oil (used externally) for treatment of joint pain and poor circulation. However, there is no meaningful scientific evidence that rosemary is effective for any of these uses. Only double-blind, placebo-controlled studies can prove that a treatment really works, and no studies of this type have found rosemary effective.

Rosemary essential oil, like many essential oils, has antimicrobial properties when it comes in direct contact with bacteria and other microorganisms. Note, however, that this does not mean that rosemary oil is an antibiotic. Antibiotics are substances that can be taken internally to kill microorganisms throughout the body. Rosemary oil, rather, has shown potential antiseptic properties.

Scientific Evidence
One animal study found evidence that rosemary might help withdrawal from narcotics. Even weaker evidence hints that rosemary or its constituents may have antithrombotic (blood-thinning), anticancer, diuretic, liver-protective, and ulcer-protective effects.

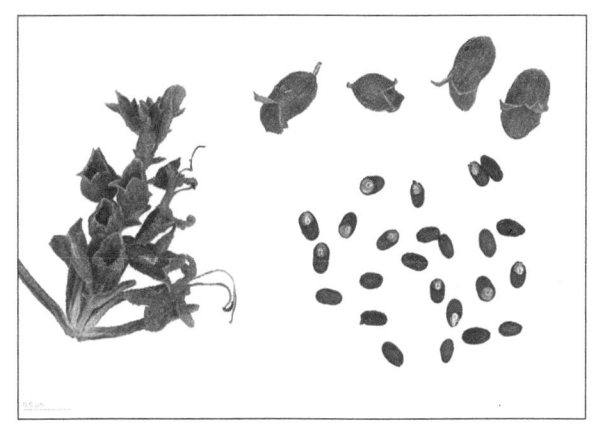

Rosmarinus officinalis. (Roger Culos via Wikimedia Commons)

Rosmarinic acid from rosemary has shown potential anti-inflammatory and antiallergic actions, but most published studies (including double-blind trials) have used a different plant source of the substance (the herb *Perilla frutescens*).

One controlled study failed to find rosemary cream protective against skin irritation caused by sodium lauryl sulfate (a common ingredient of cosmetic products).

Rosemary essential oil has been used in aromatherapy (treating conditions through scent). One controlled study evaluated rosemary aromatherapy for enhancing memory and found results that were mixed at best. Another study failed to find that rosemary aromatherapy reduced tension during an anxiety-provoking task; in fact, it appeared that the use of rosemary actually increased anxiety.

Safety Issues
Although rosemary's use in foods suggests a relatively low level of toxicity, rosemary has not undergone comprehensive safety testing. Rosemary essential oil can be toxic if taken even in fairly low doses, and the maximum safe dose is not known.

Based on its traditional use for abortion, as well as preliminary evidence showing embryotoxic effects, rosemary should not be used by pregnant women or women who wish to become pregnant.

One study suggests that rosemary may have diuretic effects. If it does, the herb could theoretically present risks in people taking the medication lithium.

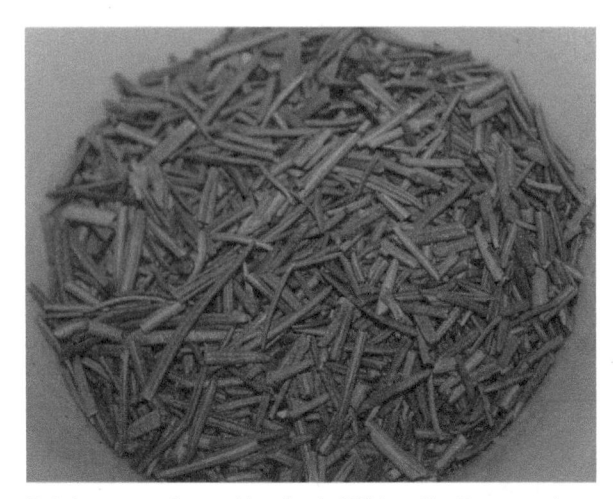

Dried rosemary leaves. (Atudu via Wikimedia Commons)

Other weak evidence hints that rosemary may enhance the liver's rate of deactivating estrogen in the body. This suggests that rosemary might present risks for females as well as for anyone who uses medications containing estrogen. Additionally, one study hints that rosemary might worsen blood sugar control in people with diabetes.

Persons who are taking lithium should use rosemary only with caution. Persons taking medications containing estrogen should be aware that rosemary may decrease the effects of such medications.

—*EBSCO CAM Review Board*

References

A.D.A.M. "Rosemary." *Milton S. Hershey Medical Center*, Penn State Hershey, 20 Jan. 2017, pennstatehershey.adam.com/content.aspx?productId=107&pid=33&gid=000271.

Fanous, Summer, and Natalie Butler. "The Health Potential of Rosemary." *Healthline*, 27 May 2016, www.healthline.com/health/rosemary-health-potential.

Hongratanaworakit, Tapanee, et al. "Development of Aroma Massage Oil for Relieving Muscle Pain and Satisfaction Evaluation in Humans." *Journal of Applied Pharmaceutical Science*, vol. 8, no. 4, 2018, pp. 126–130., doi:10.7324/japs.2018.8418.

Mirsadraei, Majid, et al. "Effects of Rosemary and Platanus Extracts on Asthmatic Subjects Resistant to Traditional Treatments." *European Respiratory Journal*, vol. 42, 2013.

Moss, Mark, et al. "Acute Ingestion of Rosemary Water: Evidence of Cognitive and Cerebrovascular Effects in Healthy Adults." *Journal of Psychopharmacology*, vol. 32, no. 12, 15 Oct. 2018, pp. 1319–1329., doi:10.1177/0269881118798339.

Oliveira, Jonatas Rafael De, et al. "Rosmarinus Officinalis L. (Rosemary) as Therapeutic and Prophylactic Agent." *Journal of Biomedical Science*, vol. 26, no. 1, 9 Jan. 2019, doi:10.1186/s12929-019-0499-8.

Shahgholian, Nahid, and Sekine Keshavarzian. "Comparison of the Effect of Topical Application of Rosemary and Menthol for Musculoskeletal Pain in Hemodialysis Patients." *Iranian Journal of Nursing and Midwifery Research*, vol. 22, no. 6, 2017, p. 436., doi:10.4103/ijnmr.ijnmr_163_16.

■ Turmeric

CATEGORY: Herbs and Supplements; Anti-Inflammatory; Functional Food
ALSO KNOWN AS: *Curcuma longa*, curcumin
ANATOMY OR SYSTEM AFFECTED: Gastrointestinal system; Immune system; Musculoskeletal system

Overview

Turmeric is a widely used tropical herb in the ginger family. Its stalk is used both in food and in medicine, yielding the familiar yellow ingredient that colors and adds flavor to, or spices, curry. In the traditional Indian system of herbal medicine known as Ayurveda, turmeric is believed to strengthen the overall energy of the body and to relieve gas, dispel worms, improve digestion, regulate menstruation, dissolve gallstones, and relieve arthritis, among other uses.

Modern interest in turmeric began in 1971 when Indian researchers found evidence suggesting that turmeric may possess anti-inflammatory properties. Much of this observed activity appeared to be caused by the presence of a constituent called curcumin. Curcumin is also an antioxidant. Many of the studies mentioned here used curcumin rather than turmeric.

Uses and Applications

Turmeric's antioxidant abilities make it a good food preservative, provided that the food is already yellow in color, and it is widely used for this purpose. Turmeric has been proposed as a treatment

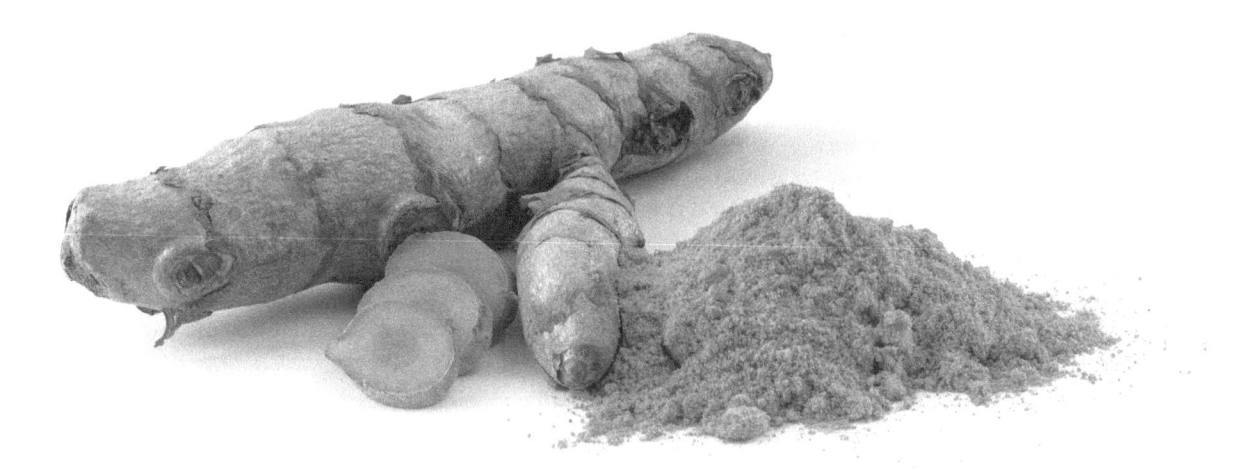

Turmeric (Curcuma longa): *fresh rhizome and powder.* (Simon A. Eugster via Wikimedia Commons)

for dyspepsia. "Dyspepsia" is a catchall term that includes a variety of digestive problems, such as stomach discomfort, gas, bloating, belching, appetite loss, and nausea. Although many serious medical conditions can cause digestive distress, the term "dyspepsia" is most often used when no identifiable medical cause can be detected.

In Europe, dyspepsia is commonly attributed to inadequate bile flow from the gallbladder. While this has not been proven, turmeric does appear to stimulate the gallbladder. More important, one double-blind, placebo-controlled study suggests that turmeric does reduce dyspepsia symptoms. Another double-blind, placebo-controlled study suggests that, when taken with standard medications, curcumin can help maintain remission in people with ulcerative colitis.

Other proposed uses of turmeric or curcumin have little supporting evidence. Based on test-tube and animal studies, and on human trials too preliminary to provide any meaningful evidence, curcumin and turmeric are frequently described as anti-inflammatory substances and are recommended for the treatment of such conditions as osteoarthritis and menstrual pain. Some advocates state that curcumin is superior to standard medications in the ibuprofen family, because, at standard doses, it does not appear to harm the stomach. However, until turmeric is actually proven to meaningfully reduce pain and inflammation, such a comparison is premature. Also, high doses of curcumin might increase the risk of ulcers, and, contrary to some reports, turmeric does not appear to be effective for treating ulcers.

Animal and test-tube studies suggest (but do not prove) that turmeric might help prevent cancer. Weak evidence hints that curcumin might help prevent the heart and kidney injury potentially caused by the chemotherapy drug doxorubicin.

Some researchers have reported evidence that curcumin or turmeric might generally help protect the liver from damage. However, other researchers have failed to find any liver-protective effects, and there are even some indications that turmeric extracts can damage the liver when taken in high doses or for an extended period.

On the basis of even weaker evidence, curcumin or turmeric has also been recommended for preventing Alzheimer's disease, cataracts, chronic anterior uveitis (an inflammation of the iris of the eye), fungal infections, and multiple sclerosis, and for treating high cholesterol.

One preliminary study failed to find curcumin helpful for lichen planus, a disease of the skin and mucous membranes. A six-month, double-blind, placebo-controlled study of thirty-six elderly persons failed to find that the consumption of curcumin (at a dose of up to 4 grams [g] daily) led to improvements in cholesterol profile.

Scientific Evidence

Dyspepsia. A double-blind, placebo-controlled study performed in Thailand compared the effects of 500 milligrams (mg) curcumin four times daily with placebo and with a locally popular over-the-counter treatment. A total of 116 people were enrolled in the study. After seven days, 87 percent of the curcumin group experienced full or partial symptom relief from dyspepsia, compared with 53 percent of the placebo group; this difference was statistically significant.

Ulcerative colitis. Ulcerative colitis is a disease of the lower digestive tract marked by alternating periods of quiescence and flare-up. Curcumin has shown some promise for helping to maintain remission and prevent relapse. In a double-blind, placebo-controlled study, eighty-nine people with quiescent ulcerative colitis were given either placebo or curcumin (1 g twice daily) with standard treatment. In the six-month treatment period, the relapse rate was significantly lower in the treatment group than in the placebo group.

Dosage

For medicinal purposes, turmeric is frequently taken in a form standardized to curcumin content, at a dose that provides 400 to 600 mg of curcumin three times daily.

Safety Issues

Turmeric is on the GRAS (Generally Recognized As Safe) list of the U.S. Food and Drug Administration, and curcumin too is believed to be fairly nontoxic. Reported side effects are uncommon and are generally limited to mild stomach distress.

However, there is some evidence to suggest that turmeric extracts can be toxic to the liver when taken in high doses or for a prolonged time. For this reason, turmeric products should probably be avoided by persons with liver disease and by those who take medications that are hard on the liver.

In addition, because of curcumin's stimulating effects on the gallbladder, persons with gallbladder disease should use curcumin only on the advice of a physician. Safety in young children, pregnant or nursing women, and those with severe kidney disease also has not been established.

—EBSCO CAM Review Board

References

Daily, James W., et al. "Efficacy of Turmeric Extracts and Curcumin for Alleviating the Symptoms of Joint Arthritis: A Systematic Review and Meta-Analysis of Randomized Clinical Trials." *Journal of Medicinal Food*, vol. 19, no. 8, 2016, pp. 717–729., doi:10.1089/jmf.2016.3705.

Gaffey, Andrew, et al. "The Effects of Curcumin on Musculoskeletal Pain: a Systematic Review Protocol." *JBI Database of Systematic Reviews and Implementation Reports*, vol. 13, no. 2, 2015, pp. 59–73., doi:10.11124/jbisrir-2015-1684.

Hewlings, Susan, and Douglas Kalman. "Curcumin: A Review of Its' Effects on Human Health." *Foods*, vol. 6, no. 10, 22 Oct. 2017, p. 92., doi:10.3390/foods6100092.

Johnson, Jon. "Turmeric for Rheumatoid Arthritis: Does It Work?" *Medical News Today*, MediLexicon International, 19 June 2019, www.medicalnewstoday.com/articles/325508.php.

Mackeen, Dawn. "What Are the Benefits of Turmeric?" *The New York Times*, 16 Oct. 2019, www.nytimes.com/2019/10/16/style/self-care/turmeric-benefits.html.

Perkins, Kimberly, et al. "Efficacy of Curcuma for Treatment of Osteoarthritis." *Journal of Evidence-Based Complementary & Alternative Medicine*, vol. 22, no. 1, 23 Mar. 2016, pp. 156–165., doi:10.1177/2156587216636747.

Sahebkar, Amirhossein, and Yves Henrotin. "Analgesic Efficacy and Safety of Curcuminoids in Clinical Practice: A Systematic Review and Meta-Analysis of Randomized Controlled Trials." *Pain Medicine*, vol. 17, no. 6, June 2016, pp. 1192–1202., doi:10.1093/pm/pnv024.

Sun, Jia, et al. "Role of Curcumin in the Management of Pathological Pain." *Phytomedicine*, vol. 48, 2018, pp. 129–140., doi:10.1016/j.phymed.2018.04.045.

Wong, Cathy. "The Health Benefits of Turmeric." *Verywell Health*, 16 Sept. 2019, www.verywellhealth.com/turmeric-for-pain-relief-can-it-help-4173236.

■ Valerian

CATEGORY: Herbs and Supplements; Sedative
ALSO KNOWN AS: *Valeriana officinalis*
ANATOMY OR SYSTEM AFFECTED: Central nervous system

Overview

More than two hundred plant species belong to the genus *Valeriana*, but the one most commonly used as an herb is *V. officinalis*. The root is used for medicinal purposes.

Galen recommended valerian for insomnia in the second century. Beginning in the sixteenth century, this herb became popular as a sedative in Europe, and it later became popular in the United States. Scientific studies on valerian in humans began in the 1970s, leading to its approval as a sleep aid by Germany's Commission E in 1985. However, the scientific evidence showing that valerian really works remains incomplete.

As with most herbs, experts are not exactly sure which ingredients in valerian are most important. Early research focused on a group of chemicals known as valepotriates, but they are no longer considered candidates. A constituent called valerenic acid has also undergone study, but its role is far from clear. Another substance in valerian, called linarin, has also attracted research interest.

The understanding of how valerian might function remains similarly incomplete. Several studies suggest that valerian affects GABA, a naturally occurring amino acid that appears to be related to the experience of anxiety. Conventional tranquilizers in the valium family are known to bind to GABA receptors in the brain, and valerian may work similarly. However, there are some significant flaws in these hypotheses, and the reality is that experts do not really know how valerian works, or, indeed, whether it does work.

Therapeutic Dosages
For insomnia, the standard adult dosage of valerian is 2 grams (g) to 3 g of dried herb, 270 to 450 mg of an aqueous valerian extract, or 600 mg of an ethanol extract, taken thirty to sixty minutes before bedtime. The same amount, or a reduced dose, can be taken twice daily for anxiety.

Because of valerian's unpleasant odor, European manufacturers have created odorless valerian products. However, these are not widely available in the United States. Valerian is not recommended for children under three years old.

Therapeutic Uses
Valerian is commonly recommended as a mild treatment for occasional insomnia. However, evidence from the best positive study on valerian suggests that it is useful only when taken over an extended period of time for chronic sleep disorders. Overall, it is not clear whether valerian is effective for sleep at all.

Like other treatments used for insomnia, valerian has also been proposed as a treatment for anxiety, but there is no reliable evidence that it is effective. Finally, valerian is sometimes suggested as a treatment for a nervous stomach; however, there is no supporting scientific evidence for this use.

Scientific Evidence
Insomnia. Overall, the evidence supporting valerian as a sleep aid remains substantially incomplete and contradictory. A systematic review published in 2007 concluded that valerian is probably not effective for treating insomnia. In a subsequent review of eighteen randomized trials, researchers found that people who took valerian did report an improvement in their sleep, but this finding was not supported by more objective measures of sleep quality.

However, there have been some positive results, both with valerian alone and with valerian combined with other herbs. The best positive study of valerian for insomnia followed 121 people for twenty-eight days. In this double-blind, placebo-controlled trial, half of the participants took 600 milligrams (mg) of an alcohol-based valerian extract one hour before bedtime, while the other half took placebo. Valerian did not work right away. For the first couple of weeks, valerian and placebo were running neck and neck. However, by day twenty-eight, valerian pulled far ahead. Effectiveness was rated as good or very good by participant evaluation in 66 percent of the valerian group and in 61 percent by doctor evaluation, whereas in the placebo group, effectiveness was so rated by only 29 percent of participants and doctors.

Although positive, these results are a bit confusing. In another large study, valerian was immediately more effective than placebo, which is more in keeping with how the herb is typically used. This trial followed 128 subjects who had no sleeping problems. On nine nonconsecutive nights, each participant took one of three treatments: valerian, a combination of valerian and the herb hops, or placebo. The results showed that on the nights they took valerian alone, participants fell asleep faster than when they were taking placebo or the combination. In contradiction to this, other studies have failed to find any immediate mental-depressant effects with valerian; most substances that rapidly induce sleep also sedate the mind.

Furthermore, the more recent and best-designed studies have generally failed to find valerian more helpful at all. One of these was a four-week study in

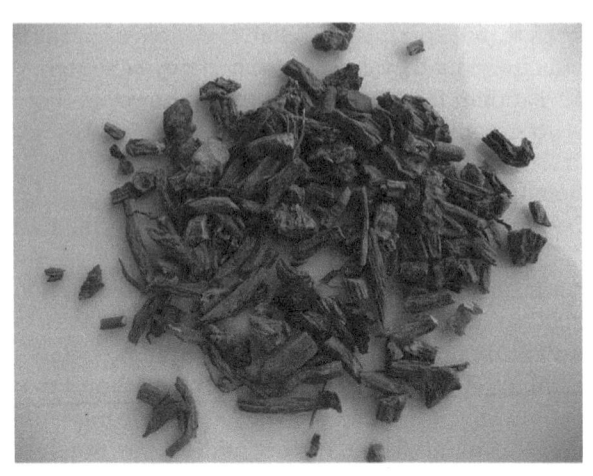

Dried valerian root. (via Wikimedia Commons)

which 135 people were given valerian and 135 were given placebo. Another was a two-week study of 405 people that found "modest benefits at most."

A six-week, double-blind study of 202 people with insomnia compared valerian extract (600 mg at bedtime) with the standard drug oxazepam (10 mg at bedtime) and found equal efficacy. Equivalent benefits were also seen in a similar study of 75 people. However, the absence of a placebo group in these two studies decreases the reliability of the results.

A study of 184 people tested a standardized combination of valerian and hops, with mixed results. Researchers tested quite a few aspects of sleep, such as time to fall asleep, length of sleep, and number of awakenings, and found evidence of benefit in only a few. This use of "multiple outcome measures" makes the results somewhat unreliable.

A much smaller study also found evidence that a combination of hops and valerian extract is more effective as a sleep aid than placebo. The results of this trial also hint that hops plus valerian is more effective than valerian alone, but this possible finding did not reach statistical significance.

A double-blind comparative study that enrolled forty-six patients compared the effects of the standard drug bromazepam to a mixture of valerian and hops with either treatment taken half an hour before bedtime. The results suggest that the two treatments were equally effective. One study found that this valerian-hops combination can antagonize the arousal produced by caffeine.

A combination of valerian and lemon balm has also been tried for insomnia. A rather poorly designed thirty-day, double-blind, placebo-controlled study of ninety-eight individuals without insomnia found marginal evidence that a valerian-lemon balm combination improved sleep quality compared with placebo. However, a double-blind crossover study of twenty people with insomnia compared the benefits of the sleeping drug Halcion (0.125 mg) against placebo and a combination of valerian and lemon balm and failed to find the herb effective. The drug, however, did prove effective. In addition, valerian has shown some promise for helping people sleep better after discontinuing conventional sleeping pills in the benzodiazepine family.

Anxiety and stress. In a double-blind, placebo-controlled study, thirty-six people with generalized anxiety disorder were given either valerian extract, Valium, or placebo for a period of four weeks. The study failed to find statistically significant differences between the groups, presumably due to its small size.

Valerian has also been tested for possible benefits during stressful circumstances. Two preliminary double-blind studies found weak evidence that valerian may produce calming effects in induced stressful situations. Another study evaluated the effects of a combination containing valerian and lemon balm taken in various doses. Some benefits were seen with doses of 600 mg or 1200 mg three times daily, but the highest dose, 1,800 mg three times daily, actually appeared to increase anxiety symptoms during a stressful situation. Furthermore, people taking the herbal treatment at any dose showed slightly decreased cognitive function compared with those given placebo.

Safety Issues

Valerian is on the U.S. Food and Drug Administration's (FDA) Generally Recognized As Safe (GRAS) list and is approved for use as a food. In animals, it takes enormous doses of valerian to produce any serious adverse effects. Valerian has shown an excellent safety profile in clinical trials.

In a suicide attempt, one young woman took approximately 20 g of valerian, twenty to forty times the recommended dose. Only mild symptoms developed, including stomach cramps, fatigue, chest tightness, tremors, and light-headedness. All of these symptoms were resolved within twenty-four hours after two treatments with activated charcoal. The woman's laboratory tests, including tests of her

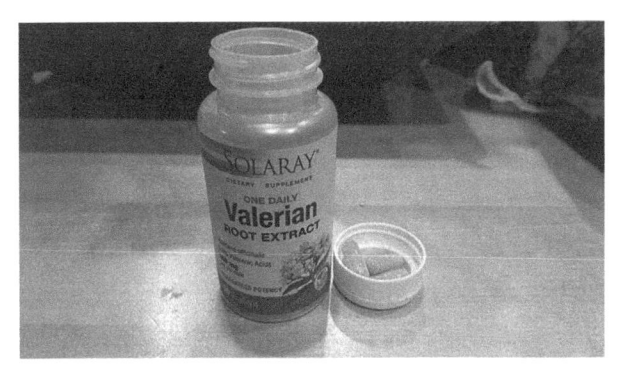

A bottle of valerian capsules. (Breawycker via Wikimedia Commons)

liver function, remained normal. However, this does not mean that people can safely exceed the recommended dose.

One report did find toxic results from herbal remedies containing valerian mixed with several other herbal ingredients, including skullcap. Four individuals who took these remedies later developed liver problems. However, skullcap products are sometimes contaminated with the liver-toxic herb germander, and this could have been the explanation.

There have also been about fifty reported cases of overdose with a combination preparation called Sleep-Qik, which contains valerian, as well as conventional medications. Researchers specifically looked for liver injury, but they found no evidence that it occurred.

There are some safety concerns about valepotriates, constituents of valerian, because in test-tube studies they have been found to affect deoxyribonucleic acid (DNA) and cause other toxic effects. However, valepotriates are not present to a significant extent in any commercial preparations.

Although no animal studies or controlled human trials have found evidence that valerian causes withdrawal symptoms when stopped, one case report is sometimes cited in support of the possibility that this might occur. It concerns a fifty-eight-year-old man who developed delirium and rapid heartbeat after surgery. According to the patient's family, he had been taking high doses of valerian root extract, about 2.5 to 10 g per day, for many years. His physicians decided that he was suffering from valerian withdrawal. However, considering the many other factors involved, such as multiple medications and general anesthesia, it is not really possible to conclude that valerian caused his symptoms.

In clinical trials, use of valerian has not been associated with any significant side effects. A few people experience mild gastrointestinal distress, and there have been rare reports of people developing a paradoxical mild stimulant effect from valerian.

Valerian does not appear to impair driving ability or produce morning drowsiness when taken at night. As noted above, most studies have failed to find any immediate sedative effect with valerian. However, one study reported finding mild impairment of attention for a couple of hours after taking valerian. For this reason, it is not a good idea to drive immediately after taking it.

There have been no reported drug interactions with valerian, and two studies found reasons to believe that valerian should not raise or lower the blood levels of too many medications. Nonetheless, there are at least theoretical concerns that valerian might amplify the effects of sedative drugs. A 1995 study was somewhat reassuring on this score because it found no interaction between alcohol and valerian. However, animal studies have found that valerian extracts may prolong the effects of some sedatives, and there have been some worrisome case reports suggesting that the combination of valerian and alcohol can lead to excessive sedation in some people. For this reason, experts recommend that people not combine valerian with central nervous system depressants, except under a doctor's supervision.

Safety in young children, pregnant or nursing women, and those with severe liver or kidney disease has not been established. People who are taking sedative drugs, such as benzodiazepines, should not take valerian in addition to them, except under physician supervision.

—*EBSCO CAM Review Board*

References

Barton, Debra L., et al. "The Use of Valeriana Officinalis (Valerian) in Improving Sleep in Patients Who Are Undergoing Treatment for Cancer: A Phase III Randomized, Placebo-Controlled, Double-Blind Study (NCCTG Trial, N01C5)." *The Journal of Supportive Oncology*, vol. 9, no. 1, 2011, pp. 24–31., doi:10.1016/j.suponc.2010.12.008.

Bauer, Brent A. "Valerian: A Safe and Effective Herbal Sleep Aid?" *Mayo Clinic*, Mayo Foundation for Medical Education and Research, 15 Feb. 2018, www.mayoclinic.org/diseases-conditions/insomnia/expert-answers/valerian/faq-20057875.

Hill, John. *Valerian. or, the Virtues of That Root in Nervous Disorders.* 2nd ed., Gale Ecco, 2018.

Moghadam, Zahra Behboodi, et al. "The Effect of Valerian Root Extract on the Severity of Pre Menstrual Syndrome Symptoms." *Journal of Traditional and Complementary Medicine*, vol. 6, no. 3, 2016, pp. 309–315., doi:10.1016/j.jtcme.2015.09.001.

Sharma, Muktika, et al. "A Comprehensive Pharmacognostic Report on Valerian." *International Journal of Pharmaceutical Sciences and Research*, vol. 1, no. 7, 1 July 2010, pp. 6–40., doi:10.13040/ijpsr.0975-8232.1(7).6-40.

Wexler, Alyse. "Valerian Root for Insomnia and Anxiety: Benefits, Dosage, and More." *Medical News Today*, MediLexicon International, 25 June 2017, www.medicalnewstoday.com/articles/318088.php.

Wong, Cathy. "The Benefits and Uses of Valerian Root." *Verywell Health*, 17 July 2019, www.verywellhealth.com/what-you-need-to-know-about-valerian-88336.

Zare, Afshin, et al. "Analgesic Effect of Valerian Root and Turnip Extracts." *World Journal Of Plastic Surgery*, vol. 7, no. 3, Sept. 2018, pp. 345–350., doi:10.29252/wjps.7.3.345.

■ White willow

CATEGORY: Herbs and Supplements; Anti-Inflammatory
ALSO KNOWN AS: *Salix alba*
ANATOMY OR SYSTEM AFFECTED: Craniofacial; Reproductive system; Musculoskeletal system

Overview

Willow bark has been used as a treatment for pain and fever in China since 500 B.C.E. In Europe, it was primarily used for altogether different purposes, such as stopping vomiting, removing warts, and suppressing sexual desire. However, in 1828, European chemists made a discovery that would bring together some of these different uses. They extracted the substance salicin from white willow, which was soon purified to salicylic acid. Salicylic acid is an effective treatment for pain and fever, but it is also sufficiently irritating to do a good job of burning off warts. Chemists later modified salicylic acid (this time from the herb meadowsweet) to create acetylsalicylic acid, or aspirin.

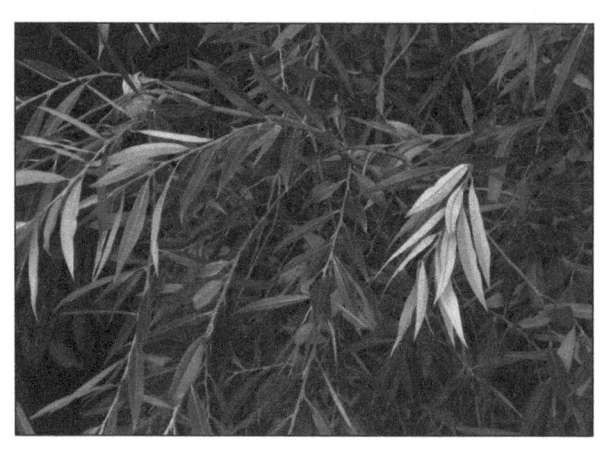

Salix alba. *The white tone of the undersides of the leaves give the white willow its name.* (via Wikimedia Commons)

Therapeutic Dosages

Standardized willow bark extracts should provide 120 to 240 milligrams (mg) of salicin daily.

Therapeutic Uses

As interest in natural medicine has grown, many people have begun to turn back to white willow as an alternative to aspirin. One double-blind, placebo-controlled trial found it effective for back pain, and another found it helpful for osteoarthritis. White willow is also used for such conditions as bursitis, dysmenorrhea, tension headaches, migraine headaches, rheumatoid arthritis, and tendonitis. However, two recent studies failed to find it effective for rheumatoid arthritis or osteoarthritis.

Aspirin and related anti-inflammatory drugs are notorious for irritating or damaging the stomach. However, when taken in typical doses, willow does not appear to produce this side effect to the same extent. This may be partly due to the fact that most of the salicylic acid provided by white willow comes from salicin and other chemicals that are converted to salicylic acid only after absorption into the body. Other evidence suggests that standard doses of willow bark are the equivalent of one baby aspirin daily, rather than a full dose.

This latter finding raises an interesting question: If willow provides only a small amount of salicylic acid, how can it work? The most likely answer seems to be that other constituents besides salicin play a role. Another possibility is that the studies finding benefit were flawed and that it actually does not work.

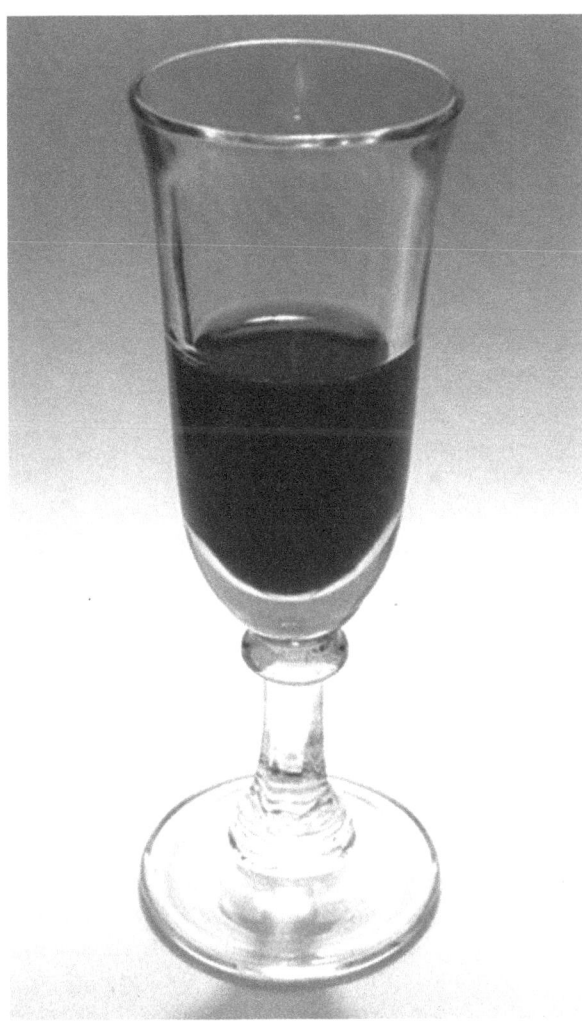

A tincture prepared from white willow bark and ethanol, containing salicin (from which salicylic acid-based products like aspirin are derived). (Badagnani via Wikimedia Commons)

Scientific Evidence

In a four-week, double-blind, placebo-controlled study of 210 individuals with back pain, two doses of willow bark extract were compared against placebo. The higher-dose group received extract supplying 240 mg of salicin daily; in this group, 39 percent were pain-free for at least five days of the last week of the study. In the lower-dose group (120 mg of salicin daily), 21 percent became pain-free. In contrast, only 6 percent of those given placebo became pain-free. Stomach distress did not occur in this study. The only significant side effect seen was an allergic reaction in one participant given willow. Benefits were also seen in a double-blind, placebo-controlled trial of seventy-eight individuals with osteoarthritis of the knee or hip.

However, two subsequent double-blind, placebo-controlled studies performed by a single research group failed to find white willow more effective than placebo. One enrolled 127 people with osteoarthritis (OA) of the hip or knee, the other 26 outpatients with active rheumatoid arthritis (RA). In the OA trial, participants received either willow bark extract (240 mg of salicin per day), the standard drug diclofenac (100 mg per day), or placebo. In the RA trial, participants received either willow bark extract at the same dose or placebo. While diclofenac proved significantly more effective than placebo in the OA trial, willow bark did not. It also failed to prove more effective than placebo in the RA study. The most likely interpretation of these conflicting findings is that willow provides at best no more than a modest level of pain relief.

Safety Issues

Evidence suggests that willow, taken at standard doses, is the equivalent of 50 mg of aspirin, a very small dose. Willow does not impair blood coagulation to the same extent as aspirin, and it also does not appear to significantly irritate the stomach. Nonetheless, it seems reasonable to suppose that if it is used over the long term or in high doses, willow could still cause the side effects associated with aspirin. All the risks of aspirin therapy potentially apply.

For this reason, white willow should not be given to children because of the risk of Reye's syndrome. It should also not be used by people with aspirin allergies, bleeding disorders, or kidney disease. In addition, white willow may interact adversely with blood thinners, other anti-inflammatory drugs, methotrexate, metoclopramide, phenytoin, probenecid, spironolactone, and valproate. Safety in pregnant or nursing women, or in those with severe liver or kidney disease, has not been established.

Important Interactions

Persons should avoid combining white willow with blood-thinning medications such as warfarin (Coumadin), heparin, clopidogrel (Plavix), ticlopidine (Ticlid), and pentoxifylline (Trental); with aspirin, methotrexate, metoclopramide, phenytoin (Dilantin), sulfonamide drugs, spironolactone and other potassium-sparing diuretics; or with valproic acid.

—*EBSCO CAM Review Board*

References

A.D.A.M. "Willow Bark." *Milton S. Hershey Medical Center*, Penn State Hershey, 5 Aug. 2015, pennstatehershey.adam.com/content.aspx?productId=107&pid=33&gid=000281.

Cheungpasitporn, Wisit, et al. "White Willow Bark Induced Acute Respiratory Distress Syndrome." *North American Journal of Medical Sciences*, vol. 5, no. 5, 2013, p. 330., doi:10.4103/1947-2714.112483.

Mahdi, Jassem G. "Medicinal Potential of Willow: A Chemical Perspective of Aspirin Discovery." *Journal of Saudi Chemical Society*, vol. 14, no. 3, 2010, pp. 317–322., doi:10.1016/j.jscs.2010.04.010.

Matyjaszczyk, Ewa, and Regina Schumann. "Risk Assessment of White Willow (Salix Alba) in Food." *EFSA Journal*, vol. 16, no. S1, 28 Aug. 2018, doi:10.2903/j.efsa.2018.e16081.

Shara, Mohd, and Sidney J. Stohs. "Efficacy and Safety of White Willow Bark (Salix Alba) Extracts." *Phytotherapy Research*, vol. 29, no. 8, 22 May 2015, pp. 1112–1116., doi:10.1002/ptr.5377.

Vlachojannis, J. E., et al. "A Systematic Review on the Effectiveness of Willow Bark for Musculoskeletal Pain." *Phytotherapy Research*, vol. 23, no. 7, 2009, pp. 897–900., doi:10.1002/ptr.2747.

Wong, Cathy. "Can Willow Bark Relieve Pain?" *Verywell Health*, 17 July 2019, www.verywellhealth.com/white-willow-bark-89085.

■ Witch hazel

CATEGORY: Herbs and Supplements; Anti-Inflammatory; Astringent
ALSO KNOWN AS: *Hamamelis virginiana*
ANATOMY OR SYSTEM AFFECTED: Skin

Overview

The bark, leaves, and twigs of the witch hazel shrub were widely used as medicinal treatments by native peoples of North America. Witch hazel was applied topically as a treatment for such conditions as skin wounds, insect bites, hemorrhoids, muscle aches, and back stiffness, and it was taken internally for colds, coughs, and digestive problems. It came into use among European colonists in the 1840s, when a businessperson named Theron Pond marketed an extract of witch hazel as Golden Treasure.

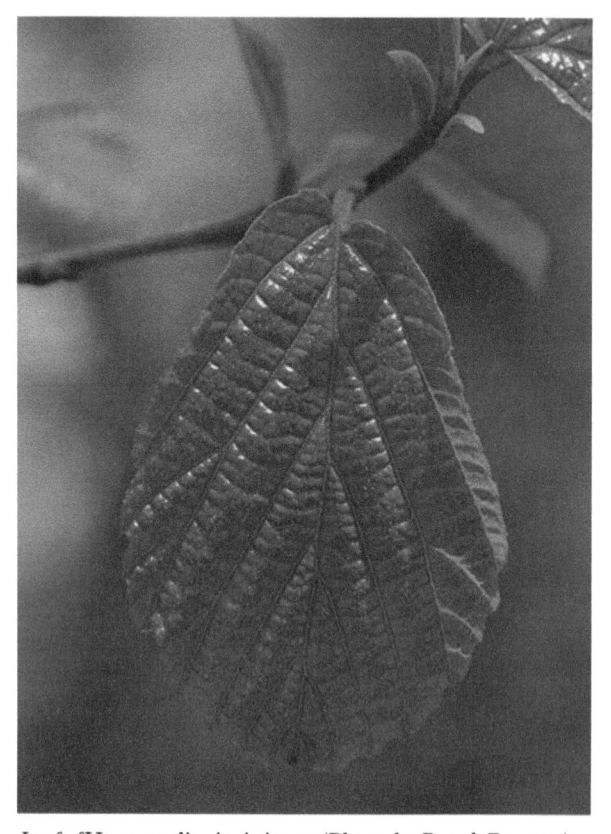

Leaf of Hamamelis virginiana. (Photo by Derek Ramsey)

The most common witch hazel product available in the United States is made from the whole twigs of the shrub. Extracts of the bark alone are used in Europe.

Therapeutic Dosages

Witch hazel preparations should be used according to label instructions.

Therapeutic Uses

Witch hazel is widely marketed for direct application to the skin to relieve pain, stop bleeding, control itching, reduce symptoms of eczema, and treat muscle aches. Pads, ointments, and suppositories containing witch hazel are used for treatment of hemorrhoids. Extracts of the bark and leaf are used in Europe to treat diarrhea, inflammation of the gums, canker sores, and varicose veins. However, there is no meaningful evidence that witch hazel is actually effective for any of these conditions.

One small double-blind study is commonly cited as evidence that witch hazel is effective for treatment of eczema. This study compared topical witch hazel ointment to the drug bufexamac and found them equally effective. However, bufexamac itself has not been shown effective for the treatment of eczema, and so this study proves little. A subsequent study failed to find witch hazel more effective than a placebo treatment for eczema.

There are no other meaningful studies of witch hazel. Extremely preliminary evidence hints that it may have anti-inflammatory properties, and even weaker evidence suggests that witch hazel may increase the contractility of veins, potentially making it useful in varicose veins. However, this evidence is far too weak to support using witch hazel for any of these conditions.

Safety Issues

Witch hazel appears to be a relatively safe substance, but comprehensive safety studies have not been performed. When applied to the skin, it may cause allergic reactions. Witch hazel contains tannins, which can upset the stomach. Safety in pregnant or nursing women, young children, and people with severe liver or kidney disease has not been established.

—*EBSCO CAM Review Board*

References

Greive, Kerryn, et al. "Evaluation of a Topical Treatment for the Relief of Sensitive Skin." *Clinical, Cosmetic and Investigational Dermatology*, vol. 8, 2015, p. 405., doi:10.2147/ccid.s87509.

Kingston University. "Age-Old Remedies Using White Tea, Witch Hazel and Rose May Be Beneficial, Study Suggests." *ScienceDaily*, 2 Dec. 2011, www.sciencedaily.com/releases/2011/12/111201132501.htm.

Thring, Tamsyn Sa, et al. "Antioxidant and Potential Anti-Inflammatory Activity of Extracts and Formulations of White Tea, Rose, and Witch Hazel on Primary Human Dermal Fibroblast Cells." *Journal of Inflammation*, vol. 8, no. 1, 2011, p. 27., doi:10.1186/1476-9255-8-27.

Trüeb, Ralphm. "North American Virginian Witch Hazel (Hamamelis Virginiana): Based Scalp Care and Protection for Sensitive Scalp, Red Scalp, and Scalp Burn-Out." *International Journal of Trichology*, vol. 6, no. 3, 2014, pp. 100–103., doi:10.4103/0974-7753.139079.

Wong, Cathy. "The Health Benefits of Witch Hazel." *Verywell Health*, 17 July 2019, www.verywellhealth.com/the-benefits-of-witch-hazel-90061.

■ Yoga

CATEGORY: Therapy or Technique; Physiotherapy; Prevention

ANATOMY OR SYSTEM AFFECTED: All

KEY TERMS

- *asana*: (in Sanskrit seat or posture); a yogic posture or position; the ability to sit unmoving with a straight spine for long periods of time
- *pranayama*: (in Sanskrit prana = energy + yama = control); type of meditation technique that involves various ways of controlling the breathing, with the goal being to withdraw ones senses from the outside world
- *vinyasa*: (in Sanskrit vi = special + nyasa = to place) movement between poses in yoga, typically accompanied by regulated breathing

Overview

Hatha yoga, commonly called yoga in the United States, is an exercise system derived from ancient traditions in India. There are many schools or varieties of yoga, but all of them involve asanas, or postures. Many asanas function as gentle stretching exercises, increasing flexibility. Others encourage the development of strength and balance.

The practice of yoga goes beyond exercise, however. Special breathing techniques are almost always part of the process; in fact, some forms of yoga focus primarily on breathing and, therefore, overlap with traditional breathing practices generally known as *pranayama*. Because yoga originated in traditional Hindu spiritual practice, it can involve meditation, chanting, and philosophical and religious introspection. However, completely secular versions of yoga are widely available.

Yoga is believed by its practitioners to provide benefits above and beyond simple exercise. For example, certain asanas are said to address specific health problems. However, there is only minimal scientific evidence that yoga actually provides any well-defined medical benefits.

Uses and Applications

There are numerous specific schools of yoga, including Iyengar yoga, Ashtanga yoga, Kriya yoga,

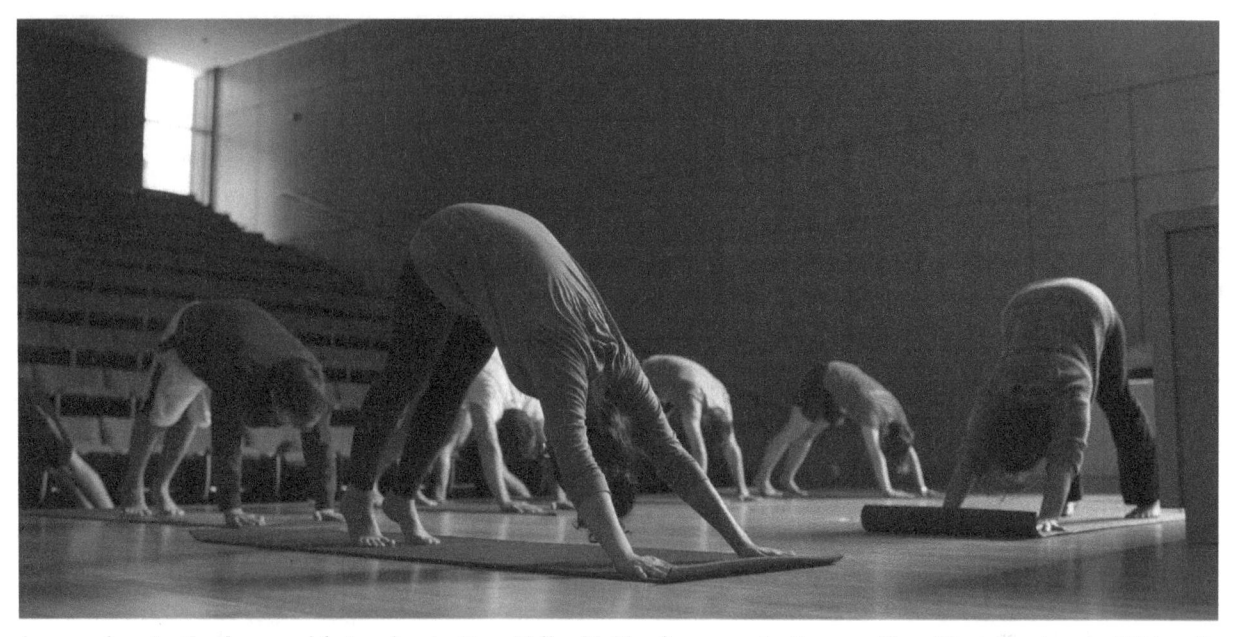

A yoga class in the downward-facing dog position (Adho Mukha Svanasana). (Jeremy Hess Photography via Wikimedia Commons)

Vini yoga, and Bikram yoga, as well as the "generic" yoga. Yoga is ordinarily learned through inexpensive group lessons, but regular at-home practice is necessary to progress in skill (and to derive potential health benefits). Lessons are commonly available at hospital wellness centers, health clubs, city recreation departments, and private yoga studios. Do-it-yourself yoga DVDs and books are available too, but most serious yoga practitioners caution against learning the technique without an instructor present.

Scientific Evidence

Although some evidence exists that yoga may offer medical benefits, this evidence, in general, is not strong. There are several reasons for this (including funding obstacles), but one is fundamental: Even with the best of intentions, it is difficult to properly ascertain the effectiveness of an exercise therapy like yoga. Only one form of study can truly prove that a treatment is effective: the double-blind, placebo-controlled trial. However, it is not possible to fit yoga into a study design of this type. While it might be possible to design a placebo form of yoga, it would be quite difficult to keep participants and researchers "in the dark" regarding who is practicing real yoga and who is practicing fake yoga.

Some compromise with the highest research standards is, therefore, inevitable. However, the compromise used in most studies is less than optimal. In these trials, yoga has been compared to no treatment. The problem with such studies is that a treatment, any treatment, frequently appears to be better than no treatment. It would be better to compare yoga to generic forms of exercise, such as daily walking, but thus far this method has not seen much use. Given these caveats, the following is a summary of what science knows about the possible medical benefits of yoga.

Possible benefits. Yoga, like Tai Chi, has been advocated as a means of increasing strength, balance, and physical function in the elderly. However, there is little scientific proof that yoga offers such benefits or that it is superior to generic exercises such as walking. There is little doubt that yoga, like any form of stretching, will increase flexibility if it is practiced consistently and over a long period of time.

Yoga is also said to relieve tension and stress. In one study of sixty-five women with depression or anxiety (or both), a two-month yoga program specifically designed to address these emotional conditions significantly reduced anxiety (but not depression) compared to enrolled women who were waiting for the program to begin. Another study found that participation in a six-week yoga program

> ## Finding the Right Type of Yoga and The Right Teacher
>
> The word "yoga" as used in the United States refers to a broad range of different kinds of mental, physical, and spiritual practices. Persons who have a desire to learn should take some time to get acquainted with the different schools and styles to appreciate what various teachers have to offer. Yoga is a most personal kind of exercise, and the benefits accrue slowly and subtly over time.
>
> Many different schools and styles of yoga are taught in the United States. Some teachers have been certified in particular traditions, others offer a synthesis based on their own practice with yoga masters. The various major traditions include the following:
>
> *Astanga yoga.* This form of yoga, developed by K. Pattabhi Jois, is a demanding form of the practice. This yoga uses a concept of "flow" that has participants moving continuously and jumping from one posture to another, building strength, flexibility, and stamina. Astanga yoga is an intense workout and is not recommended for persons looking for leisurely stretching exercises.
>
> *Integral yoga.* This form of yoga was developed by Swami Satchidananda. It relies on breathing exercises (*pranayama*) and meditation as much as on postures for the practice.
>
> *Iyengar yoga.* Iyengar yoga is a style of yoga developed by B. K. S. Iyengar, who systemized his training and certified teachers who have completed an extensive two-to-five-year training program. Iyengar practitioners use props such as blocks and belts to aid them in performing many of the more difficult postures, and great attention is paid to a precise alignment of postures.
>
> *Kripalu yoga.* This form of yoga places emphasis on "honoring the wisdom of the body" and allowing each student to develop an awareness of mind, body, emotion, and spirit. The practice is delineated into three stages: learning the postures and exploring the body's abilities, holding the postures for an extended time and developing an inner awareness, and moving from one posture to another in a spontaneous movement.
>
> *Kundalini yoga.* This form of yoga involves postures, meditation, and the coordination of breath. The practice is said to create a controlled release of kundalini energy, a creative force thought to be at the base of the spine.
>
> *Viniyoga.* Viniyoga was developed by Krishnamacharya, a teacher whose disciples have created numerous other yoga forms. Viniyoga is a gentle form of flow yoga (continuous movement) that focuses on a student's ability rather than on idealized form.
>
> *Bikram yoga.* Bikram yoga, founded by Bikram Choudhury, utilizes yoga postures practiced in a heated environment.
>
> *Sivananda yoga.* This form of yoga involves a set structure that includes relaxation, pranayama (breathing), and classic asana postures.
>
> Many excellent yoga books explain the postures and feature beautiful photographs and illustrations. Teachers, however, can impart an understanding of the poses and the practice of yoga in ways that books cannot. A teacher can also help one develop correct alignment in the various poses so that one gets the greatest benefit and so that internal stretching and healing begin.
>
> While there is still an emphasis on yoga as a physical exercise, many teachers now address the more spiritual aspects of practice too. Other teachers take a holistic or even therapeutic approach with their students, reading their yoga practice as an open book on their personality and behavior.
>
> The kind of relationship one develops with his or her yoga teacher depends on the teacher's philosophy and on what kind of response the student wants. However, certain basic rules should be followed in assessing a yoga teacher's capabilities.
>
> Upon seeing a new student in class, most teachers will acknowledge that the student is new to class and will have a short chat with the student. Teachers also might ask the student if he or she has any injuries so they can recommend alternative poses if they think some routines are too difficult. Good yoga teachers will carefully watch the new student, make adjustments to postures, and push the student beyond perceived limits.
>
> —*Reviewed by Brian Randall, M.D.*

was associated with reduced anxiety, depression, and stress in women having radiotherapy for breast cancer. Finally, a trial of 122 healthy pregnant women demonstrated that daily yoga practice incorporating deep relaxation significantly reduced self-perceived stress scores, compared to standard prenatal exercises.

Weak evidence hints that yoga may offer modest benefits for people with chronic obstructive pulmonary disease (COPD) or asthma. For example, in one controlled study, fifty-nine people with mild asthma were randomly assigned to practice yoga and attend a general class or simply to attend the general class. The results showed slight improvements in asthma in the treated group compared to the untreated group. However, even these modest benefits did not last; assessment two months later showed no difference between the groups. Furthermore, as noted, studies in which the participants in the control group do not receive placebo treatment are inherently unreliable. A small 2009 study of twenty-nine adults with COPD suggests that a twelve-week yoga program may be associated with slight improvement in timed walking distance and self-reported functional ability. A special breathing technique called yogic-style Buteyko breathing may reduce medication use and subjective symptoms, though it does not appear to actually improve lung function.

In another study, forty-two people with carpal tunnel syndrome were randomly assigned to receive either yoga or a wrist splint for eight weeks. The results indicated that the use of yoga was more effective than the wrist splint. However, participants in the control group were simply offered the wrist splint and given the choice of using it or not; it would have been preferable for them to have received a more believable placebo, like other forms of meditative exercise.

In a randomized, controlled trial, eight weeks of daily supervised yoga was modestly more effective than a similar amount of supervised physical exercise in relieving menopausal symptoms (such as hot flashes), decreasing psychological stress, and improving cognitive abilities among 120 perimenopausal women. Only weak evidence has been reported regarding the possible usefulness of yoga for depression, obsessive-compulsive disorder, low back pain, general well-being, migraine headaches, osteoarthritis, and congestive heart failure. A small trial involving fifty-four adolescents with eating disorders found that adding eight weeks of yoga twice weekly to standard therapy was associated with improved eating-disorder-related thoughts and behaviors. Yoga has also been studied for schizophrenia. In one small trial, participants who supplemented their regular treatment with a yoga program lasting four months had improved symptoms, were able to function better, and reported a better quality of life compared to those who engaged in physical therapy.

Yoga also has been promoted as a treatment for epilepsy (seizure disorder), but a review of all published scientific trials concluded that there is no meaningful evidence that it is effective. Some evidence suggests that yoga is not helpful for chemical dependency or high blood pressure.

What to Expect During Treatment
Yoga classes typically last about one to two hours. Most of that time is spent practicing various asanas; however, other activities such as breathing exercises may take place too. Yoga is generally a gentle, nonaerobic form of exercise. However, some types of yoga, such as Iyengar yoga, are more physically vigorous.

By the end of a yoga class, many people report feeling relaxed and comfortable, and they consider this a meaningful benefit in itself. However, without regular home practice, it is unlikely that performing yoga will provide any long-term benefit. For this reason, instructors generally encourage daily practice, ranging from a few minutes to an hour or more.

Safety Issues
Yoga is generally as safe as any other stretching-based exercise program. However, there are a few yoga positions, such as the headstand, that can cause injury when they are performed by a person who is not yet sufficiently advanced in yoga or who has certain health problems, such as a detached retina. A properly qualified instructor can help participants avoid injury by taking each person's individual health status into account.

—*EBSCO CAM Review Board*

References
Bergland, Christopher. "How Does Yoga Relieve Chronic Pain?" *Psychology Today*, Sussex Publishers, 27 May 2015, www.psychologytoday.com/us/blog/the-athletes-way/201505/how-does-yoga-relieve-chronic-pain.

Fishman, Loren. *Healing Yoga: Proven Postures to Treat Twenty Common Ailments – from Backache to Bone Loss, Shoulder Pain to Bunions, and More.* W.W. Norton & Company, 2015.

Florida Atlantic University. "First Study to Show Chair Yoga as Effective Alternative Treatment for Osteoarthritis." *ScienceDaily*, 11 Jan. 2017, www.sciencedaily.com/releases/2017/01/170111091417.htm.

Mayo Clinic Staff. "Yoga: Fight Stress and Find Serenity." *Mayo Clinic*, Mayo Foundation for Medical Education and Research, 19 Sept. 2019, www.mayoclinic.org/healthy-lifestyle/stress-management/in-depth/yoga/art-20044733.

Pearson, Neil, et al. *Yoga and Science in Pain Care: Treating the Person in Pain*. Singing Dragon, 2019.

Vallath, Nandini. "Perspectives On Yoga inputs in the Management of Chronic Pain." *Indian Journal of Palliative Care*, vol. 16, no. 1, 2010, pp. 1–7., doi:10.4103/0973-1075.63127.

Wise, Jacqui. "Yoga Is Reasonable Alternative to Physical Therapy for Lower Back Pain, Say Researchers." *Bmj*, 20 June 2017, doi:10.1136/bmj.j2964.

"Yoga for Pain Relief." *Harvard Health Publishing*, Harvard Medical School, Apr. 2015, www.health.harvard.edu/alternative-and-complementary-medicine/yoga-for-pain-relief.

"Yoga for Pain." *National Center for Complementary and Integrative Health*, U.S. Department of Health and Human Services, 21 Sept. 2018, nccih.nih.gov/health/providers/digest/yoga-pain.

Yuhas, Daisy. "Forget Pills and Surgery for Back Pain." *Scientific American*, 1 Oct. 2017, www.scientificamerican.com/article/forget-pills-and-surgery-for-back-pain/.

Death and Dying

■ Coping with a terminal illness

CATEGORY: Therapy or Technique; Psychological

KEY TERMS
- *death anxiety:* also known as thanatophobia, a form of anxiety characterized by a fear of one's own death or the process of dying
- *hospice:* care designed to give supportive care to people in the final phase of a terminal illness and focus on comfort and quality of life, rather than cure
- *palliative care:* a specialized medical care that focuses on providing patients relief from pain and other symptoms of a serious illness, no matter the diagnosis or stage of disease
- *thanatology:* the scientific study of death and the practices associated with it, including the study of the needs of the terminally ill and their families

Introduction

A terminal illness cannot be cured and, therefore, is recognized by the person dying as a catastrophic threat to the self, to the individual's relationships, and to the body. In terms of the model of coping proposed by Richard Lazarus and Susan Folkman, death is the perceived threat or stressor causing stress and is evaluated by primary appraisal; the response or coping strategy depends on the person's secondary appraisal of available physical, psychological, social, and spiritual resources. The relationship between the perception of threat and the coping response is dynamic in that it changes over time. For example, the threat of death varies with physical or psychological deterioration and calls for changing strategies during the period of dying.

Anxiety and fear are typical of any crisis; however, when faced with the overwhelming crisis that death poses, a dying person is flooded with death anxiety or mortal fear of dying. Two classic views of death anxiety are Freudian and existential. Sigmund Freud believed that it was impossible to imagine one's own death and that "death anxiety" is really fear of something else, whereas the existentialists believe that awareness of mortality is a basic condition of human existence and is the source of death anxiety. In 1996, Adrian Tomer and Grafton Eliason offered a contemporary "regrets" model, where death anxiety is a function of how much one regrets not having accomplished what one had hoped to accomplish in light of the time left. A major criticism of their work is that achievement takes precedence over social relationships and other sources of meaning. In 2000, Robert J. Kastenbaum proposed an edge theory, where the response to extreme danger is distinct from the ordinary awareness of mortality. He suggested that death anxiety is the consequence of a heightened awareness of potential disaster at the edge of what is otherwise known to be relatively safe.

Thanatology, the study of death and dying, focuses on the needs of the terminally ill and their survivors. Some thanatologists distinguish between fear of the process of dying and fear of the unknown at death. For example, the Collett-Lester Scale, established in 1994, operationalizes these ideas by offering four subscales: death of self, death of others, dying of self, and dying of others. A major problem with studies of death anxiety is that researchers typically employ self-report questionnaires that measure conscious attitudes. In general, the construct validity of questionnaires is reduced when anxiety is confounded with unconscious denial or when death is confounded with dying.

Hospice and Palliative Care

From the beginning of the twentieth century until the 1970s, Americans with terminal illnesses usually died in hospitals. Medical treatment focused on pathology; control of pain with narcotics was limited, as most physicians were worried about consequent drug addiction. Efforts to save lives were machine-intensive and often painful. The psychological, social, and spiritual needs of the person were not as important as the heroic effort to preserve life at any cost. When Dame Cicely Saunders,

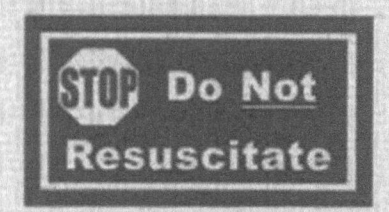

Durable Do Not Resuscitate Order

VIRGINIA DEPARTMENT OF HEALTH

Patient's Full Legal Name _____ Date _____

Physician's Order

I, the undersigned, state that I have a bona fide physician/patient relationship with the patient named above. I have certified in the patient's medical record that he/she or a person authorized to consent on the patient's behalf has directed that life-prolonging procedures be withheld or withdrawn in the event of cardiac or respiratory arrest.

I further certify [must check 1 or 2]:

☐ 1. The patient is CAPABLE of making an informed decision about providing, withholding or withdrawing a specific medical treatment or course of medical treatment. (Signature of patient is required; **see reverse**.)

☐ 2. The patient is INCAPABLE of making an informed decision about providing, withholding or withdrawing a specific medical treatment or course of medical treatment because he/she is unable to understand the nature, extent or probable consequences of the proposed medical decision, or to make a rational evaluation of the risks and benefits of alternatives to that decision.

If you checked 2 above, check A, B or C below.

☐ A. While capable of making an informed decision, the patient has executed a written advanced directive which directs that life-prolonging procedures be withheld or withdrawn.

☐ B. While capable of making an informed decision, the patient has executed a written advanced directive which appoints a "Person Authorized to Consent on the Patient's Behalf" with authority to direct that life-prolonging procedures be withheld or withdrawn. (Signature of "Person Authorized to Consent on the Patient's Behalf" is required; **see reverse**.)

☐ C. The patient has not executed a written advanced directive (living will or durable power of attorney for health care). (Signature of "Person Authorized to Consent on the Patient's Behalf" is required; **see reverse**.)

I hereby direct any and all qualified health care personnel, commencing on the effective date noted above, to withhold cardiopulmonary resuscitation (cardiac compression, endotracheal intubation and other advanced airway management, artificial ventilation, defibrillation and related procedures) from the patient in the event of the patient's cardiac or respiratory arrest. I further direct such personnel to provide the patient other medical interventions, such as intravenous fluids, oxygen or other therapies deemed necessary to provide comfort care or alleviate pain.

_____ _____ _____
Physician's Printed Name   Physician's Signature   Emergency Phone Number

Sample Virginia Durable Do Not Resuscitate Order. (Commonwealth of Virginia wia Wikimedia Commons)

a British nurse and physician, opened St. Christopher's Hospice in London in 1967, she introduced holistic reforms that treated both the dying person and his or her family and included regular administrations of morphine for the amelioration of pain. It was discovered that control of pain is better when dosing at regular intervals and that the total dosage may be less than if drugs are offered only in response to severe, acute pain. Saunders was a profound inspiration to the international hospice movement, as well as to the new field of palliative medicine. (The goal of palliative care is to relieve pain and symptoms and is different from traditional, curative care.)

Initially, hospices were based in hospitals; however, toward the end of the twentieth century, home-based care became common. A full-service program provides an interdisciplinary team of a physician, social worker, registered nurse, and pastor or counselor; round-the-clock care is available. Furthermore, after death, support services are offered to grieving families. In the United States, the National Hospice Reimbursement Act of 1983 offered financial support for full-service hospice care. A local hospice is an important coping resource for someone who chooses to forgo traditional medical treatment. It offers a means for preserving some control of the environment, as well as for maintaining personal dignity. Most important, a peaceful, pain-free death is possible.

Stages of Dying
About the time that the international hospice movement was gaining momentum, an important book titled *On Death and Dying* (1969) was published in America by the psychiatrist Elisabeth Kübler-Ross. She presented transcripts of interviews with dying patients who were struggling with common end-of-life concerns. What gripped American readers was her call for the treatment of dying people as human beings and her compelling, intellectual analysis of dying as a sequence of five stages: denial and isolation, anger, bargaining, depression, and acceptance. However, according to Robert J. Kastenbaum, there is no real empirical verification of her stage theory. Specifically, dying need not involve all stages and may not proceed in the sequence described by Kübler-Ross. Therapists point out that depression and anxiety are ever present but change in intensity—sometimes manageable, sometimes overwhelming. Although theoreticians argue about the scientific status of Kübler-Ross's stage theory, clinicians use her ideas to tailor therapeutic regimens depending on the current needs of their patients. One way to evaluate current status is in terms of how the patient is coping with various threats and challenges posed by dying.

The "stages" of dying may be thought of as emotion-focused coping behaviors for responding to death, a stressor that cannot be changed. In contrast, problem-focused coping behaviors are appropriate when an aspect of the stressor can be changed. When a dying mother is too weak to care for a child, she copes with the problem of her weakness by arranging for child care. When a husband is worried about the financial security of his wife, he draws up a will.

Denial is usually the first response to the shocking news of terminal illness. Denial of one's impending death is a way of coping with the threat of losing one's self and key relationships. The loss of one's self is characterized by the loss of what one values as personally defining. For example, death implies the ultimate loss of strength or of the capacity for meaningful work and ushers in a radical, unwanted change of self-concept. However, denial allows an acceptance of the facts at a slower, more manageable rate and is a way to cope emotionally with death anxiety.

Anger is a common venting response once denial is no longer consuming. (Other venting strategies include crying, yelling, sarcasm, and recklessness.) The private or public expression of anger is evidence that the person has moved beyond complete denial toward the recognition of death as a real threat.

Bargaining with fate or some higher power is a futile but common coping strategy, whereby the person tries desperately to restore body integrity and self-concept. The efforts are sometimes heroic, as when a person has accepted that he or she is dying but tries to maintain some version of prior meaningful activities. The scope is limited and the places may change, but relationships and activities critical to self-concept continue for as long as possible.

Depression is marked by sorrow, grief for current and future losses, and diminished pleasure. It is different from the anxiety that arises when a person fears that what is necessary for an intact self is jeopardized; in contrast, depression occurs when the dying person is certain that he or she has lost what is necessary. Depression is the most common psychological problem in palliative-care settings. However, when ordinary depression becomes major, the treatable condition is often unrecognized and patients suffer needless emotional pain. Minor depression, an expected coping behavior, may be adaptive, whereas major depression is maladaptive and requires medical intervention.

Acceptance of a terminal condition is viewed by many clinicians as a desired end-state because the possibility of a peaceful death comes with acceptance. The person has not given up emotionally but has reached a point of choosing not to struggle for survival. Therapists of various kinds interpret acceptance in the light of a particular worldview or theoretical paradigm. For example, the transpersonal counselor sees acceptance as evidence of an intrapsychic transformation of the self to a higher level of consciousness.

Other Coping Strategies

Dying presents many threats and challenges, including psychological and spiritual distress, pain, exhaustion, loss of independence, loss of dignity, and abandonment. In addition to depression and anxiety, guilt is a response to believing that one must have been a bad person to deserve such a fate or that one risked one's health in a way that brought on the illness. Sometimes people feel guilty because of anger and sarcasm vented on hapless family members, friends, helpers, or a higher power. Thoughts of suicide may occur when depression is severe enough or if the pain is intolerable. Not all people suffer all these assaults, but each requires a strategy for coping.

It is not uncommon for friends and relatives to pull away from the dying person because of their own anxiety and discomfort. Witnessing the physical and emotional distress of a valued person poses a threat to successful, day-to-day management of mortal fears; one way to cope is by ignoring the dying. Unfortunately, physical or emotional distancing causes dreadful isolation and a sense of abandonment just when social support is most critically needed. The terminally ill in such a predicament may cope by turning to a pastoral counselor, therapist, self-help group, or local hospice.

Each type of therapist has a different focus. A psychoanalyst might encourage frank discussions of fears and anxieties. A cognitive behavioral therapist might focus on changing maladaptive behavior by modifying negative thought patterns. A humanistic-existentialist might encourage a life review to help consolidate the patient's perceptions of the meaning of life and as a way to say "good-bye." A transpersonal counselor might focus on facilitating a meaningful transformation of self in preparation for death. A primary goal of therapy of any kind with dying patients is to promote physical and psychological comfort. Often, the therapist is an advocate acting as a liaison between the patient and the hospice, hospital, family, or friends. The therapist may provide helpful psychoeducational interventions, such as alleviating distress about an upcoming medical procedure by informing the patient about the rationale for the procedure, the steps involved, the predictable side effects, and the prognosis or forecast for the outcome. When the therapist also educates the family, the quality of their support is enhanced, thereby improving the well-being of the patient.

Self-Help Groups

Self-help groups provide significant mutual support to the terminally ill and to those in mourning. They are available in professional and nonprofessional settings. They are usually composed of peers who are in a similar plight and who, therefore, are familiar with the depression, anxiety, and guilt associated with dying. Access to a new, primary group counteracts common feelings of alienation and victimization by offering the opportunity for meaningful social support and information. Mutual disclosure reduces feelings of isolation and abandonment by building a community of peers. Sharing successful strategies for coping with secondary losses triggered by terminal illness restores hope. (For example, group members may know how to cope with the disfigurement of mastectomy or with confinement to a wheelchair.) Group participants also encourage one another to be active partners in their own medical care. Unreliable patterns of communication and reluctance to talk about dying are common outside the group; however, group members talk to one another openly, thereby reducing the dismay associated with patronizing exchanges with doctors and nurses or the silence of family and friends.

—*Tanja Bekhuis*

Resources

Choi, Jin Young, et al. "Factors That Affect Quality of Dying and Death in Terminal Cancer Patients on Inpatient Palliative Care Units: Perspectives of Bereaved Family Caregivers." *Journal of Pain and Symptom Management*, vol. 45, no. 4, 2013, pp. 735–745., doi:10.1016/j.jpainsymman.2012.04.010.

Iverach, Lisa, et al. "Death Anxiety and Its Role in Psychopathology: Reviewing the Status of a Transdiagnostic Construct." *Clinical Psychology Review*, vol. 34, no. 7, 2014, pp. 580–593., doi:10.1016/j.cpr.2014.09.002.

Kastenbaum, Robert J. *Death, Society, and Human Experience*. 11th ed. Pearson, 2014.

Kessler, David. *The Needs of the Dying: A Guide for Bringing Hope, Comfort, and Love to Life's Final Chapter*. New York: Harper, 2007.

Kübler-Ross, Elisabeth. *On Death and Dying*. Reprint ed. Routledge, 2009.

Kyota, Ayumi, and Kiyoko Kanda. "How to Come to Terms with Facing Death: a Qualitative Study Examining the Experiences of Patients with Terminal Cancer." *BMC Palliative Care*, vol. 18, no. 1, 4 Apr. 2019, doi:10.1186/s12904-019-0417-6.

Menzies, Rachel E., et al. "The Effects of Psychosocial Interventions on Death Anxiety: A Meta-Analysis and Systematic Review of Randomised Controlled Trials." *Journal of Anxiety Disorders*, vol. 59, 2018, pp. 64–73., doi:10.1016/j.janxdis.2018.09.004.

Miller, Glen E. *Living Thoughtfully, Dying Well: A Doctor Explains How to Make Death a Natural Part of Life*. Herald, 2014.

■ Euthanasia

CATEGORY: Procedure

KEY TERMS

- *active euthanasia*: administration of a drug or some other means that directly causes death; the motivation is to relieve patient suffering
- *durable power of attorney*: designation of a person who will have legal authority to make health care decisions if the patient becomes incapable of making decisions for himself or herself
- *living will*: a legal document in which the patient states a preference regarding life-prolonging treatment in the event that he or she cannot choose
- *nonvoluntary euthanasia*: a decision to terminate life made by another when the patient is incapable of making a decision for himself or herself
- *passive euthanasia*: ending life by refusing or withdrawing life-sustaining medical treatment
- *voluntary euthanasia*: a patient's consent to a decision which results in the shortening of his or her life

The Controversy Surrounding Euthanasia

In the past, the role of the doctor was clear: The physician should minimize suffering and save lives whenever possible. In the present, it is possible for these two goals to be at odds. Saving lives in some situations seems to prolong the misery of the patient. In other cases, procedures or treatments may only marginally postpone the time of death. Advances in medical technology enable many to live who would have died just a few years ago, and massive amounts of money are spent each year on medical research with the goal of prolonging life. Experts in US population trends indicate that by the year 2030, those over the age of sixty-five will comprise about 20 percent of the country's total population. These people will probably be healthy and alert well into their eighties; however, in the last years of their lives they will probably require significant medical care, putting financial stress on the health care system.

The complex issues surrounding death, suffering, and economics create demands for answers to difficult ethical questions. Does all life have value? Should one fight against death even when suffering is intense? Should suffering be lessened if the time of death is brought nearer? Should a patient be given the right to refuse medical treatment if the result is death? Should others be allowed to make this decision for the patient? Should other factors such as the financial or emotional burden on the family be part of the decision-making process? Once a decision has been made to terminate suffering by death, is there any ethical difference between discontinuing medical treatment and giving a lethal dosage of painkilling medication? Should laws be put into place that offer guidelines in these situations, or should each case be decided

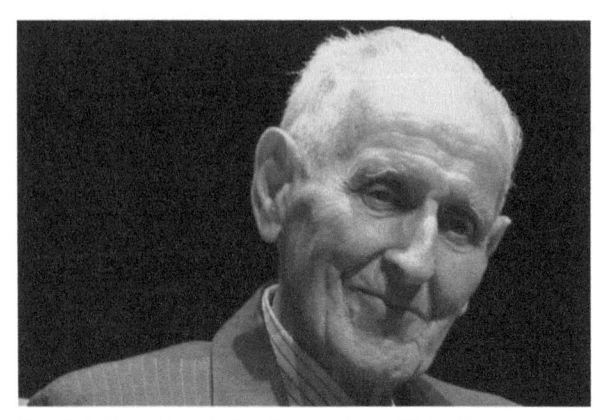

Dr. Jack Kevorkian is best known for publicly championing a terminal patient's right to die by physician-assisted suicide, embodied in his quote "Dying is not a crime". (Gevorg Gevorgyan via Wikimedia Commons)

on an individual basis? And who should decide? There is a wide range of opinion and much uncertainty involving euthanasia and what constitutes a "good" death.

Euthanasia comes from a Greek word that can be translated as "good death" and is defined in several ways, depending on the philosophical stance of the one giving the definition. Tom Beauchamp, in his book *Health and Human Values* (1983), defines euthanasia as putting to death or failing to prevent death in cases of terminal illness or injury; the motive is to relieve comatoseness, physical suffering, anxiety or a serious sense of burdensomeness to self and others. In euthanasia at least one other person causes or helps to cause the death of one who desires death or, in the case of an incompetent person, makes a substituted decision, either to cause death directly or to withdraw something that sustains life.

Most patients who express a wish to die more quickly are terminally ill; however, euthanasia is sometimes considered as a solution for nonterminal patients as well. An example of the latter would be seriously deformed or retarded infants whose futures are judged to have a poor "quality of life" and who would be a serious burden on their families and society.

When discussing the ethical implications of euthanasia, the types of cases have been divided into various classes. A distinction is made between voluntary and nonvoluntary euthanasia. In voluntary euthanasia, the patient consents to a specific course of medical action in which death is hastened. Nonvoluntary euthanasia would occur in cases in which the patient is not able to make decisions about his or her death because of an inability to communicate or a lack of mental facility. Each of these classes has advocates and antagonists. Some believe that voluntary euthanasia should always be allowed, but others would limit voluntary euthanasia to only those patients who have a terminal illness. Some, although agreeing in principle that voluntary euthanasia in terminal situations is ethically permissible, nevertheless oppose euthanasia of any type because of the possibility of abuses. With nonvoluntary euthanasia, the main ethical issues deal with when such an action should be performed and who should make the decision. If a person is in an irreversible coma, most agree that that person's physical life could be ended; however, arguments based on "quality of life" can easily become widened to include persons with physical or mental disabilities. Infants with severe deformities can sometimes be saved but not fully cured with medical technology, and some individuals would advocate nonvoluntary euthanasia in these cases because of the suffering of the infants' caregivers. Some believe that family members or those who stand to gain from the decision should not be allowed to make the decision. Others point out that the family is the most likely to know what the wishes of the patient would have been. Most believe that the medical care personnel, although knowledgeable, should not have the power to decide, and many are reluctant to institute rigid laws. The possibility of misappropriated self-interest from each of these parties magnifies the difficulty of arriving at well-defined criteria.

The second type of classification is between passive and active euthanasia. Passive euthanasia occurs when sustaining medical treatment is refused or withdrawn and death is allowed to take its course. Active euthanasia involves the administration of a drug or some other means that directly causes death. Once again, there are many opinions surrounding these two types. One position is that there is no difference between active and passive euthanasia because in each the end is premeditated death with the motive of prevention of suffering. In fact, some argue that active euthanasia is more compassionate than letting death occur naturally, which may involve suffering. In opposition, others believe that there is a fundamental difference between active and passive euthanasia. A person may have the right to die, but not the right to be killed. Passive euthanasia, they argue, is merely allowing a death that is inevitable to occur. Active euthanasia, if voluntary, is equated with suicide because a human being seizes control of death; if nonvoluntary, it is considered murder.

Passive euthanasia, although generally more publicly acceptable than active euthanasia, has become a topic of controversy as the types of medical treatment that can be withdrawn are debated. A distinction is sometimes made between ordinary and extraordinary means. Defining these terms is difficult, since what may be extraordinary for one patient is not for another, depending on other medical conditions that the patient may have. In addition, what is considered an extraordinary technique today may be judged ordinary in the future. Another way to assess whether passive euthanasia should be allowed in a particular situation is to weigh the benefits against the burdens for the patient. Although most agree that there are cases in which high-tech equipment such as respirators can be withdrawn, there is a question about whether administration of food and water should ever be discontinued. Here the line between passive and active euthanasia is blurred.

Religious and Legal Implications
Decisions about death concern everyone because everyone will die. Eventually, each individual will be the patient who is making the decisions or for whom the decisions are being made. In the meantime, one may be called upon to make decisions for others. Even those not directly involved in the hard cases are affected, as taxpayers and subscribers to medical insurance, by the decisions made on the behalf of others. In a difficult moral issue such as this, individuals look to different institutions for guidelines. Two sources of guidance are the church and the law.

In 1971, the Roman Catholic Church issued *Ethical and Religious Directives for Catholic Health Facilities*. Included in this directive is the statement that

> [I]t is not euthanasia to give a dying person sedatives and analgesics for alleviation of pain, when such a measure is judged necessary, even though they may deprive the patient of the use of reason or shorten his life.

This thinking was reaffirmed by a 1980 statement from the Vatican that considers suffering and expense for the family legitimate reasons to withdraw medical treatment when death is imminent.

Bishops from The Netherlands, in a letter to a government commission, state that

> [B]odily deterioration alone does not have to be unworthy of a man. History shows how many people, beaten, tortured and broken in body, sometimes even grew in personality in spite of it. Dying becomes unworthy of a man, if family and friends begin to look upon the dying person as a burden, withdraw themselves from him....

When speaking of passive euthanasia, the bishops state, "We see no reason to call this euthanasia. Such a person after all dies of his own illness. His death is neither intended nor caused, only nothing is done anymore to postpone it." Christians from Protestant churches may reflect a wider spectrum of positions. Joseph Fletcher, an Episcopal priest, defines a person as one having the ability to think and reason. If a patient does not meet these criteria, according to Fletcher, his or her life may be ended out of compassion for the person he or she once was. The United Church of Christ illustrates this view in its policy statement:

> When illness takes away those abilities we associate with full personhood...we may well feel that the mere continuance of the body by machine or drugs is a violation of their person.... We do not believe simply the continuance of mere physical existence is either morally defensible or socially desirable or is God's will.

These varied positions generally are derived from differing emphases on two truths concerning the nature of God and the role of suffering in the life of the believer. First is the belief that God is the giver of life and that human beings should not usurp God's authority in matters of life and death. Second, alleviation of suffering is of critical importance to God, since it is not loving one's neighbor to allow him or her to suffer. Those who give more weight to the first statement believe as well that God's will allows for suffering and that the suffering can be used for a good purpose in the life of the believer. Those who emphasize the second principle insist that a loving God would not prolong the suffering of people needlessly and that one should not desperately fight to prolong a life which God has willed to die.

C. Everett Koop, former surgeon general of the United States, differentiates between the positive role of a physician in providing a patient "all the life to which he or she is entitled" and the negative role of "prolonging the act of dying." Koop has opposed euthanasia in any form, cautioning against the possibility of sliding down a slippery slope toward making choices about death that reflect the caregivers' "quality of life" more than the patient's.

Jack Kevorkian, a Michigan physician, became the best-known advocate of assisted suicide in the United States. From 1990 to 1997, Kevorkian assisted at least sixty-six people in terminating their lives. According to Kevorkian's lawyer, many other assisted suicides have not been publicized. Kevorkian believes that physician-assisted suicide is a matter of individual choice and should be seen as a rational way to end tremendous pain and suffering. Most of the patients assisted by him spent many years suffering from extremely painful and debilitating diseases, such as multiple sclerosis, bone cancer, and brain cancer.

The American Medical Association (AMA) has criticized this view, calling it a violation of professional ethics. When faced with pain and suffering, the AMA asserts that it is a doctor's responsibility to provide adequate "comfort" care, not death. In the AMA's view, Kevorkian served as "a reckless instrument of death." Three trials in Michigan for assisting in suicide resulted in acquittals for Kevorkian before another trial delivered a guilty verdict on the charge of second-degree murder in March, 1999.

During the course of reevaluating the issues involved in terminating a life, the law has been in a state of flux. The decisions that are made by the courts act on the legal precedents of an individual's right to determine what is done to his or her own body and society's position against suicide. The balancing of these two premises has been handled legally by allowing refusal of treatment (passive euthanasia) but disallowing the use of poison or some other method that would cause death (active euthanasia). The latter is labeled "suicide," and anyone who assists in such an act can be found guilty of assisting a suicide, or of murder. Following the Karen Ann Quinlan case in 1976, in which the family of a comatose woman secured permission to withdraw life-sustaining treatment, the courts routinely allowed family members to make decisions regarding life-sustaining treatment if the patient could not do so. The area of greatest legal controversy involves the withdrawal of food and water. Some courts have charged doctors with murder for the withdrawal of basic life support measures such as food and water. Others have ruled that invasive procedures to provide food and water (intravenously, for example) are similar to other medical procedures and may be discontinued if the benefit to the patient's quality of life is negligible.

In 1994, 51 percent of the voters in Oregon passed the world's first "death with dignity" law. It allowed physician-assisted suicide. Doctors could begin prescribing fatal overdoses of drugs to terminally ill patients. The vote was reaffirmed in 1997 by 60 percent of the state's voters, despite opposition from the Catholic Church, the AMA, and various anti-abortion and right-to-life groups. The Ninth United States Circuit Court of Appeals in San Francisco then lifted a lower court order blocking implementation of the law. Doctors in Oregon became free to prescribe fatal doses of barbiturates to patients with less than six months to live. Physicians were required to file forms with the Oregon Health Division before prescribing the overdose. Then, there would be a fifteen-day waiting period between the request for suicide assistance and the approval of the prescription. Opponents of the Oregon law charged that it perverted the practice of medicine and forced many suffering people to "choose" an early death to save themselves from expensive medical care or pain that could be manageable if physicians were aware of new methods of pain control. The National Right to Life Committee indicated that it would continue to fight implementation of the law in federal courts.

Since 1999, several states, including Hawaii, Connecticut, New Hampshire, Massachusetts, and Kansas, have witnessed attempts to legalize physician-assisted suicide, but the cases have either been withdrawn or defeated by voters or in state legislature. In November 2008, Washington state passed its own death with dignity act by voter initiative, with 57.8 percent of votes cast in favor of the law. In May 2013, Vermont governor Peter Shumlin signed into law the Patient Choice and Control at End of Life Act, thereby legalizing physician-assisted suicide in the state.

Although the laws vary from state to state, most states allow residents to make their wishes known regarding terminal health care either by writing a living will or by choosing a durable power of attorney. A living will is a document in which one can state that some medical treatments should not be used in the event that one becomes incapacitated to the point where one cannot choose. Living wills allow the patient to decide in advance and protect health care providers from lawsuits. Which treatment options can be terminated and when this action can be put into effect may be limited in some states. Most states have a specific format that should be followed when drawing up a living will and require that the document be signed in the presence of two witnesses. Often, qualifying additions can be made by the individual that specify whether food and water may be withdrawn and whether the living will should go into effect only when death is imminent or also when a person has an incurable illness but death is not imminent. A copy of the living will should be given to the patient's physician and become a part of the patient's medical records. The preparation or execution of a living will cannot affect a person's life insurance coverage or the payment of benefits. Since the medical circumstances of one's life may change and a person's ethical stance may also change, a patient may change the living will at any time by signing a written statement.

A second way in which a person can control what kind of decisions will be made regarding his or her death is to choose a decision maker in advance. This person assumes a durable power of attorney and is legally allowed to act on the patient's behalf, making medical treatment decisions. One advantage of a durable power of attorney over a living will is that the patient can choose someone who shares similar ethical and religious values. Since it is difficult to foresee every medical situation that could arise, there is more security with a durable power of attorney in knowing that the person will have similar values and will therefore probably make the same judgments as the patient. Usually a primary agent and a secondary agent are designated in the event that the primary agent is unavailable. This is especially important if the primary agent is a spouse or a close relative who could, for example, be involved in an accident at the same time as the patient.

Perspective and Prospects
Although large numbers of court decision, articles, and books suggest that the issues involved in euthanasia are recent products of medical technology, these questions are not new. Euthanasia was widely practiced in Western classical culture.

The Greeks did not believe that all humans had the right to live, and in Athens, infants with disabilities were often killed. Although in general they did not condone suicide, Pythagoras, Plato, and Aristotle believed that a person could choose to die earlier in the face of an incurable disease and that others could help that person to die. Seneca, the Roman Stoic philosopher, was an avid proponent of euthanasia, stating that

> Against all the injuries of life, I have the refuge of death. If I can choose between a death of torture and one that is simple and easy, why should I not select the latter? As I choose the ship in which I sail and the house which I shall inhabit, so I will choose the death by which I leave life.

The famous Hippocratic oath for physicians acted in opposition to the prevailing cultural bias in favor of euthanasia. Contained in this oath is the statement, "I will never give a deadly drug to anybody if asked for it...or make a suggestion to this effect." The AMA has reaffirmed this position in a policy statement:

> the intentional termination of the life of one human being by another-"mercy killing"-is contrary to that for which the medical profession stands and is contrary to the policy of the American Medical Association.

The great English poet John Donne, in his *Devotions Upon Emergent Occasions*, wrote extensively on the concept of suffering in the severely ill. He wrote, "Affliction is a treasure, and scarce any man hath enough of it." In addition, Jewish and Christian theology have traditionally opposed any form of euthanasia or suicide, avowing that since God is the author of life and death, life is sacred. Therefore, a man would rebel against God if he prematurely shortens his life, because he violates the Sixth Commandment: "Thou shalt not kill." Suffering was viewed not as an evil to be avoided but as a condition to be accepted. The apostle Paul served as an example for early Christians. In 2 Corinthians, he prayed for physical healing, yet when it did not come, he accepted his weakness as a way to increase his dependence on God. This position was affirmed by Saint Augustine in his work *De Civitate Dei* (413-426; *The City of God*) when he condemned suicide as a "detestable and damnable wickedness" that was worse than murder because it left no room for repentance. These strong indictments from the Church against suicide and euthanasia were largely responsible for changing the Greco-Roman attitudes toward the value of human life. They were accepted as society's position until the advent of technologies in the late twentieth century that made it possible to extend life beyond what would have been the point of death.

Although these issues have been debated by physicians and philosophers for centuries, there remains a heightened need for thoughtful discussion and resolution. The majority of nations, as well as major medical organizations such as the AMA, oppose euthanasia as contrary to the proper role of the physician and society. However, closely related and complex issues such as the treatment of pain in the terminally ill leave much room for development in human understanding.

—*Katherine B. Frederich, Ph.D.*
—*Leslie V. Tischauser, Ph.D.*

Resources

Brazier, Yvette. "Euthanasia and Assisted Suicide: What Are They and What Do They Mean?" *Medical News Today*, MediLexicon International, 17 Dec. 2018, www.medicalnewstoday.com/articles/182951.php.

Corr, Charles A., Clyde M. Nabe, and Donna M. Corr. *Death and Dying, Life and Living*. 7th ed. Wadsworth/Cengage Learning, 2013.

Dowbiggin, Ian Robert. *A Merciful End: The Euthanasia Movement in Modern America*. Oxford University Press, 2003.

Erdek, Michael. "Pain Medicine and Palliative Care as an Alternative to Euthanasia in End-of-Life Cancer Care." *The Linacre Quarterly*, vol. 82, no. 2, 2015, pp. 128–134., doi:10.1179/2050854 915y.0000000003.

O'Rourke, Mark A., et al. "Reasons to Reject Physician Assisted Suicide/Physician Aid in Dying." *Journal of Oncology Practice*, vol. 13, no. 10, 2017, pp. 683–686., doi:10.1200/jop.2017.021840.

Rietjens, Judith A. C., et al. "Terminal Sedation and Euthanasia." *Archives of Internal Medicine*, vol. 166, no. 7, 10 Apr. 2006, p. 749., doi:10.1001/archinte.166.7.749.

Rismanchi, Mojtaba. "Chronic Pain and Voluntary Euthanasia." *Journal of Medical Ethics and History of Medicine*, vol. 2, no. 1, 19 Oct. 2008.

Ruijs, Cees Dm, et al. "Unbearable Suffering and Requests for Euthanasia Prospectively Studied in End-of-Life Cancer Patients in Primary Care." *BMC Palliative Care*, vol. 13, no. 1, 2014, doi:10.1186/1472-684x-13-62.

Sulmasy, Lois Snyder, and Paul S. Mueller. "Ethics and the Legalization of Physician-Assisted Suicide: An American College of Physicians Position Paper." *Annals of Internal Medicine*, vol. 167, no. 8, 2017, p. 576., doi:10.7326/m17-0938.

Tsu, Peter Shiu Hwa. "Pain Control and Euthanasia." *Journal of Palliative Care & Medicine*, vol. 02, no. 01, 2012, doi:10.4172/2165-7386.1000e109.

■ Hospice

CATEGORY: Therapy or Technique

Overview

Hospice is a philosophy of care directed toward persons who are dying. Hospice care uses a family-oriented holistic approach to assist these individuals in making the transition from life to death in a manner that preserves their dignity and comfort. This approach, as Elisabeth Kubler-Ross would say, allows dying patients "to live until they die." Hospice care encourages patients to participate fully in determining the type of care that is most appropriate for their comfort. By creating a secure and caring community sensitive to the needs of the dying and their families and by providing care that relieves patients of the distressing symptoms of their disease, hospice care can aid the dying in preparing mentally as well as spiritually for their impending death.

Unlike traditional health care where the patient is viewed as the client, hospice care with its holistic emphasis, treats the family unit as the client. There are usually specific areas of stress for the families of the dying. In addition to the stress of caring for the physical needs of the dying, family members often feel tremendous pressure maintaining their own roles and responsibilities within the family itself. The conflict of caring for their own nuclear families while caring for dying relatives places a huge strain on everyone involved and can be a source of anxiety and guilt for the patient as well. Another area of stress experienced by family members involves concern for themselves; that is, having to put their own lives on hold, not getting physically run down, dealing with their newly acquired time constraints, and viewing themselves as isolated from friends and family. Compounding this is the guilt that many caregivers feel over not caring for the dying relative as well or as patiently as they might, or secretly wishing for the caregiving experience to reach an end.

Due to the holistic nature of the care provided, the hospice team is actually an interdisciplinary team composed of physicians, nurses, psychologists and social workers, pastoral counselors, and trained volunteers. This medically supervised team meets weekly to decide on how best to provide physical, emotional, and spiritual support for dying patients and to assist the surviving family members in the subsequent grieving process.

This type of care can be administered in three different ways. It can be home health-agency based, delivered in the patient's own home. It can be dispensed in an institution devoted solely to hospice care. It can even be administered in traditional medical facilities (such as hospitals) that allot a certain amount of space (perhaps a wing or floor, or even a certain number of beds) to this type of care. Hospice care is designed for any patient at the end stage of life. Often, people think Hospice care is just for cancer but can be for any patient facing death from any terminal disease. Heart disease, lung disease, and amyotrophic lateral sclerosis (ALS or Lou Gehrig's Disease) are others that may involve Hospice care at end of life. Hospice is available for both adults and children. A newer approach to care for patients experiencing a life-limiting condition requiring ongoing medical care or a terminal disease is palliative care. Palliative care begins much earlier in the disease process and is designed to manage the problems and issues that impair quality of life and to assist the patient to a compassionate death. Palliative care occurs much in advance of the need for Hospice care.

Principles

Hospice care uses a team-oriented approach to provide quality, compassionate care individualized to the patient and family's needs. Hospice care focuses on managing a patient's symptoms, including pain. The principles of hospice care focus on alleviating the anxieties and physical suffering that can be associated with the dying process and to insure that the patient and family can make the most of the time that remains. The goal is to not delay the dying process by using invasive medical techniques or heroic efforts. Hospice care is also based on the assertion that dying patients have certain rights that must be respected. These rights include a right to absent themselves from social responsibilities and commitments, a right to be cared for, and the right to continued respect and status. The following seven principles are basic components of hospice care.

Hospice care provides highly personalized and holistic care of the dying, which includes treating dying patients emotionally and spiritually as well as physically. This interpersonal support, known as bonding, helps patients in their final days to live as fully and as comfortably as possible, while retaining their dignity, autonomy, and individual self-worth in a safe and secure environment. This one-on-one attention involves therapeutic communication. Knowing that someone has heard, that someone understands and is concerned can be profoundly healing.

Pain management is a critical component of Hospice care. Hospice care advocates the use of narcotics at a dosage that will alleviate suffering while still enabling patients to maintain a desired level of alertness. Efforts are made to employ the least invasive routes to administer these drugs (usually orally, if possible). In addition, pain medication is administered before the pain begins, thus alleviating the anxiety of patients waiting for pain to return. Since it has been shown that fear of pain often increases the pain itself, this type of aggressive pain management gives dying patients more time and energy to respond to family members and friends and to work through the emotional and spiritual stages of dying. Use of pain medication before the pain actually occurs has historically been a controversial element in hospice care, with some critics charging that the dying are being turned into drug addicts. Given the fact that patients are not admitted into Hospice care until death is inevitable, addiction is not a factor. Hospice care generally starts no sooner than six months before predicted death. With the advent of Palliative care, entry into Hospice care is occurring later. Maintaining the comfort of the dying patient is crucial.

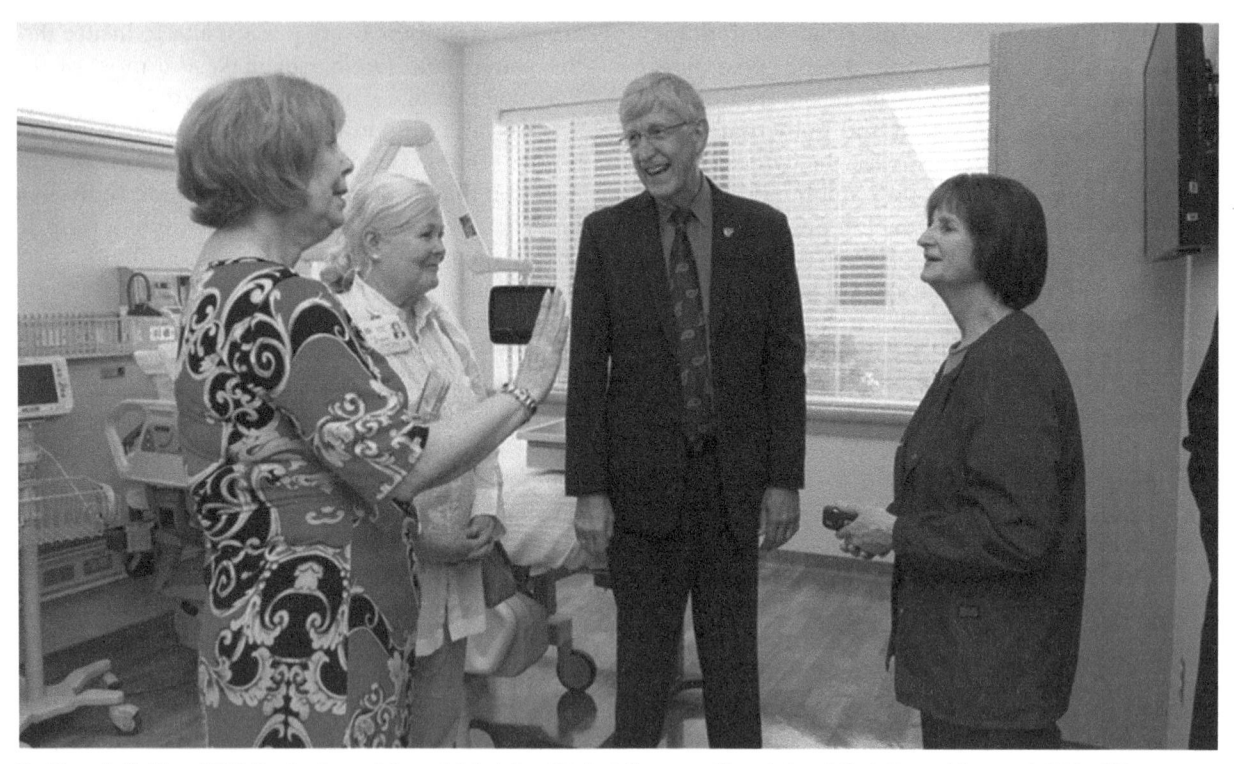

Dr. Francis Collins, NIH director (second from right), joins Clinical Center staff, and Ann Mitchell, president and CEO of Montgomery Hospice, at the opening ceremony of the Building 10 Hospice Suites. Before opening the suites, Clinical Center leaders visited local hospices, including Montgomery Hospice, to learn about their services. (National Institutes of Health)

The participation of families in caring for the dying is a cornerstone of Hospice care. Family members are trained by Hospice nurses to care for the dying patients and dispense pain medication. The aim is to prevent the patients from suffering isolation or feeling as if they are surrounded by strangers. Participation in care also helps to sustain the patients' and the families' sense of autonomy. For patients without family support, there is an increasing attention to inpatient Hospice care in either a stand-alone facility or as part of a hospital or nursing home.

Maintaining the familiarity of surroundings is a comfort measure important to the dying patient. Whenever possible, it is the goal of hospice care to keep dying patients at home. This eliminates the necessity of the dying to spend their final days in an institutionalized setting, isolated from family and friends when they need them the most. It is estimated that close to 90 percent of all hospice care days are spent in patients' own homes. When this is not possible and patients must enter institutional settings, rules are relaxed so that their rooms can be decorated or arranged in such a way as to replicate the patients' home surroundings. Visiting rules are suspended when possible, and visits by family members, children, and pets are encouraged.

Emotional and spiritual support for the family caregivers is important to better provide for the patient. Hospice volunteers are specially trained to use listening and communicative techniques with family members and to provide them with emotional support both during and after the patient's death. Because the care is holistic, the caregivers' physical needs are attended to (for example, respite is provided for exhausted caregivers), as are the caregivers' emotional and spiritual needs. This spiritual support applies to people of all faith backgrounds. In attending to the spiritual dimension, the hospice team is respectful of all religious traditions while realizing that death and bereavement have the ability to both strengthen and weaken faith. For patients and families without a professed faith, support is provided based on their needs and wants and may focus more on counseling. Support groups are often available to address the needs of family members, including children and grandchildren of patients.

Hospice services should be available twenty-four hours a day, seven days a week. Because of its reliance on the assistance of trained volunteers, round-the-clock support is available to patients and their families.

The intervention of the Hospice team does not end with the death of the patient. Bereavement counseling is provided for the survivors. At the time of death, the hospice team is available to help families take care of tasks such as planning the funeral and probating the will. In the weeks after the death, hospice volunteers offer their support to surviving family members in dealing with their loss and grief and the various phases of the bereavement process, always aware of the fact that not all bereaved need or want formal interventions. Many Hospice organizations offer support groups for families after the death of the patient. Often, family members want to become Hospice volunteers. While this is noble, many Hospices require a period of time between the death of their family member and undergoing training to become a volunteer as an objective manner is expected of volunteers.

History

The term "hospice" comes from the Latin *hospitia,* meaning "places of welcome." The earliest documented example of hospice care dates to the fourth century, when a Roman woman named Fabiola apparently used her own wealth to care for the sick and dying. In medieval times, the Catholic Church established inns for poor wayfarers and pilgrims traveling to religious shrines in search of miraculous cures for their illnesses. Such "rest homes," usually run by religious orders, provided both lodging and nursing care, since the medieval view was that the sick, dying, and needy were all travelers on a journey. This attitude also reflects the medieval notion that true hospitality included care of the mind and spirit as well as of the body. During the Protestant Reformation, when monasteries were forcibly closed, the concepts of hospice and hospital became distinct. Care of the sick and dying was now considered a public duty rather than a religious or private one, and many former hospices were turned into state-run hospitals.

The first in-patient hospice establishment of modern times (specifically called "hospice") was founded by Mary Aitkenhead and the Irish Sisters of Charity under her leadership in the 1870's in Dublin, Ireland. Cicely Saunders, a physician at St. Joseph's Hospice in London, which was founded by the English Sisters of Charity in 1908, began to adapt the ancient concept of hospice to modern palliative techniques. While there, Saunders became extremely close to a Holocaust survivor who was dying of cancer. She found that she shared his dream of establishing a place that would meet the needs of the dying. Using the money he bequeathed her at his death as a starting point, Saunders raised additional funds and opened St. Christopher's Hospice in Sydenham, outside London, in 1967. Originally it housed only cancer patients, but with the financial support of contracts with the National Health Service in England and private donations, it later expanded to meet the needs of all the dying. In fact, no patient was ever refused because of inability to pay. St. Christopher's served as a model for the hospices to be built later in other parts of the world.

Even though hospice care did not originate with Cicely Saunders, she is usually credited with founding the first modern hospice, since she introduced the concept of dispensing narcotics at regular intervals in order to preempt the pain of the dying. She was also the first to identify the need to address other, nonphysical sources of pain for dying patients.

Two years after St. Christopher's Hospice was opened, Kubler-Ross wrote *On Death and Dying,* which validated the hospice movement by relating stories of the dying and their wishes as to how they would be treated. In 1974, the United States opened its first hospice, Hospice, Inc. (later called the Connecticut Hospice), in New Haven, Connecticut. Within the next twenty-five years, over three thousand hospice programs would be implemented in the United States. In Canada, the first "palliative care" unit (as hospices are referred to in Canada) was opened in 1975 by Dr. Balfour M. Mount at the Royal Victoria Hospital in Montreal. This is considered to be the first hospital-based hospice in North America.

Cost

Because of hospice care's reliance on heavily trained volunteers and contributions, and because death is seen as a natural process that should not be prolonged by invasive and expensive medical techniques, hospice care is much less costly than traditional acute care facilities. Because hospice care is a philosophy of care rather than a specific facility, legislation to provide monetary support for hospice patients took a great deal of time to be approved. In 1982, the U.S. Congress finally added hospice care as a Medicare benefit. In 1986, it was made a permanent benefit. Medicare requires, however, that there be a prognosis of six months or less for the patient to live. Hospice care is also reimbursable by many private insurance companies.

The National Hospice and Palliative Care Organization (NHPCO) (formerly The National Hospice Organization) originated in 1977 in the United States as a resource for the many groups across the country who needed assistance in establishing hospice programs in their own communities. The purpose of this organization is to provide information about hospice care to the public, to establish conduits so that information may be exchanged between Hospice and Palliative Care organizations, and to maintain agreed-upon standards for developing hospices around the country. The NHO publishes *Guide to the Nation's Hospices* on an annual basis.

—*Mara Kelly-Zukowski, Ph.D.*
—*Marisela Fermin-Schon*
—*Patricia Stanfill Edens, RN, PhD, FACHE*

Resources

Lima, Liliana De, and Lukas Radbruch. "The International Association for Hospice and Palliative Care: Advancing Hospice and Palliative Care Worldwide." *Journal of Pain and Symptom Management*, vol. 55, no. 2, 8 Aug. 2017, doi:10.1016/j.jpainsymman.2017.03.023.

Edens, Pat Stanfill, et al. "Developing and Financing a Palliative Care Program." *American Journal of Hospice and Palliative Medicine®*, vol. 25, no. 5, 2008, pp. 379–384., doi:10.1177/1049909108319269.

"Hospice Care." *National Hospice and Palliative Care Organization*, 20 Feb. 2019, www.nhpco.org/about/hospice-care.

Kubler-Ross, Elisabeth. *On Death and Dying*. Macmillan, 1969.

Marrelli, Tina M. *Hospice & Palliative Care Handbook: Quality, Compliance, and Reimbursement*. 3rd ed., Sigma Theta Tau International, 2018.

Moments of Life: Made Possible by Hospice, National Hospice and Palliative Care Organization, moments.nhpco.org/.

Wrenn, Paula, and Jo Gustely. *Dying Well with Hospice: a Compassionate Guide to End of Life Care*. Amans Vitae Press, 2017.

■ Palliative care

CATEGORY: Therapy or Technique
SPECIALTIES AND RELATED FIELDS: Most, especially critical care, internal medicine, geriatrics, oncology, pain medicine, cardiology, pulmonary, hematology, nephrology, psychology, radiology, nursing and ethics

KEY TERMS

- *multidisciplinary care*: a comprehensive care provided by professionals from different disciplines, including doctors, nurses, pharmacists, social workers, and many others
- *hospice*: end-of-life medical care for people who are terminally ill. Similar to palliative care, the focuses are also symptom control, pain management and psychosocial support

Overview

Palliative care is a multidisciplinary medical care approach for people with serious or life-threatening illnesses. These patients often suffer from severe pain, shortness of breath, fatigue, difficulty sleeping, or other distressing physical symptoms. They and their families may also experience stress or even depression while trying to cope with the patients' illnesses. The goal of palliative care is to maximize quality of life through pain management, symptom control as well as psychosocial support. Receiving palliative care does not mean that the patient has to stop the primary curative treatment. Instead, palliative care is like another layer of support on top of the original medical treatment plan. Palliative program not only cares for

Palliative Care versus Hospice		
	Palliative Care	Hospice
Similarities	<td colspan="2"><ul><li>Improve quality of life for people with severe illness</li><li>Pain management, symptom control, psychosocial support</li><li>Patient and family-centered care</li><li>Team approach</li><li>Insurance coverage: Medicare, Medicaid, most private insurance</li></ul></td>	
Differences — Timing	• During any stage of illness, doesn't need to be terminal	• Terminal stage of illness or with limited life expectancy (generally < 6 months, varies by different hospice programs)
Location	• Hospital • Extended care facility • Nursing home • Home	• Extended care facility • Nursing home • Home
Curative or life-prolonging treatment	• Continue	• Usually stopped

the patient, but also his or her family. It designs individualized plan of care taking into consideration the patient and the family's needs, values, beliefs, and goals.

Palliative care should not be confused with hospice, which focuses on end-of-life care and comfort. Patients in hospice programs usually have stopped the curative treatments; instead, emphasis is on pain and symptom relief and how to make the most out of the last days or months of life.

Individuals who may consider palliative care includes anyone who has severe illnesses and suffers from uncontrolled pain or other distressing physical or psychological symptoms. Examples of some devastating diseases include cancer, heart disease, lung disease, kidney failure, Human immunodeficiency virus infection / acquired immunodeficiency syndrome (HIV/AIDS), Lupus, Alzheimer's, and many others. People do not need to wait until the terminal stage of his or her illness to receive palliative care. It can be started during any stage of the illness to enhance quality of life. Applying for palliative care is not difficult. Patients and families with potential needs should talk to their doctors and ask for a referral for palliative care.

Palliative care often starts in the hospital, but can be provided in various nursing facilities, outpatient clinics, hospices, or even at patients' home.

Treatment and Therapy

Palliative care is all about making the life more comfortable and meaningful for the patient and his or her loved ones. It is accomplished using a team approach. A palliative care team consists of professionals from different disciplines, including doctors, nurses, pharmacists, social workers, chaplains, nutritionists, counselors, and others. The team closely works with the patient and the family to assess their needs, values, beliefs, and goals. Patient education and counseling are also provided to help the patient better understand his or her health condition and how to more effectively cope with it. The palliative care team also works collaboratively with patient's primary health care providers to design a comprehensive and individualized treatment plan to maximize physical and emotional comfort.

The length of palliative care depends on the individual's health condition and family goals and needs. The financial aspect of the care is almost always a concern for patients and their families. The good news is that Medicare, Medicaid, and most private insurance covers all or part of palliative treatment. In instances when palliative care is not fully covered by Medicare, Medicaid, or private insurance, there may be funds available within the community or through the state to subsidize the cost.

—Zhongqi Weng

Resources

Bhatnagar, Sushma, and Mayank Gupta. "Integrated Pain and Palliative Medicine Model." *Annals of Palliative Medicine*, vol. 5, no. 3, 2016, pp. 196–208., doi:10.21037/apm.2016.05.02.

Elmokhallalati, Yousuf, et al. "Specialist Palliative Care Support Is Associated with Improved Pain Relief at Home during the Last 3 Months of Life in Patients with Advanced Disease: Analysis of 5-Year Data from the National Survey of Bereaved People (VOICES)." *BMC Medicine*, vol. 17, no. 1, 22 Mar. 2019, doi:10.1186/s12916-019-1287-8.

Goldstein, Leonard, and Scott Falkowitz. "Pain Management in a Palliative Care Setting." *Practical Pain Management*, 20 Dec. 2011, www.practicalpainmanagement.com/resources/hospice/pain-management-palliative-care-setting.

GRONINGER, HUNTER, and JAYA VIJAYAN. "Pharmacologic Management of Pain at the End of Life." *American Family Physician*, vol. 90, no. 1, July 2014, pp. 26–32.

Knaul, Felicia M, et al. "The Lancet Commission on Palliative Care and Pain Relief—Findings, Recommendations, and Future Directions." *The Lancet Global Health*, vol. 6, 1 Mar. 2018, doi:10.1016/s2214-109x(18)30082-2.

Lane, Trevor, et al. "Public Awareness and Perceptions of Palliative and Comfort Care." *The American Journal of Medicine*, vol. 132, no. 2, 2019, pp. 129–131., doi:10.1016/j.amjmed.2018.07.032.

Sholjakova, Marija, et al. "Pain Relief as an Integral Part of the Palliative Care." *Open Access Macedonian Journal of Medical Sciences*, vol. 6, no. 4, 6 Apr. 2018, pp. 739–741., doi:10.3889/oamjms.2018.163.

Wilkie, Diana J., and Miriam O. Ezenwa. "Pain and Symptom Management in Palliative Care and at End of Life." *Nursing Outlook*, vol. 60, no. 6, 2012, pp. 357–364., doi:10.1016/j.outlook.2012.08.002.

■ Palliative medicine

CATEGORY: Therapy or Technique
SPECIALTIES AND RELATED FIELDS: Anesthesiology, emergency medicine, family medicine, internal medicine, obstetrics and gynecology, pediatrics, physical medicine and rehabilitation, psychiatry and neurology, radiology and surgery

Science and Profession

While in the United States, The National Hospice and Palliative Care Organization (NHPCO) defines palliative care as: Treatment that enhances comfort and improves the quality of an individual's life during the last phase of life. No specific therapy is excluded from consideration. The test of palliative care lies in the agreement between the individual, physician(s), primary caregiver, and the hospice team that the expected outcome is relief from distressing symptoms, the easing of pain, and/or enhancing the quality of life. The decision to intervene with active palliative care is based on an ability to meet stated goals rather than affect the underlying disease. An individual's needs must continue to be assessed and all treatment options explored and evaluated in the context of the individual's values and symptoms. The individual's choices and decisions regarding care are paramount and must be followed.

Palliative medicine is a specialty that spans disciplines. The goal is to comfort and support patients as they face life-threatening illnesses, not only relieving their suffering but also addressing their emotional and spiritual needs. Although palliative medicine is typically associated with the final stages of life-threatening conditions, patients may also benefit from specialized care while they are still undergoing active treatment. In that case, symptom relief and other interventions to improve their quality of life help improve their strength and stamina to endure additional cycles of therapy.

Palliative care may be provided in a long-term care facility, a hospital, or the patient's home. Care is provided by a team consisting of primary care physicians, specialists in the patient's condition (for example, oncologists, cardiologists, or pulmonologists), palliative medicine specialist, nurses, social workers, mental health specialists (psychologists, psychiatrists, or counselors), nutritionists, and clergy. The level and type of care provided are guided by the wishes and needs of the patient. Pain management is often the greatest need, but the patient may also require relief of other symptoms associated with the condition or its treatment, such as nausea, vomiting, decreased appetite, inability to eat, dehydration, constipation or diarrhea, shortness of breath, malaise, fatigue, anxiety, depression, and altered consciousness.

Palliative medicine is recognized as a basic human right in the International Bill of Human Rights of the United Nations. The document declares that all people have the right to adequate health and medical care, and further states that patients with chronic and terminal illnesses have the right to avoid pain and die with dignity. Following these principles, Canada decreed that every citizen has the right to palliative care. The European Committee of Ministers and the South African Department of Health declared that palliative care is a right of all citizens. Palliative medicine is formally recognized as a specialty in Australia, France, Germany, Hong Kong, Ireland, New Zealand, Poland, Romania, Slovakia, Taiwan, the United States, and the United Kingdom.

Palliative medicine is an essential component of care for patients suffering from any chronic, life-threatening illness, but the specialty has taken on an added significance in the field of oncology. In the United States, the Institute of Medicine stated in 1997 that any comprehensive cancer care plan should include palliative care. A 2005 resolution of the 58th World Health Assembly to improve cancer care placed palliative medicine on equal footing with surgery, radiation, and medical oncology.

Although recognized as a medical specialty, palliative medicine relies on the unique contributions of numerous disciplines. Education in palliative techniques begins at the undergraduate level and is incorporated into the training of a number of medical specialties, such as oncology and gerontology. Continuing education programs focus on educating health care professionals in quality palliative care techniques. Other projects build on these efforts, using other health care professionals, such as nurse practitioners and physician assistants, to develop quality palliative medicine programs in their institutions.

The American Society for Clinical Oncology (ASCO) actively promotes continuing education in palliative medicine. Palliative care is incorporated into educational materials and programs developed by ASCO. The society published an educational curriculum for continuing medical education on palliative medicine, and it has a study program devoted to supportive care. Palliative medicine is included in the training for internists, as adopted by the American Board of Internal Medicine.

The National Consensus Project for Quality Palliative Care issued guidelines for palliative care to establish continuity of care across institutions. The clinical practice guidelines have been incorporated into the hospital accreditation standards of The Joint Commission (formerly the Joint Commission for the Accreditation of Hospitals). Institutions are assessed on the eight domains of palliative care: structure and process, physical aspects, psychological and psychiatric aspects, spiritual and religious aspects, cultural aspects, care of the imminently dying patient, the ethical aspects of care, and the legal aspects of care. Additionally, the Center for the Advancement of Palliative Care developed the State-by-State Report Card on Access to Palliative Care in Our Nation's Hospitals. The report card measures patient access to palliative care and to palliative medicine specialists, access of medical students to training in palliative care, and access of physicians to specialty training in palliative care. The report card emphasizes the importance of a multidisciplinary approach to palliative medicine.

Diagnostic and Treatment Techniques

Patient care is traditionally disease-oriented. Specialists in particular tend to focus narrowly on a specific organ or body system. Palliative care, however, takes a holistic, patient-centered approach. The emphasis is on communicating with the patient and family to assess the patient's specific needs and desires.

Palliative care can be divided into primary and secondary teams. The primary team, as defined by Medicare, is comprised by four core members (physician, nurse, social worker and spiritual counselor) and is responsible for assessing and managing symptoms, providing expertise regarding psychosocial services as well as communicating with the patient and family while involving the shared decision making model of care If, however, the patient's condition worsens and the primary team can no longer manage the symptoms, a palliative medicine specialist in the patient's condition is called. The palliative medicine specialist may be consulted on specific issues as needed or become a core member until the patient's death.

The whole-patient assessment begins with the patient's description of symptoms and level of function. Diagnostic tests may be used to evaluate symptom severity, but diagnosis is not the purpose. The emphasis is always on symptom relief.

Pain is a significant issue that must be managed properly. Inadequately controlled pain may reduce the effectiveness of treatment and wear the patient down psychologically. Proper pain management involves communication with and education of the patient and family members as well as continuous assessment of the effectiveness of pain medications. The World Health Organization (WHO) has developed an approach to pain for cancer patients, beginning with nonsteroidal anti-inflammatory drugs (NSAIDs), such as ibuprofen, and progressing through acetaminophen combined with an opioid medication, such as acetaminophen with codeine, and lastly to opioid medications such as morphine or oxycodone. The goal is to relieve pain while keeping the patient alert and in control.

The effect of the condition on the emotions and cognitive functioning of the patient is an important aspect of the palliative medicine assessment. Patients are facing serious issues while they battle their illnesses. They must cope with imminent death and the grief of their loved ones along with the fear of loss of control and dignity. Patients must be evaluated for depression and anxiety. Practical needs, such as relationship issues, legal affairs, and financial management, also need attention. The patient's spiritual needs should also be addressed. Spiritual counseling can be traditional religious advisement from a clergyperson or an informal discussion of personal beliefs, according to the desires of the patient.

Depression and anxiety are common among patients coping with life-threatening conditions. Feelings of sadness and depression are to be expected and should be managed appropriately even when they are not expected to be permanent. The members of the primary team who are in closest contact with the patient need to be alert for symptoms of depression that surpass the normal grieving process. Signs of major depression include persistent feelings of worthlessness, hopelessness, helplessness, and loss of self-esteem. Physical symptoms may include weight loss or changes in sleep habits, although these symptoms may also be attributed to the patient's underlying condition. Thoughts of suicide or requests by the patient to hasten death are not part of the coping process and are a sign of major depression. If the signs of depression fail to resolve after a few weeks, then the mental health specialists on the team are consulted and the depression should be treated.

Similarly, anxiety is an understandable and natural emotion as patients juggle financial concerns, family issues, medical concerns, and preparations for their own death. Anxiety may be managed through counseling or, if it is severe, with antianxiety medications.

The role of the palliative care team is not limited to the patient. The team assists family members in accepting the patient's condition, managing financial and insurance matters, and coping with grief. The health care team can advise family members on what to expect as the patient's condition deteriorates. Breathing difficulties, delirium or dementia, wasting, and incontinence can be upsetting for family members to experience if they are not properly prepared. After the patient's death, the palliative care team assists family members through the grieving process. The team follows up with the family through phone calls and home visits, providing grief counseling or referral to caregiver support groups or other mental health professionals when needed. Bereavement services often last for several months to a year after the patient's death.

Perspective and Prospects

In the span of two decades, palliative medicine progressed from haphazard training through chance experiences to a recognized specialty. A 1998 member survey by ASCO revealed 90 percent of the oncologists who responded had no formal training in palliative medicine. Rather, they indicated they learned through "trial and error." Alarmingly, more than one-third claimed that their education in palliative medicine was from a "traumatic experience" with a patient. Most had little training in how to discuss a poor prognosis with patients and their families, and only 10 percent had completed clinical training in palliative care.

Since that survey, ASCO and other professional societies have incorporated palliative medicine into their continuing education curricula. More important, national and international groups have formally recognized the importance of palliative medicine in preserving the dignity and well-being of patients nearing the end of their lives. In recent years, palliative medicine has been incorporated as a routine part of comprehensive cancer care plans in the United States.

Despite these advances, much work remains. The need for palliative medicine is increasing. The population is growing older while the prevalence of cancer is rising. Cancer treatments are becoming more effective. Although cancer death rates are declining, more people are living longer with the disease, resulting in growing numbers of people who will benefit from palliative medicine.

To meet the growing need, health care practitioners must be educated in palliative medicine. Fellowships in palliative medicine (currently 93 in the United States), continuing education, and readily available educational resources are needed now more than ever. Formal certifications and national guidelines and standards of practice have been adopted to ensure consistency in the quality of palliative medicine across states and individual institutions. The concept of palliative medicine continues to be incorporated into care plans across medical disciplines. In 2006 the American Board of Medical Specialties approved the creation of Hospice and Palliative Medicine as a subspecialty to 10 medical disciplines, and after 2013, only those who have completed an accredited fellowship program will be able to be certified and practice this discipline.

Improving end-of-life care requires more than educational and quality control initiatives; it also requires political will. Unless palliative medicine is viewed as a priority by administrators and policy makers, quality care cannot be ensured.

Pain management is an integral piece of palliative medicine. Unfortunately, misconceptions remain among health care practitioners as well as the general public regarding the use of opioid medications. The fear of addiction frequently results in less than optimal pain control and patient suffering. The need for higher doses of pain medications does not indicate addiction; it is more likely a sign the pain is inadequately controlled or the condition is progressing. The United Nations elevated effective pain control to a fundamental human right. In a formal statement, the UN equated inadequate pain control with "cruel, inhuman, and degrading treatment" and called for nations to supply adequate pain medications to patients.

Collectively, the United Nations, individual countries, and medical societies are striving to ensure that all patients suffering from terminal illnesses receive compassionate and comprehensive care. The strength of palliative medicine is in considering the patient as a whole rather than focusing exclusively on a particular diagnosis. Palliative medicine breaks from traditional medical practice and creates a multidisciplinary team to care for the patient. The direction of care is dictated by the wishes of the patient and encompasses physical, emotional, and the spiritual needs of the patient and their families.

—*Cheryl Pokalo Jones*
—*Felix Rivera, M.D.*

Resources

"Alleviating Pain & Symptoms with Palliative Medicine." *JourneyCare*, 30 July 2019, journeycare.org/alleviating-pain-symptoms-palliative-medicine/.

Chang, Victor T., et al. "Pain and Palliative Medicine." *The Journal of Rehabilitation Research and Development*, vol. 44, no. 2, 2007, p. 279., doi:10.1682/jrrd.2006.06.0067.

Fine, Perry G., et al. "Bridging the Gap: Pain Medicine and Palliative Care: Table 1." *Pain Medicine*, vol. 14, no. 9, 2013, pp. 1277–1279., doi:10.1111/pme.12187.

Martin, Laura J., et al. "Palliative Care - Managing Pain." *MedlinePlus*, U.S. National Library of Medicine, 18 Feb. 2018, medlineplus.gov/ency/patientinstructions/000532.htm.

Morrow, Angela. "Pain Management in Palliative Care." *Verywell Health*, 22 July 2016, www.verywellhealth.com/pain-management-in-palliative-care-1132349.

Piotrowski, Monica. "Frequently Asked Questions About Hospice and Palliative Care." *Palliative Doctors*, palliativedoctors.org/faq.

Psychological Pain

■ Antianxiety medications

CATEGORY: Class of Drug
ALSO KNOWN AS: Anxiolytics
ANATOMY OR SYSTEM AFFECTED: Brain, psychic-emotional system
SPECIALTIES AND RELATED FIELDS: Family medicine, forensic medicine, internal medicine, pharmacology, psychiatry

Indications and Procedures

Anxiety disorders are the most common mental health disorders. The fifth edition of the American Psychiatric Association's *Diagnostic and Statistical Manual of Mental Disorders* (2013)-the most widely used reference manual for research, clinical assessment, and insurance purposes in the field of psychiatry-lists several anxiety disorders, including generalized anxiety disorder, panic disorder, social anxiety disorder, separation anxiety disorder, agoraphobia, selective mutism, and specific phobias. Anxiety is also a pronounced symptom of other mental illnesses, such as depression, schizophrenia, avoidant personality disorder, dependent personality disorder, post-traumatic stress disorder, and obsessive-compulsive disorder.

Although the physiological responses (sympathetic nervous system activation) and behavioral tendencies (fight-or-flight reaction) are similar, fear and anxiety differ fundamentally in their causes. Anxiety is triggered by the anticipation of a future, life-altering, or adverse event (real or imagined) or the recollection of a past adverse event. Fear is triggered by an encounter with immediate danger. Worrying about an upcoming dentist's appointment is experienced as anxiety, while facing an armed robber in the hallway is experienced as fear. In both instances, people's hearts race, their pupils dilate, and their breathing accelerates. The former involves a future orientation, whereas the latter involves a present orientation. Anxiety can be elicited by an excessive concern with "worst-case-scenarios" or irrational thoughts or beliefs about performance or social acceptance. When symptoms of anxiety become distressful and cause impairment in functioning (for example, the inability to work or attend school), then diagnosis of an anxiety disorder and the use of antianxiety medications and other therapeutic interventions are indicated.

Uses and Complications

The first line of treatment for anxiety disorders is cognitive behavioral therapy, which has been shown to be as effective as medications in the treatment of anxiety. In cases where psychotherapy alone is insufficient to treat the anxiety, antianxiety medications may be prescribed to help control symptoms. Three major categories of antianxiety medications, also known as anxiolytics, are used to treat anxiety disorders, and each of these act on similar neural transmitters and pathways: benzodiazepines, selective serotonin reuptake inhibitors (SSRIs), and selective norepinephrine reuptake inhibitors (SNRIs). Tricyclic antidepressants are also used in the treatment of anxiety disorders, although SSRIs are preferred due to their greater safety and tolerability. Barbituates, which act as central nervous system depressants, were once the first line of treatment for anxiety disorders, but their clinical use in the treatment of anxiety has been phased out due to the high risk of overdose and dependence.

Selective serotonin reuptake inhibitors. Selective serotonin reuptake inhibitors (SSRIs) are the most widely prescribed medications for the treatment of anxiety. As their name suggests, SSRIs act by increasing the levels of serotonin (5-hydroxytryptamine) in the brain by preventing its reuptake by neurons. When first approved for use, SSRIs were widely acclaimed as breakthrough medications in the treatment of depression, and clinical practice soon demonstrated their effectiveness in alleviating the symptoms of anxiety as well. Medications in this class include fluoxetine (Prozac), sertraline (Zoloft), fluvoxamine

(Luvox), paroxetine (Paxil), citalopram (Celexa), and escitalopram (Lexapro).

SSRIs require four to six weeks to reach maximum efficacy and can cause withdrawal symptoms if their use is stopped abruptly. The ingestion of large doses of SSRIs can result in severe toxicity, but fatal overdoses are rare. Hence, the risk of lethality from excessive SSRI use is minimal, especially when compared to other anxiolytics. In addition, SSRIs are nonaddictive and do not cause memory impairment. However, the list of potential side effects associated with SSRI use is lengthy: anhedonia, photosensitivity, drowsiness, headache, bruxism, vivid and bizarre dreams, dizziness, fatigue, urinary retention, changes in appetite, weight gain, suicidal ideation, tremors, orthostatic hypotension, and increased sweating. In addition, the sexual side effects that stem from SSRI use include reduced libido, erectile dysfunction, anorgasmia, genital anesthesia, and premature ejaculation.

Serotonin norepinephrine reuptake inhibitors. Serotonin norepinephrine reuptake inhibitors (SNRIs) work by blocking the reuptake of serotonin and norepinephrine in the brain. Various SNRIs block the reuptake of these neurotransmitters with differing affinity ratios, so that an SNRI that causes uncomfortable side effects in a patient may be replaced with another that does not have the same negative effects. The most common side effect of SNRIs is nausea, followed by dry mouth, sweating, constipation, and heart palpitations. Medications in this class include venlafaxine (Effexor), duloxetine (Cymbalta), and desvenlafaxine (Pristiq).

Benzodiazepines. The first benzodiazepine, chlordiazepoxide (Librium), was discovered in 1955. Benzodiazepines enhance the effects of gamma-aminobutyric acid (GABA), which is the chief inhibitory neurotransmitter in the central nervous system, making them useful in the treatment of anxiety. Benzodiazepines are fast-acting and typically relieve symptoms within thirty to sixty minutes of ingestion. Although cognitive impairment and paradoxical effects such as aggression, agitation, mania, or suicidality can occasionally occur with benzodiazepine use, these drugs are generally safe and effective in the short term. Benzodiazepines possess sedative and hypnotic properties that are useful in treating agitation and insomnia. Most benzodiazepines are administered orally; however, they can also be given intravenously, intramuscularly, or rectally. Other benzodiazepines are alprazolam (Xanax), clonazepam (Klonopin), diazepam (Valium), lorazepam (Ativan), and oxazepam (Serax).

Benzodiazepines can cause many side effects, including blurred or double vision, slowed reflexes, impaired thinking and judgment, dizziness, slurred speech, and depression. These effects are especially evident with prolonged use and at higher dosages, which can lead to abuse and dependence. The fastest-acting benzodiazepines (for example, Xanax) have the greatest potential for addiction and are listed as Schedule IV controlled substances. A sudden decrease in the dosage or abrupt cessation of benzodiazepine use can result in symptoms of rebound, which is a return of anxiety but at intensities that are higher than initial levels, and of withdrawal, which causes insomnia, sweating, shaking, confusion, and tachycardia (elevated heart rate). Hence, a gradual reduction in the dosage and administration of these medications is recommended.

Tricyclic antidepressants. Antidepressants are also used in the treatment of anxiety. The first class of antidepressants prescribed as anxiolytics are known as tricyclic anti-depressants (TCAs), which are named for the chemical structure of the drugs in the class-three rings. The first TCA, imipramine (Tofranil), was discovered in the late 1950s. Other examples of tricyclic antidepressants are amitriptyline (Elavil), amoxapine (Asendin), clomipramine (Anafranil), desipramine (Norpramin), doxepin (Sinequan), nortriptyline (Pamelor), protriptyline (Vivactil), and trimipramine (Surmontil). The side effects of TCAs include hypotension (low blood pressure), blurry vision, dizziness, constipation, dry mouth, drowsiness, increased appetite, and weight gain. In addition, an overdose of TCAs can often be fatal. The severe morbidity and mortality associated with these drugs is well documented because of their cardiovascular and neurological toxicity. Due to their greater safety and tolerability, SSRIs are the preferred treatment for anxiety.

Perspective and Prospects

Anxiety disorders are among the most common types of psychiatric illnesses worldwide, with a lifetime prevalence of 15 percent and a twelve-month prevalence of more than 10 percent. Research into safer and more effective treatments for these disorders is ongoing.

—Arthur J. Lurigio, Ph.D.

References

Ananth, Kartik, et al. "Managing Chronic Pain: Consider Psychotropics and Other Non-Opioids." *Current Psychiatry*, vol. 11, no. 2, Feb. 2012, pp. 38–43.

Bandelow, Borwin, et al. "Treatment of Anxiety Disorders." *Dialogues in Clinical Neuroscience*, vol. 19, no. 2, June 2017, pp. 93–107.

Heitler, Susan. "Anxiety Treatment: Should You Be Wary of Anxiety Medication?" *Psychology Today*, Sussex Publishers, 20 Jan. 2017, www.psychologytoday.com/us/blog/resolution-not-conflict/201701/anxiety-treatment-should-you-be-wary-anxiety-medication.

Kimmel, Ryan J., et al. "Pharmacological Treatments for Panic Disorder, Generalized Anxiety Disorder, Specific Phobia, and Social Anxiety Disorder." *Oxford Clinical Psychology*, 2015, doi:10.1093/med:psych/9780199342211.003.0015.

Leonard, Jayne. "Anxiety Medication: List, Types, and Side Effects." *Medical News Today*, MediLexicon International, 13 Nov. 2018, www.medicalnewstoday.com/articles/323666.php.

Locke, Amy B., et al. "Diagnosis and Management of Generalized Anxiety Disorder and Panic Disorder in Adults." *American Family Physician*, vol. 91, no. 9, May 2015, pp. 617–624.

"Pain, Anxiety, and Depression." *Harvard Health Publishing*, Harvard Medical School, 5 June 2019, www.health.harvard.edu/mind-and-mood/pain-anxiety-and-depression.

Roy-Byrne, Peter. "What Medications Are Used to Treat Anxiety Disorders?" *Anxiety and Depression Association of America*, Feb. 2019, adaa.org/learn-from-us/from-the-experts/blog-posts/what-medications-are-used-treat-anxiety-disorders.

"Treating Generalized Anxiety Disorder in the Elderly." *Harvard Health Publishing*, Harvard Medical School, 29 May 2019, www.health.harvard.edu/mind-and-mood/treating-generalized-anxiety-disorder-in-the-elderly.

Villines, Zawn. "10 Natural Remedies for Reducing Anxiety and Stress." *Medical News Today*, MediLexicon International, 9 July 2018, www.medicalnewstoday.com/articles/322396.php.

■ Antidepressants

CATEGORY: Class of Drug
ANATOMY OR SYSTEM AFFECTED: Brain, nervous system, psychic-emotional system
SPECIALTIES AND RELATED FIELDS: Biochemistry, family medicine, neurology, psychiatry, psychology

KEY TERMS

- *bipolar disorders*: mood disorders characterized by significant swings in mood from depression to persistent feelings of elation; also known as manic-depressive illness
- *depression*: a mood disorder characterized by loss of energy, depressed mood, diminished interest in pleasurable activities, feelings of worthlessness, and difficulty in concentrating
- *fluoxetine*: the generic name for the antidepressant commonly called Prozac
- *monoamine oxidase inhibitors (MAOIs)*: a class of drugs that relieve the symptoms of depression by inhibiting the enzyme that deactivates the brain chemical monoamine oxidase
- *neurotransmitters*: chemicals produced by the brain that allow for cells to transmit electrical signals
- *obsessive-compulsive disorder*: a psychiatric disorder that causes a person to ruminate on a particular thought and then act out a ritualistic behavior
- *selective serotonin reuptake inhibitors (SSRIs)*: a class of antidepressant drugs, first introduced in 1987, that work by inhibiting the reuptake of the neurotransmitter serotonin, thus making more of it available to brain cells
- *tricyclics*: antidepressant drugs that interfere with several neurotransmitters, making more of them available to the brain

Indications and Procedures

Antidepressants are prescribed most often to individuals suffering from symptoms of clinical depression, a severe form of depression that interferes with the person's ability to function (for example, to hold down a job or to handle the responsibilities of being a student). The symptoms of depression

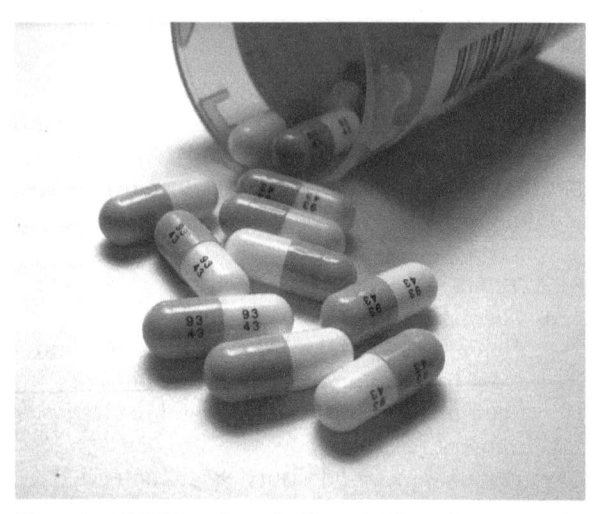

Fluoxetine HCl 20mg Capsules (Prozac). (Tom Varco via Wikimedia Commons)

must be present for at least two weeks before a diagnosis is made and treatment is recommended. Depression may be treated with antidepressant medications, brief psychotherapy, or a combination of both. Antidepressants are also used in the treatment of anxiety disorders.

Several classes of antidepressants can be considered as treatment options for depression. Each class of drugs acts on the nervous system in its own unique way, and each class produces different kinds of side effects. Monoamine oxidase inhibitors (MAOIs) and tricyclic antidepressants are regarded as two different classes of first-generation drugs. These two classes and the new-generation selective serotonin reuptake inhibitors (SSRIs), including fluoxetine (Prozac), all affect the nervous system by increasing the availability of neurotransmitters such as norepinephrine or serotonin.

Although physicians have several classes of drugs at their disposal to combat the effects of depression, no single drug or class of drugs has been found to be significantly more effective in treating symptoms. In fact, no reliable test exists to discover which antidepressant will be most effective for a particular patient. However, it is clearly the case that most patients will respond favorably to one class of drugs over the others. The effectiveness of antidepressants can be evaluated on two fronts: the degree to which symptoms of clinical depression are reduced and the pervasiveness of any adverse side effects that may result from a particular medication.

Uses and Complications

Because all antidepressant medications cause some adverse side effects, physicians attempt to determine the minimum clinically effective dose. For some patients, antidepressants may cause suicidal ideation in the first few weeks of their use. Anyone taking antidepressants should be closely monitored by a physician, especially when the medication is first prescribed. Patients should discuss how they are feeling with their doctor after a new antidepressant medication is prescribed so that the physician can evaluate the effectiveness of the antidepressant and identify any adverse side effects. Because there are several different types of antidepressants available, some experimentation may be necessary to determine which medication works best for a given patient.

In terms of specific side effects of drugs, MAOIs may produce a serious adverse side effect known as a hypertensive crisis, which results in a rapid elevation of blood pressure. This condition is caused by an interaction of the drug with foods containing tyramine, such as aged cheeses, aged meats, and red wines; thus, these foods must be avoided while MAOIs are in use. Less serious side effects produced by MAOIs include constipation, diarrhea, and difficulty falling asleep.

Tricyclic antidepressants may produce dry mouth, blurred vision, or weight gain. However, the most serious aspect of tricyclics is the danger if an overdose is taken, as fatal cardiac rhythm disturbances can occur. Given that patients suffering from depression may have thoughts of suicide, the amount of prescription given at one time must be carefully monitored and should be limited. SSRIs have fewer and more easily tolerated side effects than the first-generation antidepressants, although some patients will experience weight gain and sexual dysfunction resulting in the loss of the sexual drive.

Abruptly stopping an antidepressant prescription will lead to a range of withdrawal symptoms, from feeling more depressed to becoming irritable to developing flulike symptoms. Although the withdrawal symptoms are not dangerous, it is recommended that antidepressants be reduced in dosage over a period of several days.

Perspective and Prospects

Since the late 1980s, individuals suffering from depression have had access to medications that produce fewer adverse side effects than first-generation antidepressants. Investigators are also learning that antidepressants can help patients with other psychological conditions, such as bipolar disorders, anxiety disorders, panic attacks, and obsessive-compulsive disorder.

Despite the successes that have come with the availability of several classes of antidepressants, there still remains a group of patients suffering from depression who do not benefit from them. Investigators are continuing to look for more effective treatments, particularly ones that can alleviate the symptoms of depression more quickly. Group therapy and cognitive behavioral therapy are also effective in the treatment of depression and should be used in combination with antidepressants to improve treatment outcome.

—*Bryan C. Auday, Ph.D.*

References

Baltenberger, Elizabeth P., et al. "Review of Antidepressants in the Treatment of Neuropathic Pain." *Mental Health Clinician*, vol. 5, no. 3, 2015, pp. 123–133., doi:10.9740/mhc.2015.05.123.

Hooten, W. Michael. "Chronic Pain and Mental Health Disorders." *Mayo Clinic Proceedings*, vol. 91, no. 7, 2016, pp. 955–970., doi:10.1016/j.mayocp.2016.04.029.

Kramer, Peter D. *Ordinarily Well: the Case for Antidepressants*. Farrar, Straus & Giroux, 2017.

Lambert, Jonathan. "Antidepressants Can Interfere With Pain Relief Of Common Opioids." *National Public Radio*, 6 Feb. 2019, www.npr.org/sections/health-shots/2019/02/06/691998300/antidepressants-can-interfere-with-pain-relief-of-common-opioids.

Nekovarova, Tereza, et al. "Common Mechanisms of Pain and Depression: Are Antidepressants Also Analgesics?" *Frontiers in Behavioral Neuroscience*, vol. 8, 25 Mar. 2014, doi:10.3389/fnbeh.2014.00099.

Nordqvist, Christian. "All about Antidepressants." *Medical News Today*, MediLexicon International, 16 Feb. 2018, www.medicalnewstoday.com/kc/antidepressants-work-248320.

Riediger, Carina, et al. "Adverse Effects of Antidepressants for Chronic Pain: A Systematic Review and Meta-Analysis." *Frontiers in Neurology*, vol. 8, 14 July 2017, doi:10.3389/fneur.2017.00307.

Sheng, Jiyao, et al. "The Link between Depression and Chronic Pain: Neural Mechanisms in the Brain." *Neural Plasticity*, 2017, pp. 1–10., doi:10.1155/2017/9724371.

■ Antipsychotics

CATEGORY: Class of Drug
ANATOMY OR SYSTEM AFFECTED: Brain, Central Nervous System (CNS), Thyroid, Pituitary, Hypothalamus
SPECIALTIES AND RELATED FIELDS: Neuroscience, Neurology, Psychiatry, Psychology, Schizophrenia, Bipolar Disorder

KEY TERMS

- *central nervous system*: comprised of the brain and spinal cord. It controls thoughts, emotions and actions by electrical signals traveling though neural pathways
- *neurotransmitter*: a chemical messenger that transmits a neural signal across a synapse
- *neurons*: highly specialized cell found in the nervous system, which produces an electrical signal to transmit information
- *dopamine*: a neurotransmitter that helps send electrical signals for emotion, movement, and other processes
- *positive symptoms*: symptoms of schizophrenia that involve the production of an abnormal behavior
- *psychosis*: a mental disorder in which one's emotions and thoughts are impaired, causing a person to lose touch with reality. Primarily characterized by experience of delusions, personality shifts, discontinuous thought patterns and speech, and unrefined social behavior
- *schizophrenia*: a type of psychotic disorder involving a detachment among one's thoughts, emotions and behaviors

How are Antipsychotic Drugs Used in Medicine?

Antipsychotic drugs are most commonly used to treat schizophrenia; however, they are also used to treat other psychiatric illnesses such as bipolar disorder and depression. Additionally, recent studies indicate antipsychotic drugs can improve symptoms associated with obsessive-compulsive disorder (OCD), aggressive behavior, and cancer induced bone pain (CIPB). In extension, first-generation antipsychotics are also used to treat nausea and vomiting, to sedate patients before anesthesia, relieve sever itching, and can manage psychosis caused by drugs and alcohol.

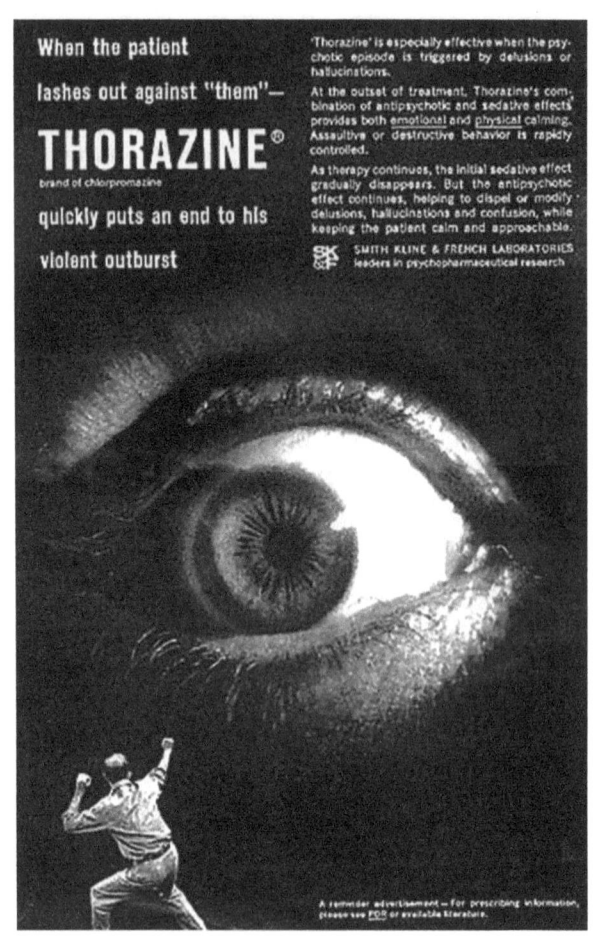

Advertisement for Thorazine (chlorpromazine) from the 1950s, reflecting the perceptions of psychosis, including the now-discredited perception of a tendency towards violence, from the time when antipsychotics were discovered. (via Wikimedia Commons)

Types of Antipsychotic Drugs
In the 1950's, researchers began using a class of drugs known as phenothiazines after recognizing its calming effects in psychiatric patients. Phenothiazines became what is commonly known today as conventional antipsychotics. Antipsychotics primarily reduce the positive symptoms of schizophrenia, a psychiatric illness that is characterized by delusions (irrational beliefs), hallucinations, and disorganized speech (incoherent speech with frequent changes of topic). Some frequently prescribed examples of first-conventional antipsychotics (these used to be called first-generation antipsychotics) include chlorpromazine, haloperidol, both in generic formulations and the brand name drugs Loxitane, Moban, Serentil, and Navane.

Beginning in the 1960's, a new class of antipsychotics was introduced as an alternative to patients who might not respond well to conventional drugs. This new class, known as atypical antipsychotics, is characterized by having fewer deleterious side effects. Some frequently prescribed examples include the brand name drugs Abilify, Clozaril, Zyprexa, and Risperdal. Both conventional and atypical antipsychotics do not produce drug dependence and it is extremely rare for patients to commit suicide using them. However, many patients may experience several unpleasant side effects. The most common side effects involve a range of movement disorders such as facial tics, hand tremors, and muscular rigidity. One of the more serious complications from using antipsychotics is tardive dyskinesia. This condition results in rhythmic, repetitive sucking and smacking movements of the lips and tongue. Usually, tardive dyskinesia appears only after using these drugs for many years, sometimes decades. Typically, this condition can be treated by early identification of the symptoms and lowering the amount of medication. Additional symptoms of these drugs can include weight gain, photosensitivity, and dry mouth. While conventional and atypical antipsychotics have been shown to be equally effective, the advantage of atypical medicines is that they have fewer incidents of adverse side effects, which allow patients to experience an overall higher quality of life.

The vast majority of antipsychotics are taken orally; however, some can be administered by intermuscular injection. Long lasting injectable antipsychotic medication have relatively fewer side effects than oral antipsychotic medications in that it is associated with less relapses and lower hospitalization. In extension, those who use long lasting injectable antipsychotic drugs are more likely to continue treatment because of the reduced undesirable side effects and patients do not have to be reminded each day to take their medication.

How do Antipsychotic Drugs Work?
Psychosis often results from an excess of the chemical dopamine. Antipsychotics primarily work by inhibiting D2 receptors in the brain to block dopamine, which in turn reduces the positive symptoms of psychosis. While blocking dopamine receptors reduces psychosis symptomology, it can lead to manifestation of abnormal motor functions

common in Parkinson's disease such involuntary tremor. Both conventional and atypical antipsychotics impact additional neurotransmitters such as serotonin and noradeline. However, the mechanism of action between the conventional and atypical antipsychotics differ in that conventional drugs primarily act by inhibiting dopaminergic receptors in four distinct dopaminergic pathways. In contrast, atypical antipsychotics block D2 receptors and a subtype serotonin receptor known as 5HT2A.

Psychedelic drugs, such as LSD, produce hallucinations comparable to those that schizophrenics experience as a result of excess serotonin secretion. Therefore, researchers reasoned that inhibiting serotonin along with dopamine would mitigate positive symptoms. Antipsychotics have an indirect effect on glutamate input and output because dopamine receptors regulate glutamine neurotransmission. Researchers further explored the relationship between glutamate delusional episodes after examining the psychedelic drug PCP that causes delusions and hallucinations by interfering with the NMDA glutamate receptor in the brain. Studying drugs that cause schizophrenia-like symptoms can shed light on the mechanism in the CNS that brings on psychosis.

Antipsychotics do not cure psychosis; rather they treat the symptoms. Therefore, a large percentage of patients will remain on medication for their entire lives. Women are more prone to adverse side effects from a lower dose of antipsychotics than men. Researchers found that in general, women are more sensitive to the total dose of antipsychotics. Therefore, lower doses should be used in women.

—*Bryan C. Auday, PhD*
—*Michelle Satava, BA*

References

Jimenez, Xavier F., et al. "A Systematic Review of Atypical Antipsychotics in Chronic Pain Management." *The Clinical Journal of Pain*, vol. 34, no. 6, 2018, pp. 585–591., doi:10.1097/ajp.0000000000000567.

Jimenez, Xavier F., et al. "A Systematic Review of Atypical Antipsychotics in Chronic Pain Management." *The Clinical Journal of Pain*, vol. 34, no. 6, 2018, pp. 585–591., doi:10.1097/ajp.0000000000000567.

Khouzam, Hani Raoul. "Psychopharmacology of Chronic Pain: a Focus on Antidepressants and Atypical Antipsychotics." *Postgraduate Medicine*, vol. 128, no. 3, 16 Feb. 2016, pp. 323–330., doi:10.1080/00325481.2016.1147925.

Kim, Young Hoon. "The Role and Position of Antipsychotics in Managing Chronic Pain." *The Korean Journal of Pain*, vol. 32, no. 1, 2019, p. 1., doi:10.3344/kjp.2019.32.1.1.

Seidel, Stefan, et al. "Antipsychotics for Acute and Chronic Pain in Adults." *Cochrane Database of Systematic Reviews*, 2013, doi:10.1002/14651858.cd004844.pub3.

■ Assimilative family therapy model

CATEGORY: Therapy or Technique; Psychotherapy

Introduction

The modern family presents many new challenges for mental and behavioral health providers because new family structures require a reformulation of strategies and interventions that differ from those employed when working with "traditional families." Traditional models of family therapy no longer adequately address the dilemmas brought to consultation rooms. A treatment model sensitive to the many unique contexts presented by the modern family is needed. A new model, the assimilative family therapy model, is an attempt to meet this need by shaping the inclusion of necessary interventions to address the specific dilemmas of a client or family. This therapy addresses the many dilemmas that are faced throughout the life cycle: differentiation of the individual, parenting and couple relationship issues, midlife issues, and caring for the elderly.

What is the assimilative family therapy model? It is an integrative, as opposed to eclectic, approach. An eclectic eater goes to a buffet and chooses several items, combining different food items at times while at other times eating one food by itself. An integrationist goes to the buffet, selects ingredients, and combines them together to create a new dish. Thus, the integrationist evaluates a client's dilemmas and combines approaches, concepts, and other variables to create the most effective treatment to enable clients to heal.

The assimilative approach falls within the field of integration. In an assimilative approach, the therapist chooses a home theory that becomes the focal therapy of the approach. Then the therapist integrates other concepts and interventions from other theories to meet the goals of the home theory and goals set by the therapist and client(s). In the assimilative family therapy model (AFT), the home theory is a systems theory. Family therapists consider clients' dilemmas from a systems point of view. They focus on the patterns of interaction of the family of origin and extended family. They also evaluate families' physical and psychological vulnerabilities, how members connect to each other and negotiate conflict, and those patterns of behavior that get transmitted from generation to generation. For example, say Bobby is a child who suffers from anxiety. His paternal family members also struggle with anxiety. Is this a pattern that has been transmitted to Bobby through genetics or is it learned by repeating his father's behaviors? The family therapist looks at an individual's or family's dilemmas by systematically considering where the behaviors and adjustments occurred in past generations.

In AFT, family therapists rely on the Bowen family systems therapy model as the home theory. They then integrate other concepts and interventions from other therapies such as psychodynamic, cognitive behavioral, communications, and other systems therapies to better meet the needs and goals of the clients. The goals of the Bowen approach are to reduce anxiety, lower emotional reactivity, and increase differentiation among all family members.

Lowering emotional reactivity is an important goal for individuals to be able to problem solve and think rationally when one is being emotionally challenged by a situation, event, feeling, or person. In the process of learning to control reactions to situations, family members also learn how to state their positions in a respectful manner even when emotions are charged or there is pressure from another to change a position. By working this way, clients' anxiety levels are lowered, enabling them to think, act, and feel in a modulated manner. In Bobby's case, the AFT therapist realizes that Bobby needs to separate his behaviors from those of his anxious father. The therapist will also incorporate mindfulness strategies and relaxation exercises to help Bobby differentiate himself from his father's behaviors and adjustments.

The individual or family context is another important concept that informs AFT therapists' work with clients. Our context sets the stage for how we view the world we live in, how we interact, and what we value. Context includes age, sex, sexual orientation, religion, spirituality, ethnicity, culture, socioeconomic level, level of attachment, and level of resilience and optimism. These contexts all contribute to clients' adjustment to life's circumstances. The more therapists understand clients' contexts, the more helpful they are in enabling them to affect change in behaviors, thinking, and actions. Because Bobby's parents come from a strict German family where children "should be seen and not heard," his level of attachment to his parents is avoidant. He does not feel safe expressing his feelings which further increases his anxiety. The family's more stoical outlook works against their ability to enjoy the positive parts of their lives which also contributes to Bobby's anxiety. If Bobby's attachment to his parents were close and warm, even though he has a genetic propensity for anxiety, he might not become symptomatic due to feeling supported. As a result, he would be more resilient and less apt to become anxious. Therefore, as therapists integrate clients' context with the theory, they begin to conceptualize the best way to help clients change their thinking, feelings, and behaviors to solve the presented dilemmas.

The assimilative family therapy model is useful in treating individuals suffering from anxiety and depression and for child and adolescent centered issues where adjustment to school, friends, or family relationships is compromised. AFT may also be effective with couple dilemmas and midlife and end of life issues and, in fact, dilemmas throughout the life cycle. The best way to understand how to use AFT is to apply it with different populations.

Many couples that come to treatment are anxious, angry, and frightened that their marriage may end, but they cannot mobilize their emotions, thoughts, and actions to do something constructive to start saving the relationship. Others enter therapy, and they desperately work at saving their relationships and are committed to each other and the process. In AFT, it is essential to help couples realize that their behaviors are most likely a repeat of their parent or family patterns in some capacity. Many clients state that they want a relationship different from their parents, but they repeat behaviors without being aware that they are doing so. The next step is enabling couples to take responsibility for their individual behaviors. With therapists' help, they jointly decide what needs to be changed within each individual and in their manner of interacting between each other. Social scientist John Gottman, who is known in family therapy circles for his work on marital stability and relational analysis, has rightly stressed the need to communicate in a more respectful manner with lowered emotional reactivity and anxiety. The couple is encouraged to develop a more differentiated stance on what each needs and wants as individuals and as a couple unit (or dyad). Once this process begins, and not until it begins, can the couple learn to create a more intimate and satisfying relationship.

Meet Kayla and Joe who have been married for six years. Kayla identified with her very strong and angry mother and was repeating these patterns when dealing with her husband. Though Joe also came from a family where his mother was dominant, he consciously decided that he would never become like his dismissed and diminished dad. When Kayla expressed anger at Joe, Joe responded with so much anger that it would exacerbate Kayla's anger. Soon, they both would be shouting at each other until battle fatigue set in and they retreated. A cessation of hostilities was achieved, but Kayla and Joe never solved their issues. At some point, they would again begin this cycle and ignite anger. Once the AFT therapist could point out patterns, it was easier and safer for Kayla and Joe to accept responsibility for their own behavior and reactions to the other. Each understood how he or she was a catalyst for the other to become increasingly angry, because each was actually, though not consciously planning to do so, repeating patterns in their family of origin. For this couple, the AFT therapist also integrated mindfulness techniques developed by Professor Emeritus of Medicine, Jon Kabatt-Zinn, who founded Mindfulness-Based Stress Reduction (MBSR). These techniques enabled each to change the way he or she reacted to the other by using role-play and other effective communication techniques (e.g., teaching them to listen, validate each other feelings by repeating them, and respond empathetically to the other) to help enable each one to feel heard and cared for. As a result, Kayla and Joe were able to change the way they viewed their own behaviors and create an identity that was different from their parents. The couple began to feel more connection and enjoyment with each other. When situations arose that ignited their mutual angers, they were able to modulate the way they interacted, avoid escalating the dilemmas, and resolve the issues presented.

A stressful time of life is midlife when caretaking responsibilities can become paramount to anything else. Many midlifers, particularly women, find themselves caring for elderly parents as well as being parents to adult children. Some midlifers become the caretakers for grandchildren as well. These midlifers are known in social science research as the "sandwich generation." The elderly population is increasing as individuals live longer and the need for informal caregiving (i.e., without pay or compensation) is growing. How the family interacted before the elderly became a pressure in the system will determine how the family is able to deal with the needs and desires of the elderly. The more connected the generations, the better they will be able to deal with the elderly member's needs and decline. Family caregivers have more mental health issues, with depression being the most common. The mortality rate of caregivers of elderly spouses (ages 66–96) is 63 percent higher than among non-caregivers in the same age bracket. The family history of elder care will likely be repeated from the previous generation with a new twist.

The therapist can help the adult children work through the mourning process of denial, bargaining, anger, depression, and acceptance. Feeling sad, helpless, and ashamed are normal feelings when interacting with our onetime strong parent who is losing his or her abilities. Adult children and elderly parents are both mourning in different ways, but both generations need to face their sadness and celebrate their function so they can establish new patterns to help the elderly and for the elderly to receive help in this difficult stage of life. In the final stage of a parent's life, the patterns that were developed over the course of a lifetime continue. Caregivers have the responsibility to change their positions within the family while working through feelings and dysfunctional individual and family patterns.

AFT also offers a practical approach to managing relationships between adult children and elderly parents. The therapy enables the caregiver and elder (if able and appropriate) to deal with feelings, identify dilemmas, and find solutions. Meet Selma, a midlife woman who has adult children and a 92-year-old mom. Selma's mom has been a widow for more than 40 years. Selma has been the backbone for her mom since her father's untimely death. Even though Grandma has been independent until the last five years, the strain of Selma's roles as an employee, wife, parent to adult married children, and caregiver of her elderly mom has taken a toll on Selma's health and sense of well-being in the form of heightened anxiety and inability to sleep. The therapist looked at the family patterns of how Selma with her siblings became the caretaker of her mom. It became obvious that this was a repeated pattern from Selma's mother's family of origin. However, today's longevity means this pattern will persist far longer and has overwhelmed Selma. The therapist was able to identify the family patterns and coach Selma to approach her siblings to ask for help in dealing with their mom. Rather than caring for her adult children, she was instructed to ask them to help with Grandma. Selma also hired some outside help within the monetary ability of Grandma's funds. Her husband, relatively absent in helping, was asked to step in. This was very difficult for Selma to learn to ask for help and let go of control as she began to take control of her own life. Along with family members, Selma needed to mourn the loss of her mother rather than avoid these feelings while caring for her. This enabled the family to be a support for Grandma who was also mourning the loss of her abilities and the eventual ending of her life. Being able to do this provided stability for the family and healthier individual functioning. By making the mourning process visible and identifiable, Selma could free her repressed anger, sadness, and energy to enable her to start caring for herself by communicating appropriately with family members, going to the doctor for check-ups, exercising, losing weight, going out with her husband, and enjoying her midlife years while at the same time continuing to balance her many responsibilities.

—*Patricia Pitta*

References

Babl, Anna, et al. "Psychotherapy Integration under Scrutiny: Investigating the Impact of Integrating Emotion-Focused Components into a CBT-Based Approach: a Study Protocol of a Randomized Controlled Trial." *BMC Psychiatry*, vol. 16, no. 1, 24 Nov. 2016, doi:10.1186/s12888-016-1136-7.

Messer, Stanley D. "Assimilative Psychotherapy Integration." *The SAGE Encyclopedia of Theory in Counseling and Psychotherapy*, 27 Sept. 2017, doi:10.4135/9781483346502.n29.

Pitta, Patricia J. *Solving Modern Family Dilemmas Assimilative Therapy*. Routledge, 2015.

Smith, Karmen R., and Kevin P. Lyness. "Solving Modern Family Dilemmas: An Assimilative Therapy Model." *Journal of Marital and Family Therapy*, vol. 42, no. 2, Apr. 2016.

Zarbo, Cristina, et al. "Integrative Psychotherapy Works." *Frontiers in Psychology*, vol. 6, 11 Jan. 2016, doi:10.3389/fpsyg.2015.02021.

■ Barbiturates

CATEGORY: Class of Drug
ANATOMY OR SYSTEM AFFECTED: Central nervous system

History of Use

In 1903, Emil Fischer and Joseph von Mering discovered an effective sedative, diethylbarbituric acid or barbital, which entered medicine under the trade name Veronal. Another barbiturate, phenobarbital (Luminal), was introduced in 1912 and continues to be used as an anticonvulsant. By the mid-twentieth century, barbiturates became the most widely used sedative-hypnotic medication and the most popular substances of misuse. Collectively referred to as "downers" because they were effective in depressing the central nervous system, barbiturates were taken alone or with alcohol (ethanol) to produce a feeling of relaxation and euphoria. In the United States, barbiturate misuse and addiction markedly increased in the 1950s and 1960s. The drugs became especially popular with people who experienced high levels of stress, anxiety, or panic attacks.

The beginning of the twenty-first century saw a modest increase in usage of barbiturates as substances of misuse. Some drug specialists attribute this increase to the desire of drug users to seek out the relaxing, calming, and disinhibiting effects of barbiturates as a means to counteract stimulant drugs such as cocaine and methamphetamines. According to a national survey on drug use and health by the US Substance Abuse and Mental

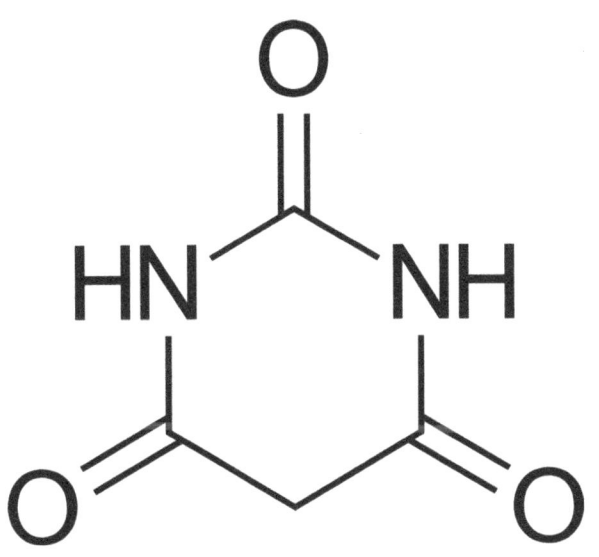

Barbituric acid, the parent structure of all barbiturates. (Manuel Almagro Rivas via Wikimedia Commons)

Health Services Administration, an estimated 3.1 million people (approximately 9%) age twelve years and older had misused barbiturates.

Barbiturates today are used clinically for treatment of seizures that last longer than five minutes or occur close together before a person regains consciousness (status epilepticus). Barbiturates are also used for anesthesia, pediatric sedation, migraines and insomnia. One particular barbiturate, pentobarbital, is the drug of choice for veterinary anesthesia and euthanasia.

Pharmacological and Psychological Effects

Barbiturates are classified according to their duration of action. The effects of ultra-short-acting drugs, such as Pentothal (used in surgical settings as an anesthesia), last less than one hour. Short-acting barbiturates (such as Nembutal and Seconal) act for three to four hours and are more likely to be taken for recreational purposes. The effects of intermediate-acting barbiturates (such as Amytal) last for six to eight hours, and the effects of long-acting barbiturates (such as Veronal and Luminal) that are taken as anticonvulsants last approximately twelve hours. Like other sedative-hypnotic drugs, barbiturates produce relaxation or sleep. Barbiturates are not analgesic. If an individual is experiencing moderate or high levels of pain, they will be less effective in producing sedation or sleep. The mechanism underlying their effect is thought to be an enhancement of the neural inhibition induced by the neurotransmitter gamma-aminobutyric acid (GABA) at the receptor. Additionally, barbiturates directly open the chloride channel on cell membranes without GABA.

Although barbiturates can produce sleep, the quality of sleep can be far from normal. The stage of sleep referred to as rapid eye movement (REM) is markedly suppressed. Since this stage is associated with dreaming, the frequency of dreams can be dramatically reduced. For individuals experiencing withdrawal, dreaming can become excessive and more vivid during this period where the brain attempts to make up for lost time spent in REM. The term "REM rebound" is used to describe this phenomenon and it can frequently bring on insomnia. However, more significant and noticeable changes brought on by barbiturates include their capacity to act as a cognitive inhibitor. Memory functioning can be compromised along with alterations of judgment, decision making, insight, and planning. An above-regular dosage of barbiturates induces a state of intoxication similar to that caused by alcohol. Mild intoxication is characterized by drunk-like behavior with slurred speech, unsteady gait, lack of coordination, abnormal eye movements, and an absence of alcohol odor. Driving prior to the drug being completely metabolized and eliminated is considered dangerous.

At regular doses, the effects of barbiturates vary depending on the user's previous experience with the drug, the setting of use, and the mode of administration. A particular dose taken in the evening, for example, may induce sleep, whereas it may produce relaxed contentment, euphoria, and diminished motor skills during the day. Some users report sedation, fatigue, unpleasant drowsiness, nausea, vomiting, and diarrhea. A paradoxical state of excitement or rage also can occur. Users may experience a "hangover" phenomenon the day after drug administration. Hypersensitivity reactions, sensitivity to sunlight (photosensitivity), decreased sexual function, and impaired memory also have been reported.

Potential Risks, Drug Misuse and Dependence

Although barbiturates have been around for over 100 years, there has been a steep and rapid decline in their clinical uses. Compared to the number of prescriptions written for barbiturates during the 1970s, today, they are rarely used. Two primary factors are responsible for the change. First, safer drug alternatives have been developed. An example of this would be the use of benzodiazepines in the treatment of anxiety disorders. Secondly, barbiturates, overall, have been found to be extremely dangerous to use effectively. They have become associated with numerous deaths, widespread dependency and misuse, and have been found to interact deleteriously with many other drugs. Barbiturates are extremely dangerous when combined with alcohol since both drugs are central nervous system depressants and they produced a synergistic, exaggerated effect when taken together.

One reason these drugs pose a significant risk is due to the fact the therapeutic dosage of any barbiturate is close to its lethal dose. Because of this narrow therapeutic window, severe intoxication or drug-induced death can easily occur. Intentional or accidental overdose results in extreme drowsiness, respiratory depression (with slow breathing), hypotension, hypothermia, renal failure, decreased reflexes, and, ultimately, coma and death. In addition, taking barbiturates over a period of months can induce tolerance whereby the sedative effects (not so much the depressant effects on respiration) diminish over time. This requires higher dosages to achieve the same clinical benefits. Eventually, the therapeutic window mentioned above is narrowed even further making barbiturate usage unacceptably dangerous.

Both physical and psychological dependence can result with normal clinical doses. This potential for misuse, particularly for short and intermediate acting barbiturates, contributed to the medical communities' movement away from using barbiturates if other drug alternatives were available. Physical dependence is characterized by withdrawal symptoms during periods of drug cessation. Withdrawal symptoms may include restlessness, disorientation, hallucinations, hyper-excitability, delirium, convulsions, and possibly death. Barbiturate dependency, followed by abrupt termination of drug use, can be extremely dangerous. Persons who want to stop taking these drugs should do so under medical supervision only.

The amount of barbiturates needed to reach a toxic dose which causes an overdose can vary considerably. However, in most circumstances, a dose of one gram of the majority of barbiturates leads to serous poisoning. Ingesting two to ten grams frequently causes death. A person with suspected barbiturate overdose should be seen by a physician without delay. In a 2016 study published about 277 people admitted to a hospital emergency room for drug overdose, investigators found that 19.5% had taken barbiturates. It was also found that these individuals needed to be monitored more closely since they had a higher risk for incurring additional medical implications. In some instances, the overdose was a deliberate attempt to die. Among advocates of euthanasia and among those who commit suicide, barbiturates remain one of the most commonly employed drugs.

—*Mihaela Avramut, MD, PhD*
—*Bryan C. Auday, PhD*

Medicines Classified as Barbiturates

- Amytal sodium
- Butisol sodium
- Luminal
- Nembutal sodium
- Phenobarbital
- Seconal sodium

References

Cordovilla-Guardia, Sergio, et al. "The Effect of Central Nervous System Depressant, Stimulant and Hallucinogenic Drugs on Injury Severity in Patients Admitted for Trauma." *Gaceta Sanitaria*, vol. 33, no. 1, 2019, pp. 4–9., doi:10.1016/j.gaceta.2017.06.006.

Davis, Kathleen. "Barbiturates: Uses, Side Effects, and Risks." *Medical News Today*, MediLexicon International, 25 June 2018, www.medicalnewstoday.com/articles/310066.php.

Gokhale, Sankalp, and Ciro Ramos-Estebanez. "An Interesting Case of Barbiturate Automatism and Review of Literature." *Case Reports in Neurological Medicine*, vol. 2013, 2013, pp. 1–2., doi:10.1155/2013/713065.

Lafferty, Keith A., et al. "Barbiturate Toxicity." *Medscape*, 14 Jan. 2017, emedicine.medscape.com/article/813155-overview.

López-Muñoz, Francisco, et al. "The History of Barbiturates a Century after Their Clinical Introduction." *Neuropsychiatric Disease and Treatment*, vol. 1, no. 4, Dec. 2005, pp. 329–343.

Oakley, Simon, et al. "Recognition of Anesthetic Barbiturates by a Protein Binding Site: A High Resolution Structural Analysis." *PLoS ONE*, vol. 7, no. 2, 16 Feb. 2012, doi:10.1371/journal.pone.0032070.

Behavioral family therapy

CATEGORY: Therapy or Technique; Psychotherapy

KEY TERMS
- *conditioning*: the process of training or accustoming a person or animal to behave in a certain way or to accept certain circumstances
- *operationalization*: a process of defining the measurement of a phenomenon that is not directly measurable, though its existence is inferred by other phenomena
- *reinforcer*: a stimulus (such as a reward or the removal of an electric shock) that increases the probability of a desired response in operant conditioning by being applied or effected following the desired response

Introduction

Behavioral family therapy is a type of psychotherapy used to treat families in which one or more members are exhibiting behavior problems. Behavioral therapy was employed originally in the treatment of individual disorders such as phobias (irrational fears). Behavioral family therapy represents an extension of the use of behavioral techniques from the treatment of individual problems to the treatment of family problems. The most common problems treated by behavioral family therapy are parent-child conflicts; however, the principles of this type of therapy have been used to treat other familial difficulties, including marital and sexual problems.

Role of Learning Theory

The principles of learning theory underlie the theory and practice of behavioral family therapy. Learning theory was developed through laboratory experimentation largely begun by Ivan Petrovich Pavlov and Edward L. Thorndike during the early 1900s. Pavlov was a Russian physiologist interested in the digestive processes of dogs. In the process of his experimentation, he discovered several properties regarding the production of behavior that have become embodied in the theory of classical conditioning. Pavlov observed that his dogs began to salivate when he entered their pens because they associated his presence (new behavior) with their being fed (previously reinforced old behavior). From this observation and additional experimentation, Pavlov concluded that a new behavior that is regularly paired with an old behavior acquires the same rewarding or punishing qualities of the old behavior. New actions become conditioned to produce the same responses as the previously reinforced or punished actions.

Another component of learning theory was discovered by Thorndike, an American psychologist. Thorndike observed that actions followed closely by rewards were more likely to recur than those not followed by rewards. Similarly, he observed that actions followed closely by punishment were less likely to recur. Thorndike explained these observations on the basis of the law of effect. The law of effect holds that behavior closely followed by a response will be more or less likely to recur depending on whether the response is reinforcing (rewarding) or punishing.

Building on the observations of Thorndike, American behaviorist B. F. Skinner developed the theory of operant conditioning in the 1930s. Operant conditioning is the process by which behavior is made to occur at a faster rate when a specific behavior is followed by positive reinforcement—the rewarding consequences that follow a behavior, which increase the rate at which the behavior will recur. An example that Skinner used in demonstrating operant conditioning involved placing a rat in a box with different levers. When the rat accidentally pushed a predesignated lever, it was given a food pellet. As predicted by operant conditioning, the rat subsequently increased its pushing of the lever that provided it with food.

Gerald Patterson and Richard Stuart, beginning in the late 1960s, were among the first clinicians to apply behavioral techniques, previously used with individuals, to the treatment of family problems. Although Patterson worked primarily with parent-child problems, Stuart extended behavioral family therapy to the treatment of marital problems.

Given the increasing prevalence of family problems, as seen by the rise in the number of divorces and cases of child abuse, the advent of behavioral family therapy has been welcomed by many therapists who treat families. The findings of a 1984 study by William Quinn and Bernard Davidson revealed the increasing use of this therapy, with more than half of all family therapists reporting the use of behavioral techniques in their family therapy.

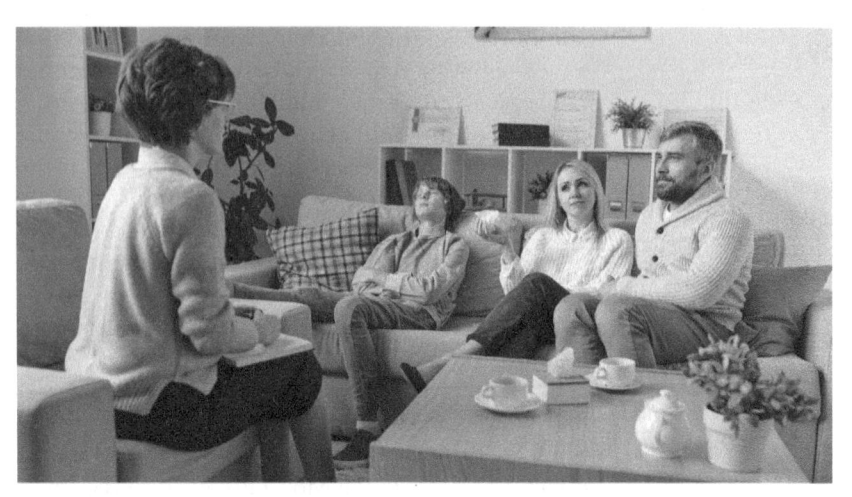

Family therapy tends to view change in terms of the systems of interaction between family members. (SeventyFour via Wikimedia Commons)

Conditioning and Desensitization

The principles of classical and operant conditioning serve to form the foundation of learning theory. Although initially derived from animal experiments, learning theory also was applied to humans. Psychologists who advocated learning theory began to demonstrate that all behavior, whether socially appropriate or inappropriate, occurs because it is either classically or operantly conditioned. John B. Watson, an American psychologist of the early twentieth century, illustrated this relationship by producing a fear of rats in an infant known as Little Albert by repeatedly making a loud noise when a rat was presented to Albert. After a number of pairings of the loud noise with the rat, Albert began to show fear when the rat was presented.

In addition to demonstrating how inappropriate behavior was caused, behavioral psychologists began to show how learning theory could be used to treat people with psychological disorders. Joseph Wolpe, a pioneer in the use of behavioral treatment during the 1950s, showed how phobias could be alleviated by using learning principles in a procedure termed systematic desensitization. Systematic desensitization involves three basic steps: teaching the phobic individual how to relax; having the client create a list of images of the feared object (for example, snakes), from least to most feared; and repeatedly exposing the client to the feared object in graduated degrees, from least to most feared images, while the individual is in a relaxed state. This procedure has been shown to be very effective in the treatment of phobias.

Behavioral family therapy makes the same assumptions regarding the causes of both individual and family problems. For example, in a fictional case, the Williams family came to treatment because their seven-year-old son, John, refused to sleep in his own bed at night. In attempting to explain John's behavior, a behaviorally oriented psychologist would seek to find out what positive reinforcement John was receiving in response to his refusal to stay in his own bed. It may be that when John was younger his parents allowed him to sleep with them, thus reinforcing his behavior by giving him the attention he desired. Now that John is seven, however, his parents believe that he needs to sleep in his own bed, but John continues to want to sleep with his parents because he has been reinforced by being allowed to sleep with them for many years. This case provides a clinical example of operant conditioning in that John's behavior, because it was repeatedly followed by positive reinforcement, was resistant to change.

Treatment Process

Behavioral family therapy is a treatment approach that includes the following four steps: problem assessment, family (parent) education, specific treatment design, and treatment goal evaluation. It begins with a thorough assessment of the presenting family problem. This assessment process involves gathering the following information from the family: what circumstances immediately precede the problem behavior; how family members react to the exhibition of the client's problem behavior; how frequently the misbehavior occurs; and how intense the misbehavior is. Behavioral family therapy differs from individual behavior therapy in that all family members are typically involved in the assessment process. As a part of the assessment process, the behavioral family therapist often observes the way in which the family handles the presenting problem. This observation is conducted to obtain firsthand information regarding ways the family may be unknowingly reinforcing the problem or otherwise poorly handling the client's misbehavior.

Following the assessment, the behavioral family therapist, with input from family members, establishes treatment goals. These treatment goals should be operationalized; that is, they should be specifically stated so that they may be easily observed and measured. In the example of John, the boy who refused to sleep in his own bed, an operationalized treatment goal would be as follows: "John will be able to sleep from 9:00 p.m. to 6:00 a.m. in his own bed without interrupting his parents during the night."

Applying Learning Theory Principles

Once treatment goals have been operationalized, the next stage involves designing an intervention to correct the behavioral problem. The treatment procedure follows from the basic learning principles previously discussed. In cases involving parent-child problems, the behavioral family therapist educates the parents in learning theory principles as they apply to the treatment of behavioral problems. Three basic learning principles are explained to the child's parents. First, positive reinforcement should be withdrawn from the unwanted behavior. For example, a parent who meets the demands of a screaming preschooler who throws a temper tantrum in the checkout line of the grocery store because he or she wants a piece of candy is unwittingly reinforcing the child's screaming behavior. Time-out is one procedure used to remove the undesired reinforcement from a child's misbehavior. Using time-out involves making a child sit in a corner or other nonreinforcing place for a specified period of time (typically, one minute for each year of the child's age).

Second, appropriate behavior that is incompatible with the undesired behavior should be positively reinforced. In the case of the screaming preschooler, this would involve rewarding him or her for acting correctly. An appropriate reinforcer in this case would be giving the child the choice of a candy bar if the child were quiet and cooperative during grocery shopping, behavior inconsistent with a temper tantrum. For positive reinforcement to have its maximum benefit, before the specific activity (for example, grocery shopping) the child should be informed about what is expected and what reward will be received for fulfilling these responsibilities. This process is called contingency management because the promised reward is made contingent on the child's acting in a prescribed manner. In addition, the positive reinforcement should be given as close to the completion of the appropriate behavior as possible.

Third, aversive consequences should be applied when the problem behavior recurs. When the child engages in the misbehavior, he or she should consistently experience negative costs. In this regard, response cost is a useful technique because it involves taking something away or making the child do something unrewarding as a way of making misbehavior have a cost. For example, the preschooler who has a temper tantrum in the checkout line may have a favorite dessert, which he or she had previously selected while in the store, taken away as the cost for throwing a temper tantrum. As with positive reinforcement, response cost should be applied as quickly as possible following the misbehavior in order for it to produce its maximum effect.

Designing Treatment Intervention

Once parents receive instruction regarding the principles of behavior therapy, they are actively involved in the process of designing a specific intervention to address their child's behavior problems. The behavioral family therapist relates to the parents as cotherapists with the hope that this approach will increase the parents' involvement in the treatment process. In relating to Mr. and Mrs. Williams as cotherapists, for example, the behavioral family therapist would have the couple design a treatment intervention to correct John's misbehavior. Following the previously described principles, the couple might arrive at the following approach: They would refuse to give in to John's demands to sleep with them; John would receive a token for each night he slept in his own bed (after earning a certain number of tokens, he could exchange them for toys); and John would be required to go to bed fifteen minutes earlier the following night for each time he asked to sleep with his parents.

Once the intervention has been implemented, the therapist, together with the parents, monitors the results of the treatment. This monitoring process involves assessing the degree to which the established treatment goals are being met. For example, in the case of the Williams family, the treatment goal was to reduce the number of times that John attempted to get into bed with his parents. Therapy progress, therefore, would be measured by counting the number of times that John attempted to get into bed with his parents. Careful assessment of an intervention's results is essential to determine whether the intervention is accomplishing its goal.

Detractions

In spite of its popularity, this type of therapy has not been without its critics. For example, behavioral family therapists' explanations regarding the causes of family problems differ from those given by the advocates of other family therapies. One major difference is that behavioral family therapists are accused of taking a linear (as compared to a circular) view of causality. From a linear perspective, misbehavior occurs because A causes B and B causes C. Those who endorse a circular view of causality, however, assert that this simplistic perspective is inadequate in explaining why misbehavior occurs. Taking a circular perspective involves identifying multiple factors that may be operating at the same time to determine the reason for a particular misbehavior. For example, from a linear view of causality, John's misbehavior is seen as the result of being reinforced for sleeping with his parents. According to a circular perspective, however, John's behavior may be the result of many factors, all possibly occurring together, such as his parents' marital problems or his genetic predisposition toward insecurity.

Integration with Other Therapies

Partially in response to this criticism, attempts have been made to integrate behavioral family therapy with other types of family therapy. Another major purpose of integrative efforts is to address the resistance often encountered from families during treatment. Therapeutic resistance is a family's continued attempt to handle the presenting problem in a maladaptive manner in spite of having learned better ways. In the past, behavioral family therapists gave limited attention to dealing with family resistance; however, behavioral family therapy has attempted to improve its ability to handle resistance by incorporating some of the techniques used by other types of family therapy.

In conclusion, numerous research studies have demonstrated that behavioral family therapy is an effective treatment of family problems. One of the major strengths of this type of therapy is its willingness to assess objectively its effectiveness in treating family problems. Because of its emphasis on experimentation, behavioral family therapy continues to adapt by modifying its techniques to address the problems of the modern family.

—*R. Christopher Qualls*

References

Crisp, Bryan, and David Knox. *Behavioral Family Therapy: An Evidence Based Approach*. Carolina Academic Press, 2009.

Friedberg, Robert D. "A Cognitive-Behavioral Approach to Family Therapy." *Journal of Contemporary Psychotherapy*, vol. 36, no. 4, 2006, pp. 159–165., doi:10.1007/s10879-006-9020-2.

Gladding, Samuel T. *Family Therapy: History, Theory, and Practice*. 7th ed., Pearson, 2019.

Goldenberg, Irene, et al. *Family Therapy: An Overview*. 9th ed., Cengage Learning, 2017.

Patterson, Terence. "A Cognitive Behavioral Systems Approach to Family Therapy." *Journal of Family Psychotherapy*, vol. 25, no. 2, 2014, pp. 132–144., doi:10.1080/08975353.2014.910023.

Tuerk, Elena Hontoria, et al. "Collaboration in Family Therapy." *Journal of Clinical Psychology*, vol. 68, no. 2, 2012, pp. 168–178., doi:10.1002/jclp.21833.

Zarnaghash, Maryam, et al. "The Influence of Family Therapy on Marital Conflicts." *Procedia - Social and Behavioral Sciences*, vol. 84, 2013, pp. 1838–1844., doi:10.1016/j.sbspro.2013.07.044.

■ Benzodiazepines

CATEGORY: Class of Drug; Muscle Relaxant; Sedative
ALSO KNOWN AS: Bars, Benzos, Blues, Chill Pills, Downers, Nerve Pills, Planks, Tranks, and Zannies
ANATOMY OR SYSTEM AFFECTED: Central nervous system

KEY TERMS

- *anticonvulsant*: a medication that prevents or relieves the spontaneous movements of convulsions
- *hypnotic*: a medication that brings about a state of partial or complete unconsciousness
- *psychotropic*: a drug that affects psychic function, behavior, or experience
- *sedative*: a medication that has a soothing or tranquilizing effect

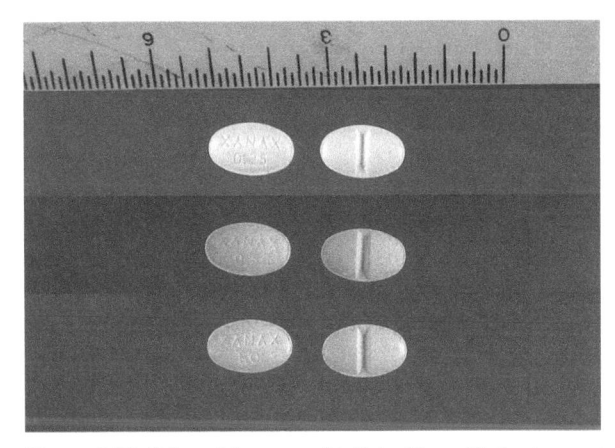

Xanax 0.25, 0.5 and 1 mg scored tablets. (Drug Enforcement Agency)

The benzodiazepines are chemically similar psychotropic medications used as muscle relaxants, sedatives, and anticonvulsants. They have potent hypnotic and sedative actions, and are used typically as anti-anxiety and sleep-inducing medications. Side effects may or may not be of importance for a particular patient. A course of treatment with benzodiazepines should not exceed four months.

Benzodiazepines

The benzodiazepines are chemically similar psychotropic medications used as muscle relaxants, sedatives, and anticonvulsants. They have potent hypnotic and sedative actions, and are used typically as anti-anxiety and sleep-inducing medications. Side effects may or may not be of importance for a particular patient. Because of their modes of action, benzodiazepine use can result in impaired psychomotor performance, the ability to carry out conscious movements and motions. This effect may remain when use of the drug is discontinued, a condition known as depressed rebound, in which the recovery of psychomotor performance is not 100 percent complete after use of the drug is discontinued. Some decreased ability continues to be observed and experienced. Benzodiazepine use may also produce amnesia and the sense of euphoria. At worst, a patient may develop dependence on benzodiazepine drugs as an addiction risk.

The risks and effects associated with the use of benzodiazepines demand that a course of treatment with benzodiazepines should not exceed four months.

Interactions

Grapefruit juice: Grapefruit juice slows the body's normal breakdown of several drugs, including some benzodiazepines, allowing them to build up to potentially dangerous levels in the blood. This effect can last for three days or more following the last glass of juice. Because of this risk, if one takes benzodiazepines, the safest approach is to avoid grapefruit juice altogether.

Hops, kava, passionflower, valerian: The herb kava (*Piper methysticum*) has a sedative effect and is used for anxiety and insomnia. Combining kava with drugs in the benzodiazepine family, which possess similar effects, could result in "add-on" or excessive physical depression, sedation, and impairment.

Experimental studies suggest that kava, similarly to benzodiazepines, exerts its sedative effects at binding sites in the brain called GABA receptors.

Other herbs with a sedative effect that might cause problems when combined with benzodiazepines include ashwagandha (*Withania somnifera*), calendula (*Calendula officinalis*), catnip (*Nepeta cataria*), hops (*Humulus lupulus*), lady's slipper (*Cypripedium*), lemon balm (*Melissa officinalis*), passionflower (*Passiflora incarnata*), sassafras (*Sassafras officinale*), skullcap (*Scutellaria lateriflora*), valerian (*Valeriana officinalis*), and yerba mansa (*Anemopsis californica*). Because of the potentially serious consequences, one should avoid combining these herbs with benzodiazepines or other drugs that also have sedative or depressant effects unless advised by one's physician.

Melatonin: Melatonin is a natural hormone that regulates sleep. Many people who take conventional sleeping pills (most of which are in the benzodiazepine family) find it difficult to quit. The reason is that when one tries to stop the medication, one may experience severe insomnia or interrupted sleep.

Warning: It can be dangerous to stop using benzodiazepines if one has taken them for a while. Consult a physician before trying melatonin to help handle benzodiazepine withdrawal or before trying to stop benzodiazepine medication under any conditions.

Pregnenolone: The hormone pregnenolone is widely sold as a kind of "fountain of youth." However, the only direct evidence that pregnenolone supplements have any effect relates to a potential interaction between the hormone and benzodiazepine drugs. Regular use of pregnenolone was found to greatly decrease the sedative effects of diazepam (Valium).

The reasons for this interaction are not known. However, people who rely upon benzodiazepine drugs may find them less effective if pregnenolone is added into the mix.

Kava (withdrawal): Although they are highly effective for anxiety, benzodiazepine drugs can cause unpleasant and dangerous withdrawal symptoms when they are discontinued. Use of kava can significantly reduce withdrawal symptoms and help to maintain control of anxiety. Close medical supervision and very gradual tapering of benzodiazepine dosages is required. Persons should not discontinue anti-anxiety medications except on the advice of a physician, as withdrawal symptoms can be life threatening.

—*Richard M. Renneboog, MSc*

References

Agarwal, Sumit D., and Bruce E. Landon. "Patterns in Outpatient Benzodiazepine Prescribing in the United States." *JAMA Network Open*, vol. 2, no. 1, 25 Jan. 2019, doi:10.1001/jamanetworkopen.2018.7399.

"Benzodiazepines (and the Alternatives)." *Harvard Health Publishing*, Harvard Medical School, 15 Mar. 2019, www.health.harvard.edu/mind-and-mood/benzodiazepines_and_the_alternatives.

Cheatle, Martin D., and Rachel Shmuts. "The Risk and Benefit of Benzodiazepine Use in Patients with Chronic Pain." *Pain Medicine*, vol. 16, no. 2, 2015, pp. 219–221., doi:10.1111/pme.12674.

Cunningham, Julie, et al. "Benzodiazepine Use in Patients with Chronic Pain in an Interdisciplinary Pain Rehabilitation Program." *Journal of Pain Research*, vol. 10, 2017, pp. 311–317., doi:10.2147/jpr.s123487.

Gauntlett-Gilbert, Jeremy, et al. "Benzodiazepines May Be Worse Than Opioids." *The Clinical Journal of Pain*, vol. 32, no. 4, 2016, pp. 285–291., doi:10.1097/ajp.0000000000000253.

Nordqvist, Joseph. "Benzodiazepines: Uses, Types, Side Effects, and Risks." *Medical News Today*, MediLexicon International, 7 Mar. 2019, www.medicalnewstoday.com/articles/262809.php.

Rapaport, Lisa. "Use of Benzodiazepines for Pain Rising in US." *Psychiatry & Behavioral Health Learning Network*, 1 Feb. 2019, www.psychcongress.com/news/use-benzodiazepines-pain-rising-us.

St. Michael's Hospital. "Dangerous Increases in Patients Mixing Opioids, Benzodiazepines or Z-Drugs." *ScienceDaily*, 17 Jan. 2019, www.sciencedaily.com/releases/2019/01/190117090455.htm.

■ Bupropion

CATEGORY: Antidepressant
ALSO KNOWN AS: Wellbutrin; Zyban

History of Use

Bupropion is a widely prescribed antidepressant, at one time the fourth-most prescribed antidepressant in the United States. It was invented in 1969 by GlaxoSmithKline (then Burroughs Wellcome) and was designed and synthesized by Nariman Mehta. It was approved as an antidepressant in 1985 by the US Food and Drug Administration, withdrawn in 1986 because of concerns over seizures, and reintroduced to the market in 1989, after the maximum dosage was adjusted. Bupropion was approved in 1997 as an aid for smoking cessation (under the name Zyban). Under the name Wellbutrin XL, it has also been approved to treat seasonal affective disorder, a mood disorder prevalent in either the winter or the summer months.

Treatment

Patients are instructed to start taking bupropion one week before they plan to stop smoking. It takes about one week for this medication to reach adequate levels in a person's system, and patients are instructed to target a specific quit date during the second week that they are taking bupropion. If a dose is missed, patients are instructed to skip it and to stay with their regular dosing schedule. Taking too much bupropion at one time can cause seizures.

Effects and Potential Risks

Most people do not have side effects from taking bupropion for smoking cessation. If side effects do occur, they can usually be minimized. In addition, side effects are most often temporary, lasting only as long as one is taking the medication.

There are rare but serious side effects that patients should be aware of. In some people, medications like bupropion may cause severe mood and behavior changes, including suicidal thoughts. Young adults may be more at risk for these side effects.

Other side effects include anxiety; buzzing or ringing in the ears; headache (severe); and skin rash, hives, or itching. Side effects that may occur frequently or become bothersome include abdominal pain, constipation, decrease in appetite,

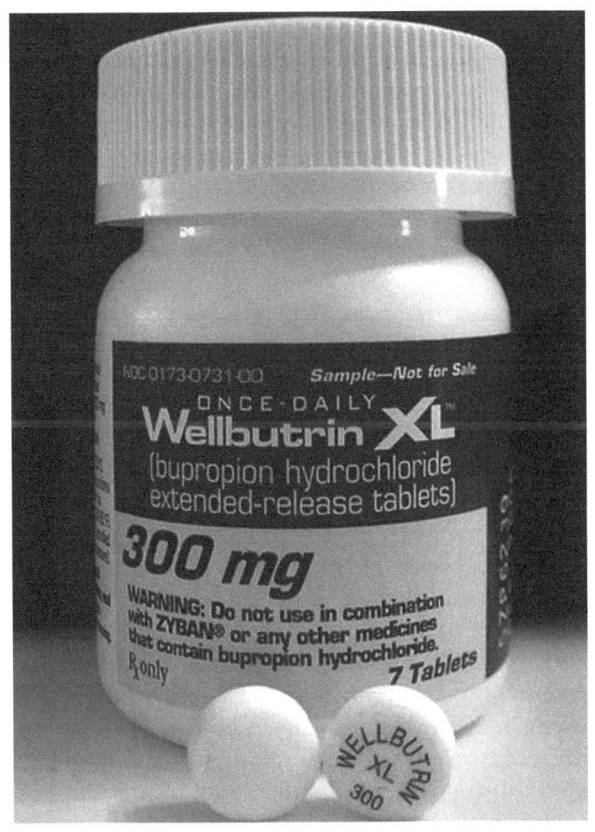

The antidepressant Wellbutrin XL (bupropion HCl, 300mg): bottle and tablets. (via Wikimedia Commons)

dizziness, dry mouth, increased sweating, nausea or vomiting, trembling or shaking, insomnia, and weight loss.

Symptoms of an overdose may be more severe than side effects seen at regular doses, or two or more side effects may occur together. They include fast heartbeat, hallucinations, loss of consciousness, nausea or vomiting (or both), and seizures.

Bupropion should not be combined with other medications that lower the threshold for seizures. These medications include theophylline, antipsychotic medications, antidepressants, Tramadol (Ultram), Tamoxifen, steroids, diabetes drugs, and Ritonavir.

—Karen Schroeder Kassel, MS, RD, Med

References

Ahmadi, Jamshid, et al. "A Randomized Clinical Trial on the Effects of Bupropion and Buprenorphine on the Reduction of Methamphetamine Craving." *Trials*, vol. 20, no. 1, 30 July 2019, doi:10.1186/s13063-019-3554-6.

Blokdijk, G. J. *Bupropion: 523 Questions to Ask That Matter to You*. CreateSpace Independent Publishing Platform, 2018.

Bortolato, Beatrice, et al. "Cognitive Remission: a Novel Objective for the Treatment of Major Depression?" *BMC Medicine*, vol. 14, no. 1, 22 Jan. 2016, doi:10.1186/s12916-016-0560-3.

"Bupropion: MedlinePlus Drug Information." *MedlinePlus*, U.S. National Library of Medicine, 15 Feb. 2015, medlineplus.gov/druginfo/meds/a695033.html.

Li, Dian-Jeng, et al. "Significant Treatment Effect of Bupropion in Patients With Bipolar Disorder but Similar Phase-Shifting Rate as Other Antidepressants." *Medicine*, vol. 95, no. 13, Mar. 2016, doi:10.1097/md.0000000000003165.

Patel, Krisna, et al. "Bupropion: a Systematic Review and Meta-Analysis of Effectiveness as an Antidepressant." *Therapeutic Advances in Psychopharmacology*, vol. 6, no. 2, 2016, pp. 99–144., doi:10.1177/2045125316629071.

Rzepa, Ewelina, et al. "Bupropion Administration Increases Resting-State Functional Connectivity in Dorso-Medial Prefrontal Cortex." *International Journal of Neuropsychopharmacology*, vol. 20, no. 6, 11 Mar. 2017, pp. 455–462., doi:10.1093/ijnp/pyx016.

Tort, Sera, and Adrian Preda. "How Does Bupropion Compare with Placebo for Preventing Seasonal Affective Disorder (SAD)?" *Cochrane Clinical Answers*, 2019, doi:10.1002/cca.2226.

Yasin, Waqas, et al. "Does Bupropion Impact More than Mood? A Case Report and Review of the Literature." *Cureus*, vol. 11, no. 3, 19 Mar. 2019, doi:10.7759/cureus.4277.

■ Chronic pain management: psychological impact

CATEGORY: Physiotherapy; Psychotherapy

Introduction

A pain free life is something that most of us take for granted. Pain is a phenomenon that we experience in episodes such as falling off a ladder, breaking an arm, or waking up with a headache from too much champagne the previous night. Most experiences of pain are short lived and diminish quickly over time. Our ideas of health and wellness often revolve around the absence of pain; therefore overall well-being can be quantified by the level of pain experienced on a daily basis.

With lack of pain topping the list of what defines a healthy life, those who suffer from chronic pain may struggle with even the most mundane of tasks. It has been estimated that 1.5 billion people suffer from chronic pain conditions in the world on a daily basis. In the United States, chronic pain has been suggested to be the top cause of people seeking medical attention, costing an annual average of $100 billion in health care. The magnitude of this problem is vast and can be extremely complicated due to the challenge in understanding the cause, diagnosis, and methods to treat chronic pain. It is necessary for knowledge to spread in order to support those around us who battle pain every day of their lives.

Chronic Pain

Chronic pain can be described as mild to severe pain which has been present for six months or longer. This pain can be due to an injury, illness, or a specific chronic pain diagnosis such as fibromyalgia. It has been estimated that approximately 100 million American adults are living with chronic pain. The impact of chronic pain can vary as much as the severity from something as mild as a headache or as severe as debilitating, widespread pain. People dealing with these symptoms often experience an overall change or challenge to their abilities and functioning level. This impact also will vary with the severity and frequency that the person experiences the pain symptoms. Chronic headaches may occur once a month and require the person to take the day off work, while a person with fibromyalgia or lupus may be rendered disabled. Because pain is a non-tangible, subjective, and personal experience it can be challenging to determine the necessary treatment and level of disability. This is the reason that chronic pain is often undiagnosed, misdiagnosed, or ignored for long periods of time.

Types and Sources of Chronic Pain

As previously stated, chronic pain ranges in severity, frequency, and duration. The source of pain may be known as in the instance of injury. It could be the result of an illness that was either cured or uncured. Diabetes is a common cause of chronic pain affecting 25 million Americans. In other instances such as chronic joint pain or headaches, the root of the pain may not be identified. Regardless of whether the cause of the chronic pain is known or unknown, it can be classified by the level of disturbance to one's overall functioning and ability to participate in previously enjoyable activities. People often seek medical attention when pain becomes overwhelming or negatively impacts their lives, such as difficulty performing work requirements or household tasks.

Diagnosis

Because pain is a subjective experience, medical professionals often find it a challenge to accurately diagnosis chronic pain. Medical professionals must rely on the patient's self-description of pain to determine how to explore causes and treatments. Because each person will have different ways in which he or she experiences and describes pain, diagnosing chronic pain is often a difficult task. It may take many years to arrive at an accurate diagnosis and correct treatment. For patients suffering from widespread chronic pain like fibromyalgia, this is a common occurrence. These individuals often tell stories of many years of seeking out numerous doctors and specialists without any relief. Each doctor may have a different option or hypothesis of what is causing the pain which leads down different diagnostic and treatment paths. Exploring these different avenues can take months or even years to rule out specific disorders and may cause increased stress on the person who is experiencing chronic pain. Due to the burden of searching for help, including the variety of interventions and treatments attempted, the person may even give up before finding any relief.

Psychological Impact

Chronic pain is linked to many psychological issues, especially depression and anxiety. People suffering from long lasting pain may experience intense emotional distress based on both physical and emotional impacts. The physical experience of pain links to the stress of a constant search for a cure, doctor's appointments, and the participation in both Western medicine and/or Eastern holistic treatments. The management of care can itself cause extensive emotional stress including time and financial burden. Even the least invasive of treatments can be pricey, leaving people with chronic pain constantly paying for care, and the cost of medical bills alone can put people into financial hardship, adding further stress and forcing the need to make difficult decisions regarding how to manage care.

Based on the severity and frequency of the chronic pain the person may have difficulty keeping regular employment, and chronic pain is a common reason people file for disability.

The emotional strife of dealing with chronic pain can lead to further and more severe mental struggles. Depression, anxiety, and long-lasting fatigue can decrease the body's ability to produce natural painkillers. Therefore, the experience of chronic pain coupled with psychological struggle can exacerbate pain's severity, frequency, and duration. As chronic pain adds to emotional turmoil, it also leads to a breakdown of the immune system needed to fight disease. Those suffering with chronic pain are more susceptible to other common illnesses such as cold or flu. As this negative cycle continues, the person dealing with chronic pain is apt to become even more depressed, anxious, angry, and fatigued. The psychological impact of chronic pain will vary for each person based on many biopsychosocial factors. Unfortunately for those experiencing chronic pain, the physical pain and emotional strife seem to influence the other, and as the physical pain worsens the psychological struggle may also worsen.

Psychological Treatment
Although chronic pain patients are often in search of a cure to their suffering, most treatment plans only have the ability to stabilize and manage the pain. As this news often comes with extreme disappointment and sadness, emotional support and mental health counseling can be very beneficial. Coping with the loss of living a pain-free life can put the chronic pain sufferer into an intense depression accompanied with anger and anxiety. Because chronic pain is an invisible ailment it is often overlooked or not understood by others. Even people closest to the individual experiencing chronic pain may not be able to understand the extent of struggle the person is experiencing. This may come across as invalidating or hurtful to the person suffering and may create further difficulties. On the other hand, even if family, friends, and employers are supportive they may still not have the ability to fully comprehend the limitations that the person is feeling. It can be hard to quantify the level of debilitation that chronic fatigue or headaches may cause. A person experiencing chronic pain may feel very alone in his or her suffering. Therefore, having a therapist, counselor, or support group is very important. Finding others to share the struggle greatly alleviates the emotional turmoil these people are feeling. Moreover, support groups are know to be beneficial because having the ability to discuss and process the challenge of managing chronic pain validates the chronic pain experience and serves as a source of pain management solutions. Thus, in addition to any medical or holistic treatment options offered, mental health support is also recommended as part of treatment. Taking an all-encompassing holistic approach is the most inclusive arena for helping the person suffering with chronic pain.

Because chronic pain is generally not a curable condition, the treatment goal revolves around helping the person return to a normal level of functioning. This includes being able to manage daily routines such as work, household management, and recreational activities. Again this will vary for each person and will be measured by the individual experiencing the pain.

Medications and Surgery
Common treatments of chronic pain include pain medications and nerve-blocking medications. Medical professionals may recommend anything from aspirin to prescription narcotics. Nerve-blocking medications are often used to treat fibromyalgia which is known to cause overactive and oversensitive nerves resulting in chronic pain. Often people who experience migraines or suffer from diabetes are on a regiment of medications to manage symptoms. In some cases surgeries or electrical stimulations are used when medications do not prove to be effective. These more invasive options range in effectiveness and may leave the individual deeply disappointed if they do not alleviate symptoms.

Surgery is a common option for those experiencing chronic back pain. These invasive surgeries can result in pain and long recoveries; however, the possibility of reduced pain motivates many individuals to choose this option.

Holistic Treatments

Many people in the United States begin their treatment with traditional Western medicine options. Along with medication or surgery, rehabilitation such as physical therapy are often the next prescribed treatment. Physical therapy is most common when suffering occurs from a known injury that precipitates the chronic pain. Physical therapy may include stretching, strengthening, muscle stimulation, and other types of rehabilitation.

Another avenue often explored by those suffering with chronic pain is Eastern or holistic medicine. Treatments include acupuncture, acupressure, biofeedback, chiropractic manipulation, massage therapy, and relaxation therapies. These alternative treatments are often used in conjunction with Western treatments. Other areas often explored are nutritional and exercise impacts and benefits. Meeting with nutritionists and exercise specialists can be extremely beneficial in managing chronic pain. Dietitians create diet plans for individuals experiencing chronic pain by including and excluding certain foods that may impact pain levels. Exercise is also suggested based on the person's mobility. Low impact exercise such as swimming, walking, or Thai Chi may be recommended. Overall, health care professionals agree that maintaining health, including a balanced body weight and nutrition, has a large impact on the management of chronic pain.

Self-Management

As an individual journeys from being diagnosed with chronic pain to managing a treatment plan, he or she will need to take the driver's seat. It is very important for these individuals to self-manage care, because chronic pain is a unique and individual experience for each person. Doctors and health care professionals may have a variety of ideas to assist their patients, but a patient must be assertive in what has worked and what has not. Chronic pain sufferers also need to advocate for themselves through research and willingness to try different avenues of pain management. It is important to be educated in their unique issues and keep track of how different treatments, foods, exercise, and medication impact pain level. As their own self-care managers, patients have the ability to join a community of others who also experience and understand chronic pain, increase their knowledge of chronic pain, and find the best options for managing levels of pain and psychological distress.

—*Kimberly Ortiz*

References

"Chronic Pain and Mental Health: Mental Health America." *Mental Health America*, 2019, www.mhanational.org/chronic-pain-and-mental-health.

Crofford, Leslie J. "Psychological Aspects of Chronic Musculoskeletal Pain." *Best Practice & Research Clinical Rheumatology*, vol. 29, no. 1, 2015, pp. 147–155., doi:10.1016/j.berh.2015.04.027.

Duenas, María, et al. "A Review of Chronic Pain Impact on Patients, Their Social Environment and the Health Care System." *Journal of Pain Research*, vol. 9, 2016, pp. 457–467., doi:10.2147/jpr.s105892.

Fine, Perry G. "Long-Term Consequences of Chronic Pain: Mounting Evidence for Pain as a Neurological Disease and Parallels with Other Chronic Disease States." *Pain Medicine*, vol. 12, no. 7, 2011, pp. 996–1004., doi:10.1111/j.1526-4637.2011.01187.x.

Kaplan, Gary, and Donna Beech. *Total Recovery: Solving the Mystery of Chronic Pain and Depression: How We Get Sick, Why We Stay Sick, How We Can Recover.* Rodale Books, 2015.

Moyle, Sally. "The Emotional and Psychological Impacts of Chronic Pain." *Ausmed*, 2 Feb. 2016, www.ausmed.com/cpd/articles/chronic-pain-emotional-psychological-impacts.

Shuchang, He, et al. "Emotional and Neurobehavioural Status in Chronic Pain Patients." *Pain Research and Management*, vol. 16, no. 1, 2011, pp. 41–43., doi:10.1155/2011/825636.

Turk, Dennis C., et al. "Assessment of Psychosocial and Functional Impact of Chronic Pain." *The Journal of Pain*, vol. 17, no. 9, 2016, doi:10.1016/j.jpain.2016.02.006.

Cognitive Behavior Therapy (CBT)

CATEGORY: Therapy or Technique; Psychotherapy

Introduction

The cognitive behavior therapies are not a single therapeutic approach, but rather a loosely organized collection of therapeutic approaches that share a similar set of assumptions. At their core, cognitive behavior therapies share three fundamental propositions: Cognitive activity affects behavior; cognitive activity may be monitored and altered; and desired behavior change may be effected through cognitive change.

The first of the three fundamental propositions of cognitive behavior therapy suggests that it is not the external situation that determines feelings and behavior, but rather the person's view or perception of that external situation that determines feelings and behavior. For example, if a person has failed the first examination of a course, that individual could appraise it as a temporary setback to be overcome or as a horrible loss. Although the situation remains the same, the thinking about that situation is radically different in the two examples cited. Each of these views will lead to significantly different emotions and behaviors.

The third cognitive behavioral assumption suggests that desired behavior change may be effected through cognitive change. Therefore, although cognitive behavior theorists do not reject the notion that rewards and punishment (reinforcement contingencies) can alter behavior, they are more likely to emphasize that there are alternative methods for behavior change, one in particular being cognitive change. Many approaches to therapy fall within the scope of cognitive behavior therapy as it is defined here. Although these approaches share the theoretical assumptions described, a review of the major therapeutic procedures subsumed under the heading of cognitive behavior therapy reveals a diverse amalgam of principles and procedures, representing a variety of theoretical and philosophical perspectives.

Rational emotive therapy, developed by psychologist Albert Ellis, is regarded by many as one of the premier examples of the cognitive behavioral approach; it was introduced in the early 1960s. Ellis proposed that many people are made unhappy by their faulty, irrational beliefs, which influence the way they interpret events. The therapist interacts with patients, attempting to direct patients to more positive and realistic views. Cognitive therapy, pioneered by Aaron T. Beck, has been applied to such problems as depression and stress. For stress reduction, ideas and thoughts that are producing stress in the patient are identified, and the therapist then gets the patient to examine the validity of these thoughts. Working together, they restructure thought processes so that the situations seem less stressful. Cognitive therapy has been found to be quite effective in treating depression, as compared with other therapeutic methods. Beck held that depression is caused by certain types of negative thoughts, such as devaluing the self or viewing the future in a consistently pessimistic way.

Rational behavior therapy, developed by psychiatrist Maxie Maultsby, is a close relative of Ellis's rational emotive therapy. In this approach, Maultsby combines several approaches to include rational emotive therapy, neuropsychology, classical and operant conditioning, and psychosomatic research; however, Maultsby was primarily influenced by his association with Ellis. In this approach, Maultsby attempts to couch his theory of emotional disturbance in terms of neuropsychophysiology and learning theory. Rational behavior therapy assumes that repeated pairings of a perception with evaluative thoughts lead to rational or irrational emotive and behavioral reactions. Maultsby suggests that self-talk, which originates in the left hemisphere of the brain, triggers corresponding right-hemisphere emotional equivalents. Therefore, to maintain a state of psychological health, individuals must practice rational self-talk that will, in turn, cause the right brain to convert left-brain language into appropriate emotional and behavioral reactions.

Rational behavior therapy techniques are quite similar to those of rational emotive therapy. Both therapies stress the importance of monitoring one's thoughts to become aware of the elements of the emotional disturbance. In addition, Maultsby advocates the use of rational emotive imagery, behavioral practice, and relaxation methods to minimize emotional distress.

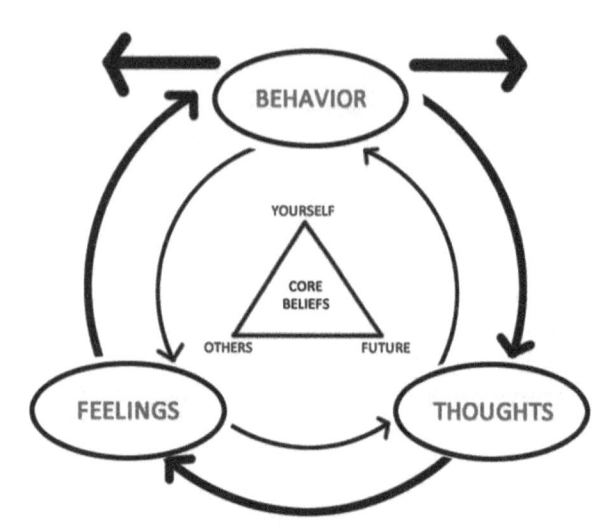

In couples therapy, the practitioner evaluates the couple's personal and relationship story as it is narrated, interrupts wisely, facilitates both de-escalation of unhelpful conflict and the development of realistic, practical solutions. (fizkes via iStock)

Self-Instructional Training

Self-instructional training was developed by psychologist Donald Meichenbaum in the early 1970s. In contrast to Ellis and Beck, whose prior training was in psychoanalysis, Meichenbaum's roots were in behaviorism and the behavioral therapies. Therefore, Meichenbaum's approach is heavily couched in behavioral terminology and procedures. Meichenbaum's work stems from his earlier research in training schizophrenic patients to emit "healthy speech." By chance, Meichenbaum observed that patients who engaged in spontaneous self-instruction were less distracted and demonstrated superior task performance on a variety of tasks. As a result, Meichenbaum emphasizes the critical role of "self-instructions"—simple instructions such as "Relax... Just attend to the task"—and their noticeable effect on subsequent behavior.

Meichenbaum developed self-instructional training to treat the deficits in self-instructions manifested in impulsive children. The ultimate goal of this program was to decrease impulsive behavior. The way to accomplish this goal, as hypothesized by Meichenbaum, was to train impulsive children to generate verbal self-commands and to respond to their verbal self-commands and to encourage the children to self-reinforce their behavior appropriately.

The specific procedures employed in self-instructional training involve having the child observe a model performing a task. While the model is performing the task, he or she is talking aloud. The child then performs the same task while the model gives verbal instructions. Subsequently, the child performs the task while instructing himself or herself aloud, then while whispering the instructions. Finally, the child performs the task while silently thinking the instructions. The self-instructions employed in the program included questions about the nature and demands of the task, answers to these questions in the form of cognitive rehearsal, self-instructions in the form of self-guidance while performing the task, and self-reinforcement. Meichenbaum and his associates have found that this self-instructional training program significantly improves the task performance of impulsive children across a number of measures.

Systematic Rational Restructuring

Systematic rational restructuring is a cognitive behavioral procedure developed by psychologist Marvin Goldfried in the mid-1970s. This procedure is a variation on Ellis's rational emotive therapy; however, it is more clearly structured than Ellis's method. In systematic rational restructuring, Goldfried suggests that early social learning experiences teach individuals to label situations in different ways. Further, Goldfried suggests that emotional reactions may be understood as responses to the way individuals label situations, as opposed to responses to the situations themselves. The goal of systematic rational restructuring is to train clients to perceive situational cues more accurately.

The process of systematic rational restructuring is similar to systematic desensitization, in which a subject is to imagine fearful scenes in a graduated order from the least fear-provoking to the most fear-provoking scenes. In systematic rational restructuring, the client is asked to imagine a hierarchy of anxiety-eliciting situations. At each step, the client is instructed to identify irrational thoughts associated with the specific situation, to dispute them, and to reevaluate the situation more rationally. In addition, clients are instructed to practice rational restructuring in specific real-life situations.

Stress Inoculation

Stress inoculation training incorporates several of the specific therapies already described. This procedure was developed by Meichenbaum. Stress inoculation training is analogous to being inoculated against disease. That is, it prepares clients to deal with stress-inducing events by teaching them to use coping skills at low levels of the stressful situation and then gradually to cope with more and more stressful situations. Stress inoculation training involves three phases: conceptualization, skill acquisition and rehearsal, and application and follow-through.

In the conceptualization phase of stress inoculation training, clients are given an adaptive way of viewing and understanding their negative reactions to stressful events. In the skills-acquisition and rehearsal phase, clients learn coping skills appropriate to the type of stress they are experiencing. With interpersonal anxiety, the client might develop skills that would make the feared situation less threatening (for example, learning to initiate and maintain conversations). The client might also learn deep muscle relaxation to lessen tension. In the case of anger, clients learn to view potential provocations as problems that require a solution rather than as threats that require an attack. Clients are also taught to rehearse alternative strategies for solving the problem at hand.

The application and follow-through phase of stress inoculation training involves the clients practicing and applying the coping skills. Initially, clients are exposed to low levels of stressful situations in imagery. They practice applying their coping skills to handle the stressful events, and they overtly role-play dealing with stressful events. Next, clients are given homework assignments that involve gradual exposure to actual stressful events in their everyday life. Stress inoculation training has been effectively applied to many types of problems. It has been used to help people cope with anger, anxiety, fear, pain, and health-related problems (for example, cancer and hypertension). It appears to be suitable for all age levels.

Problem-Solving Therapy

Problem-solving therapy, as developed by psychologists Thomas D'Zurilla and Goldfried, is also considered one of the cognitive behavioral approaches. In essence, problem-solving therapy is the application of problem-solving theory and research to the domain of personal and emotional problems. Indeed, the authors see the ability to solve problems as the necessary and sufficient condition for emotional and behavioral stability. Problem solving is, in one way or another, a part of all psychotherapies.

Cognitive behavior therapists have taught general problem-solving skills to clients with two specific aims: to alleviate the particular personal problems for which clients have sought therapy and to provide clients with a general coping strategy for personal problems.

Clients are given steps of problem solving that they are taught to carry out systematically. First, clients need to define the dilemma as a problem to be solved. Next, they must select a goal that reflects the ultimate outcome they desire. Clients then generate a list of many different possible solutions, without evaluating their potential merit (a kind of brainstorming). They then evaluate the pros and cons of each alternative in terms of the probability that it will meet the goal selected and its practicality, which involves considering the potential consequences of each solution to themselves and to others. They rank the alternative solutions in terms of desirability and practicality and select the highest one. Next, they try to implement the chosen solution. Finally, clients evaluate the therapy, assessing whether the solution alleviated the problem and met the goal, and if not, what went wrong—in other words, which of the steps in problem solving needs to be redone.

Problem-solving therapies have been used to treat a variety of target behaviors with a wide range of clients. Examples include peer relationship difficulties among children and adolescents, examination and interpersonal anxiety among college students, relapse following a program to reduce smoking, harmony among family members, and the ability of chronic psychiatric patients to cope with interpersonal problems.

Self-Control Therapy

Self-control therapy for depression, developed by psychologist Lynn Rehm, is an approach to treating depression that combines the self-regulatory notions of behavior therapy and the cognitive focus of the cognitive behavioral approaches. Essentially, Rehm believes that depressed people show deficits in one or some combination of the following areas: monitoring (selectively attending to negative events), self-evaluation (setting unrealistically high goals), and self-reinforcement (emitting high rates of self-punishment and low rates of self-reward). These three components are further broken down into a total of six functional areas.

According to Rehm, the varied symptom picture in clinically depressed clients is a function of different subsets of these deficits. Over the course of therapy with clients, each of the six self-control deficits is described, with emphasis on how a particular deficit is causally related to depression, and on what can be done to remedy the deficit. A variety of clinical strategies are employed to teach clients self-control skills, including group discussion, overt and covert reinforcement, behavioral assignments, self-monitoring, and modeling.

Structural Psychotherapy

Structural psychotherapy is a cognitive behavioral approach that derives from the work of two Italian mental health professionals, psychiatrist Vittorio Guidano and psychologist Gianni Liotti. These authors are strongly influenced by cognitive psychology, social learning theory, evolutionary epistemology, psychodynamic theory, and cognitive therapy. Guidano and Liotti suggest that for an understanding of the full complexity of an emotional disorder and subsequent development of an adequate model of psychotherapy, an appreciation of the development and the active role of an individual's knowledge of self and the world is critical. In short, to understand a patient, one must understand the structure of that person's world.

Guidano and Liotti's therapeutic process uses the empirical problem-solving approach of the scientist. Indeed, the authors suggest that therapists should assist clients in disengaging themselves from certain ingrained beliefs and judgments, and in considering them as hypotheses and theories subject to disproof, confirmation, and logical challenge. A variety of behavioral experiments and cognitive techniques are used to assist patients in assessing and critically evaluating their beliefs.

Other Therapies

The area of cognitive behavior therapy involves a wide collection of therapeutic approaches and techniques. Other cognitive behavioral approaches include anxiety management training, which comes from the work of psychologist Richard Suinn, and personal science, from the work of psychologist Michael Mahoney.

The cognitive behavioral approaches are derived from a variety of perspectives, including cognitive theory, classical and operant conditioning approaches, problem-solving theory, and developmental theory. All these approaches share the perspective that internal cognitive processes, called thinking or cognition, affect behavior, and that behavior change may be effected through cognitive change.

These approaches have several other similarities. One is that all the approaches see therapy as time limited. This is in sharp distinction to the traditional psychoanalytic therapies, which are generally open-ended. The cognitive behavior therapies attempt to effect change rapidly, often with specific, preset lengths of therapeutic contact. Another similarity among the cognitive behavior therapies is that their target of change is also limited. For example, in the treatment of depression, the target of change is the symptoms of depression. Therefore, in the cognitive behavioral approaches to treatment, one sees a time-limited focus and a limited target of change.

Evolution

Cognitive behavior therapy evolved from two lines of clinical and research activity: First, it derives from the work of the early cognitive therapists (Ellis and Beck); second, it was strongly influenced by the careful empirical work of the early behaviorists.

Within the domain of behaviorism, cognitive processes were not always seen as a legitimate focus of attention. In behavior therapy, there has always been a strong commitment to an applied science of clinical treatment. In the behavior therapy of the 1950s and 1960s, this emphasis on scientific methods and procedures meant that behavior therapists focused on events that were directly observable and measurable. Within this framework, behavior was seen as a function of external stimuli that determined or were reliably associated with observable responses. Also during this period, there was a deliberate avoidance of such "nebulous" concepts as thoughts, cognitions, or images. It was believed that these processes were by their very nature vague, and one could never be confident that one was reliably observing or measuring these processes.

It is important to note that by following scientific principles, researchers developed major new treatment approaches that in many ways revolutionized clinical practice (among them are systematic desensitization and the use of a token economy). Yet during the 1960s, several developments within behavior therapy had emphasized the limitations of a strict conditioning model to understanding human behavior.

In 1969, psychologist Albert Bandura published his influential volume Principles of Behavior Modification. In this volume, Bandura emphasized the role of internal or cognitive factors in the causation and maintenance of behavior. In response, behavior therapists who were dissatisfied with the radical behavioral approaches to understanding complex human behavior began actively to seek and study the role of cognitive processes in human behavior.

Criticisms and Questions

In the case of depression, cognitive behavior therapy holds that patients' excessive self-criticism and self-rejection are the causes of their depression. However, other psychologists argue that the patients' negative thoughts are the result of their depression, and that these patients are better helped through pharmacological means. Other criticisms are that cognitive behavior therapy, because it holds that people's perceptions of events, rather than events cause their emotions and feelings, does not delve deeply enough when causes of mental illness are deeply rooted in childhood abuse or trauma.

Cognitive behavior therapy has been used in combination with drug therapy in the treatment of schizophrenia and bipolar disorder, with some success. It has been suggested by some psychologists that the best use of cognitive behavior therapy is in combination with other therapies.

—Donald G. Beal

References

American Pain Society. "Cognitive Behavioral Therapy Improves Functioning for People with Chronic Pain, Study Shows." *ScienceDaily*, 11 July 2017, www.sciencedaily.com/releases/2017/07/170711125851.htm.

"Cognitive-Behavioral Therapy Skills for Modern Pain Care Practitioners." *Integrative Pain Science Institute*, 31 Aug. 2019, www.integrativepainscienceinstitute.com/cognitive-behavioral-therapy/.

Mayo Clinic Staff. "Cognitive Behavioral Therapy." *Mayo Clinic*, Mayo Foundation for Medical Education and Research, 16 Mar. 2019, www.mayoclinic.org/tests-procedures/cognitive-behavioral-therapy/about/pac-20384610.

Schubiner, Howard. "Mindfulness, CBT and ACT for Chronic Pain." *Psychology Today*, 8 Dec. 2014, www.psychologytoday.com/us/blog/unlearn-your-pain/201412/mindfulness-cbt-and-act-chronic-pain.

Song, Man-Kyu, et al. "Effects of Cognitive-Behavioral Therapy on Empathy in Patients with Chronic Pain." *Psychiatry Investigation*, vol. 15, no. 3, 2018, pp. 285–291., doi:10.30773/pi.2017.07.03.

Sturgeon, John. "Psychological Therapies for the Management of Chronic Pain." *Psychology Research and Behavior Management*, vol. 7, 2014, pp. 115–124., doi:10.2147/prbm.s44762.

■ Companionship

CATEGORY: Therapy or Technique; Prevention
ANATOMY OR SYSTEM AFFECTED: All

Companionship is one of the most sought-after states in human existence. The very first instance was mentioned in the Bible, when God had created Adam and declared, "It is not good for the man to be alone. I will make a helper suitable for him" Genesis 2:18 (New International Version). Thus, the woman Eve was created, and Adam had a companion by the name of Eve. Although this was a marriage relationship, we can see the deep longing Adam must have felt when looking out amongst all the animals and finding no helper for him. It is fair to say that we have a companion-shaped hole in us that needs to be filled. A companion can be another human being, but an effective form of companionship can also be found in the form of animals as well. Walking programs established for the elderly tout companionship as a draw for participants to their program, and this has proved successful. Loneliness is a prevalent issue in many developed countries, with as much as 75% of persons reporting loneliness and over half of these people have never talked about it with anyone. Companionship can be present in many forms, including the presence of another human being – this can include a spouse or other close family member, a friend, or even an animal. Emotional attachments are formed that when broken due to death or separation, leave lasting emotional scars and impede coping mechanisms with ongoing stress. Many people report that having a friend or animal companion reduces stress, helps them feel calm, provides a purpose for life, and emotional stability.

Mechanisms of Action
Companionship provides a sense of calm, lowers blood pressure, and lowers perceived stress levels and pain perception. A study of older adults said that their pets help them enjoy life (88%), make them feel loved (86%), reduce stress (79%), provide a sense of purpose (73%), and help them stick to a routine (62%). Having companionship either through a person or an animal fosters a sense of peace and well-being, which can contribute to a different perception of pain when it occurs.

Uses and Applications
Amongst human-human companionship, the marital union is the primary example used to display the complete concept of companionship. Many older couples, finding themselves alone at the end of their lives (most frequently due to death of their spouse) enjoy being with other people and perhaps finding a new spouse to alleviate loneliness. If this is not the most feasible way for a lonely person to have a companion, the next most logical step is to have an animal companion. Although most animal companions are dogs ("man's best friend"), cats and even other small animals including birds and fish have been designated as "buddies." Having someone or something to care for, enjoy activities with, and even talk to (97% of pet owners admit talking to their animals), can bolster self-esteem and foster serenity in an otherwise chaotic world.

Scientific Evidence
In a recent study done at the University of Michigan, older adult respondents reported that their pets "connect them with other people (65%), help them be physically active (64% overall and 78% among dog owners), and help them cope with physical and emotional symptoms (60%), including taking their mind off pain (34%).". Individuals in a treatment group became more socially active, found new friends, and experienced an increase in feeling needed.

Finding Ways to Connect
Connecting with others can occur in a myriad of ways. A lot of people use social media for contacts with others, some prefer person-to-person contacts such a mall walking groups, places of worship, activities near their residences, neighbors, and the like. For those without a lot of people contact, getting a dog or other pet can be very rewarding, especially if these animals come from a shelter or are older animals themselves. However, a companion is found, their benefits can be rewarding in lifelong ways.

—*Mary Nuckols, RN, BSN, CCM*

References
Farren, Laura, et al. "Mall Walking Program Environments, Features, and Participants: A Scoping Review." *Preventing Chronic Disease*, vol. 12, 13 Aug. 2015, doi:10.5888/pcd12.150027.

Hawkley, Louise C., and John T. Cacioppo. "Loneliness Matters: A Theoretical and Empirical Review of Consequences and Mechanisms." *Annals of Behavioral Medicine*, vol. 40, no. 2, 22 Oct. 2010, pp. 218–227., doi:10.1007/s12160-010-9210-8.

Janevic, Mary, et al. "National Poll on Healthy Aging: How Pets Contribute to Healthy Aging." *National Poll on Healthy Aging*, University of Michigan, 3 Apr. 2019, hdl.handle.net/2027.42/148428.

Siddique, Haroon. "Three-Quarters of Older People in the UK Are Lonely, Survey Finds." *The Guardian*, 21 Mar. 2017, www.theguardian.com/society/2017/mar/21/three-quarters-of-older-people-in-the-uk-are-lonely-survey-finds.

■ Coping strategies

CATEGORY: Therapy or Technique; Psychotherapy

Introduction
The word "cope" is derived from the Latin word *colpus*, meaning "to alter," and, as defined in Webster's Dictionary, is usually used in the psychological paradigm to denote "dealing with and attempting to overcome problems and difficulties." In psychology, the word "coping," in addition to this behavioral application, has been used as a broad heuristic in several other domains, including as a thought process, as a personality characteristic, and in social context.

The concept of coping can be traced back to the defense mechanisms described in the psychoanalytical model by the famous Austrian neurologist Sigmund Freud. Freud described several methods that a person's mind uses to protect itself: introjection, isolation, projection reversal, reaction formation, regression, repression, sublimation, turning against the self, and undoing. While defining all these terms is beyond the scope of the present discussion, it is worth noting that, according to Freud, mechanisms of defense are the devices that the mind uses in altering one's perception to situations disturbing the internal milieu or mental balance. He applied the concept in identifying sources of anxiety through free association.

One of Freud's associates, Austrian physician Alfred Adler, disagreed with Freud and described defense mechanisms as protective against external threats or challenges. Sigmund Freud's daughter, Anna Freud, herself a renowned psychologist, included both of these viewpoints and underscored the role of defense mechanisms as protective against both internal and external threats. She also extended the repertoire of defense mechanisms to include denial, intellectualization, ego restriction, and identification with the aggressor. Therefore, it appears that the concept of defense mechanisms was very similar to the present understanding of coping at the thought process level and preceded the concept of coping. However, psychologist Norma Haan, in her book *Coping and Defending* (1977), clearly distinguishes defense mechanisms from coping. She contends that coping is purposive and involves choices, while defense mechanisms are rigid and set. Coping, according to Haan, is more focused on the present, while defense mechanisms are premised on the past and distort the present.

Psychologist Robert White, in *Stress and Coping: An Anthology* (1991), contends that coping is derived from the larger biological concept of adaptation. The origin of all species is a result of adaptation mediated through the process of natural selection. This concept of adaptation is extended in the behavioral realm to include dealing with minor problems and frustrations, such as waiting in the grocery line, as well as more complex difficulties, such as dealing with the death of a spouse. In this context, coping is essentially an adaptation under more difficult conditions. White also talks about the term "mastery," which he contends is quite unpopular with psychologists because of its connotation with "superiority" and "winning and losing." However, mastery is another way of describing the concept of coping, whereby the anxiety or danger is mastered.

Perhaps the greatest impetus to the contemporary understanding of coping has come from the work of the American psychologist Richard Lazarus, an emeritus professor at the University of California at Berkeley, and his colleagues. Lazarus introduced the transactional model of stress and coping in his 1966 book *Psychological Stress and the Coping Process*. He elaborated this concept further in 1984 in the book *Stress, Appraisal, and Coping* (with coauthor Susan Folkman).

According to the transactional model, stressful experiences are perceived as person-environment transactions. In these transactions, the person undergoes a four-stage assessment known as appraisal. When confronted with any possible stressful situation, the first stage is the primary appraisal of the event. In this stage, based on one's previous experience, knowledge about oneself, and knowledge about the event, the person internally determines whether he or she is in trouble. If the event is perceived to be threatening or has caused harm or loss in the past, then the stage of secondary appraisal occurs. If, on the other hand, the event is judged to be irrelevant or poses no threat, then stress does not develop and no further coping is required. The secondary appraisal determines how much control one has over the situation or the event. Based on this understanding, the individual ascertains what means of control are available. This is the stage known as coping. Finally, the fourth stage is the stage of reappraisal, in which the person determines whether the original event or situation has been effectively negated. The primary focus of Lazarus's conceptualization of coping is on coping as an application of thought processes and behavioral efforts to combat demands that exceed a person's resources. The hallmarks of this conceptualization are its focus on the process of coping as opposed to personality traits; the importance of specific stressful situations in inducing coping as opposed to a general physiological response; and a lack of reference to the outcome (whether positive or negative), as opposed to the mastery concept, which emphasizes only the positive aspects.

Coping Strategies

According to the transactional model, there are two broad categories of coping. The first one is called problem-focused coping, and the second one is called emotion-focused coping. Problem-focused coping is based on one's capability to think about and alter the environmental event or situation. Examples of this strategy at the thought-process level include utilization of problem-solving skills, interpersonal conflict resolution, advice seeking, time management, goal setting, and gathering more information about what is causing one stress. Problem solving requires thinking through various solutions, evaluating the pros and cons of different solutions, and then implementing a solution that seems most advantageous to reduce the stress. Examples of this strategy at the behavioral or action level include activities such as joining a smoking-cessation program, complying with a prescribed medical treatment, adhering to a diabetic diet plan, or scheduling and prioritizing tasks for managing time.

In the emotion-focused strategy, the focus is inward on altering the way one thinks or feels about a situation or an event. Examples of this strategy at the thought-process level include denying the existence of the stressful situation, freely expressing emotions, avoiding the stressful situation, making social comparisons, or minimizing (looking at the bright side of things). Examples of this strategy at the behavioral or action level include seeking social support to negate the influence of the stressful situation; using exercise, relaxation, or meditation; joining support groups; practicing religious rituals; and escaping through the use of alcohol and drugs.

Several predictive empirical studies done using this model have generally shown that problem-focused strategies are quite helpful for stressful events that can be changed, while emotion-focused strategies are more helpful for stressful events that cannot be changed. Some of these coping strategies are healthy, such as applying problem-solving skills; some are neither inherently healthy nor unhealthy, such as practicing some religious rituals; and some are unhealthy or maladaptive, such as denying the existence of a stressful situation or escaping through the use of drugs.

Choice of coping strategy is influenced by the quantity and quality of available resources for coping that may be available to a person. These resources include knowledge (for example, knowledge of the functioning at a workplace), skills (such as analytical skills), attitudes (for example, self-efficacy or confidence in one's ability to perform a specific behavior), social resources (people with whom a person can exchange information), physical resources (health and stamina), material resources (money), and societal resources (policies and laws).

Measurement of Coping Strategies

Self-reported, paper-and-pencil tools are commonly used in measuring coping strategies. A popular assessment tool for measuring coping strategies is the Ways of Coping (WOC) Checklist developed by Lazarus and Folkman, which contains sixty-eight different items. These responses have been divided into eight categories: accepting of responsibility (such as criticizing or lecturing oneself), confrontational coping (expressing anger), distancing (trivializing the situation), escape avoidance (wishing that the situation would go away), planned problem solving (making a plan of action and following it), positive reappraisal (changing or growing as a person in a good way), seeking of social support (talking to someone to find out about more about the situation), and self-controlling (keeping feelings to oneself). A further revision of this scale, the Ways of Coping Checklist-Revised, contains a list of forty-two coping behaviors.

American psychologist Charles S. Carver and his colleagues have designed the Coping Orientations to Problems Experienced (COPE) scale. The COPE scale has twelve component scales for types of coping strategies that include acceptance, active coping, denial, disengagement, humor, planning, positive reframing, religion, restraint, social support, self-distraction, and suppression of competing activities. Carver has also designed and tested a brief version of the COPE scale for use with other large protocols that has been found to be efficacious. Other scales have been developed to measure the daily utilization of coping.

Personality Traits and Coping

The relationship between personality trait characteristics and coping has been suggested and studied by several researchers. American psychologist Suzanne Kobasa, in her 1977 University of Chicago doctoral dissertation, studied the role of personality and coping. Specifically, she examined the characteristics of highly stressed people among those who remained healthy and those who did not manifest any illness following stressful times. She coined the term "hardiness" to depict the personality profile of people who remained healthy. Her research found three general characteristics of hardiness: the belief of control or the ability to influence the events of one's experience, commitment to activities in life or a feeling of deep involvement, and challenge to further development or anticipation of change.

Israeli medical sociologist Aaron Antonovsky described the concept of "sense of coherence," also related to personality traits, as being central to coping. He described three components as being representative of this concept: comprehensibility, meaningfulness, and manageability. Comprehensibility means that the person believes that the world around him or her is making some sense, there is some set structure, and there is some level of predictability. Manageability implies the faith that a person has in his or her ability to meet the various demands in life in one way or another. Meaningfulness implies the belief that whatever one does has a purpose in life. Antonovsky proposed that people who possess a higher sense of coherence tend to cope better in life.

Another personality characteristic that has been studied in relation to coping is optimism. Optimism is the tendency to look at the brighter side of things and to expect positive outcomes from one's actions. Research has shown that optimism improves effective coping. Carver and his colleagues studied the effects of optimism in patients suffering from breast cancer, heart rehabilitation patients, and people in other stressful situations and found the beneficial effect of optimism on coping.

American cardiologists Meyer Friedman and Ray Rosenman, in their observations of heart disease patients, described two types of personalities: Type A and Type B. People with type A behavior pattern are characterized by time urgency impatience, competitiveness, and hostility. Those with type B show the opposites of these characteristics, exemplified by no time urgency and being cooperative and patient in their disposition. Type A personalities have been found to demonstrate negative coping styles in terms of showing more negative physiological and psychological outcomes.

Social Environment and Coping

Coping does not occur in vacuum. Most stressful situations entail involvement with people. Therefore, social environment influences stress and coping. Social environment can be conceptualized at a broader level as the social structure, and it can also be conceptualized in a specific, narrow way as close social relationships. The latter are often described as social support and depict the most common way researchers have studied the social relationship in the context of coping. The broader effect of social structure on coping is rather obvious. For example, a person on the higher rung of the social ladder would have access to greater resources and thus would be able to apply a variety of coping resources, while a person at the bottom of the social ladder, living in poverty, would have fewer resources at his or her disposal.

Social support has been conceptualized from different perspectives. American sociologist James House defined social support as the "aid and assistance that one receives through social relationships and interpersonal exchanges" and classified it into four types. The first is emotional social support, or the empathy, love, trust, and caring that one receives from others. The second kind is instrumental social support, or the tangible aid and service that one receives from others. The third type is informational social support, or the advice, suggestions, and information that one receives from others. The fourth type is appraisal social support, or the information that one receives for self-assessment. Social support has a direct effect on lowering stress levels and improving effective coping, as well as providing stress "buffering effects," or what statisticians call effect modulation. For example, a person undergoing stress may talk to a friend, who may provide a tangible aid to cope (direct effect), may modify the receiver's perception of the stressful event, or may enhance the receiver's belief that he or she can cope with the stressful event (buffering effect).

—*Manoj Sharma*

References

Booth, Jessie W., and James T. Neill. "Coping Strategies and the Development of Psychological Resilience." *Journal of Outdoor and Environmental Education*, vol. 20, no. 1, 2017, pp. 47–54., doi:10.1007/bf03401002.

Health.com. "Real Life Strategies for Coping with Chronic Pain." *Health.com*, 29 Feb. 2016, www.health.com/health/condition-article/0,20189626,00.html.

Heffer, Taylor, and Teena Willoughby. "A Count of Coping Strategies: A Longitudinal Study

Investigating an Alternative Method to Understanding Coping and Adjustment." *Plos One*, vol. 12, no. 10, 5 Oct. 2017, doi:10.1371/journal.pone.0186057.

Litt, Mark D, and Howard Tennen. "What Are the Most Effective Coping Strategies for Managing Chronic Pain?" *Pain Management*, vol. 5, no. 6, 2015, pp. 403–406., doi:10.2217/pmt.15.45.

Maeng, S., et al. "Changes In Coping Strategy With Age." *Innovation in Aging*, vol. 1, no. suppl_1, 30 July 2017, pp. 897–897, doi:10.1093/geroni/igx004.3218.

Morales-Rodríguez, Francisco Manuel, and José Manuel Pérez-Mármol. "The Role of Anxiety, Coping Strategies, and Emotional Intelligence on General Perceived Self-Efficacy in University Students." *Frontiers in Psychology*, vol. 10, 7 Aug. 2019, doi:10.3389/fpsyg.2019.01689.

■ Couples therapy

CATEGORY: Therapy or Technique; Psychotherapy

Introduction

Traditionally, marriage vows have represented pledges of mutual love and enduring commitment. Since the 1960s, however, marital relationships have changed dramatically. In fact, while more than 90 percent of the United States population will marry at least once in their lifetime, the US Census Bureau estimated in 2009 that approximately 40 percent of all first marriages and approximately 60 percent of all second marriages end in divorce. Moreover, while the average first marriage in the United States will last approximately eight years, second marriages typically endure for approximately the same time period at 8.5 years. It appears that a repetitive pattern of marriage, distress, and divorce has become commonplace. Such a cycle often results in considerable pain and psychological turmoil for the couple, their family, and their friends. These statistics dramatically indicate the need for effective ways to help couples examine and reapproach their relationships before deciding whether to terminate them.

Interpersonal relationships are a highly complex yet important area of study and investigation. The decision to marry (or at least to commit to a serious intimate relationship) is clearly one of the most significant choices many people make in their lives. Fortunately, advances in couples therapy have led to increased knowledge about interpersonal relationships and methods for improving relationship satisfaction. These advances have been documented in the scientific literature, and they extend to the treatment of cohabitating partners, premarital couples, remarried partners, married and premarital same-sex couples, separating or divorced couples, and stepfamilies. Moreover, couples-based treatment programs have shown effectiveness in the treatment of depression, anxiety disorders, domestic violence, sexual dysfunction, and a host of other problems.

Communication and Conflict Resolution

Often, partners who seek couples therapy or counseling have problems in two areas: communication and conflict resolution. These are the two major difficulties that most often lead to divorce. It has been shown that communication skills differentiate satisfied and dissatisfied couples more powerfully than any other factor. Indeed, communication difficulties are the most frequently cited complaint among partners reporting relationship distress.

Psychologist John M. Gottman, in *Marital Interaction: Experimental Investigations* (1979) and the co-written *A Couple's Guide to Communication* (1976), is one of many researchers who have highlighted the importance of communication problems within distressed relationships. Many characteristic differences between distressed and satisfied couples have been noted. Partners in distressed couples often misperceive well-intended statements from their partners, whereas satisfied couples are more likely to rate well-intended messages as positive; distressed partners also engage in fewer rewarding exchanges and more frequent punishing interactions than nondistressed couples. A partner in a distressed relationship is more immediately reactive to perceived negative behavior exhibited by his or her partner. There is generally a greater emphasis on negative communication strategies between distressed partners.

Distressed couples appear to be generally unskilled at generating positive change in their relationship. Gottman also reported that distressed couples are often ineffectual in their attempts to resolve conflicts. Whereas nondistressed couples

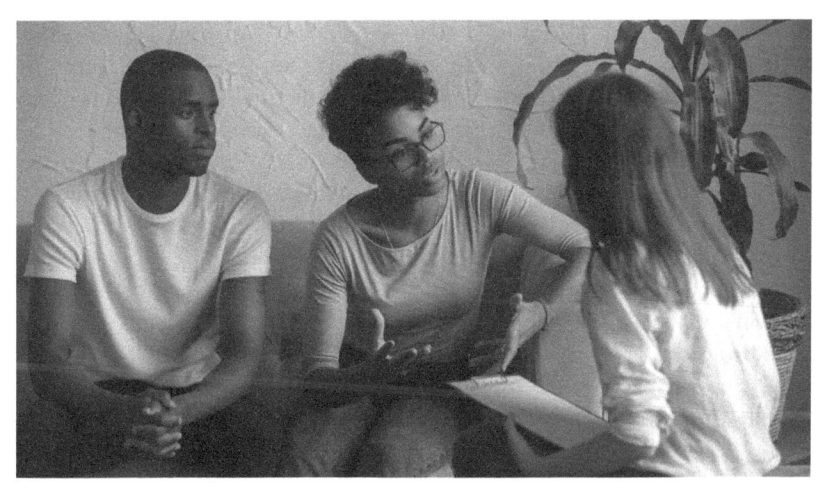

In couples therapy, the practitioner evaluates the couple's personal and relationship story as it is narrated, interrupts wisely, facilitates both de-escalation of unhelpful conflict and the development of realistic, practical solutions. (fizkes via iStock)

employ "validation loops" during problem-solving exercises (one partner states the conflict and the other partner expresses agreement or support), distressed couples typically enter into repetitive, cross-complaining loops. These loops can be described as an interactional sequence wherein both individuals describe areas of dissatisfaction within the relationship yet fail to attend to their partners' issues. Moreover, as one spouse initiates aversive control tactics, the other spouse will typically reciprocate with similar behavior.

Therapy Formats

Couples therapy attempts to alleviate distress, resolve conflicts, improve daily functioning, and prevent problems via an intensive focus on the couple as a unit and on each partner as an individual. Couples therapists are faced with a variety of choices regarding treatment format and therapeutic approach. Individual therapy focuses treatment on only one of the partners. Although generally discouraged by most practitioners, individual treatment of one partner can provide greater opportunities for the client to focus on his or her own thoughts, feelings, problems, and behaviors. Clients may feel less hesitant in sharing some details they would not want a spouse to hear, and individual treatment may encourage the client to take greater personal responsibility for problems and successes. In general, these advantages are outweighed by the difficulties encountered when treating relationship problems without both partners being present. In particular, interpersonal interactions are complex phenomena that need to be evaluated and treated with both partners present.

Concurrent therapy involves both partners being seen in treatment separately, either by the same therapist or by two separate but collaborating therapists. Advantages of the concurrent format include greater individual attention and opportunities to develop strategies to improve relationship skills by teaching each partner those techniques separately. Concurrent treatment, however, does not allow the therapist(s) to evaluate and treat the nature of the interpersonal difficulties with both partners present in the same room.

Conjoint format, on the other hand, involves both partners simultaneously in the therapy session. Conjoint treatment is widely used and generally recommended because it focuses intensively on the quality of the relationship, promotes dialogue between the couple, and can attend to the needs and goals of each partner as well as the needs and goals of the couple. The history of conjoint marital therapy begins, ironically, with Sigmund Freud's failures in this area. He believed firmly that it was counterproductive and dangerous for a therapist ever to treat more than one member of the same family. In fact, in 1912, after attempting to provide services simultaneously to a husband and wife, Freud concluded that he was at a complete loss about how to treat relationship problems within a couple. He also added that he had little faith in individual therapy for them.

Conjoint treatment is designed to focus intensively on the relationship to effect specific therapeutic change for that particular couple. Interventions can be tailor-made for the couple seeking treatment, regardless of the nature of the problem the couple describes (such as sexual relations, child rearing, or household responsibilities). Moreover, couples are constantly engaged in direct dialogue, which can foster improved understanding and resolution of conflict. As compared with other approaches, conjoint marital therapy can focus on each of the specific needs and goals of the individual couple.

Group couples treatment programs have received increased attention and have shown very good to excellent treatment success. Advantages of group treatment for couples include opportunities for direct assessment and intervention of the relationship within a setting that promotes greater opportunity for feedback and suggestions from other couples experiencing similar difficulties. In fact, group therapy may promote positive expectations through witnessing improvements among other couples as well as fostering a sense of cohesiveness among couples within the group. In the group format, each partner has the opportunity to develop improved communication and conflict resolution approaches by learning relationship skills via interaction with the therapist(s), his or her spouse, and other group members. In addition, the cost of individual, concurrent, and conjoint therapy, in terms of time as well as dollars, has prompted several researchers and clinicians to recommend group couples therapy.

Therapeutic Approaches
There are numerous approaches to the treatment of relationship problems practiced in the United States. Psychodynamic therapy focuses attention on the unconscious needs and issues raised during an individual's childhood. Phenomenological therapists focus on the here-and-now experiences of being in a relationship and have developed a variety of creative therapeutic techniques. Systems therapists view interpersonal problems as being maintained by the nature of the relationship structure, patterns of communication, and family roles and rules.

Behavioral marital therapy, however, is the most thoroughly investigated approach within the couples therapy field. Starting from a focus on operant conditioning (a type of learning in which behaviors are altered primarily by the consequences that follow them— reinforcement or punishment), behavioral marital therapy includes a wide range of assessment and treatment strategies. The underlying assumption that best differentiates behavioral treatments for distressed couples from other approaches is that the two partners are viewed as ineffectual in their attempts to satisfy each other.

Thus, the goal of therapy is to improve relationship satisfaction by creating a supportive environment in which the skills can be acquired. Behavioral marital therapy incorporates strategies designed to improve daily interactions, communication patterns, and problem-solving abilities and to examine and modify unreasonable expectations and faulty thinking styles.

Behavioral-Exchange Strategies
Psychologists Philip and Marcy Bornstein, in their book *Marital Therapy: A Behavioral-Communications Approach* (1986), described a sequential five-step procedure in the treatment of relationship dysfunction. These steps include intake interviewing, behavioral exchange strategies, communication skills acquisition, training in problem solving, and maintenance and generalization of treatment gains.

Intake interviewing is designed to accomplish three primary goals: development of a working relationship with the therapist, collection of assessment information, and implementation of initial therapeutic regimens. Because spouses entering treatment have often spent months, if not years, in conflict and distress, the intake procedure attempts to provide a unique opportunity to influence and assess the couple's relationship immediately. Because distressed couples often devote a considerable amount of time thinking about and engaging in discordant interpersonal interactions, it naturally follows that they will attempt to engage in unpleasant interactions during initial sessions. Information about current difficulties and concerns is clearly valuable, but improved communication skills and positive interactions appear to be of even greater merit early in treatment. Thus, couples are discouraged from engaging in cross-complaining loops and are encouraged to develop skills and implement homework procedures designed to enhance the relationship.

Skill Training
Building a positive working relationship between partners is viewed as essential in couples treatment programs. During training in behavioral exchange strategies, couples are aided in specifying and pinpointing behaviors that tend to promote increased harmony in their relationship. Couples engage in contracting and compromise

activities to disrupt the downward spiral of their distressed relationship.

Training in communication skills focuses on practicing the basics of communication (such as respect, understanding, and sensitivity) and of positive principles of communication (timeliness, marital manners, specification, and "mind reading"), improving nonverbal behaviors, and learning "molecular" verbal behaviors (such as assertiveness and constructive agreement). Improved communication styles are fostered via a direct, active approach designed to identify, reinforce, and rehearse desirable patterns of interactions. Clients are generally provided with specific instructions and "practice periods" during sessions in which partners are encouraged to begin improving their interactional styles. It is common for these sessions to be audiotaped or videotaped to give couples specific feedback regarding their communication style.

Training in problem solving is intended to teach clients to negotiate and resolve conflicts in a mutually beneficial manner. Conflict resolution training focuses on learning, practicing, and experiencing effective problem-solving approaches. Couples receive specific instruction on systematic problem-solving approaches and are given homework assignments designed to improve problem-solving skills. Because the value of couples therapy lies in the improvement, maintenance, and use of positive interaction styles over time and across situations, treatment often aims to promote constructive procedures after the termination of active treatment. Thus, people are taught that it is generally easier to change oneself than one's partner, that positive interaction styles may be forgotten or unlearned if these strategies are not regularly practiced, and that new positive interactions can continue to develop in a variety of settings even as treatment ends.

Comparative Research

To highlight further the utility and effectiveness of behavioral-communications relationship therapy, Philip Bornstein, Laurie Wilson, and Gregory L. Wilson conducted an empirical investigation in 1988 comparing conjoint and behavioral-communications group therapy and group behavioral-communications therapies to a waiting-list control group (couples who were asked to wait two months prior to beginning treatment). Fifteen distressed couples were randomly assigned to experimental conditions and offered eight sessions of couples therapy. At the conclusion of treatment (as well as six months later), the couples in active treatment revealed significant alleviation of relationship distress. The conjoint and group couples revealed similar levels of improvement in communication skills, problem-solving abilities, and general relationship satisfaction. The waiting-list couples, on the other hand, revealed no improvement while they waited for treatment, indicating that relationship distress does not tend to improve simply as the result of the passage of time.

Prevention and Disorders

Another line of couples research has focused on the utility of premarital intervention and distress- and divorce-prevention programs. Unlike treatment programs, prevention programs intervene before the development of relationship distress. Prevention efforts are focused on the future and typically involve the training of specific skills that are viewed as useful in preventing relationship distress. Three major approaches to premarital intervention include the Minnesota Couples Communication Program, Bernard Guerney's relationship enhancement approach, and the Premarital Relationship Enhancement Program. Research is generally supportive of the effectiveness of these programs in helping partners learn useful skills that translate into improved relationships for at least three to eight years following the program. In addition, some evidence indicates that the alarming divorce rate in the United States can be decreased if partners participate in prevention programs before marriage; prevention programs that emphasize communication and conflict-resolution skills seem most advantageous.

Improving Treatment

Researchers and clinicians have witnessed large increases in the numbers of couples seeking treatment from therapists. The Bureau of Labor Statistics reported the employment rate for marriage and family therapists to grow an estimated 29 percent from 2012 to 2022, which is a much faster-than-average growth rate than is predicted in other occupations. As the demand for couples treatment increases, more time and effort is devoted to improving treatment methods. The behavioral approach has been shown to be highly effective in reducing relationship distress and preventing divorce; however, many believe that cognitive components such as causal attributions and expectations are strongly related to satisfaction in the relationship. Moreover, it has been argued that dysfunctional cognitions may interfere with both the establishment and maintenance of positive behavior change. Evidence has prompted some researchers and practitioners to advocate a more systematic inclusion of strategies of cognitive behavior therapy within the behavioral marital therapy framework. Specifically, it is possible that the combination of cognitive and behavioral approaches will demonstrate increased utility if the two treatments are presented together in a singular, integrated treatment intervention. Such treatment would afford couples the opportunity to benefit from either one or both of the complementary approaches, depending on their own unique needs, at any time during the course of treatment. Moreover, such an integration of cognitive and behavioral tactics would parallel effective approaches already employed with depressed or anxious clients.

—*Gregory L. Wilson*

References

Cano, Annmarie, et al. "A Couple-Based Psychological Treatment for Chronic Pain and Relationship Distress." *Cognitive and Behavioral Practice*, vol. 25, no. 1, 2018, pp. 119–134., doi:10.1016/j.cbpra.2017.02.003.

Gillihan, Seth J. "What Happens When Partners Fight Chronic Pain Together?" *Psychology Today*, 19 June 2017, www.psychologytoday.com/us/blog/think-act-be/201706/what-happens-when-partners-fight-chronic-pain-together.

Kindt, Sara, et al. "Helping Motivation and Well-Being of Chronic Pain Couples." *Pain*, vol. 157, no. 7, 2016, pp. 1551–1562., doi:10.1097/j.pain.0000000000000550.

Kindt, Sara, et al. "Helping Your Partner with Chronic Pain: The Importance of Helping Motivation, Received Social Support, and Its Timeliness." *Pain Medicine*, vol. 20, no. 1, Jan. 2019, pp. 77–89., doi:10.1093/pm/pny006.

Richeimer, Steven. "Couples-Based Therapy May Help with Chronic Pain." *Medium*, 25 May 2018, medium.com/@stevenricheimer/couples-based-therapy-may-help-with-chronic-pain-138d1cafa681.

Smith, Shannon M., et al. "Couple Interventions for Chronic Pain." *The Clinical Journal of Pain*, vol. 35, no. 11, 2019, pp. 916–922., doi:10.1097/ajp.0000000000000752.

Suso-Ribera, Carlos, et al. "Empathic Accuracy in Chronic Pain: Exploring Patient and Informal Caregiver Differences and Their Personality Correlates." *Medicina*, vol. 55, no. 9, 27 Aug. 2019, p. 539., doi:10.3390/medicina55090539.

Williams, Amy M., and Annmarie Cano. "Spousal Mindfulness and Social Support in Couples With Chronic Pain." *The Clinical Journal of Pain*, vol. 30, no. 6, 2014, pp. 528–535., doi:10.1097/ajp.0000000000000009.

■ Dialectical behavioral therapy

CATEGORY: Therapy or Technique; Psychotherapy

Introduction

In 1987, psychologist Marsha M. Linehan published her method for treating patients with borderline personality disorder (BPD), which she called dialectical behavioral therapy. Borderline personality disorder is one of more serious and treatment-resistant personality disorders, characterized by dysregulation of emotions (an inability to regulate and control emotional responses), as well as of thoughts, behaviors, and interpersonal relations, including how a person relates to the self. People with this personality configuration experience affective instability, difficulty managing their anger, random impulsivity, proclivity for self-harm, paranoia, extreme fear of abandonment, uncertainty about who they are, and chronic emotional emptiness.

Traditional treatments assumed that therapists could not avoid rejecting patients' self-destructive behaviors and attitudes. These approaches were change-oriented and, though well intentioned, frequently put the therapist at odds with the patient. In developing dialectical behavioral therapy, Linehan enumerated strategies that allowed therapists to accept patients where they were, promoting acceptance-oriented skills in addition to traditional

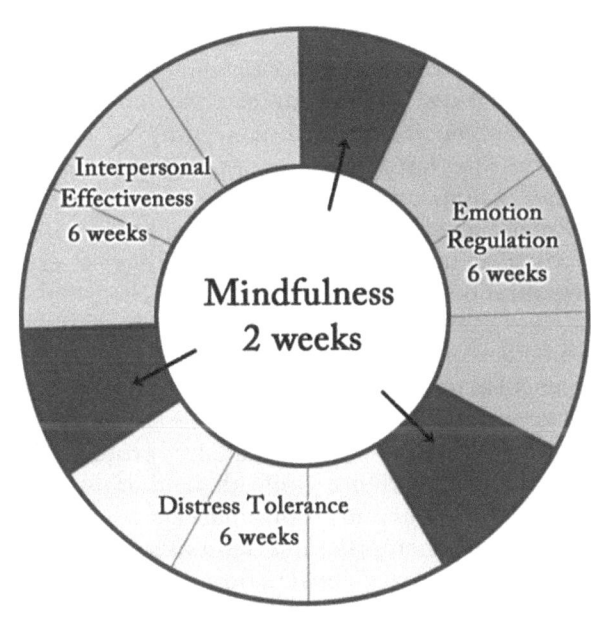

The stages used in dialectical behavior therapy. (MargaritaJP via Wikimedia Commons) *media Commons*)

change-oriented skills. An accepting attitude toward patients affirms the worldview inherent in their feelings, attitudes, thoughts, and behavior. It promotes the rectitude of patients' experiences and all aspects of their personal worlds. It also maintains that, however patients are being in the moment, it is the best that they are able to be at that time.

Underlying dialectical behavioral therapy is a constellation of worldviews that highlights the importance of dialectic and the acceptance of life as it is. Acceptance draws heavily from Zen principles; dialectic has its philosophical roots in the work of Immanuel Kant, Frederick Shelling, and, most of all, Georg Hegel. Dialectic is the synthesizing of point and counterpoint. For every stance or particular behavioral occurrence, there is an equally valid, but opposite, stance or occurrence. The therapist supports the patient's moving toward a healthier integration of these ostensibly irreconcilable positions. In practice, dialectical behavioral therapy strategies draw heavily from traditional cognitive and behavioral therapy techniques and process approaches well known in person-centered and emotion-focused therapies.

Before dialectical behavioral therapy, patients with borderline personality disorder were considered almost impossible to treat effectively beyond varying levels of therapeutic stabilization. People with borderline personality disorder are emotionally flammable and fragile, unable to reliably regulate their inner states, have conflict-ridden relationships, frequently consider suicide, and often engage in self-harming behaviors such as cutting. They were raised in and typically perpetuate an invalidating environment, a social environment that actively opposes acceptance of patients' perceptions, feelings, judgments, attitudes, and behaviors. This toxic climate perpetuates pervasive criticism, denigration, trivializing, and random social reinforcement. People in this environment are denied genuine attention, respect, understanding from others, and positive regard for who they are and what they are experiencing. Stress and perceived abandonment or rejection overwhelm the ability of people with borderline personality disorder to self-regulate, and they remain chronically, recurrently, emotionally vulnerable. Therapists were often frustrated (and sometimes intimidated) by these patients' volatility and high degree of risk. Dialectical behavioral therapy became a road map for therapists who trained in it.

How the Therapy Works

Patients who undertake dialectical behavioral therapy begin with "pretreatment," a series of psychotherapy sessions in which the therapist and patient establish a shared understanding of dialectical behavioral therapy's rationale, agreements about what each expects of the other, the levels of dialectical behavioral therapy interventions and treatment targets, and perhaps most important, the commitment to be in treatment. In pretreatment, patients agree to stay in therapy for a specified period, most commonly a year, to come to all therapy sessions, to come on time, to work toward ending all self-harming behaviors, to undertake interpersonal skills training, and to pay fees in a timely manner. Therapy is usually discontinued if four consecutive sessions are missed. Therapists promise to maintain their own ongoing and professionally supportive training, to be available for weekly sessions and phone consultations, to demonstrate positive regard and nonjudgmental attitudes, maintain confidentiality, and obtain additional consultation as would benefit the therapy.

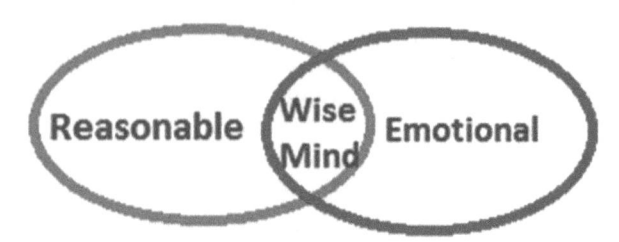

A diagram used in DBT, showing that the Wise Mind is the overlap of the emotional mind and the reasonable mind. (Mmm Daffodils via Wikimedia Commons) taJP via Wikimedia Commons) media Commons)

Levels of Treatment

Level I of treatment establishes a target hierarchy that includes reduction of self-harming behaviors such as cutting or burning oneself, of behaviors and barriers that interfere with treatment, and of behaviors that interfere with establishing a healthier quality of life. Patients at the early stages of dialectical behavioral therapy treatment are usually highly distressed, bordering on hopelessness, and at the mercy of the enigmatic flow of their own emotional surges. Self-injury, drug abuse, depression, and suicidal thinking are the norm at this state.

Level II begins when the skills developed in Level I are sufficient to contain self-harming patterns. The therapist begins to presumptively treat patients with post-traumatic stress interventions, as these enhance their ability to experience aversive emotions without being undone by them. As progress is made, other emotionally difficult, even overwhelming targets are identified. The emotional and psychological commitments to remaining in treatment at these early stages can result in patients' working against their goals, as in missing therapy appointments, showing up late, and not completing agreed-on homework; it can also result in psychological regression, wherein patients at Level II treatment exhibit Level I functioning (for example, burning or cutting themselves or engaging in other dangerous behaviors). Patients at these levels of care must be closely monitored. Once the functional goals of Level II are reliably sustained, the majority of patients leave treatment. They have expended a great effort at much personal cost to have gotten this far.

For patients proceeding to Level III, the targets of treatment are similar to those of typical psychotherapy in that they aim at reducing or eliminating behaviors that are not debilitating but interfere with experiencing ordinary pleasure, happiness, fulfillment, and personal meaning.

Level IV targets higher-order psychological values: a functional application of one's philosophy of person, integration, and the blending of spiritual elements with those of psychological self-actualization.

Modalities of Treatment

Dialectical behavioral therapy uses four modes of treatment that are not commonly found together in other therapeutic approaches: group-skills training for patients, individual therapy for patients, telephone consultations between patients and therapists, and therapists' participation in an ongoing consultation team. Many of the ways borderline personality disorder patients regress are through perceived, and thus experienced, negative social interactions. These are most effectively worked through and improved by training in a group setting. Individual therapy is typically weekly and involves working toward the established and mutually agreed-on targets during pretreatment. Because the inner life of patients with borderline personality disorder can be so tumultuous, telephone consultations are routinely used to bolster patients and review how to apply the concepts and skills discussed in individual and group training. Because this is such a challenging patient population, the standard practice of dialectical behavioral therapy requires its practitioners to meet regularly with other dialectical behavior therapists for case presentation, honing of dialectical behavioral therapy therapeutic skills, and peer consultation.

Future

Though Linehan focused her earlier work on patients with borderline personality disorder, and dialectical behavioral therapy is the therapy of first choice in their treatment, the principles and techniques have been applied to other often hard-to-treat patient groups such as those with eating disorders, bipolar disorder (in conjunction with targeted psychopharmacology), histrionic personality disorder, a history of sexual and violent assault, and a variety of diagnoses among the elderly. Though it requires a high degree of patient commitment and specific training that implies lifelong learning, it is the most powerful and effective intervention available to a patient group that had often been considered nearly impossible to treat effectively.

—Paul Moglia

References

Flynn, Daniel, et al. "Dialectical Behaviour Therapy for Treating Adults and Adolescents with Emotional and Behavioural Dysregulation: Study Protocol of a Coordinated Implementation in a Publicly Funded Health Service." *BMC Psychiatry*, vol. 18, no. 1, 26 Feb. 2018, doi:10.1186/s12888-018-1627-9.

Linton, Steven J. "Applying Dialectical Behavior Therapy to Chronic Pain: A Case Study." *Scandinavian Journal of Pain*, vol. 1, no. 1, 2010, pp. 50–54., doi:10.1016/j.sjpain.2009.09.005.

May, Jennifer M, et al. "Dialectical Behavior Therapy as Treatment for Borderline Personality Disorder." *Mental Health Clinician*, vol. 6, no. 2, 2016, pp. 62–67., doi:10.9740/mhc.2016.03.62.

Reddy, M. S., and M. Starlin Vijay. "Empirical Reality of Dialectical Behavioral Therapy in Borderline Personality." *Indian Journal of Psychological Medicine*, vol. 39, no. 2, 2017, p. 105., doi:10.4103/ijpsym.ijpsym_132_17.

Sysko, Helen, et al. "Dialectical Behavior Therapy for Chronic Pain in Gastrointestinal Disorders." *Inflammatory Bowel Diseases*, vol. 22, Mar. 2016, doi:10.1097/01.mib.0000480106.40651.21.

■ Equine-assisted therapy

CATEGORY: Therapy or Technique; Physiotherapy; Psychotherapy

KEY TERMS

- *equine-facilitated learning (EFL)*: using horses to promote learning experiences that develop skills intended for real-world environments
- *equine-facilitated psychotherapy (EFP)*: follows a psychoanalytic approach by using the human-horse interactions as a tool for a therapist to gauge and discuss about their patients reactions and intentions
- *heart rate variability*: interval of time in-between heart beats that changes correlates to a changes in emotional states
- *hippotherapy*: using horses for occupational, physical or speech therapy
- *therapeutic horseback riding*: recreational horseback riding for disabled individuals

Why Horses?

Horses are highly sensitive animals. Whether it due to the centuries of interacting with humans or an individual horse's experience, research has shown horses have the ability to detect human emotional states. A study done at the University of Sussex reveals horses have the ability to distinguish between a 'happy' and 'angry' human face. 28 horses were shown photos of humans with positive and negative human facial features. When shown a photo of a person with negative facial features, the horse's heart rate increased. They also were more likely to move their head to look at the faces with their left eye. This behavior has been found in many species to reflect the processing of threatening stimuli. For many species, the left eye collects threatening information due to the specialization right brain's hemisphere.

When shown a positive facial expression horses have less of a reaction. Their heart rate did not increase and they did not look with their left eye. This could be because they know a positive human face does not indicate a possible negative interaction so it does not increase their state of arousal. Professor Karen McComb, an author of the study, notes the result could be due to the individual experience of each horse of their lifetime, or an "ancestral ability" that allows horses to read facial cues as an adaptive trait to appropriately respond.

Another study done by Dr. Ellen Kaye Gehrke at the Institute of HeartMath, uses heart rate variability (HRV) as a measure to study emotional states in humans and horses. The HRV is useful because of its sensitivity to emotional states and is under the control of the autonomic nervous system. It is an unconscious response that both humans and animals have developed to acclimate to an ever-changing environment. It is separate from heart rate and measures the time in-between heart beats. When negative emotions are experienced, HRV is irregular and inconsistent. She first proved that horses have similar HRV patterns in humans by using an ECG holster monitor during activities like riding and grooming. Then, she monitored horses over a 24 hour period and found that their HRV patterns were consistent.

Dr. Gehrke then studied different pairs of horses known to have different relationships to see the reaction in the HRV's. She found that horses that were labeled as 'close friends' had overlapping HRV's, two horses that rarely interact, did not have a significant HRV relationship. When separated, close pairs showed a strong stress reactions. This proved that horses are conscious of each other and have an emotional response. This consciousness transfers to their interactions with humans.

When interacting with both familiar and unfamiliar humans, Dr. Gehrke found that the horses HRVs did not differ. It was not the novelty of the stimuli the horses responded to, but actually the HRV of the human themselves. If a person had a balanced HRV, the horse was more interested in an interaction. To further explore this exchange Dr. Ann Baldwin joined the study. Together, they found that throughout the interactions between 7 human-horse pairs, 6 of their human subject's HRVs synchronized to the horses' specific HRV cycle. It even synchronized for some due to mere exposure to horse and not consciously expressing positive feelings.

All together the research provides evidence a relationship between horses and human emotional states. Horses are sentient creatures that have an emotional reaction to separation and interaction with each other. And most importantly for therapy, a horse's HRV can influence a humans. There are many benefits from this finding. Potentially a much stressed person can be calmed by a relaxed horse. Also research hints that if a person projects positive emotions, the horse can detect them. Making the horse more likely to respond positively, to approach and begin a mutual trust between them.

This emotional consciousness and capacity, whatever the cause may be, can be utilized for therapeutic treatments. Although other animals have been used for therapy, the benefit of horses is the ability to ride them and experience the simultaneous physical benefits from their movements as well as the psychological. Several therapies have been developed to engage the human-horse interaction that benefit patients with a variety of issues from autism, PTSD, depression, and many different physical, mental and emotional disabilities.

Equine-facilitated Psychotherapy (EFP)

Equine-facilitated psychotherapy, EFP, also known as Equine-assisted psychotherapy, utilizes the horses ability to detect and reflect human's emotional states for psychological benefits. This follows a psychoanalytic approach to uncovering a patient's problems and patterns and interpreting them. It requires a mental health professional to monitor the patient, and a horse specialist to monitor the therapy horse. The two professionals address the psychotherapy goals through the patient's relationship and interactions with the horse. The idea is that the horse can aid to unveil deeper issues that a therapist alone cannot. EFP can be used for patients with a variety of health needs. It can benefit people with anxiety, mood disorders, eating disorders, PTSD, schizophrenia, patients going through major life changes like grief or divorce and a variety of problems. Though each specific case will vary, EFP works on a number of levels and begins through building a relationship between patient and horse.

Patients learn the basic needs for a horse. They learn to care for them and through grooming, walking, riding, feeding, and even playing games, the patient develops a bond and relationship to the therapy horse. The horse is a nonjudgmental creature that can promote healthy relationship skills for patients without the fear of disproval or rejection. Fostering a bond to a non-human can help patients who have had negative experiences and have a hard time trusting people. It is an easy way to build trust without making the patient feel too vulnerable.

EFP puts people in a situation that can promote discussion about the individual problems they face. Therapy horses have an unbiased, accurate understanding of patients' emotional states before the patient. Their responses reflect the interaction. Therapists can use the response of a horse to a human can shed light on insecurities, emotions and deeper problems.

Therapists and patients can discuss the patients' reactions to the horse and analyze it. It can be used to interpret their patients' reactions in real-world situations. Discussing what the patient interpreted about the horse's behavior and in turn their own reaction to it can promote self-awareness, and can uncover a patients thinking pattern. This unique method allows people to learn about themselves, promotes social and psychological understanding and growth and can help people heal.

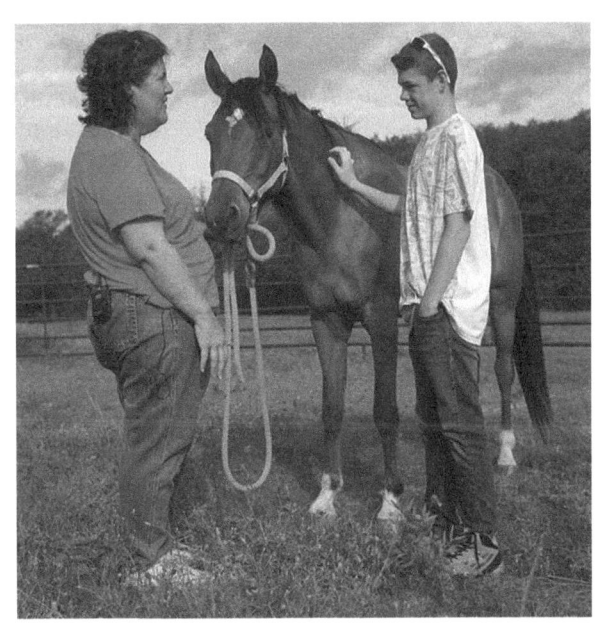

Donna Otabachian, the executive director of the Star Healing With Horses ranch, conducts an equine therapy session with Roger Flores-Hoops, 14, who suffers from secondary PTSD. Secondary PTSD is suffered mainly by the children of service members who have PTSD, as they can be traumatized by changes in their parents' personalities and the conflicts that result from those changes. (U.S. Army photo by Sgt. Ken Scar, 7th Mobile Public Affairs Detachment)

In a case study done by Krista M. Meinersmann, PhD, RN; Judy Bradberry, PhD, RN; and Florence Bright Roberts, PhD, RN, five adult female survivors of abuse were selected for EFP treatment and studied over four thinking patterns.

The first was 'I Can Have Power.' Through EFP, the women interacted and interpreted their experiences with the therapist. They did not need to feel powerless. They learned how to control this big animal, to move the horse around the stalls and get the horses to do certain things. When they learned how to control and manage these horses, they gained confidence in their abilities and realized they had power. Whether it was over the horse or themselves.

The next pattern was 'Doing It Hands On' where the women learned from the physical, visual and kinesthetic experiences with the horses. One women learned to focus her breathing with the horse, saying if she didn't she would fall off. One woman learned she could cry on the horse, and another learned to stay in her own body.

The third pattern is 'Horses as Co-Therapist' where they were able to trust the horses more easily, respect and work with them. The bond facilitated creates an honest relationship. The women claimed the horses mirrored their emotions. If they entered the stall with frustration and an energy they may have thought they weren't projecting, they would notice the horse back away and ignore them immediately. It creates a nonjudgmental mirror that makes one more self-aware and conscious. It makes patients feel safe because they do not worry about rejection and helped them learn to trust.

The last conversation pattern discussed how EFP 'Turned My Life Around' where one woman said she was no longer suicidal and made her want to live. She took a trip alone that she would've never taken, one woman was able to go back to work. It felt to those patients more intimate and more intense than traditional therapy solutions.

Equine-facilitated Learning (EFL)

Equine-facilitated learning, EFL, also known as Equine-assisted learning uses a similar interaction as EFP but focuses on education, professional development and personal development. It, highlights the emotional, spiritual and cognitive influence of the human-horse interaction and is geared towards learning through experiences. It is typically done in group settings and does not typically use riding, as the work is done on the ground. EFL focuses less on personal issues and more on principles and concepts.

In EFL, experiences with horses teach patients concepts like cooperating, working together and learning boundaries for both themselves and the horse. Patients gain insight on ways to manage their behaviors to achieve a goal. In one study done in 2016 by Beth Saggers & Jill Strachan, EFL was used for students in danger of school failure and drop out by using EFL to foster social-emotional leaning and resilience in the at-risk students. Eleven students, 5 boys and 6 girls from ages 10-13 from a primary school in Brisbane, Australa. They were chosen to participate because of their "at-risk" status as determined by the schools welfare team. The students worked with the horses 2 hours a week for 8 weeks, where each week had a different focus. For example, week two's lesson was teaching the students about the horses' needs, week five's lessons included putting a bridle on the horse as a team and week seven was trust building exercises on horseback.

The participants were interviewed before and after EFL. Their post-interviews revealed that they felt more confident, thought positive thoughts, found ways to cope with stress, and learned more effective communication skills. They had taught them to think about why the horses reacted in certain ways as a way to think about their own behavior. They then learned to regulate their behaviors, form a bond with the horse through positive interactions, think of not only their goals but how to accomplish them and experience success. All of the interactions helped foster their abilities to be respectful, mindful, observant and better at working as a team. It increased their capacity to self-regulate and encouraged them to engage in school. EFL utilized the interactions of the students and horses to teach them skills they could apply to school, to their social and home life and to their future careers.

Hippotherapy
Hippotherapy is a form of equine therapy used by occupation, speech, or physical therapists. It assists patients with mental and physical disabilities through the movements of the horse. Hippotherapy helps patients a variety of patients from people who have had a stroke, to patients with cerebral palsy or multiple sclerosis. The horse's movement can enhance functional activities and improve motor skills. Participants can improve things like their balance and can learn to control posture. The different movements of the horse and rider, such as bouncing or holding a position, provides the brain with stimuli that teaches the body to react to complex motor tasks.

Different activities can help with different problems. For example, because a horse's gait is similar to a humans, a therapist can teach someone who can't walk or walks irregularly what his or her gait should feel like. Riding provides joints and muscles with pressure and stimulation they may not normally feel. So slow, rhythmic movements of the horse can help with spasticity. Quick, erratic motions can help heighten attention and make the patient more conscious of their posture. Using the reins helps patients who struggle with right/left coordination.

In one study done by Eun Sook Park, Dong-Wook Rha, Jung Soon Shin, Soohyeon Kim, and Soojin Jung, 34 children with spastic cerebral palsy has 45-minute sessions twice a week for 8 weeks. The study used the GMFM to score the capacity of gross motor function. GMFM-88 breaks movement into five dimensions including, lying and rolling, sitting, crawling and kneeling, standing, and walking, running and jumping. The GMFM-66 measures these tasks based on difficulty. Although both the control and hippotherapy groups improved over the 8-week period, the GMFM-66 scores were significantly greater than the control group. The GMFM-88 scores in sitting increased in both groups, but the other GMFM-88 scores were significantly higher in the hippo therapy group and especially in the walking, running and jumping dimension, thus providing evidence of the benefits of hippotherapy for children with spastic CP.

Therapeutic Riding
Therapeutic riding is horseback riding lessons that are adapted for people with disabilities. It is conducted by a certified therapeutic horseback riding instructor rather than a therapist. It benefits a variety of issues. In TR, someone on the autism spectrum engage in activity that foster awareness about the horses and about. Someone with an eye disorder can benefit from the physical enhancement of fine motor control because TR requires attention to sequencing. For all participants it helps socially because it creates an environment which riders, instructors and volunteers communicate and interact in a fun, recreation activity.

One study showed the significant effects of TR in 20 breast cancer survivors done by Claudia Cerulli, PhD,1 Carlo Minganti, PhD,1 Chiara De Santis, DR,2 Eliana Tranchita, MD,1 Federico Quaranta, MD,1 and Attilio Parisi, MD1. These women who had a mastectomy at the Belcolle Hospital in Viterbo, Italy were selected to participate in therapeutic riding sessions for two hours over a 16-week period. After the study the women had a significant increase in strength, quality of life and aerobic capacity.

Perspective and Prospects
As early as 460 BC the benefits of human-horse interactions have been recorded. Hippocrates found the physical benefits of riding as a natural form of exercise that helps strengthen muscles. In 600 BC horses were used in ancient Greece for therapeutic riding. In 1875, Charles Chassaignac, a French neurologist, used horses to treat patients with a variety of disorders including his paraplegic patients. Today, the

benefits of horses are being utilized for many treatment options. The versatility of these programs can be applied to such a vast range of issues and benefit patients from all walks of life. Because of the fluidity of the programs, its potential is limitless.

—Nancy W. Comstock, Briana Moglia

References

Angoules, Antonios, et al. "A Review of Efficacy of Hippotherapy for the Treatment of Musculoskeletal Disorders." *British Journal of Medicine and Medical Research*, vol. 8, no. 4, Apr. 2015, pp. 289–297., doi:10.9734/bjmmr/2015/17023.

Dreher, Diane. "Why Do Horses Help Us Heal?" *Psychology Today*, 6 Jan. 2018, www.psychologytoday.com/us/blog/your-personal-renaissance/201801/why-do-horses-help-us-heal.

Håkanson, Margareta, et al. "The Horse as the Healer—A Study of Riding in Patients with Back Pain." *Journal of Bodywork and Movement Therapies*, vol. 13, no. 1, 2009, pp. 43–52., doi:10.1016/j.jbmt.2007.06.002.

Kinney, Adam R., et al. "Equine-Assisted Interventions for Veterans with Service-Related Health Conditions: a Systematic Mapping Review." *Military Medical Research*, vol. 6, no. 1, 29 Aug. 2019, doi:10.1186/s40779-019-0217-6.

Lieber, Mark. "Equine Therapy May Help Autism, PTSD and Pain." *CNN*, Cable News Network, 10 July 2018, www.cnn.com/2018/06/18/health/equine-assisted-therapy-cfc/index.html.

Macguire, Eoghan. "Equine-Assisted psychotherapy: Horses as healers." CNN, Cable News Network, 30 Nov. 2015, www.cnn.com/2015/11/30/sport/horse-psychotherapy-otra-mas/index.html.

Naste, Tiffany M., et al. "Equine Facilitated Therapy for Complex Trauma (EFT-CT)." *Journal of Child & Adolescent Trauma*, vol. 11, no. 3, 17 Aug. 2017, pp. 289–303., doi:10.1007/s40653-017-0187-3.

Romaniuk, Madeline, et al. "Evaluation of an Equine-Assisted Therapy Program for Veterans Who Identify as 'Wounded, Injured or Ill' and Their Partners." *Plos One*, vol. 13, no. 9, 27 Sept. 2018, doi:10.1371/journal.pone.0203943.

Wollenweber, Vanessa, et al. "Study of the Effectiveness of Hippotherapy on the Symptoms of Multiple Sclerosis – Outline of a Randomised Controlled Multicentre Study (MS-HIPPO)." *Contemporary Clinical Trials Communications*, vol. 3, 2016, pp. 6–11., doi:10.1016/j.conctc.2016.02.001.

■ Faith healing

CATEGORY: Therapy or Technique

KEY TERMS
- *intercessory prayer*: the act of praying to a deity on behalf of others
- *psychic healing*: the process of sending healing energy by one or more persons to another person in order to re-energize him or her

Overview

The practice of faith healing is common to most if not all religions. Examples of faith healing include the Buddhist focus on healthy karma created by mind/body balance, the practice of Ruqya in Islam, the Zohar of Jewish mysticism, and the Christian belief that adherents may claim physical health as a benefit of salvation.

While occurring throughout history and in all societies, faith healing in Western culture may be more expressive of the individualistic nature of postmodern society. Religious meaning is increasingly found within the context of personal faith and encounter as opposed to the inclusive experience offered by institutions. Practitioners of faith healing also tend to be individual charismatic healers operating either in a religious context or in New Age and mentalist constructs of paranormal healing through the forces of nature.

Faith healing differs from more general exercises in prayer. It is intensely personal and more individualistic than group or shrine contexts, in which healing is experienced through a holy place, through a saint, or through intercessory prayer.

Issues

Medical analyses of faith healing have not produced any final results concerning its effectiveness. Studies devoted to the general issues of spirituality and health, or the relation of prayer to healing, have focused upon selected recipients, such as ethnic groups, religious congregations, or medical groupings. Faith healing is more difficult to isolate in that it occurs within an intensely personal and often independent context. The most prominent faith healers in contemporary American and European societies operate as independent entities. While these figures may host large meetings, the groups themselves are not expressive of any one culture or religious tradition.

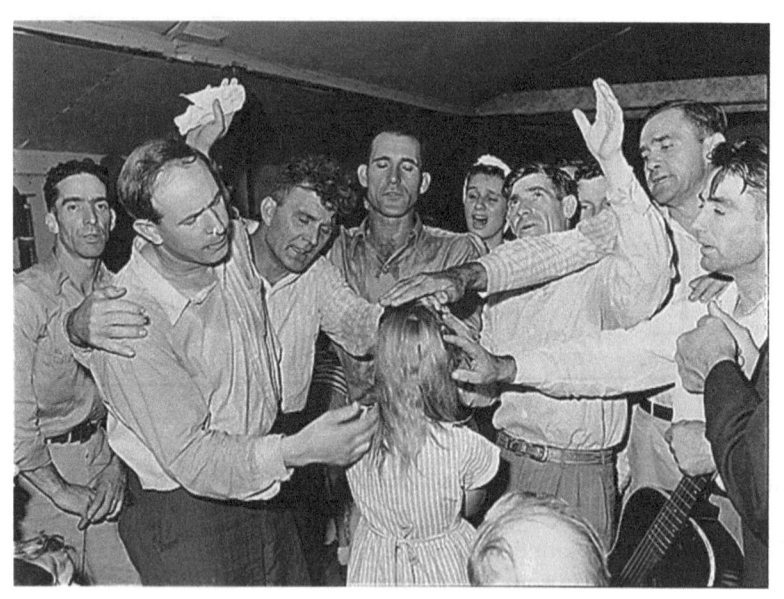

Members of the Pentecostal Church of God in Lejunior, Kentucky pray for a girl in 1946. (Russell Lee via National Archives and Records Administration)

The importance of the entire issue of spirituality and health is demonstrated by the creation of a number of medical centers devoted to investigating the relationship between healing and prayer. These centers include the Center for Spirituality, Theology, and Health at Duke University; the Benson-Henry Institute for Mind Body Medicine at Massachusetts General Hospital; and the George Washington Institute for Spirituality and Health.

Two primary challenges faced by researchers as they study the spectrum of faith/prayer and healing are the problem of establishing basic parameters under which the studies can be conducted and the issues of verification and falsification. At the same time, the medical community has willingly joined forces with the religious in asserting the value of positive attitudes and the exercise of faith in obtaining physical and emotional healing.

—*James F. Breckenridge, Th.D.*

References

Andrade, Chittaranjan, and Rajiv Radhakrishnan. "Prayer and Healing: A Medical and Scientific Perspective on Randomized Controlled Trials." *Indian Journal of Psychiatry*, vol. 51, no. 4, 2009, p. 247., doi:10.4103/0019-5545.58288.

Cook, Gareth. "The Science of Healing Thoughts." *Scientific American*, 19 Jan. 2016, www.scientificamerican.com/article/the-science-of-healing-thoughts/.

Dedeli, Ozden, and Gulten Kaptan. "Spirituality and Religion in Pain and Pain Management." *Health Psychology Research*, vol. 1, no. 3, 23 Sept. 2013, p. 29., doi:10.4081/hpr.2013.e29.

Jantos, Marek, and Hosen Kiat. "Prayer as Medicine: How Much Have We Learned?" *Medical Journal of Australia*, vol. 186, no. S10, 2007, doi:10.5694/j.1326-5377.2007.tb01041.x.

Nita, Maria. "'Spirituality' in Health Studies: Competing Spiritualities and the Elevated Status of Mindfulness." *Journal of Religion and Health*, vol. 58, no. 5, 26 Feb. 2019, pp. 1605–1618., doi:10.1007/s10943-019-00773-2.

Siddall, Philip J., et al. "Spirituality: What Is Its Role in Pain Medicine?" *Pain Medicine*, vol. 16, no. 1, 2015, pp. 51–60., doi:10.1111/pme.12511.

■ Group therapy

CATEGORY: Therapy or Technique; Psychotherapy

Introduction

Society to a greater or lesser degree always forms itself into groupings, whether they are for economic stability, religious expression, educational endeavor, or simply a sense of belonging. Within the field of psychotherapy, many theories and practices have been developed that deal with specific problems facing individuals as they try to relate to their environment as a whole and to become valuable members of society. Available approaches range from psychoanalysis to transpersonal therapy. Taking advantage of the natural tendency for people to form groups, therapists, since the years following World War II, have developed various forms of group therapy. Therapy groups, although they do not form "naturally," are most frequently composed of people with similar problems.

Immediately after World War II, the demand for therapeutic help was so great that the only way to cope with the need was to create therapeutic groups. Group therapy did not boast any one particular founder at that time, although among the first counseling theorists to embrace group therapy actively were Joseph Pratt, Alfred Adler, Jacob Moreno, Trigant Burrow, and Cody Marsh. Psychoanalysis, so firmly placed within the schools for individual psychotherapy, nevertheless became one of the first therapeutic approaches to be applied to group therapy. Gestalt psychology and transactional analysis have proved extremely successful when applied to the group dynamic. Fritz Perls was quick to apply his Gestalt theories to group therapy work, although he usually worked with one member of the group at a time. Gestalt group therapists aim as part of their treatment to try to break down the numerous denial systems that, once overcome, will bring the individual to a new and more unified understanding of life. Eric Berne, the founder of transactional analysis, postulated that the group setting is the ideal therapeutic setting.

Types and Advantages of Group Counseling
Among the different types of group counseling available are those that focus on preventive and developmental aspects of living. Preventive group counseling deals with enhancing the individual's understanding of a specific aspect of life. These aspects range from simple job-seeking skills to more complex studies of career changes in midlife. Developmental groups are composed of well-adjusted people who seek to enhance their social and emotional skills through personal growth and transformation. Conversely, group therapy is concerned with remedial help. The majority of people entering group therapy are aware that they have dysfunctional components in their life; they are seeking group work as a possible way of resolving those problems. The size of most groups ranges from five to fifteen participants. Sometimes all the members in the group belong to one family and the group becomes a specialized one with the emphasis on family therapy. Treating the problems of one family member in the larger context of the whole family has proved successful.

There are as many approaches to therapy as there are therapists; thus, the direction that any given group takes will be dependent on the group leader. Group leadership is probably the one factor that is vital in enabling a group to succeed in reaching both individual and group goals. A leader is typically a qualified and trained therapist whose work is to lead the group through the therapeutic process. Often there will be two therapists involved with the one group, the second therapist sometimes being an intern or trainee.

There are definite advantages, both economic and therapeutic, to group therapy. The economic burden of paying for therapy does not fall solely on one person's shoulders; moreover, the therapist can use his or her time economically, helping a larger number of people. More important, group work may be much more beneficial than individual therapy for certain people. For some, it can be less intimidating than the one-on-one interaction that characterizes individual therapy. Often, the group setting will produce conditions similar to those the member faces in real life and can thus offer an opportunity to face and correct the problem.

Stages of Group Sessions
In group therapy, a "session" consists of a number of meetings; the number is specific and is usually determined at the beginning by the group leader. Flexibility is a key concept in counseling, however, and if a group requires more time and all the participants agree, then the number of sessions can usually be extended. In closed groups, all members start the session together whereas in open group therapy, new participants can join whenever. Therapists have generally come to accept five stages as being necessary for a group to complete a therapy session. These five stages do not have definite boundaries; indeed, if a group experiences problems at any stage, it may return to earlier stages.

Orientation is a necessary first step in establishing a sense of well-being and trust among the group's members. A therapy group does not choose its own members; it is a random and arbitrary gathering of different people. Each member will assess the group critically as to whether this group will benefit him or her. One way for participants to discover the sincerity of the membership of the group is to reveal something of the problem that brought them to the group in the first place, without going into a full disclosure (the point at which a member of a group will share private feelings and concerns). An individual can then assess from the responses of the other members of the group whether they are going to be empathetic or critical. After the orientation stage comes the transitional stage, in which

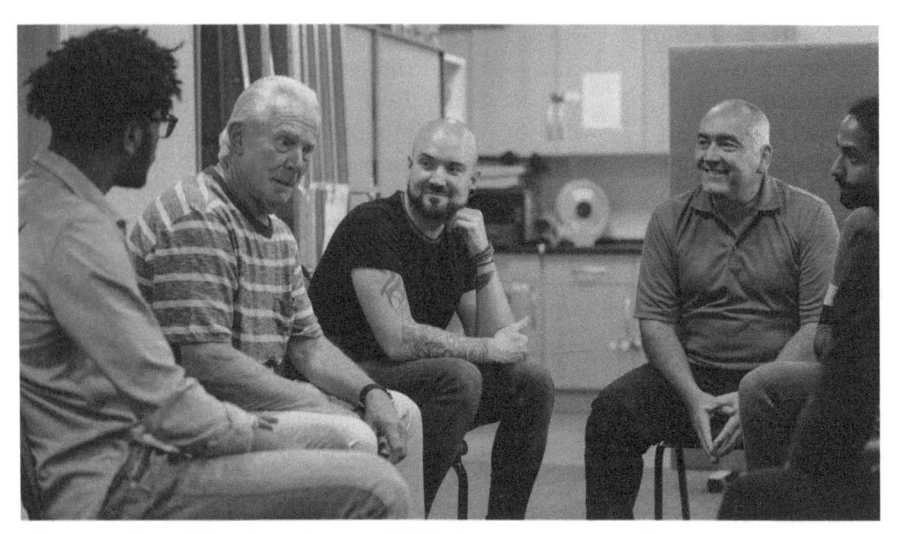

The recognition of shared experiences and feelings among group members and that these may be widespread or universal human concerns, serves to remove a group member's sense of isolation, validate their experiences, and raise self-esteem. (SolStock via iStock)

more self-revelation is required on the part of the individual members. This is usually a time of anxiety for members of the therapy group. Yet despite this anxiety, each member must make a commitment to the group and must further define the problem that has brought him or her to the group in the first place.

When the transitional stage has proved successful, the group will be able to begin the third stage, which involves a greater sense of cohesiveness and openness. This sense of belonging is a necessary and important aspect of group therapy. Without this feeling, the subsequent work of resolving problems cannot be fully addressed. By this time, each member of the group will have disclosed some very personal and troubling part of their lives. Once a group cohesiveness has been achieved, the fourth stage—actually wanting to work on certain behavior-modifying skills—becomes dominant. At this point in the therapeutic continuum, the group leader will play a less significant role in what is said or the direction taken. This seeming withdrawal on the part of the leader allows the group participants to take the primary role in creating changes that will affect them on a permanent basis.

As with all therapeutic methods and procedures, regardless of school or persuasion, a completion or summation stage is vital. The personal commitment to the group must be seen in the larger context of life and one's need to become a part of the greater fabric of living. By consciously creating a finale to the therapy sessions, members avoid being limited in their personal growth through dependence on the group. This symbolic act of stepping away from the group reaffirms all that the group work achieved during the third and fourth stages of the therapeutic process.

Group Dynamics

Group work offers participants an opportunity to express their feelings and fears in the hope that behavioral change will take place. Group therapy takes on significance and meaning only when the individual members of the group want to change their old behavioral patterns and learn a new behavioral repertoire. Most individuals come from a background in which they have experienced difficulties with members of their immediate family. Whether the problem has been a spousal difficulty or a parental problem, those who enter into therapy are desperately looking for answers. The very fact that there is more than one person within the group who can understand and sympathize with another's problem begins the process of acceptance and change. The group dynamic is thus defined as the commonality of purpose that unites a group of people and their desire to succeed.

A group will very quickly become close, intimate, and in some ways self-guarding and self-preserving. Through continually meeting with one another in an intense emotional environment, members begin to look on the group as a very important part of their lives. When one member does not come to a meeting, it can create anxiety in others, for the group works as a whole; for one person not to be present undermines the confidence of those who already lack self-esteem. There are also those who come to group meetings and express very little of what is actually bothering them. While even coming into the therapeutic process is one large step, to disclose anything about themselves is too painful. For those who remain aloof and detached, believing that they are the best judge of their own problems, the group experience will be a superficial one.

Emotional Involvement and Cohesiveness

According to Irvin D. Yalom, therapy is "an emotional and a corrective experience." The corrective aspect of therapy takes on a new meaning when placed in a group setting. There is general agreement that a person who seeks help from a therapist will eventually reveal what is truly troubling him or her. This may take weeks or even months of talking—generally talking around the problem. This is equally true of group participants. Since many difficulties experienced by the participants will be of an interpersonal nature, the group acts as a perfect setting for creating the conditions in which those behavioral problems will manifest. One major advantage that the group therapist has over a therapist involved in individual therapy is that the conditions that trigger the response can also be observed.

For those people who believe that their particular problem inhibits them from caring or even thinking about others, particularly those with a narcissistic or schizoid personality disorder, seeing the distress of others in the group often evokes strong sympathy and caring. The ability to be able to offer some kind of help to another person often acts as a catalyst for a person to see that there is an opportunity to become a whole and useful member of the greater community. For all of its limitations, the group reflects, to some degree, the real-life situations that each of its members experiences every day.

The acknowledgment of another member's life predicament creates a cohesiveness among the members of the group, as each participant grapples with his or her own problems and with those of the others in the group. As each member becomes supportive of all other members, a climate of trust and understanding comes into being. This is a prerequisite for all group discovery, and it eventually leads to the defining of problems and thus to seeking help for particular problems shared by members. Respecting each member's right to confidentiality is another important component to building and maintaining trust. When the individual members of a group begin to care and respond to the needs of the other members, a meaningful relationship exists that allows healing to take place. Compassion, tempered by understanding and acceptance, will eventually prove the ingredients of success for participating members.

Assessing Effectiveness

Group therapy has not been fully accepted in all quarters of the therapeutic professions. Advocates of group therapy have attempted to show, through research and studies, that group therapy is equally effective as individual therapy, but this claim has not settled all arguments. In fact, what has been shown is that if the group leader shows the necessary warmth, understanding, and empathy with the members, then success is generally assured. If, however, the group leader is more on the offensive—even taking on an attacking position—then the effects are anything but positive.

Group therapy continues to play an important role within the field of professional care. There is increasing systematized study and research into the effectiveness of group therapy, especially as far as feedback from the participants of the group therapy experience is concerned. The findings of such studies may led psychologists and counselors to assess more closely the type of therapy that is being offered.

—*Richard G. Cormack*

References

Friedman, Robi. "Individual or Group Therapy? Indications for Optimal Therapy." *Group Analysis*, vol. 46, no. 2, 22 Apr. 2013, pp. 164–170., doi:10.1177/0533316413483691.

Kaklauskas, Francis J., and Les R. Greene. *Core Principles of Group Psychotherapy: a Training Manual for Theory, Research, and Practice.* Routledge, 2019.

Keefe, Francis J., et al. "Group Therapy for Patients with Chronic Pain." *Psychological Approaches to Pain Management: a Practitioner's Handbook*, edited by Dennis C. Turk and Robert J. Gatchel, 3rd ed., The Guilford Press, 2018, pp. 205–229.

Thimm, Jens C, and Liss Antonsen. "Effectiveness of Cognitive Behavioral Group Therapy for Depression in Routine Practice." *BMC Psychiatry*, vol. 14, no. 1, 21 Oct. 2014, doi:10.1186/s12888-014-0292-x.

Whitman, Sarah M. "Group Psychotherapy for Chronic Pain Patients." *Practical Pain Management*, 16 May 2011, www.practicalpainmanagement.com/treatments/psychological/group-psychotherapy-chronic-pain-patients.

Ketamine

CATEGORY: Addiction Risk; Anesthetic; Antidepressant
ALSO KNOWN AS: K; Special K; Vitamin K
ANATOMY OR SYSTEM AFFECTED: Brain; Nervous system

History of Use

Ketamine was first synthesized in 1962 in the laboratories of the Parke-Davis pharmaceutical company. It was developed as an alternative to phencyclidine (PCP) for use as an anesthetic. Clinical use in short-term surgery in humans was initiated in 1975. Many patients began reporting hallucinations while under the drug's influence. Its use is now limited in humans, but it has more widespread applications in veterinary medicine. The drug was soon diverted from hospitals, medical offices, and medical supply houses.

Ketamine became a popular drug for recreational use among teenagers and young adults in the club scene. The US Drug Enforcement Administration added ketamine to its list of emerging drugs of misuse in the mid-1990s. It was classified as a schedule III controlled substance in 1999.

Since the early 2000s, various institutions have been conducting studies to determine whether ketamine can safely be used as an antidepressant and mood stabilizer. With one of the first small studies conducted at the National Institutes of Health, other larger studies have been performed by scientists at Yale University and Mount Sinai Hospital. It is believed that ketamine could relieve depression within hours, and researchers have continued to test the drug's effect on depression on patients for whom other medications have not worked; however, as of 2015, the US Food and Drug Administration had not approved ketamine for the treatment of depression.

Effects and Potential Risks

Primary side effects of ketamine observed in medical settings include increased heart rate and blood pressure, impaired motor function and memory, numbness, nausea, and vomiting. While sedated, patients are unable to move or feel pain. Once the drug wears off, patients have no memory of what occurred while they were sedated.

In unmonitored situations, ketamine produces a dose-related progression of serious adverse effects from a state of dreamy intoxication to hallucinations and delirium. A "trip" on ketamine has been described as being cut-off from reality—"going down into a K hole"—and as an out-of-body or near-death experience. Users may be unable to interact with others around them or even see or hear them. Ketamine has been used as a date rape agent because the victim has no memory of what occurred.

Because misusers feel no pain, they may injure themselves without realizing they are doing so. Chronic use can lead to panic attacks, rage, and paranoia. High doses or prolonged dosing can lead to respiratory depression or arrest and even death. Ketamine is often mixed with heroin, cocaine, or ecstasy. Any of these combinations can be lethal.

—*Ernest Kohlmetz, MA*

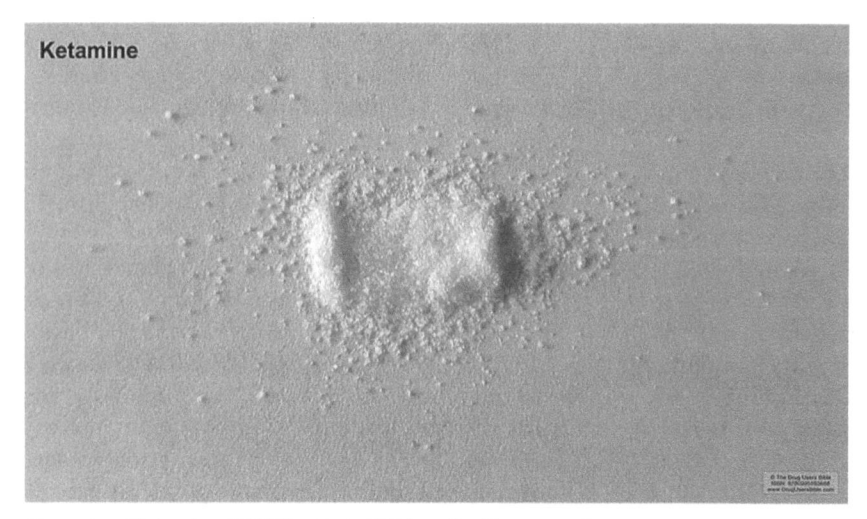

Granules of ketamine. (DMTrott via Wikimedia Commons)

References

Bell, Rae Frances, and Eija Anneli Kalso. "Ketamine for Pain Management." *PAIN Reports*, vol. 3, no. 5, 2018, doi:10.1097/pr9.0000000000000674.

Gass, Natalia, et al. "Differences between Ketamine's Short-Term and Long-Term Effects on Brain Circuitry in Depression." *Translational Psychiatry*, vol. 9, no. 1, 28 June 2019, doi:10.1038/s41398-019-0506-6.

Grady, Sarah E., et al. "Ketamine for the Treatment of Major Depressive Disorder and Bipolar Depression: A Review of the Literature." *Mental Health Clinician*, vol. 7, no. 1, 2017, pp. 16–23., doi:10.9740/mhc.2017.01.016.

Jonkman, Kelly, et al. "Ketamine for Pain." *F1000Research*, vol. 6, 20 Sept. 2017, p. 1711., doi:10.12688/f1000research.11372.1.

Meisner, Robert C. "Ketamine for Major Depression: New Tool, New Questions." *Harvard Health Blog*, Harvard Medical School, 20 May 2019, www.health.harvard.edu/blog/ketamine-for-major-depression-new-tool-new-questions-2019052216673.

Orhurhu, Vwaire, et al. "Ketamine Infusions for Chronic Pain." *Anesthesia & Analgesia*, vol. 129, no. 1, 2019, pp. 241–254., doi:10.1213/ane.0000000000004185.

Parsaik, Ajay K., et al. "Efficacy of Ketamine in Bipolar Depression." *Journal of Psychiatric Practice*, vol. 21, no. 6, 2015, pp. 427–435., doi:10.1097/pra.0000000000000106.

Serafini, Gianluca, et al. "The Role of Ketamine in Treatment-Resistant Depression: A Systematic Review." *Current Neuropharmacology*, vol. 12, no. 5, 12 Sept. 2014, pp. 444–461., doi:10.2174/1570159x12666140619204251.

Wadehra, Sunali, and Charles F. van Gunten. "Ketamine for Chronic Pain Management." *Practical Pain Management*, 4 Dec. 2018, www.practicalpainmanagement.com/patient/treatments/medications/ketamine-chronic-pain-management-current-role-future-directions.

Light therapy

CATEGORY: Therapy or Technique; Psychotherapy
ANATOMY OR SYSTEM AFFECTED: Brain, nervous system, psychic-emotional system, skin
SPECIALTIES AND RELATED FIELDS: Dermatology, gerontology, oncology, ophthalmology, psychiatry, psychology

Indications and Procedures

Light therapy, or phototherapy, treats a variety of disorders. By exposing individuals to different kinds of light (for example, monochromatic, polychromatic, ultraviolet), symptoms can often be delayed, reduced, and eradicated. Immunological, neurotransmitter, and neuroendocrine systems play key roles in response to this type of treatment.

Best known in psychiatry, light therapy serves as a treatment for seasonal affective disorder (SAD), or winter depression; bulimia nervosa; sleep disorders; and "sundowner's syndrome," the late afternoon confusion and agitation sometimes accompanying Alzheimer's disease. Shift workers can also experience difficulties related to light exposure, and light therapies may provide some relief. Reduced environmental light is a factor in the etiology, onset, or maintenance of these problems. Thus, treatment involves exposing individuals to bright, full-spectrum light for specific time periods. Duration of exposure and light intensity vary by the disorder and the individual treated.

In dermatology and oncology, light therapy treats psoriasis, skin ulcers, tumors, and esophageal cancers. The type of light and the intensities used, however, vary considerably from those applied for the treatment of psychiatric disorders.

Uses and Complications

The side effects of light therapy are best documented in psychiatry: insomnia, mania, and (less frequently) morning hot flashes have been noted. Persons with other sensitivity to light, such as those prone to migraines, may also need to exercise caution with light therapy in order to avoid undesirable effects. Careful monitoring by medical providers of the patient's response to treatment is necessary. Additionally, professionals advise morning administrations of light therapy.

Users of light therapy must also be cautioned to adhere closely to recommended doses and intensity of exposure to light. Use of light outside prescribed parameters may be damaging to the eyes.

Light therapy is not effective universally; some patients may experience no improvement. For seasonal affective disorder, evidence suggests that younger individuals whose depression involves weight gain and increased sleep may be most likely to respond to treatment. For psoriasis, complementary treatments, such as psychotherapy, may facilitate a response to treatment.

Perspective and Prospects

Light and dark cycles are a biological reality; thus, it is no surprise that light affects physical,

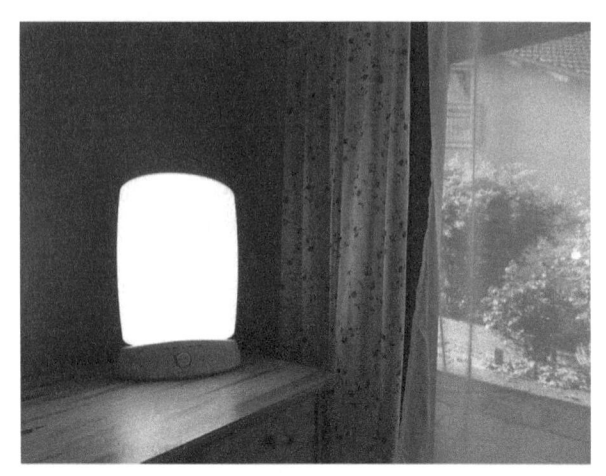

The brightness and color temperature of light from a light box are quite similar to daylight. (Slllu via Wikimedia Commons)

emotional, and mental well-being. As the interest in noninvasive interventions increases, the attention given to environmental treatments such as light therapy is likely to increase as well. Recent developments in the use of light therapy for sleep and behavioral disorders are fueling clinical, research, consumer, and other business interests in this procedure. Experimentation with different frequencies or colors of light, doses, intensities, and sites on the body for the application of light are ongoing and likely to increase the diversity of uses for this type of treatment. Additionally, applications of light-based interventions in the workplace and elsewhere may prove useful in preventing disorders related to light deprivation and in helping to affect productivity, directly and indirectly.

—*Nancy A. Piotrowski, Ph.D.*

References

Cafasso, Jacqueline, and Cynthia Cobb. "Red Light Therapy Benefits." *Healthline*, 11 May 2018, www.healthline.com/health/red-light-therapy.

Huang, S., et al. "The Effectiveness of Bright Light Therapy on Depressive Symptoms in Older Adults with Nonseasonal Depression." *International Journal of Evidence-Based Healthcare*, vol. 14, 2016, doi:10.1097/01.xeb.0000511626.75195.51.

Mayo Clinic Staff. "Light Therapy." *Mayo Clinic*, Mayo Foundation for Medical Education and Research, 8 Feb. 2017, www.mayoclinic.org/tests-procedures/light-therapy/about/pac-20384604.

Oakes, Kari. "Green Light Therapy: A Stop Sign for Pain?" *MDedge Neurology*, 15 May 2019, www.mdedge.com/neurology/article/200743/pain/green-light-therapy-stop-sign-pain.

Reeves, Gloria M., et al. "Improvement in Depression Scores After 1 Hour of Light Therapy Treatment in Patients With Seasonal Affective Disorder." *The Journal of Nervous and Mental Disease*, vol. 200, no. 1, 2012, pp. 51–55., doi:10.1097/nmd.0b013e31823e56ca.

University of Arizona. "Promise in Light Therapy to Treat Chronic Pain." *ScienceDaily*, 28 Feb. 2017, www.sciencedaily.com/releases/2017/02/170228185325.htm.

■ Meditation and relaxation

CATEGORY: Therapy or Technique
ANATOMY OR SYSTEM AFFECTED: Brain

Introduction

Forms of meditation have been practiced in many cultures throughout the ages. Traditionally, meditation techniques have been used to cultivate self-realization or enlightenment, in which higher levels of human potential are said to be realized. Traditional meditation techniques as well as modern techniques of relaxation are often used today for more limited purposes—to combat stress and specific problems of physical and mental health. There is also growing interest, however, in the greater purpose of meditation to achieve higher states of human development.

Techniques

The various techniques of meditation practiced today derive from diverse sources. Some, such as yoga and Zen Buddhism, come from ancient traditions of India and other Asian countries, having been introduced in the West by traditional teachers and their Western students. Others originate in Western traditions such as Christianity. Some relaxation techniques taught today were adapted from these traditions, whereas others were invented independently of meditative traditions. For example, Edmund Jacobson introduced a progressive relaxation technique in 1910

> ## HOW TO MEDITATE
>
> There are many different types of meditation, but there is no "right" technique for every person. Most types of meditation include the following basic elements: position, focus, attitude, and breathing.
>
> *Position.* Before engaging your mind, you should follow these guidelines to make your body comfortable: Sit in a comfortable position on the floor or in a chair. If you choose a chair, keep your knees comfortably apart and rest your hands in your lap. If you sit on the floor, choose one of these poses: tailor fashion (cross-legged), with a cushion under your buttocks; Japanese fashion (on your knees, with your big toes touching and your buttocks resting on the soles of your feet), with a cushion between your feet and buttocks; the yoga full lotus position (not recommended for beginners), in which you keep your spine straight and vertical, but not rigid, and then briefly rock from side to side and from front to back until you feel comfortable and balanced on your hips.
>
> *Focus.* To direct your thoughts, close your eyes (unless the focus of attention is an object). Focus attention on a silent thought, word, or prayer, or on a mental image. Focus on the sensation of each breath during inhaling and exhaling, or on an object such as a candle flame, flower, painting, or bare wall.
>
> *Attitude.* It is important to maintain a gentle and nonjudgmental attitude while you meditate. This will help you to relax. Do not be concerned about your goals or whether or not you are meditating correctly. As a beginner, it is natural for your attention to wander frequently. When your attention wanders, gently redirect it back. Do not try to force attention. Meditation should not be stressful.
>
> *Breathing.* Proper breathing can enhance your experience. Breathe through your nose, if possible. Place your tongue on the ridge behind your upper teeth. Focus your attention on your stomach and diaphragm rather than your nostrils and chest. Place your hand on your stomach and feel the sensations as you inhale and exhale. Your stomach should rise when you inhale and should fall when you exhale. Be attentive to your breathing, but stay relaxed and breathe naturally.
>
> *Progress.* Meditation should become easier with regular practice. You should experiment to find out what technique works best for you, and you should consider taking a meditation class. Many different techniques are taught. Some have a spiritual focus and others are more focused on stress reduction.
>
> —*Amy Scholten, M.P.H.; reviewed by Brian Randall, M.D.*

and advocated its use to the medical profession and the public for more than fifty years. His research found progressive relaxation helpful for a variety of stress-related problems. Jacobson's rather elaborate procedure, which could require up to six months of training, was adapted and shortened by Joseph Wolpe in his book *Psychotherapy by Reciprocal Inhibition* (1958). Later, Douglas A. Bernstein and Thomas D. Borkovec, in *Progressive Relaxation Training: A Manual for the Helping Professions* (1973), further adapted progressive relaxation. These programs require a qualified therapist to teach the relaxation technique. A different approach, autogenic training, derived from self-hypnotic techniques by Johannes Schultz, has been used widely, especially in Europe, since the 1930s.

The approaches of various meditation techniques differ greatly. Most techniques involve sitting quietly with the eyes closed. In some techniques, however, the eyes are kept open, or partially open, as in Zazen practice of Zen Buddhism. Other "meditative" techniques, among them tai chi and hatha-yoga, involve physical movement. Techniques of meditation may be classified according to the way in which mental attention is used during the practice. In some techniques, one focuses or concentrates attention on a specific thought, sensation, or external object. Such concentration techniques train the mind to ignore extraneous thoughts and sensations to remain quiet and focused, as in the Theravadin Buddhist tradition's second stage of practice. Other techniques, such as mindfulness or insight meditation, allow the mind to experience all thoughts and perceptions without focusing on a specific object. In these techniques, the goal is to remain aware of the present moment without judging or reacting to it. Both concentration and mindfulness techniques may be employed in different Buddhist practices. In another approach, contemplative meditation, one thinks about a philosophical question or a pleasant concept such as "love," contemplating the meaning of the thought. This technique is employed, for example, in some Christian practices to produce tranquillity in the mind.

Relaxation techniques take various forms. In progressive relaxation (PR), muscles are consciously tensed and relaxed in a systematic manner. PR is often combined with pleasant mental imagery in a directed manner called guided imagery to produce physical relaxation and a calm mind. Relaxation strategies are often employed in programs of systematic desensitization relaxation techniques to reduce stress responses to frightful or anxiety-producing situations. Autogenic training, another major approach to relaxation, employs an adaptation of self-hypnosis to change the body's functioning. This self-regulation can be very effective, as can biofeedback, which uses scientific instruments to reveal specific physiologic information. While observing signals from the instruments, one consciously manipulates bodily functions to achieve more normal states. In clinical settings, biofeedback is more effective when combined with relaxation and psychotherapeutic techniques than when used alone. Relaxation techniques such as these produce physical and mental relaxation and give the individual some control over physiological processes such as breathing and heart rate. They also result in lower levels of stress hormones such as adrenaline.

Though often confused with these approaches, transcendental meditation, commonly called TM, involves different mechanics. In TM, one uses a sound without meaning, selected for its soothing influence on the mind. This process does not involve concentration, because the sound is used effortlessly. This use of a sound allows one's awareness to shift from the surface level of thinking to subtler levels of the thinking process, and ultimately to transcend thinking and experience a state of silent, restful alertness without thoughts, bodily sensations, or emotions. This inner wakefulness is called transcendental consciousness or pure consciousness. TM is taught in accord with the ancient Vedic tradition of India. Each tradition of meditation has its own understanding of the goals of long-term practice. Though the theme of gaining pure consciousness is shared by several meditative traditions, it cannot be assumed that all techniques of meditation produce the same results.

Potential Benefits

There has been considerable controversy over the years about whether meditation and relaxation techniques differ significantly in the relaxation they produce or in the cumulative effects of their long-term practice. The use of meta-analysis—statistical comparison of the results of many studies—has produced interesting results in this area. Meta-analyses can reveal trends not observed in individual studies and can control for effects of such variations in methods as sample size, study period, and observer bias by combining results from different sources. Because meditation techniques differ and because most meditation studies have been done on TM, these meta-analyses have tended to focus on potential differences between TM and relaxation.

In the mid-1980s, some researchers asked whether simply relaxing with the eyes closed would produce the same level of physiological rest as meditation. A meta-analysis of thirty-one studies showed significantly deeper rest during TM than during eyes-closed rest as indicated by breath rate, basal skin resistance (a measure of stability of the autonomic nervous system), and plasma lactate (a chemical in the blood related to stress).

Individuals practice meditation or relaxation techniques for many different reasons, particularly for relief from anxiety and stress. Both scientific research and anecdotal evidence on some of these techniques indicate that they may produce significant benefits to physical and mental health and to the quality of life as a whole.

Applications

People often use relaxation techniques to relieve specific problems. For example, progressive relaxation has been demonstrated to reduce high blood pressure, headaches, insomnia, and anxiety; to improve memory; to increase internal locus of control (being in control of oneself); and to facilitate positive mood development in

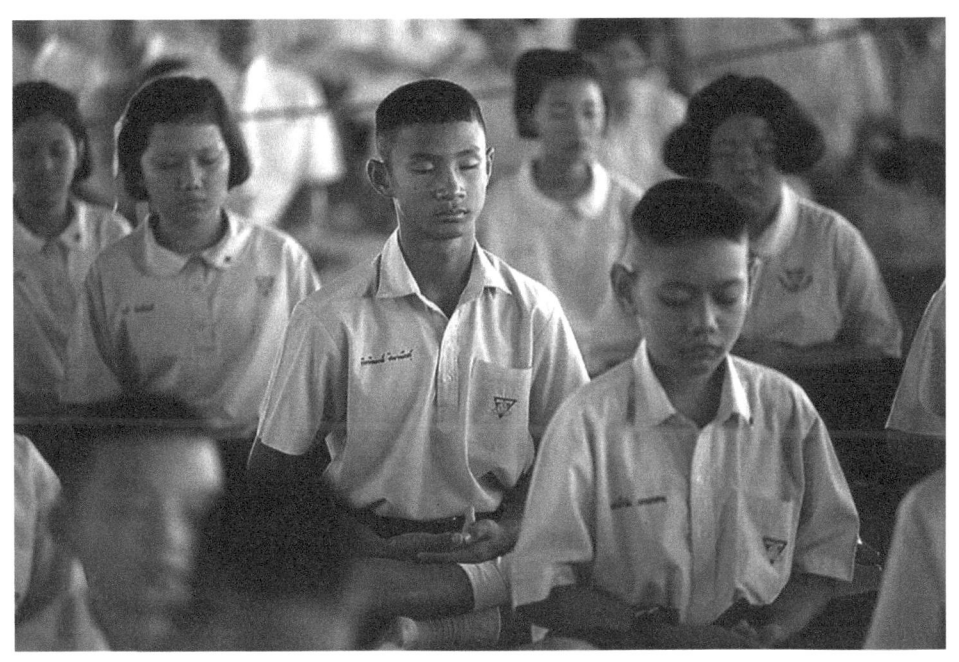

Thai school children meditating as part of organized activities at school. (Kochphon (Honey) Onshawee via Wikimedia Commons)

some people. When used in conjunction with muscle biofeedback, progressive muscle relaxation (PMR) has been effective in treating alcoholism. Autogenic training has also been shown to be effective in many of these areas. These techniques find wide application in psychologists' offices, in hospitals, in schools, and in institutions. For example, medical practitioners teach relaxation techniques to patients for pain management and anxiety reduction, for the control of asthma symptoms, and for treating migraine headaches. Studies have also shown that relaxation improves the concentration abilities of severely intellectually disabled adults and increases academic performance among grade school children.

Of the various meditation techniques, transcendental meditation is the most widely practiced in the West. The standardized method of teaching and uniform method of practicing TM make it particularly suitable for scientific study, and more than five thousand studies have delineated the effects of TM. In a study of health insurance statistics published in 1987 in *Psychosomatic Medicine*, for example, two thousand TM meditators showed 50 percent less serious illness and use of health care services than did nonmeditators over a five-year period. Risk factors for disease, such as tobacco and alcohol use, high blood pressure, and high cholesterol levels, also have been found to decrease among TM meditators. In 1994, psychologist Charles Alexander found that TM proved to be an effective treatment for substance dependence.

There is also some evidence suggesting that meditation is more effective than relaxation techniques. For example, a meta-analysis of 144 independent findings published in the *Journal of Clinical Psychology* in 1989 indicated that the effect of TM on reducing trait anxiety (chronic stress) was approximately twice as large as that produced by progressive relaxation, other forms of relaxation, or other forms of meditation. This was the case even when researchers statistically controlled for differences among studies in subject expectancy, experimenter bias, or quality of research design.

Although meditation is usually considered an activity that affects only the individual practitioner, studies have been performed that suggest that the influence of meditation can extend beyond the meditator to the environment. Such findings are controversial, with many scientists summarily dismissing the possibility of any correlation between meditation and external events. Respected journals have published such studies, however, because the methodologies used were deemed scientifically sound. More than forty studies have found improvements in social conditions and prosperity when a small proportion of the population involved practices TM. For example, in 1999, British researchers Guy Hatchard, Ashley Deans, Kenneth Cavanaugh, and David Orme-Johnson reported that crime rates in Merseyside, England, dropped by 13 percent when the local TM group grew to a certain size. This drop in crime was sustained for the following four years of the study.

Scientific Research on Meditation
Meditation has its origins in spirituality, but is now of particular interest to those wishing to improve psychological and physical health. Decades of research have left little doubt that meditation can be of benefit in the alleviation of stress and anxiety. Other firm conclusions concerning the possible benefits of meditation are difficult to draw, as various forms of meditation are examined in different studies, with a variety of practitioners and a variety of outcome variables.

A number of researchers have examined the physiological effects of meditation. Foremost among these is Richard Davidson of the University of Wisconsin. Davidson has emphasized the ability of the mind to change itself as the result of experience. For example, he has found that meditators with more than 10,000 hours of practice experience sustained attention, but show less activation in attention related areas in the brain than novice meditators. They seem to be able to sustain attention with less effort than novices. They also seem to be both more mindful and less reactive to sensory stimuli, as indicated by imaging of the amygdala and insular cortex, two areas of the brain associated with arousal. In other research, after an eight-week training program in mindfulness, participants experienced an enhanced positive response to an influenza vaccine, in comparison with participants who did not have meditation training.

Research involving the Shamatha project, a longitudinal study involving experienced meditators centered at the University of California, Davis, has found evidence for lowered cortisol, a stress hormone, in meditators as opposed to control participants. Research with participants in this project, has found increased telomerase activity, which is a measure of cell viability.

Much research has suggested that there are psychological benefits of meditation, but the specific nature and potency of these benefits has not been clear. Neither has the "active ingredient" that accounts for these benefits, as the experience of meditation is confounded with specific methods, teachers, and participant characteristics. Meta-analyses, which statistically combine the results of many individual studies are helpful in overcoming some of the difficulties of assessing individual studies, but they too are dependent upon the particular subset of studies included in the meta-analysis.

A meta-analysis of the results of studies using kindness based meditation (including loving kindness meditation and compassion meditation) found that meditators reported less depression and more compassion, self-compassion, and positive emotions than control groups of participants. Other meta-analyses examining a variety of meditative techniques in non-clinical populations found widespread positive effects on emotional variables such as lowered anxiety, increased positive emotions, and decreased neuroticism.

In summary, there is evidence that meditation can produce positive outcomes in terms of stress reduction. Relatively short-term meditators can experience relaxation and increased compassion from meditation, and long-term meditators may experience stronger health benefits mediated by brain changes that occur with practice.

Meditation and the Science of Psychology
The field of psychology was born with the hope that it would someday provide a complete account of human nature. William James, the founder of American psychology, in seeking ways to promote psychological growth, attempted to study elevated states of consciousness and suggested that meditation might be a means to cultivate their development. Few psychologists pursued this direction, however, until advances in bioengineering and the introduction of standardized forms of meditation and relaxation allowed psychologists to study consciousness in the laboratory.

Studies of self-actualization conducted by Abraham Maslow also renewed interest in meditation. According to Maslow, self-actualizing persons are individuals who display high levels of creativity, self-esteem, capacity for intimacy, and concern for the well-being of the world community. They seem to have mastered living happily in a complex world. Maslow believed that self-actualization was the pinnacle of psychological development, and he found that some adults spontaneously had "peak" or transcendental experiences. Sometimes these experiences produced abrupt changes in people's self-perception and significantly advanced their psychological development. Recognizing that meditation might produce such transcendental experiences, Maslow strongly encouraged research on meditation as a means for developing self-actualization.

With the recent development of appropriate scientific methods, alternative states of consciousness such as meditation and relaxation have once again become the focus of much research. Meditation and relaxation are the subject of thousands of studies each year. These studies investigate a wide range of psychological variables, from social development and self-actualization to brain activity.

The various types of meditation are based in ancient systems of philosophy or religion and therefore have ultimate purposes beyond those of strictly psychological approaches to personal development. Whereas self-actualization typically refers to the development of one's unique individual self, Vedic philosophy describes the potential for realizing a transcendental self in the growth of "higher states of consciousness" beyond self-actualization. Through repeated transcendence, one is said to experience this transcendental self as a limitless field of intelligence, creativity, and happiness at the source of the individual mind. In higher states of consciousness, the transcendental self comes to be fully realized and permanently maintained in daily life. In the Vedic tradition, the enlightened are said to enjoy freedom from stress and to find life effortless and blissful.

—*Charles N. Alexander,*
David Sands, Cynthia
McPherson Frantz, Susan E. Beers

References

Blödt, Susanne, et al. "Effectiveness of App-Based Relaxation for Patients with Chronic Low Back Pain (Relaxback) and Chronic Neck Pain (Relaxneck): Study Protocol for Two Randomized Pragmatic Trials." *Trials*, vol. 15, no. 1, 2014, doi:10.1186/1745-6215-15-490.

Cour, Peter La, and Marian Petersen. "Effects of Mindfulness Meditation on Chronic Pain: A Randomized Controlled Trial." *Pain Medicine*, vol. 16, no. 4, 2015, pp. 641–652., doi:10.1111/pme.12605.

Hilton, Lara, et al. "Mindfulness Meditation for Chronic Pain: Systematic Review and Meta-Analysis." *Annals of Behavioral Medicine*, vol. 51, no. 2, 22 Sept. 2016, pp. 199–213., doi:10.1007/s12160-016-9844-2.

Jacob, Julie A. "As Opioid Prescribing Guidelines Tighten, Mindfulness Meditation Holds Promise for Pain Relief." *Jama*, vol. 315, no. 22, 14 June 2016, p. 2385., doi:10.1001/jama.2016.4875.

Penman, Danny. "Can Mindfulness Meditation Really Reduce Pain and Suffering?" *Psychology Today*, 9 Jan. 2015, www.psychologytoday.com/us/blog/mindfulness-in-frantic-world/201501/can-mindfulness-meditation-really-reduce-pain-and-suffering.

Zeidan, Fadel, and David R. Vago. "Mindfulness Meditation-Based Pain Relief: a Mechanistic Account." *Annals of the New York Academy of Sciences*, vol. 1373, no. 1, 2016, pp. 114–127., doi:10.1111/nyas.13153.

■ Mirtazapine

CATEGORY: Antidepressant, Antiemetic, Anxiolytic, Sedative, Appetite Stimulant
ALSO KNOWN AS: Remeron
ANATOMY OR SYSTEM AFFECTED: Sympathetic nervous system

KEY TERMS
- *FDA:* U.S. Food and Drug Administration, a federal agency that provides safety, efficacy, and protection from biologicals
- *major depressive disorder:* mental health disorder characterized by persistent

depressed mood and loss in interest of social activities
- *serotonin syndrome*: a condition that results from the release of high levels of serotonin into the body, causing agitation, confusion, dilated pupils, and muscle twitching
- *MAOI inhibitors*: class of drugs that stop the activity of monoamine oxidase enzymes, and includes such antidepressants such as selegiline *(Eldepry, Emsam, Zelapar)*, phenelzine *(Nardil)*, isocarboxazid *(Marplan)*, tranylcypromine *(Parnate)*

Introduction

Mirtazapine is a central alpha-2 antagonist that is FDA-approved for the treatment of Major Depressive Disorder (MDD). Mirtazapine promotes the release of the neurotransmitters noradrenaline and serotonin, which enhances serotonin neurotransmission. Increased serotonin neurotransmission has both analgesic (pain-relieving) and soporific (improves sleep patterns) effects. Due to its sedative, antinausea, anxiolytic, and appetite stimulant effects, mirtazapine has also been used off-label to assist in the treatment of insomnia, post-traumatic stress syndrome, gastrointestinal distress, and generalized anxiety disorder. Currently, there is available evidence to show that mirtazapine is effective for all stages of depression as well as a range of conditions associated with depression.

How Anti-Depressant Medications Work

Mirtazapine is part of the tetracyclic antidepressant group and works by antagonizing centrally-located pre-synaptic alpha-2 adrenergic receptors. Because activation of alpha-2 adrenergic receptors decreases the release of specific neurotransmitters, alpha-2 receptor antagonists increase the quantities of neurotransmitters released by these neurons. Mirtazapine, therefore, promotes the release of serotonin and norepinephrine and activates the sympathetic nervous system. This increases the appetite and energy level of the patient. About 85% of the drug is attached to plasma proteins that circulate throughout the bloodstream. Mirtazapine is rapidly absorbed into the body and metabolized by the liver. Approximately 15% of the drug is then excreted through feces, while 75% is excreted through the urinary system.

It is important for dosing to be reviewed and changed as appropriate to a patient's renal function. For example, elderly patients or those with significantly impaired hepatic or renal function should have their drug clearance rates regularly ascertained and their dosages adjusted accordingly. Patients should also have their lipid profiles regularly checked, and be monitored for depression, signs or symptoms of serotonin syndrome, weight gain, and a blood condition called agranulocytosis.

Side Effects

Common side effects for mirtazapine (meaning that these adverse effects occur in more than 10% of the population) include drowsiness, weight gain, constipation, serum lipid level increases, and increased appetite.

In a double-blind, placebo-controlled study in Japan, mirtazapine, dosed at 30mg daily, was both safe and effective in the treatment of fibromyalgia, a chronic pain condition that affects the nervous system. Mirtazapine proved more useful in providing a greater analgesic effect as well as improving a patient's quality of life from the social standpoints of job ability, mood, and role functioning.

Clinical trials have established the increased safety and efficacy of selective serotonin reuptake inhibitors (SSRIs) and serotonin/norepinephrine reuptake inhibitors (SNRIs) relative to classic tricyclic antidepressants. Other studies have demonstrated that, when used as directed, all the antidepressants seem to be equally safe. Mirtazapine is one of the medications along with SSRIs that rarely increase the incidence of suicidal ideations. Consequently, mirtazapine does come with a black-box warning.

Contraindications

Any allergic reaction or sensitivity to mirtazapine should prompt the patient to immediately stop using the medication and seek professional guidance.

The concomitant use of MAO inhibitors and mirtazapine is contraindicated. Both mirtazapine and MAO inhibitors increase serotonin neurotransmission in the brain, and concurrent use of these medications that lead to serotonin overload in the brain, which results in a condition called "serotonin syndrome." Since MAO inhibitors are used to treat depression, patients may have prescriptions for mirtazapine and a MAO inhibitor at the same time. However, patients using either medication should wait 14 days after stopping one of these them before beginning the other. This two-week waiting period reduces the risk of serotonin syndrome.

Mirtazapine should be used cautiously in women who are breastfeeding, since metabolites of the medication are secreted into breastmilk, although adverse effects in breastfed babies have been reported only rarely.

—*Shauna Bumford, RN*

References

Brannon, Guy. E. and Karen D. Stone. "The Use of Mirtazapine in a Patient with Chronic Pain." *Journal of Pain and Symptom Management*, vol. 18, no. 5, 1999. pp. 382-385.

Han, Da Hee. "Mirtazapine for Fibromyalgia: An Effective Treatment Option?" *MPR*, 5 June 2018, www.empr.com/home/news/mirtazapine-for-fibromyalgia-an-effective-treatment-option/.

IBM Micromedex. "Mirtazapine (Oral Route) Side Effects." *Mayo Clinic*, Mayo Foundation for Medical Education and Research, 1 Nov. 2019, www.mayoclinic.org/drugs-supplements/mirtazapine-oral-route/side-effects/drg-20067334?p=1.

Jilani, Talha N., and Abdolreza Saadabadi. "Mirtazapine." *StatPearls*, 9 Oct. 2019.

Kenji, M., et al. "Efficacy of Mirtazapine for the Treatment of Fibromyalgia without Concomitant Depression: A Randomized, Double-Blind, Placebo-Controlled Phase IIa Study in Japan." The *Journal of the International Association for the Study of Pain*, vol. 157, no. 9, 2016, pp. 2089-2096. doi: 10.1097/j.pain.0000000000000622

Riediger, C., et al. "Adverse Effects of Antidepressants for Chronic Pain: A Systematic Review and Meta-Analysis." *Frontiers in Neurology*, vol. 8, 2017, p. 307. doi: 10.3389/fneur.2017.00307

■ Music, dance, and theater therapy

CATEGORY: Therapy or Technique; Physiotherapy; Psychotherapy

Introduction

Music, dance, and theater therapies employ a wide range of methods to accomplish the goal of successful psychotherapy. "Psychotherapy" is a general term for the wide variety of methods psychologists and psychiatrists use to treat behavioral, emotional, or cognitive disorders. Music, dance, and theater therapies are not only helpful in the observation and interpretation of mental and emotional illness but also useful in the treatment process. Many hospitals, clinics, and psychiatrists or therapists include these types of therapy in their programs. They are not limited to hospital and clinical settings, however; they also play important roles in a wide variety of settings, such as community mental health programs, special schools, prisons, rehabilitation centers, nursing homes, and other settings.

Music, dance, and theater therapies share a number of basic characteristics. The therapies are generally designed to encourage expression. Feelings that may be too overwhelming for a person to express verbally can be expressed through movement, music, or the acting of a role. Loneliness, anxiety, and shame are typical of the kinds of feelings that can be expressed effectively through music, dance, or theater therapy. These therapies share a developmental framework. Each therapeutic process can be adapted to start at the patient's physical and emotional level and progress from that point onward.

Music, dance, and theater therapies are physically integrative. Each can involve the body in some way and thus help develop an individual's sense of identity. Each therapy is inclusive and can deal with either individuals or groups and with verbal or nonverbal patients in different settings. Each is applicable to different age groups (children, adolescents, adults, the elderly) and to different diagnostic categories, ranging from mild to severe. Although music, dance, and theater therapies share these common characteristics, however, they also differ in important respects.

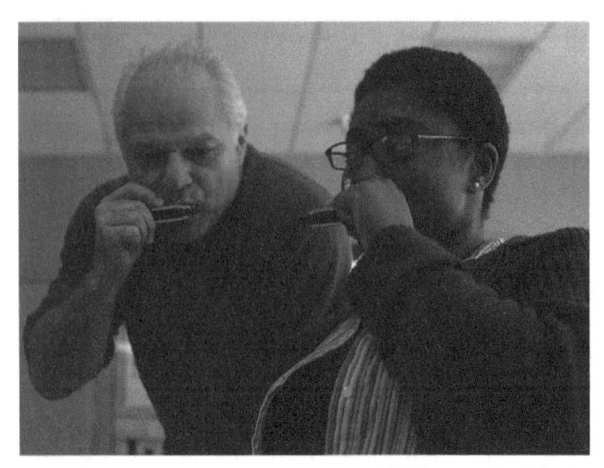

Rand De Mattei, a music instructor with Blues in the Schools, gets in tune with Petty Officer 2nd Class Tyreen S. McRae, a participant in neurologic music therapy. (Lance Cpl. Lisa M. Tourtelot via Wikimedia Commons)

Dance Therapy

Dance therapy does not use a standard dance form or movement technique. Any genre, from ritual dances to improvisation, may be employed. The reason for such variety lies in the broad spectrum of persons who undergo dance therapy: Neurotics, psychotics, schizophrenics, the physically disabled, and geriatric populations can all benefit from different types of dance therapy. Dance therapy may be based on various philosophical models. Three of the most common are the human potential model, the holistic health model, and the medical model. The humanistic and holistic health models have in common the belief that individuals share responsibility for their therapeutic progress and relationships with others. By contrast, the medical model assumes that the therapist is responsible for the treatment and cure.

Dance therapy is not a derivative of any particular verbal psychotherapy. It has its own origin in dance, and certain aspects of both dance and choreography are important. There are basic principles involving the transformation of the motor urge and its expression into a useful, conscious form. The techniques used in dance therapy can allow many different processes to take place. During dance therapy, the use of movement results in a total sensing of submerged states of feeling that can serve to eliminate inappropriate behavior. Bodily integration is another process that can take place in dance therapy. The patient may gain a feeling of how parts of the body are connected and how movement in one part of the body affects the total body. The therapist can also help the patient become more aware of how movement behavior reflects the emotional state of the moment or help the patient recall earlier emotions or experiences. Dance therapy produces social interaction through the nonverbal relationships that can occur during dance therapy sessions.

Music Therapy

Music therapy is useful in facilitating psychotherapy because it stimulates the awareness and expression of emotions and ideas on an immediate and experiential level. When a person interacts musically with others, he or she may experience (separately or simultaneously) the overall musical gestalt of the group, the act of relating to and interacting with others, and his or her own feelings and thoughts about self, music, and the interactions that have occurred. The nonverbal, structured medium allows individuals to maintain variable levels of distance from intrapsychic (within self) and interpersonal (between people) processes. The abstract nature of music provides flexibility in how people relate to or take responsibility for their own musical expressions. The nonverbal expression may be a purely musical idea, or it may be part of a personal expression to the self or to others.

After the activity, the typical follow-through is to have each client share what was seen, heard, or felt during the musical experience. Patients use their musical experiences to examine their cognitive and affective reactions to them. It is then the responsibility of the music therapist to process with the individual the reactions and observations derived from the musical experience and to help the person generalize them—that is, determine how they might be applied to everyday life outside the music therapy session. Group musical experiences seem to stimulate verbal processing, possibly because of the various levels of interaction available to the group members.

Theater Therapy

Theater therapy, or drama therapy, uses either role-playing or improvisation to reach goals similar to those of music and dance therapy. The aims of the drama therapy process are to recognize experience, to increase one's role repertoire, and to learn how to play roles more spontaneously and competently.

The key concepts of drama therapy are the self and roles. Through role taking, the processes of imitation, identification, projection, and transference take place. Projection centers on the concept that inner thoughts, feelings, and conflicts will be projected onto a relatively ambiguous or neutral role. Transference is the tendency of an individual to transfer his or her feelings and perceptions of a dominant childhood figure—usually a parent—to the role being played.

Uses and Goals of Psychotherapies

New approaches and applications of music, dance, and theater therapies have been and are being developed as these fields grow and experiment. The goal of theater or drama therapy is to use the universal medium of theater as a setting for psychotherapeutic goals. Opportunities for potential participants include forms of self-help, enjoyment, challenge, personal fulfillment, friendship, and support. The theater setting helps each individual work with issues of control, reality testing, and stress reduction.

David Johnson and Donald Quinlan conducted substantial research into the effects of drama therapy on populations of schizophrenics. Their research addressed the problem of the loss of the self and the potential of drama therapy in recovering it. They found that paranoid schizophrenics create more rigid boundaries in their role-playing, while nonparanoid schizophrenics create more fluid ones. They concluded that improvisational role-playing is an effective means to assess boundary behaviors and differentiate one diagnostic group of schizophrenics from another. Subtypes of schizophrenia diagnosis, however, are no longer included in the American Psychiatric Association's *Diagnostic and Statistical Manual of Mental Disorders*, which was published in its fifth addition in 2013.

Drama therapy has also been used in prison environments to institute change and develop what has been termed a therapeutic community. The Geese Theatre Company, founded in the United States in 1980, works to change the institutional thinking, metaphors, responses, and actions unique to the prison environment, to allow both staff and prisoners to change and convert prisoner images and metaphors. The therapists found that drama therapy, or role-play, intensifies the affect necessary to challenge beliefs. The method requires strong support from the staff and the institution. Drama therapy, they point out, provides an unexpected format, action-based, and driven by people in relationship with one another. Their work in prison settings in both Australia and Romania helped in continuing development of process and principles for transforming prison cultures into effective therapeutic communities.

Dance therapy has been found to be extremely useful in work with autistic children as well as with children with minimal brain dysfunction (MBD). The symptoms of a child with MBD may range from a behavioral disorder to a learning disability. Though the symptoms vary, and some seem to vanish as the child matures, the most basic single characteristic seems to be an inability to organize internal and external stimuli effectively. By helping the child with MBD to reexperience, rebuild, or experience for the first time those elements on which a healthy body image and body scheme are built, change can be made in the areas of control, visual-motor coordination, motor development, and self-concept.

The goals of dance therapy with a child with MBD are to help the child identify and experience his or her body boundaries, to help each child master the dynamics of moving and expressing feelings with an unencumbered body, to focus the hyperactive child, to lessen anxiety and heighten the ability to socialize, and to strengthen the self-concept.

Music therapy has been used successfully with patients who have anorexia nervosa, an eating disorder that has been called self-starvation. Anorexia nervosa represents an attempt to solve the psychological or concrete issues of life through direct, concrete manipulation of body size and weight. Regardless of the type or nature of the issues involved, which vary greatly among anorectic clients, learning to resolve conflicts and face psychological challenges effectively without the use of weight control is the essence of therapy for these clients. To accomplish this, anorectics must learn to divorce their eating from their other difficulties, stop using food as a tool for problem solving, face their problems, and believe in themselves as the best source for solving those problems. Music therapy has provided a means of persuading clients to accept themselves and their ability to control their lives, without the obsessive use of weight control, and to interact effectively and fearlessly with others.

Many health professionals have acknowledged the difficulty of engaging the person with anorexia in therapy, and music has been found to work well. Because of its nonverbal, nonthreatening, creative characteristics, music can provide a unique, experiential way to help clients acknowledge psychological and physical problems and resolve personal issues.

Music and dance therapies are being used to improve quality of life for older victims of dementias, including Alzheimer's disease. The number of cases of Alzheimer's is expected to increase as the population ages. It has been found that both music and movement can be used to reach these patients when other methods fail. The keys to this therapy include song preference of the client and the use of music specific to the client's life and youth. This music has been most effective if presented live, using the same rhythms and syncopations as the original music. Such therapy can be used to support and encourage behaviors that allow patients with dementia access to a higher quality of life, and to the expression of feelings and enjoyment.

Dynamic play therapy is another approach that combines concepts and techniques of drama and dance improvisation. It has been used in clinical settings involving foster, adoptive, and birth families with troubled children. This type of family play therapy emerged from sessions that often included adult caretakers of foster children and addressed specific problems concerning abuse and family-related expressive activities.

Interdisciplinary Relationships
The interdisciplinary sources of dance, music, and drama therapies bring a wide range of appropriate research methodologies and strategies to the discipline of psychology. These therapies tend to defy conventional quantification. Attempts to construct theoretical models of these therapies draw on the disciplines of psychology, sociology, medicine, and the arts. There is no unified approach to the study and the practice of these therapies.

Dance therapy has its roots in ancient times, when dance was an integral part of life. It is likely that people danced and used body movement to communicate long before language developed. Dance could express and reinforce the most important aspects of a culture. Societal values and norms were passed down from one generation to another through dance, reinforcing the survival mechanism of the culture.

The direct experience of shared emotions on a preverbal and physical level in dance is one of the key influences in the development of dance or movement therapy. The feelings of unity and harmony that emerge in group dance rituals provide the basis of empathetic understanding between people. Dance, in making use of natural joy, energy, and rhythm, fosters a consciousness of self. As movement occurs, body sensations are often felt more clearly and sharply. Physical sensations provide the basis from which feelings emerge and become expressed. Through movement and dance, preverbal and unconscious material often crystallizes into feeling states of personal imagery. It was the recognition of these elements, inherent in dance, that led to the eventual use of dance or movement in psychotherapy.

Wilhelm Reich was one of the first physicians to become aware of and use body posturing and movement in psychotherapy. He coined the term "character armor" to describe the physical manifestation of the way an individual deals with anxiety, fear, anger, and similar feelings. The development of dance into a therapeutic modality, however, is most often credited to Marian Chace, a former dance teacher and performer. She began her work in the early 1940s with children and adolescents in special schools and clinics. In the 1950s and 1960s, other modern dancers began to explore the use of dance as a therapeutic agent in the treatment of emotional disturbances.

There is a much earlier history of music therapy; the use of music in the therapeutic setting dates back to the 1700s. The various effects of different types of music on emotions were recognized. Music could be used to restrain or inflame passions, as in examples of martial, joyful, or melancholic music. It was therefore concluded that music could also have positive healing effects, although these would vary from person to person. Early research showed music therapy to be useful in helping mental patients; people with physical disabilities; children with emotional, learning, or behavioral problems; and people with a variety of other difficulties. Music could be used to soothe and to lift the spirits, but it required experimentation and observation.

Although its theatrical roots are ancient, drama or theater therapy is still in early stages of professional development. The field developed out of clinical experience in the 1920s, and its use and its value as a psychotherapeutic tool is well documented. As a profession, drama therapy now requires the articulation and documentation of theories and methods as well as intensive case studies as support. Four challenges have been identified for the field: to develop new university programs and to increase the supply of students, to expand opportunities for advanced learning and to use mentors to help internalize a professional identity, to produce books and texts to attract new students and to establish the field academically, and to participate with other creative arts therapy organizations to protect legislatively professional interests and the needs of clients. All these forms of therapy can thus be best understood in terms of their backgrounds, relationships, and individual contributions to therapeutic applications in both mental and physical healing.

—Robin Franck
—Martha Oehmke Loustaunau

References

Brazier, Yvette. "Drama Therapy: Unlocking the Door to Change." *Medical News Today*, MediLexicon International, 30 Mar. 2016, www.medicalnewstoday.com/articles/308452.php#1.

Harari, Michal Doron. "'To Be On Stage Means To Be Alive' Theatre Work with Education Undergraduates as a Promoter of Students' Mental Resilience." *Procedia - Social and Behavioral Sciences*, vol. 209, 2015, pp. 161–166., doi:10.1016/j.sbspro.2015.11.272.

Ho, Rainbow T H, et al. "Psychophysiological Effects of Dance Movement Therapy and Physical Exercise on Older Adults With Mild Dementia: A Randomized Controlled Trial." *The Journals of Gerontology: Series B*, 2018, doi:10.1093/geronb/gby145.

Karkou, Vicky, et al. "Effectiveness of Dance Movement Therapy in the Treatment of Adults With Depression: A Systematic Review With Meta-Analyses." *Frontiers in Psychology*, vol. 10, 3 May 2019, doi:10.3389/fpsyg.2019.00936.

Koch, Sabine C., et al. "Effects of Dance Movement Therapy and Dance on Health-Related Psychological Outcomes. A Meta-Analysis Update." *Frontiers in Psychology*, vol. 10, 20 Aug. 2019, doi:10.3389/fpsyg.2019.01806.

Leggieri, Melissa, et al. "Music Intervention Approaches for Alzheimer's Disease: A Review of the Literature." *Frontiers in Neuroscience*, vol. 13, 12 Mar. 2019, doi:10.3389/fnins.2019.00132.

Leubner, Daniel, and Thilo Hinterberger. "Reviewing the Effectiveness of Music Interventions in Treating Depression." *Frontiers in Psychology*, vol. 8, 7 July 2017, doi:10.3389/fpsyg.2017.01109.

Ml, Montánchez Torres, et al. "Benefits of Using Music Therapy in Mental Disorders." *Journal of Biomusical Engineering*, vol. 04, no. 02, 2016, doi:10.4172/2090-2719.1000116.

■ Pet therapy

CATEGORY: Therapy or Technique

According to a 2018 survey conducted by the American Veterinary Medical Association, nearly 70% of households in the United States have at least one companion animal. For the past several decades, it has become widely accepted that pets enhance the psychological and physical well-being of their owners. Psychologically, companion animals can be a source of unconditional love and acceptance, and provide a source of purpose, security, belonging, and identity. Pet owners typically report greater levels of self-esteem, social and emotional support and lower levels of anxiety and depressive symptoms compared to non-pet owners. Companion animals have positive effects on how individuals regulate emotions, deal with trauma, and relate to others. Physically, pet ownership correlates with improved cardiovascular health, fewer doctor visits and hospitalizations, and an overall increase in daily activity and exercise. Companion animals serve as a buffer against several of the physiological aspects of stress by decreasing activation of the sympathetic nervous system, which results in lowered blood pressure, heart rate, and production of stress hormones.

More recently, health care professionals recognize the role of companion animals in pain management. Mainly, Animal-Assisted Therapy (AAT) is being used in combination with traditional pharmaceuticals for pain relief. While most of the research has been conducted on AAT programs that use specially trained dogs, there is evidence that suggests similar effects are obtained from other animals such as cats, rabbits, birds, horses, and even fish.

Mechanisms of Action

Pet therapy seems to relieve pain by increasing the production of endogenous opioids and other pain-relieving molecules in pet owners. Studies have shown that even a 10-minute interaction with a companion animal can increase the production of beta-endorphin (an endogenous opioid), the hormones oxytocin and prolactin, and the pleasure-promoting neurotransmitter dopamine. The same 10-minute interaction with pets also decreases levels of the stress hormone cortisol. The adrenal glands secrete cortisol, and cortical levels are consistently higher in patients with chronic pain disorders.

Neurologically, the chemical basis for the human-animal bond is the hormone oxytocin. Oxytocin is released by the posterior lobe of the pituitary gland during labor, delivery, and breastfeeding in women. More commonly, however, oxytocin is responsible for pair bonding between couples and between humans and their animal companions. Therefore, the same hormone that allows a mother to bond to her newborn baby is used by the brains of pet owners and their companion animals to form a durable social bond. Individuals with higher levels of oxytocin are more apt to engage in social interactions. The closer the bond between the pet owner and their companion animal, and the more the pet owner touches their companion animal, the more oxytocin is released. Oxytocin decreases pain by influencing the periaqueductal grey region in the midbrain, a region of the brain known to downregulate pain perception. In the spinal cord, oxytocin has the effect of an endogenous opioid.

Psychologically, oxytocin acts on the amygdala to reduce anxiety. It counteracts the activity of the hypothalamus-pituitary-adrenal-axis by decreasing the secretion of the stress hormone cortisol. Oxytocin helps improve the symptoms of depression and depression-related health problems. Patients with major depressive disorders and some types of autism spectrum disorder consistently possess lower blood levels of oxytocin. Increased levels of oxytocin during therapy for depression correlate positively with recovery. Activation of the oxytocin system requires physical touch and influences the dopamine-based reward circuit, which is mediated by the mesolimbic system.

Other studies have demonstrated reductions in cardiovascular stress (decreased blood pressure and heart rate) when pet owners interact with their animals. Human-animal interactions reduce stress-related indicators such as epinephrine and norepinephrine, improve immune system functioning and pain management, decrease aggression, augment empathy, increase the trustworthiness of and trust toward other persons, and improve learning.

Uses and Applications

Pet therapy can help reduce pain in three different groups of clients. The first group is service dog owners who have dogs trained to do specialized tasks for their disabled owners. There are eight main categories of service dogs: guide dogs, hearing dogs, diabetic alert dogs, mobility assistance dogs, seizure response dogs, autism support dogs, allergy detection dogs, and psychiatric service dogs. Second are those individuals who have access to an animal through an AAT program. These animals, typically dogs, are certified through programs like Therapy Dogs International or Animal Assistance Therapy. Third, pet owners can reap some of the pain-reducing effects of pet therapy by only interacting at home with their pets.

Scientific Evidence

The professional literature is replete with evidence for the positive impact of Animal-Assisted Therapy on hospitalized patients and individuals who have appointments at outpatient clinics. For example, even though it is not an AAT program, when dogs visit patients who have had a total joint replacement procedure, they have decreased postoperative pain. They also report significant pain reductions in their initial physical therapy sessions. Other studies have demonstrated that the more time total joint replacement patients spent with dogs, postoperatively, the less they used prescribed pain relievers.

Similarly, patients with fibromyalgia who spent 10-15 minutes with a therapy dog while waiting for their medical appointment reported less pain, fatigue, and emotional distress compared to patients in the control group who had no such animal interaction. These positive results were independent of how the individuals initially felt about dogs.

Using AAT in conjunction with traditional pharmaceutical agents also seems to have a positive impact on children. Children hospitalized for various illnesses and procedures, including cancer and cancer treatments, reported less physical pain and emotional distress when they participated in interactive sessions with a service dog as part of the hospital's AAT program.

The post-surgical recovery of pet owners compared to the recovery of non-pet owners has yet to be rigorously studied and awaits further research.

Safety Issues

Because animals can carry diseases, infection is a potential concern for people participating in pet therapy and pet owners in general. However, several studies have failed to demonstrate greater rates of infection among pet owners versus non-pet owners, and participants in AAT programs do not show higher rates of disease. Animals can also bite or scratch their owners, but the proper training of both dogs and their handlers can virtually eliminate this risk. Nevertheless, inadvertent injuries caused by any animal should be immediately disinfected and bandaged, and, if necessary, patients should seek further medical attention.

While gazing into the eyes of a companion animal can increase the production of oxytocin and enhance the bonding process, care must be taken not to stare or make direct contact in any way that the animal might perceive as intimidating or threatening. When interacting with a companion animal, any person who does not have a high-quality, trusting relationship with the animal should avoid direct eye contact at first. Also, people should avoid any gestures that animals may potentially perceive as threatening, such as invading the animal's space or pulling on their tail, fur, or ears should be avoided.

—*Terri Pardee Ph.D. and Michael A. Buratovich Ph.D.*

References

Braun, Carie, et al. "Animal-Assisted Therapy as a Pain Relief Intervention for Children." *Complementary Therapies in Clinical Practice*, vol. 15, no. 2, 2009, pp. 105-109.

Harper, Carl M., et al. "Can Therapy Dogs Improve Pain and Satisfaction after Total Joint Arthroplasty? A Randomized Controlled Trial." *Clinical Orthopaedics and Related Research*, vol. 473, no. 1, 2015, pp. 372-9. doi:10.1007/s11999-014-3931-0.

Harvey, Julia, et al., "The Effect of Animal-Assisted Therapy on Pain Medication Use After Joint Replacement." *Anthrozoös*, vol. 27, no. 3, 2014, pp. 361-369, doi:10.2752/175303714X13903827487962

Marcus, Dawn W., et al. "Animal-Assisted Therapy at an Outpatient Pain Management Clinic." *Pain Medicine*, vol. 13, no. 1, 2012, pp. 45-57. doi:10.1111/j.1526-4637.2011.01294.x.

——. "Impact of Animal-Assisted Therapy for Outpatients with Fibromyalgia." *Pain Medicine*, vol. 14, no. 1, 2013, pp. 43-51. doi:10.1111/j.1526-4637.2012.01522.x.

Odendaal, JS, and R. A. Meintjes. "Neurophysiological Correlates of Affiliative Behaviour Between Humans and Dogs." *Veterinary Journal*, vol. 165, no. 3, 2003, pp. 296-301.

Sobo, Elisa, Eng, Brenda, and Nadine Kassity-Krich. "Canine Visitation (Pet) Therapy: Pilot Data on Decreases in Child Pain Perception." *Journal of Holistic Nursing*, vol. 24, no. 1, 2006, pp. 51-57.

Urbanski, Beth L., and Mark Lazenby. "Distress Among Hospitalized Pediatric Cancer Patients Modified by Pet-Therapy Intervention to Improve Quality of Life." *Journal of Pediatric Oncology Nursing*, vol. 29, no. 5, 2012, pp. 272-82. doi: 10.1177/1043454212455697.

Wu, Adam S., Niedra, Ruta, Pendergast, Lisa, and Brian W. McCrindle. "Acceptability and Impact of Pet Visitation on a Pediatric Cardiology Inpatient Unit." *Journal of Pediatric Nursing*, vol. 17, no. 5, 2002, pp. 354-362.

■ Play therapy

CATEGORY: Therapy or Technique; Psychotherapy

Introduction

Children of all ages learn about their environment, express themselves, and develop relationships with others through their play activity. Play is an integral part of childhood, an activity that must be allowed to facilitate a child's development. In fact, play is seen as such an important aspect of a child's life that the United Nations made the right to play an inalienable right for children across the world. Some adults have labeled play a child's "work," and this may be an appropriate way of looking at children's play. Just as work fosters self-esteem for adults, so does play enhance the self-esteem of children. Just as adults learn to solve problems through their work, children learn to cope with and invent solutions to problems through their play.

Growth through Play
Through play, children grow and learn in a number of ways. First, play helps children grow emotionally; children learn to express their feelings, understand their feelings, and control their emotions through play by acting out a variety of situations and roles. They learn to share and cooperate with other children as well as language, they learn to think in symbols, and they learn that the same object can have different functions and that things can break and be repaired. They also act out rules and regulations in play with other children. They learn that some things hurt other people and should therefore not be done, and they realize that rules often serve a purpose of protection or safety. All these growth processes are extremely important by-products of play, but perhaps the most important aspect of play is that of communication, defined here as the sharing of information with other people, either through language or through other ways of interacting. Children tell about themselves and their lives through play. Even when they do not yet have language skills, they possess the ability to play.

Role of Therapist and Setting
This aspect of communication through play is perhaps the most important element of play therapy. In play therapy, a therapist uses children's play to understand them and to help them solve problems, feel better about themselves, and express themselves better. Children often have difficulty telling adults what they feel and experience, what they need and want, and what they do not want and do not like. Often, they lack the language skills to do so, and sometimes they are too frightened to reveal themselves for fear of punishment or rejection.

In play therapy, however, the therapist is an adult who is empathic, sensitive, and—above all—accepting and nonthreatening. The child is made to feel comfortable in the room with this adult and quickly recognizes that this person, despite being quite old (at least from the child's perspective), understands the child and accepts his or her wishes and needs. Children learn to play in the presence of this therapist or with the therapist, and through this play, they communicate with the therapist. They reveal through their activity what they have experienced in life, how they feel, what they would like to do, and how they feel about themselves.

The toys and activities that play therapists use vary significantly, though therapists take great care to equip the room in which they work with the child in such a way as to allow maximum freedom and creativity on the child's part. Therapists generally have art supplies such as clay, crayons, and paints; toy kitchen appliances and utensils; baby items such as bottles and rattles; a variety of dolls and dollhouses; toy guns and soldiers; toy cars and boats; blocks and erector sets; and stuffed animals. All these materials share several important traits: They foster creativity, have many different uses, are safe to play with, and can easily be used by the child for communication. On the other hand, therapists rarely have things such as board games or themed toys (for example, television action heroes), because these toys have a definite use with certain rules and restrictions, are often used merely to re-create stories observed on television, or are not very handy for getting children to express themselves freely. Most of the time, the toys are kept in an office that is specifically designed for children, not a regular doctor's office. As such, the room generally has a child-size table and chairs but no adult-size desk. It usually has no other furniture but may have some large cushions that the child and therapist can sit on if they want to talk for a while. Often the room has a small, low sink for water play, and sometimes even a sandbox. Floor and wall coverings are constructed of easily cleaned materials so that spills are not a problem. The room is basically a large play area; children generally like the play therapy room because it is unlike any other room they have ever encountered and because it is equipped specifically with children in mind.

Therapeutic Process
There are many reasons a child may be seen in play therapy. For example, a referral may come from a teacher who is concerned about a drop in the child's academic performance; from day-care personnel who are concerned about the child's

inability to relate to other children; from the child's pediatrician, who believes the child is depressed but cannot find a physical cause; or from parents who think the child is aggressive or withdrawn. Whatever the reason, therapy begins with an intake interview. The intake is a session during which the therapist meets not only with the child but also with the parents and siblings in an attempt to find out as much about the child as possible to gain an understanding of what is wrong.

Once the therapist knows what is happening with the child, recommendations for treatment are made. Sometimes the recommendation is for the entire family to be seen in family therapy. Sometimes the recommendation is for the parents to be seen. Sometimes the recommendation is for play therapy for the child.

Once a child enters play therapy, the child meets with the therapist once weekly for fifty or sixty minutes (sometimes, for very young children, sessions can be as short as thirty minutes) for several weeks or months. During the sessions, the child decides what to play with and how, and the therapist is there to understand the child, help the child solve problems, and facilitate growth and self-esteem. The therapist never recommends toys or activities to the child nor speculates aloud what the child's play might symbolize; instead, the child self-directs his or her play activity without guidance from the therapist. Often, while the child is being seen, the parents are also in some type of therapy session themselves. Children's problems often arise because of problems in the family, which is why it is rare that only the child is in treatment. Parents are often seen so that they can work on their relationship either with each other or with the whole family, or to learn parenting skills.

The first thing that happens in play therapy is that the therapist and the child get to know each other and develop a positive relationship. Once the child begins to trust the therapist, the child starts to reveal his or her needs, wishes, concerns, fears, and problems through play. The therapist observes and interacts with the child to help the individual work out problems, deal with strong feelings, accept needs, and learn to deal with often difficult family or environmental circumstances. All this work is done through the child's play in much the same way as children use play while growing up. In addition to using play activity, however, the therapist uses the trusting relationship with the child. Play

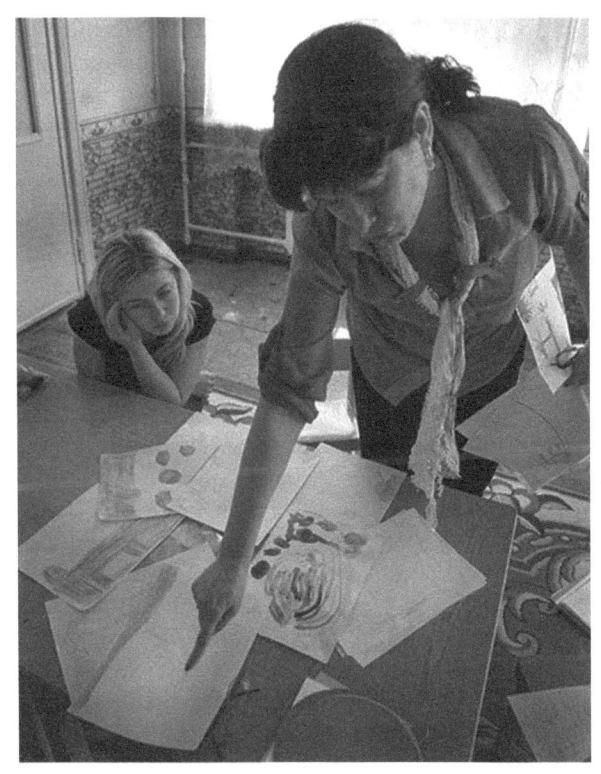

Volunteer psychologists Valentina Nikolaeva (right) *and Evgeniya Doronina show how drawings can reveal the mental condition of children.* (UNICEF Ukraine via Wikimedia Commons)

therapy fosters open and voluntary communication, promotes creative problem-solving, and builds trust and mastery.

Example of Therapy

The process of play therapy is best demonstrated by an example of an actual play therapy interaction between a child and therapist. A nine-year-old boy was referred by his teacher because he was depressed and frightened, had difficulty making friends, and was not able to trust people. In the intake interview, the therapist found out that the boy had been severely physically abused by his father and that he was abandoned by his birth mother at the age of two. His stepmother had brought three children of her own into the blended family and did not have much time for this child. In fact, it appeared as though he was left to his own devices most of the time. The family had a number of other problems but refused family therapy. Thus, the child was seen in play therapy. He had considerable difficulty trusting the therapist and showed this reluctance in his play. He would often start to play, then check with the therapist for approval, and then stop before he became too involved in any one activity. After six weeks, he realized that the therapist was there to help him, and he began to communicate about his family through play.

The following exchange is a good example of what happens in play therapy. One day, the boy picked up a large wooden truck and two small ones. He proceeded to smash the large truck into the small red one over and over. He took the other small truck and put it between the large one and the small red one, as if to protect the red truck from being hit by the large one. In the process, the small blue truck was hurt badly and had to retreat. The boy repeated this activity several times. The therapist picked up a toy truck of her own and drove between the large truck and both of the small trucks, indicating that she had a truck that was tough enough to stop the large truck from hurting the small ones. The child was visibly relieved and turned to another activity.

What had happened? Before the session, the therapist had received a call from the child's social worker, who told her that the night before, the boy's father was caught sexually abusing his four-year-old stepdaughter, who shared this boy's room. The boy had awakened and unsuccessfully tried to stop his father. He ran to a neighbor's house, and this woman called the police. The father was arrested but threatened to get revenge on both children before he was taken away. The boy had play-acted this entire scene with the toy trucks. The father was the large truck; the red truck, his sister; the blue one, himself. The relief sensed by the boy after the therapist intervened is understandable, as her truck communicated to the boy that he would be protected from his father.

Evolution of Play Therapy

Children use their play in play therapy not only to communicate but also to solve problems and deal with overwhelming feelings. How this happens has been explained and described by many different therapists and theorists since play came to be viewed as an acceptable means of conducting therapy in the early 1930s, based on the work of Melanie Klein, Hug Hellmuth, and Anna Freud. These three psychologists developed theories and play therapy methods that were based on Sigmund Freud's earlier psychoanalytic theories. In this approach, free play was considered most important, and the therapist did not generally become engaged at all in the play. The therapist merely reflected back to the child what was seen and occasionally interpreted to the child what the play may have meant.

In the 1940s, Virginia Axline developed her approach to play therapy, which was similar to Klein's and Freud's. Axline also believed in free play and did not play with the child. She interpreted and emphasized an environment that put no limits or rules on the child. She introduced the idea that children in play therapy need to experience unconditional acceptance, empathic concern, and a nondirective atmosphere. In other words, Axline's approach to play therapy was to sit and observe and not be involved with the child.

Types of Play Therapists

Since then, the lack of limit setting (imposing rules or regulations on another person and then enforcing them in a predictable way), as well as the lack of active involvement with children in play therapy, has been criticized by play therapists. Nowadays, play therapists are more likely to get involved in play and to respond to children through play activity (as in the example), as opposed to using language to communicate with them. There are two major groups of therapists who use play therapy. Traditional psychoanalytic or psychodynamic therapists who are followers of Klein or Axline make up one group; however, even within this group, there is much diversity with regard to how involved the therapist becomes with the child's play. The second group is composed of therapists who focus on the human interaction that takes place—that is, humanistic therapists.

Regardless of which group a play therapist belongs to, however, the primary ingredients that were proposed many years ago remain intact. Free play is still deemed important, and empathy is stressed in the relationship with the child. Many therapists believe that the interpersonal matrix—the environment and the relationship between two or more people who spend time together—that exists between the child and the therapist is critical to changes noted in the child. A national center for play therapy has been created at the University of North Texas, and the field is represented by the Association for Play Therapy, located in Fresno, California, which publishes three major quarterly periodicals: *The International Journal of Play Therapy, The Association for Play Therapy Newsletter,* and *Play Therapy.*

Recent trends in the field include the incorporation of play therapy by elementary school counselors and early childhood educational entities; the incorporation of play therapy in family therapy, in the form of filial therapy, where parents are trained to use techniques with their children; and the application of play therapy theory to children with special needs or disabilities and children with limited language skills (such as children with severe autism). Overall, a primary focus remains on the symbolism (the use of indirect means to express inner needs or feelings; a way of sharing oneself without doing so directly or in words) and metaphor expressed by children through play.

—Christiane Brems

References

He, Hong-Gu, et al. "The Effectiveness of Therapeutic Play Intervention in Reducing Perioperative Anxiety, Negative Behaviors, and Postoperative Pain in Children Undergoing Elective Surgery: A Systematic Review." *Pain Management Nursing*, vol. 16, no. 3, 2015, pp. 425–439., doi:10.1016/j.pmn.2014.08.011.

Li, William H. C., et al. "Play Interventions to Reduce Anxiety and Negative Emotions in Hospitalized Children." *BMC Pediatrics*, vol. 16, no. 1, 11 Mar. 2016, doi:10.1186/s12887-016-0570-5.

Mountain, Vivienne. "Play Therapy – Respecting the Spirit of the Child." *International Journal of Children's Spirituality*, vol. 21, no. 3-4, 30 Sept. 2016, pp. 191–200., doi:10.1080/1364436x.2016.1228616.

Scarponi, Dorella, and Andrea Pession. "Play Therapy to Control Pain and Suffering in Pediatric Oncology." *Frontiers in Pediatrics*, vol. 4, 8 Dec. 2016, doi:10.3389/fped.2016.00132.

Schottelkorb, April A., et al. "Effectiveness of Play Therapy on Problematic Behaviors of Preschool Children With Somatization." *Journal of Child and Adolescent Counseling*, vol. 1, no. 1, 2 May 2015, pp. 3–16., doi:10.1080/23727810.2015.1015905.

Swan, Karrie L., and Dee C. Ray. "Effects of Child-Centered Play Therapy on Irritability and Hyperactivity Behaviors of Children With Intellectual Disabilities." *The Journal of Humanistic Counseling*, vol. 53, no. 2, 2014, pp. 120–133., doi:10.1002/j.2161-1939.2014.00053.x.

Trice-Black, Shannon, et al. "Play Therapy in School Counseling." *Professional School Counseling*, vol. 16, no. 5, 2013, doi:10.1177/2156759x1201600503.

■ Psychoanalysis

CATEGORY: Therapy or Technique; Psychotherapy

KEY TERMS

- *countertransference:* the emotional reaction of the analyst to the subject's contribution
- *free association:* the mental process by which one word or image may spontaneously suggest another without any apparent connection
- *overdetermination:* the idea that a single observed effect is determined by multiple causes at once (any one of which alone might be enough to account for the effect)
- *transference*: a patient's displacement or projection onto the analyst of those unconscious feelings and wishes originally directed toward important individuals, such as parents, in the patient's childhood

Introduction

Psychoanalysis began as a method for treating emotional suffering. Sigmund Freud, the founder of psychoanalysis, working at the beginning of the twentieth century, made many discoveries by studying patients with symptoms such as excessive anxiety (fear that is not realistic) or paralysis for which no physical cause could be found. He became the first psychoanalyst (often called analyst) when he developed the method of free association, in which he encouraged his patients to say whatever came to mind about their symptoms and their lives. He found that by talking in this way, his patients discovered feelings and thoughts they had not known they had. When they became aware of these unconscious thoughts and feelings, their symptoms lessened or disappeared.

Psychoanalysis as a form of psychotherapy continues to be an effective method for treating certain forms of emotional suffering, such as anxieties and inhibitions (inner constraints) that interfere with success in school, work, or relationships. It is based on the understanding that each individual is unique, that the past shapes the present, and that factors outside people's awareness influence their thoughts, feelings, and actions. As a comprehensive treatment, it has the potential to change many areas of a person's functioning. Although modern psychoanalysis is different in many ways from what was practiced in Freud's era, talking and listening remain important. Psychoanalytic psychotherapy is a modified form of psychoanalysis, usually with less frequent meetings and more modest goals.

From the beginning, psychoanalysis was more than just a treatment. It was, and continues to be, a method for investigating the mind and a theory to explain both everyday adult behavior as well as child development. Many of Freud's insights, which seemed so revolutionary at the beginning of the twentieth century, are now widely accepted by various schools of psychological thought and form the basis for several theories of psychological motivation, most theories of child development, and all forms of psychodynamic psychotherapy. Some of Freud's ideas, such as his theories about women, turned out to be wrong and were revised by other psychoanalysts during the 1970's and 1980's. Other ideas, such as those about the nature of dreams, although rejected by some scientists during the 1980's and 1990's, were returned to by other scientists by the beginning of the twenty-first century. Psychoanalytic ideas and concepts are used in communities to solve problems such as bullying in schools and can be applied in many other fields of study.

In the early years of psychoanalysis, Freud trained most psychoanalysts. Later, different schools of psychoanalytic thought branched out from this original source. Groups of psychoanalysts joined together in organizations, and each organization developed its own standards for training psychoanalysts. There were no nationally accepted standards for psychoanalytic training in the United States until the beginning of the twenty-first century, when several of these groups joined together to establish the Accreditation Council of Psychoanalytic Education. This council agreed to core standards for psychoanalytic institutes (schools that train psychoanalysts). Psychoanalytic psychotherapy, while practiced by trained psychoanalysts, is also practiced by psychotherapists who are not trained as psychoanalysts.

Psychoanalytic Treatment
Psychoanalysis is a method for helping people with symptoms that result from emotional conflict. Common symptoms in the modern era include anxiety (fear that is not realistic), depression (excessive sadness that is not due to a current loss), frequent unhealthy choices in relationships, and trouble getting along well with peers or family members. For example, some people may feel continuously insecure and worried about doing well in school or work despite getting good grades or reviews. Other people may be attracted to sexual and emotional partners who treat them poorly. Others may experience loneliness and isolation because of fears about close relationships. Others may sabotage their success by always changing direction before reaching their goals. Children may have tantrums beyond the age when these are normal, or be afraid of going to sleep every night, or feel unhappy with their maleness or femaleness.

The same symptom can have several different causes, an etiology Freud termed overdetermination. For example, depression may be due to inner emotional constraints that prevent success, to biological vulnerability, or to upsetting events (such as the death of a loved one), or it may result from a combination of these. Therefore, most psychoanalysts believe in meeting with a person several times before deciding on the best treatment. Psychoanalysis is not for everyone who has a symptom. Sometimes psychoanalysis is not needed because the problems can be easily helped by other, less intensive forms of therapy. Sometimes biological problems or early childhood experiences leave a person too vulnerable to undertake the hard work of psychoanalysis. When psychoanalysis is not necessary, or not the best treatment for a particular person, a psychoanalyst may recommend psychoanalytic psychotherapy, a treatment that is based on the same principles as psychoanalysis but with less ambitious goals and, usually, less frequent sessions.

Psychoanalysis can treat specific emotional disorders, as described in the *Diagnostic and Statistical Manual of Mental Disorders: DSM-V-TR* (rev. 5th ed., 2013), but can also help with multiple sets of problematic symptoms, behaviors, and personality traits (such as being too perfectionistic or rigid). Since psychoanalysis affects the whole person rather than just treating symptoms, it has the potential to promote personal growth and development. For adults, this can mean better

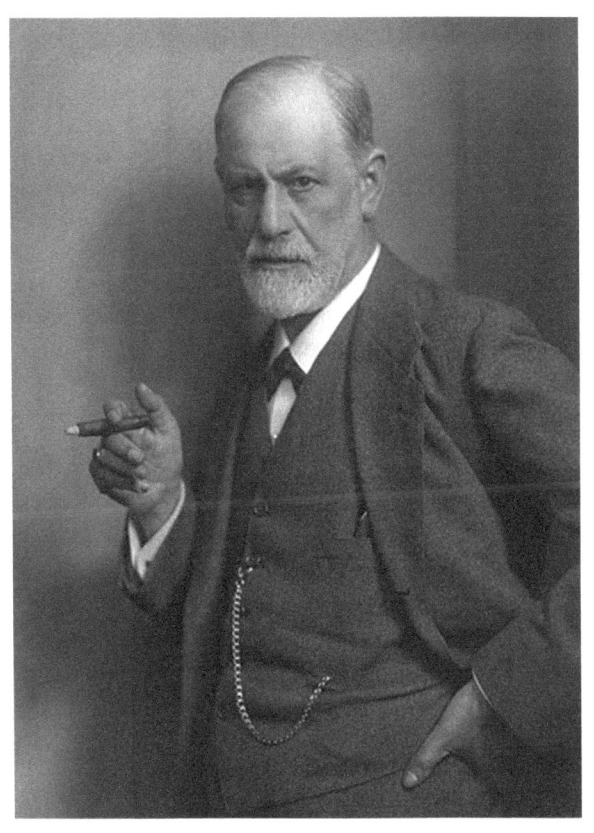

Sigmund Freud by Max Halberstadt, c. 1921. (via Wikimedia Commons)

relationships or marriages, jobs that feel more satisfying, or the ability to enjoy free time when this was difficult before. Children may do better in school after fears about competition and success diminish, or they may have more friends and get along better with parents after they begin to feel better about themselves.

Because psychoanalysis is a very individual treatment, the best way to determine whether it would be beneficial for an individual is through consulting an experienced psychoanalyst. In general, people who benefit from psychoanalysis have some emotional sturdiness. They tend to be capable of understanding themselves and learning how to help themselves. Usually, they have had important accomplishments in one or more areas of their lives before seeking psychoanalytic treatment. Often, they have tried other forms of treatment that may have been helpful but have not been sufficient to deal with all their difficulties. Sometimes they are people who work with others (therapists, rabbis, teachers) whose emotions have been interfering with their ability to do their jobs as well as possible. Whatever the problems, psychoanalysts understand them in the context of each individual's strengths, vulnerabilities, and life situation.

Method of Treatment in Psychoanalysis

A person who goes to a psychoanalyst for consultation usually meets with the analyst at least three times face-to-face before the analyst recommends psychoanalysis. Sometimes the patient and analyst meet for several weeks, months, or years in psychoanalytic psychotherapy; they decide on psychoanalysis if they identify problems that are unlikely to be solved by less intensive treatment.

Once they begin psychoanalysis, the analyst and patient usually meet four or five times per week for fifty-minute sessions, as this creates the intensive personal relationship that plays an important role in the therapeutic process. The frequent sessions do not mean that the patient is very sick; they are necessary to help the patient reach deeper levels of awareness. (People with the severest forms of mental illness, such as schizophrenia, are not usually treated with psychoanalysis.) Often the adult patient lies on a couch, as this may make it easier to speak freely. The couch is not essential, and some patients feel more comfortable sitting up.

By working together to diminish obstacles to free expression in the treatment sessions, the analyst and patient come to understand the patient's worries and learn how the patient's mind works. The patient learns about thoughts and feelings he or she has kept out of awareness or isolated from each other. Through the intensity that comes from frequent meetings with the analyst, the patient often experiences the analyst as if the analyst were a parent or other important person from the past. This is called transference. Eventually, the patient has a chance to see these feelings from a more mature point of view. Although the patient may experience intense emotions within the analytic sessions, the anxieties and behaviors that brought him or her to treatment gradually diminish and feel more under control. The patient feels freer and less restricted by worries and patterns that belong to the past.

For example, a patient may be very fearful of angry feelings and avoid telling the analyst about them, expecting punishment or rejection. As a result, the patient may turn the anger on himself or herself in a form of self-sabotage. Often this is the way the patient dealt with angry feelings toward significant people while growing up. Over time, as the patient and analyst understand this behavior, the patient feels freer to express angry feelings directly and eventually feels less need to sabotage or self-punish.

Gradually, in the course of the intensive analytic relationship, the patient learns more about his or her maladaptive ways of dealing with distressing thoughts and feelings that have developed during childhood. By understanding them in adulthood or (for a child) at a later age, the patient gains a different perspective and is able to react in a more adaptive way. Rigid personality traits that had been used to keep the childhood feelings at a distance are no longer necessary, and the patient is able to react to people and situations in a more flexible way.

During the course of the treatment, the analyst will often have strong feelings toward the patient, called countertransference. Well-trained analysts are required to undergo psychoanalysis themselves before treating patients. In their own analysis, they learn how to cope with their countertransference feelings in ways that will not hurt the patient. For example, they learn not to take the patient's expressions of anger personally but to help the patient express the emotion more fully and understand where it originates.

Children and adolescents can be treated with psychoanalysis or psychoanalytic psychotherapy by using methods suitable for their ages. Most children play with toys, draw, or explore the room, in addition to talking, during their sessions with the analyst, and these activities provide ways to explore inner thoughts and feelings. The analyst meets with the parents before the treatment starts and continues to do so regularly during the course of the child's therapy or analysis. Adolescents usually sit face-to-face or draw or write about their feelings and worries. Occasionally, older adolescents want to lie on the couch. Adolescents often prefer that the analyst not meet with the parents on a regular basis. Instead, the analyst and adolescent usually develop some way to keep the parents informed about what they might need to know about the treatment.

Psychoanalytic Psychotherapy
Psychoanalytic psychotherapy is more varied than psychoanalysis. It may be very intensive, or it may be focused on a specific problem, such as a recent loss or trouble deciding about a job. In psychoanalytic psychotherapy, the patient and therapist usually sit face-to-face and approach the patient's problems, whatever they are, in a more interactive way. Most often, patient and therapist meet twice per week in fifty-minute sessions. Once per week is also common but not considered to be as helpful. More frequent meetings (three to five times per week) may be necessary if the patient is in crisis or has chronic problems that are not treatable with psychoanalysis.

Although psychoanalysts are well trained to practice psychoanalytic psychotherapy, this treatment is also practiced by psychotherapists who are not psychoanalysts. Some of these therapists have taken courses at psychoanalytic institutes.

Medication and Confidentiality Issues
In the early days of psychoanalysis, analysts believed that treatment with medication would interfere with psychoanalysis. Most modern psychoanalysts believe that, although medicine can sometimes interfere, there are times when it can be used in a helpful way in combination with psychoanalytic psychotherapy or even with psychoanalysis.

"Confidentiality" is the term used to describe the privacy necessary for individuals to be able to speak freely about all their thoughts and feelings. Responsible psychoanalysts and psychotherapists agree to keep private everything about their patients, including the fact that the patient has come for treatment, unless the patient gives permission to release some specific information. One exception is when patients are at risk for hurting themselves or someone else.

—*Judith M. Chertoff*

References

"About Psychoanalysis." *APsaA*, American Psychoanalytic Association, apsa.org/content/about-psychoanalysis.

Ackerman, Courtney E. "Psychoanalysis: A Brief History of Freud's Psychoanalytic Theory [2019]." *PositivePsychology.com*, 27 Oct. 2019, positivepsychology.com/psychoanalysis/.

Cherry, Kendra. "How Psychoanalysis Influenced the Field of Psychology." *Verywell Mind*, 13 Oct.

2019, www.verywellmind.com/what-is-psychoanalysis-2795246.

Giacolini, Teodosio, and Ugo Sabatello. "Psychoanalysis and Affective Neuroscience. The Motivational/Emotional System of Aggression in Human Relations." *Frontiers in Psychology*, vol. 9, 14 Jan. 2019, doi:10.3389/fpsyg.2018.02475.

Johnson, Brian, and Daniela Flores Mosri. "The Neuropsychoanalytic Approach: Using Neuroscience as the Basic Science of Psychoanalysis." *Frontiers in Psychology*, vol. 7, 13 Oct. 2016, doi:10.3389/fpsyg.2016.01459.

Moccia, Lorenzo, et al. "The Experience of Pleasure: A Perspective Between Neuroscience and Psychoanalysis." *Frontiers in Human Neuroscience*, vol. 12, 2018, doi:10.3389/fnhum.2018.00359.

Novotney, Amy. "Not Your Great-Grandfather's Psychoanalysis." *Monitor on Psychology*, American Psychological Association, Dec. 2017, www.apa.org/monitor/2017/12/psychoanalysis.

Paris, Joel. "Is Psychoanalysis Still Relevant to Psychiatry?" *The Canadian Journal of Psychiatry*, vol. 62, no. 5, 31 Jan. 2017, pp. 308–312., doi:10.1177/0706743717692306.

■ Reminiscence therapy

CATEGORY: Therapy or Technique; Psychotherapy
ANATOMY OR SYSTEM AFFECTED: Memory
SPECIALTIES AND RELATED FIELDS: Gerontology, psychology

Overview

At its most basic, *reminiscence therapy* involves listening to a patient and encouraging the individual to share his or her memories. The listener may ask directed questions to encourage further sharing. Reminiscence therapy is most beneficial in treating individuals with memory disorders such as dementia, as well as anxiety and depression, and may be useful as an alternative to drug therapies for challenging patients.

Persons benefit from knowing their experience is valued by others. Many times, older individuals feel marginalized. They may have mobility issues that prevent them from seeking out company, or they may be intimidated by technology—cell phones and computers, for example—and therefore feel isolated. Individuals with cognitive challenges such as dementia may find the modern world confusing and lonely. They often lose *short-term memory*—memory of what has happened very recently—and may feel disoriented and frightened. Such feelings of isolation often lead to depression. Caregivers may be older individuals' only source of companionship. By encouraging persons to share stories and actively listening to these tales, caregivers often can help these individuals to feel connected to the modern world.

Persons with dementia generally retain their earliest memories for the longest time. Reminiscence therapy has been found to be most beneficial to individuals with mild to moderate dementia. According to the Institute for Research and Innovation in Social Services (IRISS) in Scotland, several 2009 studies found that patients who participated in reminiscence therapy had better relationships with caregivers and families, had improved cognitive abilities and mood, functioned better, and had reduced symptoms of depression. A 2010 study in Taiwan found that aged persons without dementia also benefited from reminiscence therapy, according to IRISS. They were less depressed, more sociable, and generally in better mental health than individuals in the control group. The studies found no negative effects from reminiscence therapy.

Reminiscence therapy provides both *therapeutic*, or healing, benefits and pleasure. Recalling happier times reinforces the individual's connection to the world and may increase feelings of self-worth. Memories of difficult experiences such as loss or tragedy may help individuals process feelings and gain a better understanding of both events and themselves. Reminiscence therapy can improve cognitive ability among patients by providing stimulation.

Working with Patients

Reminiscence therapy may be conducted one-on-one or in group settings with a therapist who facilitates discussion and encourages all participants to share stories. Reminiscence activities have an overall positive effect when conducted with groups of aged populations. Therapists may use items, such as photos, or play music to spark memories. At times, therapists may use one-on-one sessions to collect information and create a book of an individual's life history (*life story work*), which may further help a patient who struggles to maintain his or her identity as cognitive function fails. Such information also aids caregivers. For example, reminiscence therapy and life story work may reveal and document favorite or hated foods and activities such as hobbies and lifestyles—information that enables care homes and caregivers to provide appropriate opportunities. A patient who once enjoyed outdoor activities may benefit from regular walks outside, for instance. A person who once practiced needlepoint may be encouraged to try painting. Family members may even develop life stories for individuals as they prepare to move to care facilities to aid the transition and help the patient hold on to his or her identity. Both music therapy and reminiscence therapy are currently being used to increase aspects of wellbeing in older people, including those with memory diseases such as dementia, as alternatives to pharmacological treatments. There is growing evidence that combining these therapies in a focused way would provide unique wellbeing outcomes for this population.

Though sad memories of difficult times may bring tears, they can be therapeutic. Listeners must respect the memories and experiences of the patient and allow them to feel their emotions. Silence, too, is important—while at times a listener may need to ask questions or share appropriate stories, at other times it is best to sit in silence together.

Reminiscence may be encouraged at all times of the day, and nurses and other caregivers may be best positioned to facilitate such talk. Patients in care facilities might be open to talking about the past during meals, while receiving physical therapy, or while walking with assistance. Reminiscence also may be used as an aid to encouraging relationships with caregivers and developing friendships with other patients. This therapy may help patients transition from their home environment to an institutional setting or when moving between institutions. Caregivers such as nurses are encouraged to see patients as individuals (to see beyond the diagnosis) and be sensitive to their culture and background to deliver *person-centered care*, which focuses on treating patients with dignity and respect and ensuring they have personal choice and a sense of community and security. Reminiscence therapy has been shown to benefit both patients and caregivers.

For late-stage dementia patients, who often are unable to communicate well or to even speak, stimulation such as music is likely to trigger memories. By providing music associated with happy times or events, caregivers can improve patients' moods. This outcome may provide a long-lasting effect, because moods often last longer than memories.

Caregivers can provide reminiscence therapy by encouraging communication using many methods, including the following:

Ask open-ended questions. How did you learn to paint? What were you doing when (the first astronauts went to space, World War II ended, etc.)?

Take cues from the patient's possessions. Ask questions about photographs and souvenirs: Who are the people in the photo? Is this memento from a trip? What was it like?

Stimulate the senses. Music, dancing, food, and smells, for example, may trigger memories.

Turn to literature. Read an excerpt from a book set in an earlier time or an account of some event or activity from decades ago, and ask the individual to comment.

—*Josephine Campbell*
—*Geraldine Marrocco*

References

Huang, Hui-Chuan, et al. "Reminiscence Therapy Improves Cognitive Functions and Reduces Depressive Symptoms in Elderly People With Dementia: A Meta-Analysis of Randomized Controlled Trials." *Journal of the American Medical Directors Association*, vol. 16, no. 12, 2015, pp. 1087–1094., doi:10.1016/j.jamda.2015.07.010.

Klever, Sandy. "Reminiscence Therapy." *Nursing*, vol. 43, no. 4, 2013, pp. 36–37., doi:10.1097/01.nurse.0000427988.23941.51.

Li, Mo, et al. "The Clinical Efficacy of Reminiscence Therapy in Patients with Mild-to-Moderate Alzheimer Disease." *Medicine*, vol. 96, no. 51, 2017, doi:10.1097/md.0000000000009381.

Lök, Neslihan, et al. "The Effect of Reminiscence Therapy on Cognitive Functions, Depression, and Quality of Life in Alzheimer Patients: Randomized Controlled Trial." *International Journal of Geriatric Psychiatry*, vol. 34, no. 1, 2018, pp. 47–53., doi:10.1002/gps.4980.

Woods, Bob, et al. "Reminiscence Therapy for Dementia." *Cochrane Database of Systematic Reviews*, 1 Mar. 2018, doi:10.1002/14651858.cd001120.pub3.

Serotonin-norepinephrine reuptake inhibitors

CATEGORY: Class of Drug
ALSO KNOWN AS: SNRIs
ANATOMY OR SYSTEM AFFECTED: Nervous system

KEY TERMS

- *discontinuation syndrome*: a condition caused by the abrupt discontinuation of antidepressant or antipsychotic medications
- *5-Hydroxytryptamine*: also known as 5-HT; another name for the neurotransmitter serotonin
- *ligand-gated ion channel*: proteins embedded in the membranes of neurons that are permeable to specific ions, but whose permeability is regulated by the binding of small molecules (ligands) that include neurotransmitters.
- *neurotransmitter*: small molecules released by neurons to either activate or inhibit neighboring neurons
- *norepinephrine*: a hormone released by the adrenal glands; a neurotransmitter released by sympathetic nerves in response to stress, and by clusters of neurons in the brain to enhance alertness, attention, memory formation and retrieval, processing of sensory inputs, and adaptation to changing environments
- *norepinephrine* reuptake transporter: a protein embedded in the membrane of the axon terminus of a presynaptic neuron that decreases the concentration of norepinephrine in the synaptic cleft by effecting norepinephrine reuptake in the presynaptic neuron
- *serotonin*: a neurotransmitter released by neurons in the gastrointestinal tract and central nervous system that regulates appetite, sleep, emotional states, motor function, cognition and many other neurological and physiological functions
- *serotonin reuptake transporter*: a protein embedded in the membrane of the axon terminus of a presynaptic neuron that decreases the concentration of serotonin in the synaptic cleft by effecting serotonin reuptake in the presynaptic neuron

Mental health providers use serotonin-norepinephrine reuptake inhibitors (SNRIs) to treat major depression and anxiety disorders. However, they are also used to treat chronic pain syndromes, including diabetic peripheral neuropathy, fibromyalgia, and chronic musculoskeletal pain. SNRIs are used to treat body dysmorphic disorder, obsessive-compulsive disorder, and posttraumatic stress syndrome. Other conditions that often respond to SNRIs include menopausal hot flashes, urinary incontinence, and vulvodynia (chronic pain or discomfort around the opening of the vagina).

How SNRIs Receptor Antagonists Work

Neurons communicate with each other by releasing small molecules called neurotransmitters. Neurotransmitters bind to ligand-gated ion channels embedded in the cell membranes of neurons and induce these ion channels to either open or close. The influx of positively-charged (e.g., sodium and calcium) ions into neurons activates them, but the influx of negatively-charged (e.g., chloride) ions into neurons inhibits them. Therefore, neurotransmitters can stimulate or inhibit neighboring neurons according to the receptors they bind, and the biological effects those receptors elicit within the neuron.

Neurons also regulate the quantity of neurotransmitters to which they are exposed. The first regulatory mechanism involves enzymes that degrade neurotransmitters once nearby neurons release them. For example, the enzyme monoamine oxidase (MAO) degrades the neurotransmitters dopamine, serotonin, and norepinephrine. Another enzyme, catechol-O-methyltransferase (COMT), chemically modifies and inactivates the neurotransmitters dopamine, norepinephrine, and epinephrine. These enzymes limit the activity of neurotransmitters and prevent neurons from overdosing on them. Both enzymes are the target of antidepressants and drugs that treat Parkinson's disease.

A second mechanism by which neurons limit their exposure to neurotransmitters is through reuptake transporters. The serotonin transporter (SERT) recycles the neurotransmitter serotonin from the synaptic cleft back into the neuron that released it, which limits the duration of serotonin activity. A second reuptake transporter, the norepinephrine transporter (NET), recycles norepinephrine from the synaptic cleft.

Drugs that inhibit neurotransmitter reuptake transporters can increase the efficacy and biological activity of specific neurotransmitters. Since some psychiatric and pain disorders are associated with a deficit in serotonin and norepinephrine neurotransmission, drugs that inhibit both these neurotransmitter reuptake transporters can potentially ameliorate the symptoms of these conditions. A class of drugs called serotonin-norepinephrine reuptake inhibitors (SNRIs) consists of chemically unrelated but mechanistically similar agents that treat pain and psychiatric conditions.

The SSRIs include venlafaxine (Effexor) and the very similar desvenlafaxine (Pristiq), duloxetine (Cymbalta), and milnacipran (Savella) and the closely-related compound levomilnacipran (Fetzima).

Clinical Uses of SNRIs

Venlafaxine is FDA-approved for the treatment of major depression and anxiety disorders, including generalized anxiety disorder, social anxiety disorder, and panic disorder. Off-label uses of venlafaxine include posttraumatic stress syndrome, for which it is an effective treatment and acute and chronic diabetic neuropathic pain. Desvenlafaxine is FDA-approved for major depression and is not used off-label for other indications.

Duloxetine is FDA-approved for the treatment of major depression, anxiety, stress incontinence, painful diabetic neuropathy, fibromyalgia, chronic lower back pain, and osteoarthritis. It is especially useful for patients with chronic pain that also suffer from depression since duloxetine can effectively treat both ailments.

Milnacipran is FDA-approved for fibromyalgia. Although it is not FDA-approved for depression, clinical trials have shown that it is just as effective against major depression as other SNRIs. Levomilnacipran is FDA-approved for major depression and is not used off-label for other indications.

Side Effects

SNRIs commonly cause nausea, sweating, and dizziness. Nausea diminishes with time and abates if patients take these medicines with food. SNRIs can also raise blood pressure, but the extent to which they raise blood pressure is dose-dependent. Nevertheless, any patient on an SSRI should have their blood pressure checked routinely. Abruptly discontinuing an SNRI can also cause "discontinuation syndrome." This condition is a type of antidepressant withdrawal syndrome that causes flu-like symptoms, insomnia, nausea, poor balance, sensory changes, and anxiety. Therefore, patients should never discontinue or reduce the dose of their SNRI without their physician's supervision. Patients with angle-closure glaucoma, kidney disease, or high blood pressure should avoid SNRIs.

Venlafaxine has five times the affinity for the SERT than for the NET. Therefore, at lower doses (75 mg/day), venlafaxine has a side effect profile associated with increased serotonin levels, such as nausea, insomnia, tremor, and sexual dysfunction. At higher doses (150-225 mg/day), venlafaxine functions as a dual SERT/NET inhibitor and additionally causes hypertension, dry mouth, and sweating. Dizziness and constipation are also occasionally reported adverse effects of venlafaxine. Desvenlafaxine has a very similar adverse effect profile, but its main side effects are nausea, dizziness, sweating, constipation, and anorexia (appetite loss). It also causes less sexual dysfunction than venlafaxine.

Duloxetine causes nausea, dry mouth, constipation, insomnia, dizziness, fatigue, diarrhea, sleepiness, sweating, and anorexia. Sexual dysfunction is also common with duloxetine.

Milnacipran causes nausea, headache, dry mouth, abdominal pain, constipation, and insomnia. Levomilnacipran causes the same side effects as milnacipran, except that levomilnacipran increases heart rate and causes dizziness, sweating, and sexual dysfunction.

—*Michael A. Buratovich, Ph.D.*

References

Hayashida, Ken-ichiro, and Hideaki Obata. "Strategies to Treat Chronic Pain and Strengthen Impaired Descending Noradrenergic Inhibitory System." *International Journal of Molecular Science*, vol. 20, no. 4, 2019, p. e822. doi:10.3390/ijms20040822.

Jordan, Ann Westcot. Antidepressants: *History, Science, and Issues.* Greenwood, 2018.

Khawam, Elias A., Laurencic, Georgia, and Donald A. Malone, Jr. "Side Effects of Antidepressants: An Overview." *Cleveland Clinic Journal of Medicine*, vol. 73, no. 4, 2006, pp. 351-353, 356-361.

Sadock, Benjamin J., Sadock, Virginia A., and Pedro Ruiz, eds. *Kaplan and Sadock's Comprehensive Textbook of Psychiatry*, 10th ed. Lippincott, Williams, & Wilkins, 2017.

Schatzberg, Alan F., and Charles B. Nemeroff, eds. *Essentials of Clinical Psychopharmacology*, 3rd ed. CBS Publishing, Pub, 2017.

Stahl, Stephen M. *The Prescriber's Guide*, 6th ed. Cambridge University Press, 2017.

Shock therapy

CATEGORY: Therapy or Technique; Psychotherapy
ALSO KNOWN AS: Electroshock, shock treatment, electroconvulsive therapy (ECT)
ANATOMY OR SYSTEM AFFECTED: Brain, nerves, nervous system, psychic-emotional system
SPECIALTIES AND RELATED FIELDS: Neurology, psychiatry

KEY TERMS

- *anesthetic*: any of a variety of drugs used to cause a patient to become unconscious and amnesiac for a brief period of time; very short-acting anesthetics, such as methohexital, thiamylal sodium, thiopental sodium, and etomidate, are often used in conjunction with electroconvulsive therapy
- *convulsion*: an instance of high-frequency and amplitude-random electrical activity in the brain; electroconvulsive therapy causes a convulsion in the brain, which is believed to be related to its mechanism of action
- *electrocardiogram*: a recording of the electrical activity of the heart; used during electroconvulsive therapy to monitor changes in heart rate, rhythm, and conduction, any or all of which may be temporarily affected by this procedure
- *electroencephalogram*: a brain wave trace used to monitor the onset, termination, and duration of the convulsion or seizure
- *mood disorders*: any of a number of mental conditions characterized by a primary disturbance of mood as distinct from thinking or behavior
- *muscle relaxant*: any of a number of medications used to paralyze the muscles of the patient temporarily before delivering the electrical stimulus; the main medication used for this purpose is succinylcholine
- *organic brain syndrome (organicity)*: changes in memory, orientation, and perception that occur as a side effect of electroconvulsive therapy
- *psychotic disorder*: a psychiatric condition in which an individual's mental state is out of touch with reality, as displayed by abnormal and bizarre perceptions, thoughts, behavior, judgment, and reasoning
- *seizure*: used interchangeably with the term "convulsion"

Introduction

Electroconvulsive therapy (ECT), also known as shock therapy, is a somatic, or physical, form of therapy that is used for some individuals who suffer from severe mental disorders. It involves the direct application of an electric current to the brain. Typically, this current lasts for up to one second at a rate of 140 to 170 volts. The purpose of this electrical charge is to induce a grand mal seizure that will usually last for thirty to sixty seconds. The seizure that is induced is similar to those experienced in some types of epilepsy. It is through this grand mal seizure that ECT has its beneficial effect in reducing the symptoms of the patient.

The use of electrical charges as a medical treatment has been reported for centuries. As early as 47 C.E., Scribonius Largus used an electric eel to treat headaches. During the sixteenth century, Ethiopians were reported to have used electric catfish to expel evil spirits from the bodies of the mentally ill. Direct electric charges for the treatment of nervous complaints were also reported during the eighteenth century in Europe.

The modern application of electric current for the treatment of individuals with mental disorders began in 1938. It was at this time that two Italians, Ugo Cerletti, a psychiatrist, and Lucio Bini, a neuropathologist, invented the first ECT machine for use on humans. Cerletti and Bini first used their newly developed ECT machine to induce convulsions for the treatment of schizophrenic patients, and they reported that the treatment was a success.

ECT was introduced into the United States in 1940, at which time it quickly became the major somatic treatment for all severely disturbed individuals, regardless of mental disorder. By the mid-1950's, its use began to decline rapidly for several reasons, including the introduction of psychotropic medications, increasing demands for civil rights for the mentally ill, and concerns about potential adverse effects of ECT. Subsequently, however, a growing body of research has indicated that ECT is an effective treatment for some severe mental disorders. This research has led to a gradual increase in the acceptance of its use, particularly in the treatment of severely depressed individuals.

When ECT was first used for the treatment of mental disorders, the patient would be strapped to a table and, without any medications or other medical safeguards, would be administered the electrical

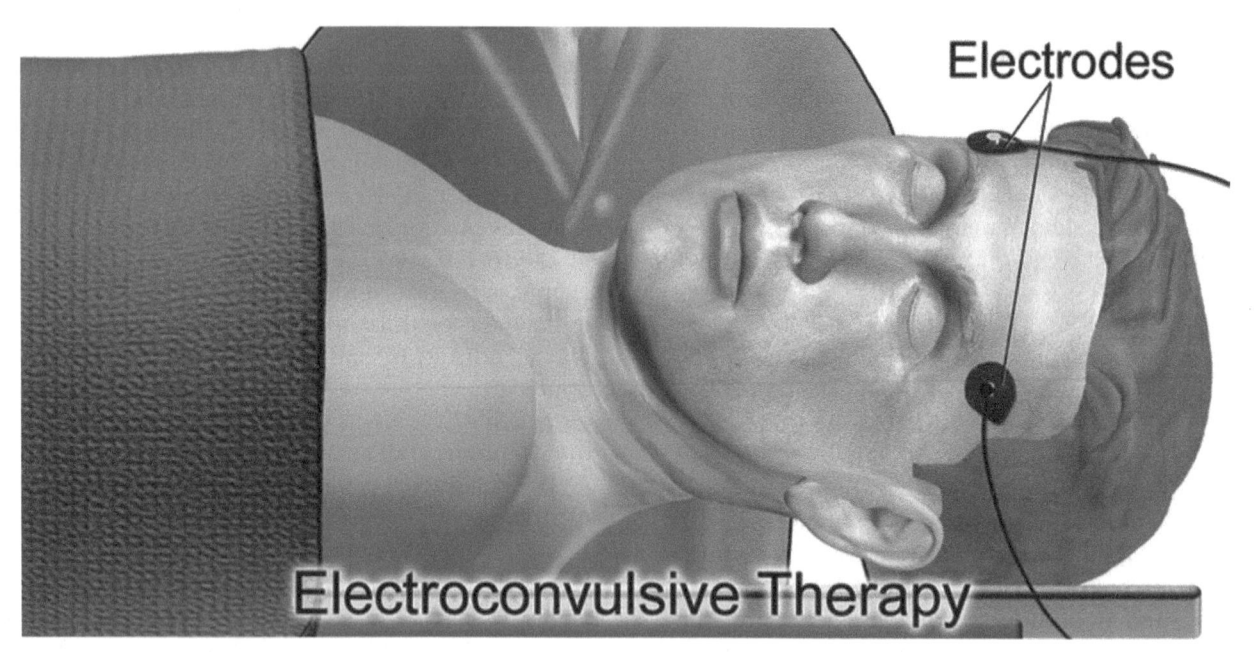

An illustration depicting electroconvulsive therapy. (BruceBlaus via Wikimedia Commons)

current and sent into a convulsion. During this convulsion, the patient would thrash around on the table, often being left with broken limbs and other physical complications. In its later use, prior to administration of the ECT, the patient is given a muscle relaxant, which completely immobilizes the body, and anesthesia, which makes the patient completely unconscious. The result of these safeguards has been a much safer treatment of the patient.

Theories of Efficacy

Although ECT has been demonstrated to be an effective treatment, it is not known how and why ECT works. The theoretical basis of the original use of ECT had to do with the observation that schizophrenia and epilepsy rarely occur together, suggesting that the two are mutually exclusive. Based on this observation, it was hypothesized that, if a seizure could be induced in a schizophrenic, the schizophrenic symptoms could be eliminated. Physicians had tried previously to induce such seizures by means of injections of insulin, camphor, and other chemicals, but these approaches proved to have more disadvantages relative to ECT.

Although this early theory of the mechanics of ECT has been refuted, there still is little knowledge of how and why ECT actually works. The only fact that has been firmly established is that it is the seizure that ECT induces that creates any positive changes in the patient's symptoms. There is no clear-cut explanation, however, of how the seizure creates the changes. Several theories have been developed to explain the process, most of which center on ECT's effect on neurotransmitters.

Neurotransmitters are chemicals that are used in the brain to transmit messages from one cell to another. One well-accepted theory holds that abnormalities in the level and utilization of certain neurotransmitters lead to the development of mental disorders such as depression, schizophrenia, and mania. Consequently, it is thought that ECT, through the creation of a seizure, somehow affects the level and utilization of some of these neurotransmitters, and that it is this process that reduces the patient's symptoms of mental disorder. While research to investigate how ECT works continues, it is important to remember that, as with all somatic treatments, ECT does not cure the disorder; it provides only temporary relief from the symptoms.

Despite its reported effectiveness, ECT remains a controversial treatment for mental disorders. Opponents point to potential adverse effects that ECT can cause, particularly the possibility of permanent brain damage resulting from the induced seizure. These opponents, who highlight the negative effects that ECT can have on a patient's memory, prefer the use of alternative treatment methods. The public media have served to exacerbate negative perceptions of ECT by depicting it as an inhumane treatment that is used only to control and punish malcontents, not to help the severely disturbed. There is perhaps no better example of the media's distorted depiction of ECT than that found in the film *One Flew Over the Cuckoo's Nest* (1975), in which ECT was used as a brutal method to control and manage the main character. As a result of these misunderstandings and distorted perceptions, ECT is often not used when it might be helpful.

Uses

It has been estimated that each year 60,000 to 100,000 people in the United States receive electroconvulsive therapy. This form of treatment has been used to treat a variety of mental disorders, including severe major depression, schizophrenia, and mania. Several surveys have indicated that more than three-fourths of individuals who receive ECT have been diagnosed as suffering from severe major depression. The second-largest group of individuals receiving ECT consists of those who have been diagnosed as schizophrenic. While there is substantial evidence that ECT is effective in the treatment of severe major depression, the evidence supporting the use of ECT to treat other disorders is not as strong.

Generally speaking, ECT is not seen as a treatment of choice. It will most likely not be the first treatment given to someone suffering from a severe mental disorder. Instead, it is typically viewed as the treatment of last resort and is used primarily to treat individuals who do not respond to any other treatments. For example, a typical course of treatment for an individual suffering from debilitating severe major depression would be talking therapy and one of the many antidepressant medications. For most people, it takes two to four weeks to respond to such medications. If the patient does not respond to the medication, another antidepressant medication may be tried. If, after several trials of medication, the patient still does not respond and continues to be severely depressed, ECT might be considered a viable option.

There are a few individuals for whom ECT might be considered the treatment of choice. These individuals include those who are in life-threatening situations, such as those who show symptoms of severe anorexia or strong suicidal tendencies, or those for whom medications would be damaging. ECT might be used to treat pregnant women, for example, since it presents fewer risks for a fetus than medication does, or individuals with heart disease, for whom medications can cause severe complications.

Because of the stigma attached to ECT as a result of its historical misuse and its characterization in the popular media, many physicians believe that ECT is not used as widely as it could and should be. Often, ECT is suggested as the treatment of choice, but because of its stigma, other approaches are tried first. The effect of this decision is to deprive the patient of an effective treatment and delay or prevent remission.

Techniques and Effects

When ECT is indicated for the treatment of a mental disorder, it usually involves five to ten applications of ECT administered at a rate of two or three per week. The number of ECT treatments given, however, will vary depending on the individual's medical history and the severity of the presenting symptoms. ECT is always administered by a physician; it cannot be ordered by a psychologist. When ECT is applied, many medical safeguards are used to prevent or minimize adverse effects. They include the use of a muscle relaxant, anesthesia, and oxygen. These medical procedures have made the use of ECT much safer than it was during the days when the patient would thrash about the table, breaking bones.

Additional refinements in the use of ECT have made it even safer. One such refinement is the application of unilateral, rather than bilateral, ECT. In unilateral ECT, the electric shock is sent through only one of the brain's two hemispheres. Usually, the shock is sent through the right hemisphere, which controls abstract thinking and creativity, rather than the left hemisphere, which controls language and rational thinking. While usually as effective as bilateral ECT, in which the shock goes through the entire brain, unilateral ECT has been shown to cause fewer adverse side effects.

Despite the refinements in ECT and the caution exercised in its use, there are several documented potential adverse side effects. Although most research indicates that these effects are temporary, some researchers suggest that ECT can cause permanent

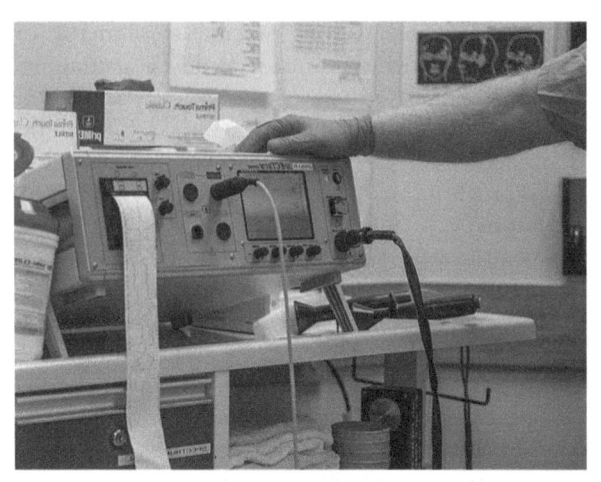

MECTA spECTrum 5000Q with electroencephalography (EEG) in a modern ECT suite. (via Wikimedia Commons)

brain damage. The major adverse effects of ECT relate to how well the patient's brain functions after the treatment. The most common effect is extreme confusion and disorientation in the patient on awakening after an ECT treatment. Generally, this confusion will last for only a few minutes to a few hours.

Another serious concern about ECT's effects on the cognitive functioning of the patient has to do with the patient's memory. ECT can cause retrograde amnesia, the inability to remember things from the past, and anterograde amnesia, the inability to memorize new material. Both forms of amnesia are most noticeable in the first days and weeks after the ECT treatments have stopped. With the passage of time, the patient will slowly remember more from the past and will regain or strengthen the ability to remember new material. In most patients, this recovery of memory will take no more than two to six months. The patient may, however, permanently lose memories of events that occurred immediately before the ECT treatments or while the patient was hospitalized for the treatments. The degree of memory loss appears to be related to the number of ECT treatments the patient received.

Research investigating permanent brain damage from the use of ECT has been mixed. Some research has indicated that any application of ECT will cause brain damage and that more brain damage will occur as more treatments are applied. Long-term impairment in the patient's memory is one effect that has thus been identified as permanent. Other researchers, however, have reported that ECT does not cause permanent brain damage. In the meantime, ECT is used cautiously, and research continues into its potential adverse effects.

Changing Attitudes

Before the advent of psychotropic medications, there were few effective treatments for the severely mentally ill. Numerous treatment methods were attempted to help relieve the symptoms of mental illness. Among these methods were bloodletting, the use of leeches, and immersion in water. Perhaps the most common approach was the permanent institutionalization of severely mentally ill individuals. This was done not only to control patients but also to protect others, since patients were viewed as a threat to others and themselves.

As a result of the ineffectiveness of these treatments and the growing concern about the institutionalization of the mentally ill, a number of new treatment approaches were developed and applied. Among these new approaches was electroconvulsive therapy. Electroconvulsive shock therapy was first used on schizophrenic patients, and the treatment met with some success. It was also tried on depressed and manic patients, with even greater success. As a result of these successes and the lack of other effective treatment approaches, ECT quickly came to be a commonly used treatment for individuals who suffered from a variety of mental disorders.

Many factors caused ECT to fall out of favor during the late 1950's. First, the earlier applications of ECT held significant dangers for the patient. The risk of death was approximately one in one thousand, and the risk of physical damage, such as broken bones, was even greater—in fact, such damage was noted in up to 40 percent of the patients. Concerns about complications continue today, and their focus is the impact of ECT on cognitive functioning.

Another factor that led to the decline in the use of ECT was the development and introduction of psychotropic shock therapy versus medications. These medications revolutionized the treatment of the mentally ill and led to thousands of patients being deinstitutionalized. In terms of both effectiveness and safety, it soon became evident that the use of these medications was substantially preferable to the use of ECT.

A third major influence on the decline of ECT's use was the growing civil rights movement for the mentally ill. Many community and religious leaders began to advocate the fair and humane treatment of the seriously mentally ill. These individuals saw ECT as an undesirable treatment method, used as an instrument for controlling and punishing individuals who could not defend themselves. This view of ECT as inhumane soon came to be widely held. ECT was perceived as a method to control, rather than help, patients—as a punishment rather than a therapy.

These and other factors led to the substantially decreased use of ECT. Subsequently, however, well-designed research has begun to define ECT as a relatively safe treatment method that may be the best therapy in certain situations. Additionally, refinements in the application of ECT have increased its effectiveness and reduced its complications. As a result of not only the ambiguity about its potential adverse effects but also the emotional issues related to its use, the controversy about ECT and its relative risks and benefits is likely to continue for many years.

—*Mark E. Johnson*

References

Kerner, Nancy, and Joan Prudic. "Current Electroconvulsive Therapy Practice and Research in the Geriatric Population." *Neuropsychiatry*, vol. 4, no. 1, 2014, pp. 33–54., doi:10.2217/npy.14.3.

Lilienfeld, Scott O. "The Truth about Shock Therapy." *Scientific American*, 1 May 2014, www.scientificamerican.com/article/the-truth-about-shock-therapy/.

Mayo Clinic Staff. "Electroconvulsive Therapy (ECT)." *Mayo Clinic*, Mayo Foundation for Medical Education and Research, 12 Oct. 2018, www.mayoclinic.org/tests-procedures/electroconvulsive-therapy/about/pac-20393894.

Read, John, et al. "Should We Stop Using Electroconvulsive Therapy?" *BMJ*, 30 Jan. 2019, doi:10.1136/bmj.k5233.

Sackeim, Harold A. "Modern Electroconvulsive Therapy." *JAMA Psychiatry*, vol. 74, no. 8, 1 Aug. 2017, p. 779., doi:10.1001/jamapsychiatry.2017.1670.

Singh, Amit, and Sujita Kumar Kar. "How Electroconvulsive Therapy Works?: Understanding the Neurobiological Mechanisms." *Clinical Psychopharmacology and Neuroscience*, vol. 15, no. 3, 31 Aug. 2017, pp. 210–221., doi:10.9758/cpn.2017.15.3.210.

Wells, Karen, et al. "Decision Making and Support Available to Individuals Considering and Undertaking Electroconvulsive Therapy (ECT): a Qualitative, Consumer-Led Study." *BMC Psychiatry*, vol. 18, no. 1, 24 July 2018, doi:10.1186/s12888-018-1813-9.

Zilles, David. "Beneficial Effects of Electroconvulsive Therapy in Elderly People." *The Lancet Psychiatry*, vol. 5, no. 9, 2018, pp. 697–698., doi:10.1016/s2215-0366(18)30264-5.

■ Transcranial Magnetic Stimulation (TMS)

CATEGORY: Procedure
ANATOMY OR SYSTEM AFFECTED: Brain; nervous system; skull
SPECIALTIES AND RELATED FIELDS: Neuroscience, Psychology, Neurology, Psychiatry

KEY TERMS

- *central nervous system*: comprised of the brain and spinal cord
- *cerebral cortex*: the outer covering of the brain that is comprised of neurons and glia cells
- *neurons*: highly specialized cell found in the nervous system that produces an electrical signal to transmit information
- *peripheral nervous system*: refers to all of the neurons in the body located outside the brain and spinal cord

How Does TMS Work?

Since the brain is made up of many distinct neuroanatomical structures that are integrated and interlinked, neuroscientists are interested in studying the functional properties of these brain sites to learn more about their role in perceptual, emotional, and cognitive processing. Transcranial magnetic stimulation (TMS) is a technology that applies a strong magnetic field to a particular focal region of the brain, just beneath the skull, causing the functional properties of a specific area to be malfunction. The interference is brought on by artificially stimulating neurons in a brain structure, which causes it to stop working normally. This effect has been described as the application of a "virtual lesion" to the brain, since the disabling influence is temporary and reversible. By temporarily knocking

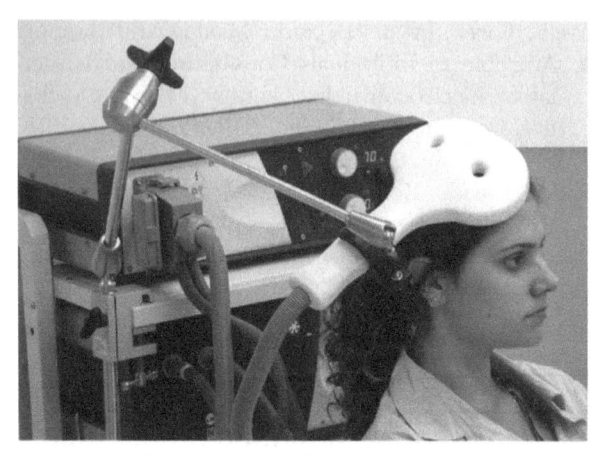

A magnetic coil is positioned at the head of the patient. (Baburov via Wikimedia Commons)

out an area of the brain, investigators are able to use TMS to determine what role it plays in normal brain functioning.

The magnetic field is applied to the scalp using a hand-held coil that is typically in the shape of a figure-eight. A high-voltage current passes through the coil in pulses. Each electrical pulse produces a rapid increase, then a decrease, in the magnetic field around the coil. The coil can be controlled to emit a single pulse that lasts for 1 millisecond, or it can be programmed to send repetitive pulses as rapid as 50 times per second. Using a train of pulses is referred to as *repetitive TMS* and designated as *rTMS*. The number of pulses is dependent on the length of time that an investigator wants to disable a brain region. At low levels, TMS can stimulate a specific region providing more information about its relative importance. High levels of pulsating can shut down a focal region. TMS has been used by neurosurgeons to map the outer layer of the brain prior to removing abnormal tissue. The mapping gives them information regarding the functional properties of the tissue they are working near. If a particular area is involved in critical functions, such as language processing, neurosurgeons will avoid permanently damaging those sites.

Research Applications

As a research tool, TMS has a number of advantages over organic lesion techniques used in the past. First, since the effects of activating or disabling brain tissue using TMS is short-lived and reversible, investigators do not have to worry about the brain reorganizing itself and changing how it processes information. Traditional lesion techniques required a surgeon to permanently destroy brain tissue, which usually sets in motion compensatory changes. Second, TMS allows for the virtual lesion to be moved within the same subject. This affords the advantage of studying the interplay of multiple brain sites that are adjacent to each other. For example, if a neuroscientist wanted to investigate moral decision-making, she could have a participant solve ethical dilemmas while TMS is applied to different areas of the cerebral cortex. This type of study might reveal that several different brain regions—each with its own unique specialized functionality—contribute to how a person engages in moral decision-making. Third, when TMS is combined with functional magnetic imaging (fMRI), the functional integration of brain structures can be studied.

TMS has some disadvantages when compared to traditional lesion techniques. One major limitation is that TMS only affects only the brain tissue directly under the skull. This rules out any investigation into subcortical brain structures, since they are too deep to be impacted. Also, organic lesions created by surgery or by injury can be precisely localized; however, the exact boundaries of the virtual lesion created using TMS is less clear.

—*Bryan C. Auday, PhD*

References

Bermudes, Richard A., et al. *Transcranial Magnetic Stimulation: Clinical Applications for Psychiatric Practice.* American Psychiatric Association Publishing, 2018.

Hardy, Sheila, et al. "Transcranial Magnetic Stimulation in Clinical Practice." *BJPsych Advances*, vol. 22, no. 6, 2016, pp. 373–379., doi:10.1192/apt.bp.115.015206.

Janicak, Philip, and Mehmet E. Dokucu. "Transcranial Magnetic Stimulation for the Treatment of Major Depression." *Neuropsychiatric Disease and Treatment*, 2015, p. 1549., doi:10.2147/ndt.s67477.

Kar, Sujita Kumar. "Predictors of Response to Repetitive Transcranial Magnetic Stimulation in Depression: A Review of Recent Updates." *Clinical Psychopharmacology and Neuroscience*, vol. 17, no. 1, 28 Feb. 2019, pp. 25–33., doi:10.9758/cpn.2019.17.1.25.

Mayo Clinic Staff. "Transcranial Magnetic Stimulation." *Mayo Clinic*, Mayo Foundation for Medical

Education and Research, 27 Nov. 2018, www.mayoclinic.org/tests-procedures/transcranial-magnetic-stimulation/about/pac-20384625.

Saini, Rajivkumar, et al. "Transcranial Magnetic Stimulation: A Review of Its Evolution and Current Applications." *Industrial Psychiatry Journal*, vol. 27, no. 2, 2018, p. 172., doi:10.4103/ipj.ipj_88_18.

Singh, Aditya, et al. "Personalized Repetitive Transcranial Magnetic Stimulation Temporarily Alters Default Mode Network in Healthy Subjects." *Scientific Reports*, vol. 9, no. 1, 4 Apr. 2019, doi:10.1038/s41598-019-42067-3.

Voigt, Jeffrey, et al. "A Systematic Literature Review of the Clinical Efficacy of Repetitive Transcranial Magnetic Stimulation (RTMS) in Non-Treatment Resistant Patients with Major Depressive Disorder." *BMC Psychiatry*, vol. 19, no. 1, 8 Jan. 2019, doi:10.1186/s12888-018-1989-z.

Pain and Addiction

■ Anesthesia misuse

CATEGORY: Addiction
ANATOMY OR SYSTEM AFFECTED: Brain, muscles, musculoskeletal system, nerves, nervous system, psychic-emotional system, skin, spine

Causes
As with any addiction, biological and environmental factors contribute to anesthesia abuse. Addicts have a genetic predisposition and a chronic, compulsive need for the substance of choice. For the anesthesia abuser, these substances include a variety of potentially addictive agents. Generally, insatiable cravings compel chronic use (abuse) of a particular drug, which results in damage to internal organs. However, because many anesthesia drugs have the potential to cause apnea or paralysis within seconds, abuse of anesthetic agents can lead to death.

Risk Factors
Although laypersons abuse anesthesia drugs, the most frequently cited anesthesia abusers are anesthesia providers such as certified registered nurse anesthetists, medical residents, and anesthesiologists. Easy access to anesthetic medications enables anesthesia providers to experiment with controlled substances such as fentanyl and other opioids, which are highly addictive.

Anesthesia providers often work long and irregular hours under stressful conditions with access to anesthetic agents. Propofol abuse is increasingly popular because the substance has a short half-life and is quickly eliminated from the body. Nitrous oxide, commonly known as laughing gas, is an inhaled anesthetic that also is abused. The primary risk of inhaled nitrous oxide is hypoxia, which results from inadequate oxygen supply to the body's tissues and particularly the brain.

Symptoms
A variety of symptoms occur from using common anesthetic medications. These symptoms (and their symptom-producing medications) include amnesia and anxiolysis (midazolam), pain relief (opioids), and sedation and apnea (opioids and propofol). Abusers experience impaired functioning because of these drugs. The dose associated with abuse is often less than that required for general anesthesia. However, the effects of anesthetic medications are dose dependent and may also lead to dysphoria and mood changes. Therefore, abusers may exhibit behavioral changes; may appear fatigued, irritable, euphoric, dysphoric, drowsy, or depressed; or may simply appear out of character. Recognition of these signs is imperative to protect the abuser and to aid health care providers who have a legal responsibility to report colleagues known or suspected of chemical dependency. This not only protects the abusers but also the patients under their care.

Screening and Diagnosis
The screening test commonly used to confirm drug use is typically a urine drug screen. However, many anesthetic medications (such as fentanyl, propofol, naltrexone, and ketamine) are not included in standard drug screens and must be specifically requested. Because of the short half-lives of these anesthesia drugs, many are quickly eliminated from the body and, therefore, are difficult to detect. In some cases, the metabolites of these drugs can be detected in urine samples, while hair samples fulfill other testing needs. Although more expensive than urine testing, hair-sample testing can detect chronic exposure to certain drugs; urine drug screens are limited to detecting drug use only within hours or days of use.

Treatment and Therapy
The American Association of Nurse Anesthetists and the American Society of Anesthesiologists are two national organizations that govern the practice of anesthesia providers. These organizations and many others not affiliated with medical and nursing personnel recommend inpatient treatment for persons with chemical dependency.

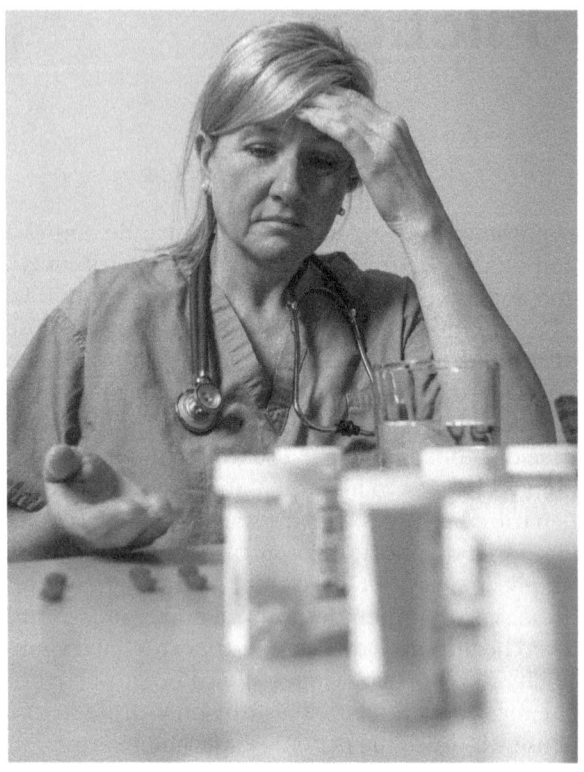

Rates of addiction are high for nurse anesthetists, due to the stressful nature of the job and the availability of the drugs. (Fertnig via iStock)

Short- and long-term therapy combined with support-group attendance and abstinence monitoring offer the highest success rates. Various peer assistance groups are available to monitor and assist those undergoing treatment. Narcotics Anonymous offers a twelve-step program that protects anonymity and offers the addict a structured plan for recovery that includes admitting loss of control over the compulsion (the repeated use of anesthetics) and the aid of a sponsor to evaluate mistakes made by the addict. In return, the addict offers help to others who have the same type of addiction.

Prevention

The US Drug Enforcement Administration (DEA) establishes standards and substance schedules and enforces these standards to prevent and control drug abuse. The DEA has plans to treat propofol as a controlled substance, and doing so would institute more accountability and address the overwhelming availability of the drug to anesthesia providers. Random drug screening in accordance with the US Substance Abuse Mental Health Services Administration's guidelines and employing the proper chain of custody are two methods that various organizations use to deter and detect drug abusers, including anesthesia abusers.

—*Virginia C. Muckler, CRNA, MSN, DNP*

References

Bryson, Ethan O., and Jeffrey H. Silverstein. "Addiction and Substance Abuse in Anesthesiology." *Anesthesiology*, vol. 109, no. 5, 2008, pp. 905–917., doi:10.1097/aln.0b013e3181895bc1.

Earley, Paul H., and Torin Finver. "Addiction to Propofol." *Journal of Addiction Medicine*, vol. 7, no. 3, 2013, pp. 169–176., doi:10.1097/adm.0b013e3182872901.

Lee, Sangseok. "Guilty, or Not Guilty?: a Short Story of Propofol Abuse." *Korean Journal of Anesthesiology*, vol. 65, no. 5, 2013, p. 377., doi:10.4097/kjae.2013.65.5.377.

Luo, Ailin, et al. "Sevoflurane Addiction Due to Workplace Exposure." *Medicine*, vol. 97, no. 38, 2018, doi:10.1097/md.0000000000012454.

Wang, Sicong, and Qing Quan Lian. "Addictions and Stress: Implications for Propofol Abuse." *Neuropsychiatry*, vol. 07, no. 05, 2017, doi:10.4172/neuropsychiatry.1000260.

Xiong, Ming, et al. "Neurobiology of Propofol Addiction and Supportive Evidence: What Is the New Development?" *Brain Sciences*, vol. 8, no. 2, 22 Feb. 2018, p. 36., doi:10.3390/brainsci8020036.

■ Benzodiazepine misuse

CATEGORY: Addiction

ANATOMY OR SYSTEM AFFECTED: Central nervous system

Causes

Benzodiazepines ("benzos") such as Valium, Xanax, Ativan and Klonopin are primarily used as anti-anxiety and anti-insomnia sedatives (tranquilizers) because of their rapid inhibitory effect. They bind to receptors for the inhibitory neurotransmitter gamma-aminobutyric acid (GABA) receptors in the central nervous system (CNS) resulting in enhancement of GABA activity.

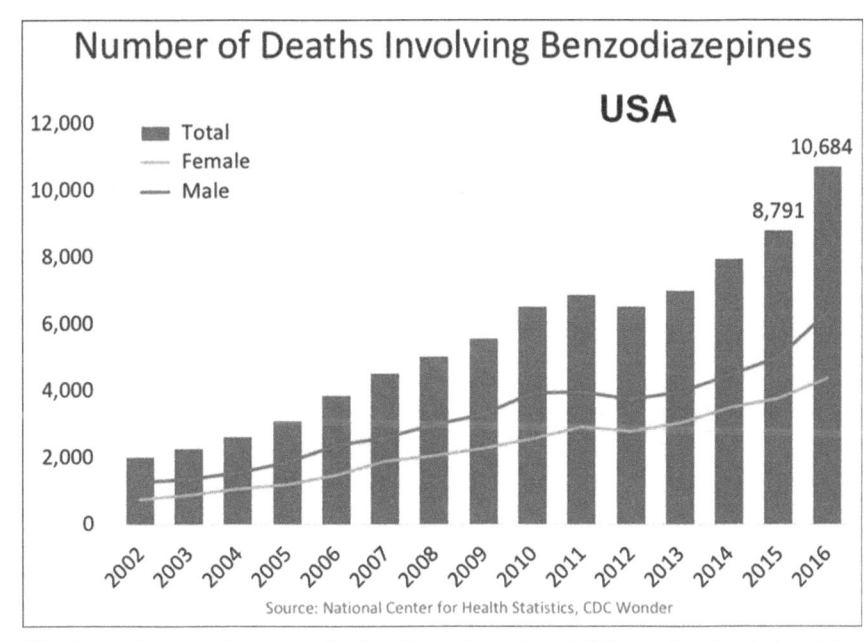

The figure above is a bar chart showing the total number of U.S. overdose deaths involving benzodiazepines from 2002 to 2016. (National Institute on Drug Abuse)

Benzodiazepines provide relaxation and hypnotic effects therapeutically and can be misused to get high or to come down from the effects of stimulants. Benzodiazepine misuse may be acute (for example, illegal use or accidental overdose from prescription) or may be chronic (for example, repeatedly and deliberately combining with cocaine or alcohol to get high or to self-medicate during alcohol withdrawal). Also, chronic misuse of prescribed benzodiazepines by increasing the dose, duration, or number of prescriptions can result in drug dependency.

Although newer CNS agents for anxiety treatment, such as selective serotonin reuptake inhibitors, are available, benzodiazepines can be taken as needed for sporadic anxiety-inducing circumstances and to quickly relieve acute anxiety. However, these uses can cause benzodiazepine misuse. The widespread availability of the drug makes accessibility for nonprescription users easier. Benzodiazepines have been used as date rape drugs, which impair function and, thus, resistance to sexual assault, especially since the drug is difficult to taste when dissolved in a drink.

Risk Factors

Although benzodiazepines have lower misuse potential than do older psychotropic drugs, opioids, and stimulants, benzodiazepines remain popular for misuse in combination. Benzodiazepines with rapid onset, such as diazepam, are the most likely to be misused, although short- or intermediate-acting agents, such as alprazolam or lorazepam, may be misused too. Longer-acting agents, such as clonazepam, are associated with fewer cases of rebound anxiety or misuse.

Longer duration of prescription use (more than four weeks) and higher prescribed dosages (greater content or multiple daily doses) both increase the risk of physical dependence and withdrawal symptoms upon drug discontinuation. As tolerance develops to the prescribed dosages, abusive self-medicating behaviors such as increasing the number of pills or increasing the times a pill is taken without consulting a physician can occur.

Additional risk factors for misuse of a benzodiazepine prescription are combining controlled substance prescriptions, particularly prescribed drugs that have similar CNS activity, and having a history of legal or illegal drug use. For example, methadone users often combine diazepam with methadone to increase the effect of the latter drug.

Symptoms

Acute symptoms of benzodiazepine misuse are less likely to be fatal than benzodiazepine misuse in combination with alcohol. Prominent acute symptoms of misuse are mood changes, increased sleep with trouble awakening, unusual behaviors, and poor focus. With high doses, possible symptoms include confusion, blurred vision, dizziness, weakness, slurred speech, poor coordination, shallow breathing, and even coma.

Chronic symptoms of benzodiazepine use disorder are more difficult to identify. Signs of addiction to a prescribed product include requests for increased doses to provide the same anxiety-relieving effects (drug tolerance) and the use of multiple prescriptions and doctors for the same

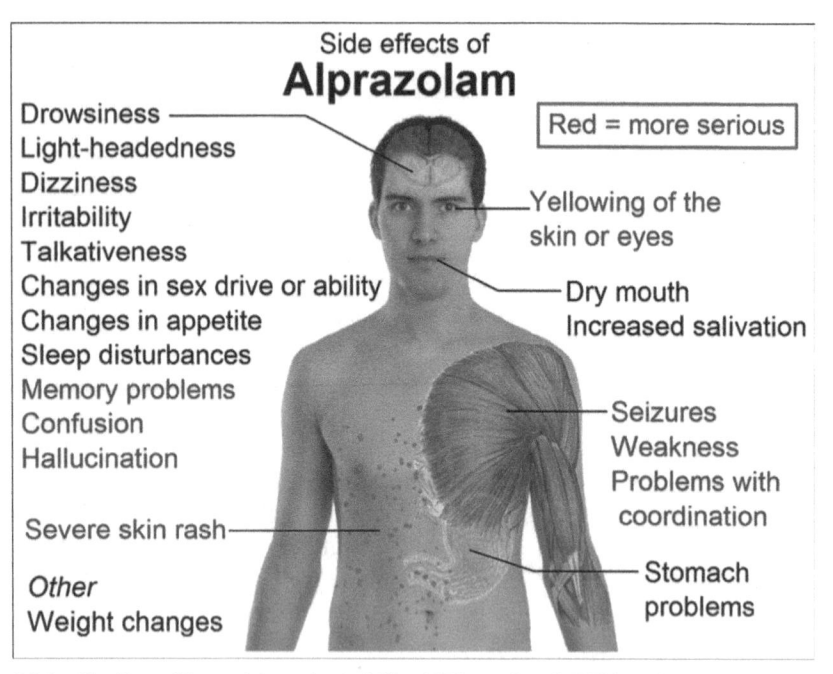

Main side effects of Xanax (alprazolam). (Mikael Häggström via Wikimedia Commons)

drugs (drug-seeking behavior). Persons who misuse benzodiazepines chronically may have a changed appearance, changed behaviors, or changed mood, and they may regularly display poor performance at work or home. At times, these symptoms may mimic anxiety disorders themselves.

Long-term benzodiazepine use may lower cognition permanently with only partial recovery of cognitive abilities upon discontinuation of the benzodiazepine. Seizure risk exists during withdrawal especially with drugs (such as alprazolam) in the class that have short half-lives.

Screening and Diagnosis

Except for acute overdose presenting in an emergency room, screening for benzodiazepine use disorder requires subtle observation by family and health care providers. Chronic misuse may lead users to stop performing their normal duties at home and work. Those struggling with benzodiazepine use disorder will increasingly neglect themselves and others. Misusers may take benzodiazepines even in unsafe circumstances, such as before driving a vehicle, and may experience legal or family problems. Repeated requests for prescriptions, early pharmacy refills, and hiding medications in different locations are signs of addiction and drug-seeking behavior.

Dependence may be identified as an aid to diagnosing benzodiazepine use disorder. When benzodiazepines are used regularly for more than two to three weeks, even at low doses, they begin to lose their inhibitory GABA effects, and higher doses are required to relieve anxiety or to obtain a high. Once this tolerance develops, withdrawal symptoms upon drug discontinuation are also likely and may occur within days of stopping the benzodiazepine.

Withdrawal symptoms also may contribute to a diagnosis of benzodiazepine use disorder because they differ from rebound anxiety symptoms and appear similar to the symptoms of alcohol withdrawal. Tremor, insomnia, sweating, and nausea and vomiting are possible. Sensitivity to light and sound are common and directly distinguish withdrawal from symptoms of an underlying anxiety disorder. More severe withdrawal symptoms include agitation, confusion, myoclonic jerks, and seizures.

Treatment and Therapy

Acute overdose treatment in an emergency room depends upon the amount of time passed since the benzodiazepine was ingested. Within one to two hours of a lethal dose, gastric lavage may be used to flush the stomach. Alternatively, one dose of activated charcoal can be given within four hours of ingestion to bind the drug in the stomach. Severe cramps and nausea are possible, and vomiting is a risk. Flumazenil provides an antidote to the sedative effects of benzodiazepines in cases of severe overdose and coma risk; however, its use may cause seizures when given to people who misuse benzodiazepines chronically and who may have become dependent.

Treating chronic benzodiazepine use disorder is multifactorial and gradual. A slow tapering of dosage is key to avoiding rebound anxiety or withdrawal symptoms which may take three to four days after drug discontinuation to begin. At the physician's discretion, a short-acting benzodiazepine

> **Common Benzodiazepines**
>
> The following common benzodiazepines are used to treat acute mania, alcohol dependence, seizures, anxiety, insomnia, and muscular disorders:
>
> **TRADE NAME : GENERIC NAME**
>
> | | |
> |---|---|
> | Ativan : lorazepam | Mogadon : nitrazepam |
> | Dalmane : flurazepam | ProSom : estazolam |
> | Dormicum : midazolam | Restoril : temazepam |
> | Halcion : triazolam | Rohypnol : flunitrazepam |
> | Klonopin : clonazepam | Sedoxil : mexazolam |
> | Lexotanil : bromazepam | Serax : oxazepam |
> | Librium : chlordiazepoxide | Valium : diazepam |
> | Loramet : lormetazepam | Xanax : alprazolam |

such as triazolam may be replaced with longer-acting agents in the class, such as chlordiazepoxide (Librium), or with a prescription agent from another class with a similar mechanism, such as gabapentin (an antiseizure drug). Either replacement may be more safely tapered and stopped.

In some persons with chronic anxiety disorder, benzodiazepines cannot be fully discontinued. These persons may remain on very low dosages of the misused drug or another benzodiazepine, under strict observation, to avoid withdrawal and rebound risks and to minimize tolerance or misuse, which are likely with higher dosages, without sacrificing anti-anxiety therapy.

Prevention

The key to prevention of acute or chronic benzodiazepine misuse is to lower its availability in prescribed and nonprescribed forms. The drug should be replaced as a prescription with safer and newer anti-anxiety agents. Physical dependence and acute misuse are less likely to occur if longer-acting or alternatively acting agents are prescribed for short time periods with careful physician supervision.

—*Nicole M. Van Hoey, PharmD,*
Charles L. Vigue, Ph.D.

References

Brett, Jonathan, and Bridin Murnion. "Management of Benzodiazepine Misuse and Dependence." *Australian Prescriber*, vol. 38, no. 5, 1 Oct. 2015, pp. 152–155., doi:10.18773/austprescr.2015.055.

Fluyau, Dimy, et al. "Challenges of the Pharmacological Management of Benzodiazepine Withdrawal, Dependence, and Discontinuation." *Therapeutic Advances in Psychopharmacology*, vol. 8, no. 5, 9 Feb. 2018, pp. 147–168., doi:10.1177/2045125317753340.

Liebrenz, Michael, et al. "High-Dose Benzodiazepine Dependence: A Qualitative Study of Patients' Perceptions on Initiation, Reasons for Use, and Obtainment." *Plos One*, vol. 10, no. 11, 10 Nov. 2015, doi:10.1371/journal.pone.0142057.

Nordqvist, Joseph. "Benzodiazepines: Uses, Types, Side Effects, and Risks." *Medical News Today*, MediLexicon International, 7 Mar. 2019, www.medicalnewstoday.com/articles/262809.php.

Reichel, Chloe. "Benzodiazepines: Another Prescription Drug Problem." *Journalist's Resource*, 30 May 2019, journalistsresource.org/studies/society/public-health/benzodiazepines-what-journalists-should-know/.

Schmitz, Allison. "Benzodiazepine Use, Misuse, and Abuse: A Review." *Mental Health Clinician*, vol. 6, no. 3, 2016, pp. 120–126., doi:10.9740/mhc.2016.05.120.

Soyka, Michael. "Treatment of Benzodiazepine Dependence." *New England Journal of Medicine*, vol. 376, no. 12, 23 Mar. 2017, pp. 1147–1157., doi:10.1056/nejmra1611832.

■ Center for Substance Abuse Treatment (CSAT)

CATEGORY: Therapy or Technique

Background

For 18 years, the Center for Substance Abuse Treatment (CSAT) was a program of the National Institute on Drug Abuse (NIDA), which was responsible both for overseeing research related to substance use disorders and for delivery of services to patients. When NIDA became part of the National Institutes of Health in 1992, its focus shifted entirely to research. CSAT and the Center for Substance Abuse Prevention became responsible for delivering services to patients.

Mission and Goals

CSAT's initiatives and programs are based on research findings and the general consensus of experts in the field of addiction. For most people, treatment and recovery work best in a community-based, coordinated system of comprehensive services. Because no single treatment approach is effective for everyone, CSAT supports efforts to provide multiple treatment modalities, evaluate treatment effectiveness, and use evaluation results to enhance treatment and recovery approaches.

Advisors

CSAT's national advisory council was established under Section 502 of the Public Health Service Act (1944) and was originally chartered on December 9, 1992, in keeping with public law. The council advises, consults with, and offers recommendations to the US Secretary of Health, the SAMHSA (Substance Abuse and Mental Health Services Administration) administrator, and the CSAT director concerning issues relating to the activities done by and through the center and to the policies related to such events.

The advisory council can, on the basis of evidence provided, make recommendations to the director of CSAT concerning actions conducted there. The council reviews applications submitted for grants and cooperative agreements for activities requiring council permission; it also recommends for approval applications for projects that show promise of making valuable contributions to CSAT's mission. Furthermore, the council can consider any grant proposal made by the organization itself.

The advisory council collects material about studies and services that are ongoing in the United States or other countries that relate to the issues of substance misuse and mental illness. The council also examines material on issues linked to diseases, disorders, or other aspects of human health that relate to the mission of SAMHSA and its programs.

The director of CSAT permits the council to make such information available through publications for the benefit of public and private health entities, health professions personnel, and the general public. The council may appoint subcommittees and convene workshops and conferences. Management and support services for the council are provided by the center.

Programs

CSAT programs include a treatment helpline (1-800-662-HELP) and National Recovery Month, which promotes the societal benefits of treatment for substance use and mental disorders, celebrates people in recovery, lauds the contributions of treatment providers, and promotes the message that recovery is possible. National Recovery Month spreads the message that behavioral health is essential to overall health, that prevention works, that treatment is effective, and that people can and do recover.

Another CSAT service is the Behavioral Health Treatment Services Locator, an online resource for locating drug and alcohol use disorder treatment programs. The locator lists private and public facilities that are licensed, certified, or otherwise approved for inclusion by their respective state's substance use disorders agency. It also lists treatment facilities administered by the US Department of Veterans Affairs, the US Indian Health Service, and the US Department of Defense.

—*Margaret Ring Gillock, MS,*
Marianne Moss Madsen, MS

References

Center for Substance Abuse Treatment. *Substance Abuse and Mental Health Services Administration*, 23 Aug. 2017, www.samhsa.gov/about-us/who-we-are/offices-centers/csat.

■ Narcotics and opioid misuse

CATEGORY: Addiction
ANATOMY OR SYSTEM AFFECTED: Brain, spinal cord and peripheral nerves

Causes

Narcotics produce their effect by binding to opioid receptors in the central nervous system. The human body contains opioid receptors to respond to naturally occurring opioids in the body known as endorphins. Endorphins serve to block or suppress the feeling of pain, having an analgesic and sedative effect. Narcotics lead to euphoria and sedation, produced by stimulation of the opioid receptors.

Risk Factors

The type of narcotic misused can be a factor in addiction potential. Heroin can cause addiction after one use; second in potency is morphine.

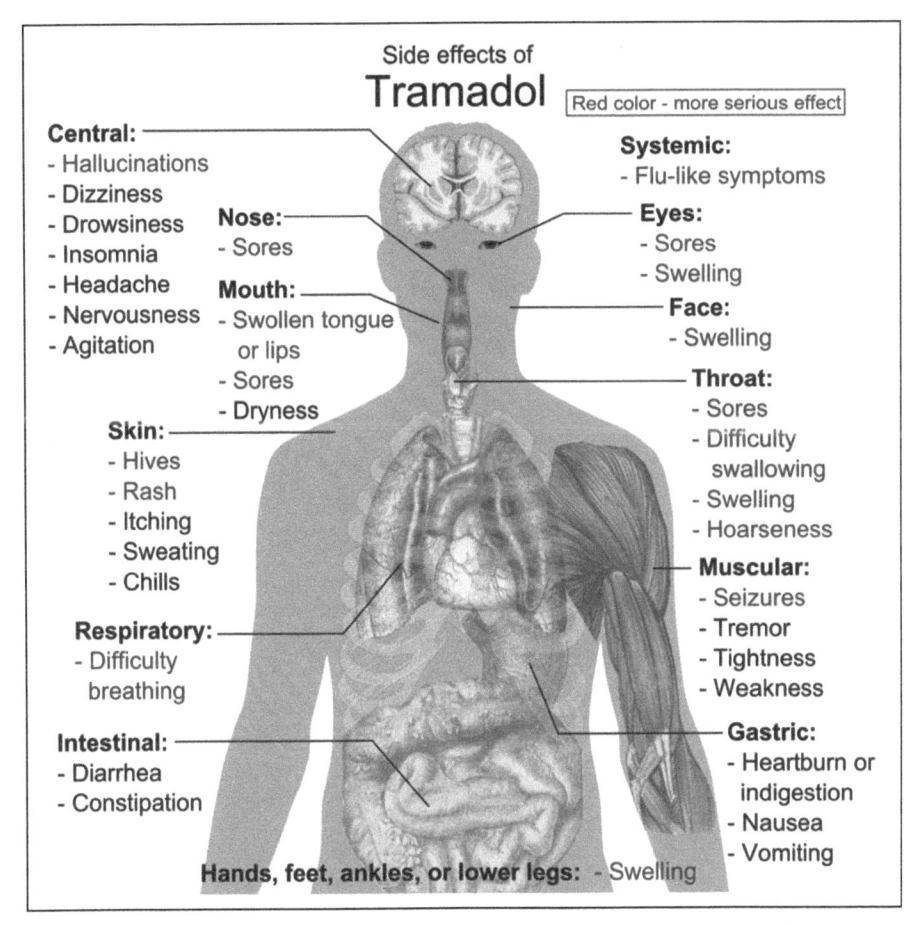

Main side effects of tramadol. (Mikael Häggström via Wikimedia Commons)

Other risk factors for narcotics misuse include psychological mind-sets such as antisocial attitudes and sensation-seeking during adolescence. Environmental risk factors include dysfunction family relationships, poverty, gang membership, urban living, disposable income, family history of substance misuse, and low self-esteem.

Symptoms

Narcotics intoxication may include sensations such as euphoria, a rush of pleasure, relaxation, and drowsiness, followed by sedation or sleep. Users report feeling free from cares and worries, a lessening of anxiety and tension, and a sense of escapism from life. The feeling is so pleasurable that the user often develops an irresistible urge to use again, an urge that may eventually develop into an addiction.

Some of the negative effects of narcotics misuse are sleep disturbances, sexual dysfunctions, anxiety, drowsiness, inability to concentrate, apathy, lethargy, flushing of the face and neck, constipation, nausea, and vomiting. A person prescribed a narcotic may develop some withdrawal symptoms over time if use is suddenly interrupted. Generally, if narcotics are prescribed for a longer time for pain relief, the dosage is progressively lowered through the weeks to prevent withdrawal symptoms.

Withdrawal symptoms for narcotics and opioids are some of the worst exhibited for any misused substance. Early symptoms of withdrawal may appear within a few hours, but typically appear within six to thirty-six hours of the last dose. Symptoms of withdrawal are typically the reverse of the pleasurable effects produced by the narcotic and include anxiety, irritability, loss of appetite, tremors, salivation, yawning, flu-like symptoms, and sweating. More serious withdrawal symptoms include abdominal cramping, fever, gooseflesh, gastrointestinal upset, confusion, and convulsions. Less acute withdrawal symptoms, which may persist for months after the last dose, include anhedonia, insomnia, and drug craving. The severity of symptoms is proportionate to dosage and duration of misuse.

Screening and Diagnosis

Persons suspected of narcotics overdose require immediate emergency medical attention. With an unconscious person suspected of narcotics overdose, doctors will look for physical signs of overdose, such as shallow breathing and small pupils. Patients are then administered naloxone, an opioid antagonist, to reverse the possibility of coma (which can occur in as quickly as one minute).

THE OPIOID EPIDEMIC BY THE NUMBERS

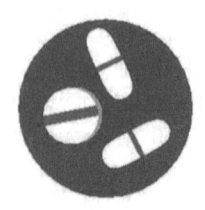

130+ People died every day from opioid-related drug overdoses[3] (estimated)

10.3 m People misused prescription opioids in 2018[1]

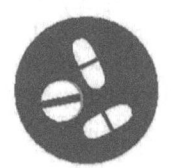

47,600 People died from overdosing on opioids[2]

2.0 million People had an opioid use disorder in 2018[1]

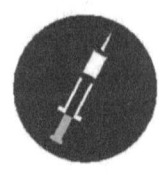

81,000 People used heroin for the first time[1]

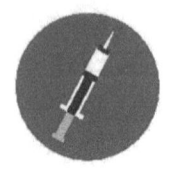

808,000 People used heroin in 2018[1]

2 million People misused prescription opioids for the first time[1]

15,349 Deaths attributed to overdosing on heroin (in 12-month period ending February 2019)[2]

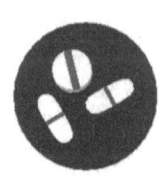

32,656 Deaths attributed to overdosing on synthetic opioids other than methadone (in 12-month period ending February 2019)[2]

SOURCES

1. 2019 National Survey on Drug Use and Health. Mortality in the United States, 2018
2. NCHS Data Brief No. 329, November 2018
3. NCHS, National Vital Statistics System. Estimates for 2018 and 2019 are based on provisional data.

Updated October 2019. For more information, visit: http://www.hhs.gov/opioids/

HHS.GOV/OPIOIDS

Source: U.S. Department of Health and Human Services

To diagnose misuse, a doctor will question a person about his or her history of drug use, including use under dangerous conditions, and will ask about failures to meet obligations, legal problems, and impairments of social or occupational functioning caused by narcotics use.

Treatment and Therapy

Treating people who are addicted to narcotics is difficult, mainly because of denial and the severity of withdrawal symptoms. Detoxification is the first step, and the most common long-term treatment is to substitute methadone (a synthetic narcotic with less addictive potential) for the misused drug, followed by weaning the misuser off the methadone. Buprenorphine is another medicine that can be used in the same manner for detoxification. The drug clonidine is also sometimes used to help alleviate some of the symptoms of withdrawal, particularly salivation, runny nose, sweating, abdominal cramping, and muscle aches. Also, recovery groups such as Narcotics Anonymous provide an important source of community support for persons who are overcoming narcotics addiction.

Prevention

To prevent possible addiction and dependence, it is important to use opioid medications only at the prescribed dosages, or to avoid narcotics altogether. A recovering addict must deal with the intense, long-term psychological dependence on narcotics. Counseling, self-help groups, halfway houses, and group therapy may help recovering addicts maintain abstinence.

—*Eugenia M. Valentine, PhD*

References

Brady, Kathleen T., et al. "Prescription Opioid Misuse, Abuse, and Treatment in the United States: An Update." *American Journal of Psychiatry*, vol. 173, no. 1, 2016, pp. 18–26., doi:10.1176/appi.ajp.2015.15020262.

Cicero, Theodore J. "No End in Sight: The Abuse of Prescription Narcotics." *Cerebrum*, 1 Sept. 2015.

Dirks, April. "The Opioid Epidemic: Impact on Children and Families." *Journal of Psychiatry and Psychiatric Disorders*, vol. 02, no. 01, 2018, pp. 9–11., doi:10.26502/jppd.2572-519x0035.

Lyapustina, Tatyana, and G. Caleb Alexander. "The Prescription Opioid Addiction and Abuse Epidemic: How It Happened and What We Can Do about It." *The Pharmaceutical Journal*, vol. 294, no. 7866, 11 June 2015, doi:10.1211/pj.2015.20068579.

Mchugh, R. Kathryn, et al. "Prescription Drug Abuse: from Epidemiology to Public Policy." *Journal of Substance Abuse Treatment*, vol. 48, no. 1, 2015, pp. 1–7., doi:10.1016/j.jsat.2014.08.004.

NIDA. "Misuse of Prescription Drugs." *National Institute on Drug Abuse*, Dec. 2018, www.drugabuse.gov/publications/misuse-prescription-drugs/overview.

■ Prescription drug misuse

CATEGORY: Addiction

Risk Factors

According to the Substance Abuse and Mental Health Services Administration (SAMHSA), 1.9 million people in the United States age twelve years and older misused or were dependent on prescription pain relievers in 2009. An additional 481,000 persons misused or depended on tranquilizers, 371,000 persons misused or depended on stimulants, and 147,000 misused or depended on sedatives.

Anyone can become addicted to prescription scheduled drugs, but some persons have a greater risk. For example, alcoholics or persons who misuse illegal drugs have an elevated risk for dependence on prescribed drugs. Alcoholics may misuse drugs such as benzodiazepines to potentiate (increase) the effects of alcohol, while others addicted to stimulants such as methamphetamine or cocaine may use benzodiazepines as sedatives to fall asleep. Misuse can escalate into an addiction.

In general, women have a higher risk for prescription drug misuse and addiction than men. For example, about 55 percent of those who use prescription pain relievers for no medical reason are women, according to SAMHSA. In addition, incarcerated persons of both genders, particularly those in prison or on parole, have a higher risk for drug misuse and dependence than those not incarcerated or on parole.

According to an analysis by researcher Li-Tzy Wu and colleagues, adolescents aged twelve to seventeen years misuse prescription pain relievers, but only about 1 percent of this group is addicted. This research also indicates female adolescents have a higher risk for addiction to opiates than males. Other risk factors for addiction among adolescents include the misuse of multiple illicit drugs and the sale of illegal drugs to others. Adolescents who misuse or depend on prescription pain relievers are significantly more likely than others to have emotional or health problems and to have problems with family or friends.

An early nonmedical use of prescription drugs is predictive of adult prescription drug misuse and dependence, according to research by Sean E. McCabe and colleagues. The researchers found that nonmedical prescription drug misuse before age thirteen years was predictive for misuse and dependence of prescription drugs at age twenty-one years and older. Among early users, 25 percent became dependent on prescription drugs later in life, compared with 7 percent who initiated their prescription drug use at or older than age twenty-one years and then became misusers or addicts.

Obtaining Drugs of Dependence
Some persons initially obtain dangerous prescription drugs from their physician because of a valid medical problem involving pain or a diagnosis of a psychiatric disorder. These persons may exceed the dosage recommended by the physician. To support this increased dosage, these users may seek a greater quantity of drugs from their doctors; if their doctor refuses, they often seek prescriptions through multiple physicians. This practice is referred to as doctor shopping.

In 2009 about one-half of persons who misused narcotics or psychiatric medications obtained these drugs from a friend or relative with that person's permission. Others obtain their drugs from the Internet or from drug dealers, or they steal drugs from friends and family members. Some addicts steal prescription pads from doctors and write their own prescriptions, while some with legitimate prescriptions are altered to obtain a greater quantity than ordered by the doctor. For this reason, doctors who prescribe pain medications often photocopy their original prescription.

Prescribed drugs are also stolen from pharmacies. For example, between January 2000 and June 2003, about 1.4 million OxyContin tablets were stolen from pharmacies. About two-thirds of these losses were attributed to break-ins or robberies, and 16.5 percent were attributed to employee theft.

Drug dealers also sell prescription drugs. A 2008 study of prescription opioid misuse among persons taking street drugs found that, based on a sample of 586 illicit heroin users in New York City, methadone was sold to them by 64.7 percent of drug dealers and OxyContin was sold by 41.4 percent. One-half of the drug dealers selling heroin and cocaine also sold prescription opioids and 25 percent of the drug dealers sold prescription opioids only.

Some people hire patients already legitimately receiving Medicare or Medicaid to complain to their doctors about pain to obtain drugs for diversion. Doctors who participate in this type of scam (and who receive illicit payments for their participation) give the patient a prescription for a large quantity of opiates. These prescriptions are then filled, given to the person who initially hired the patient, and then retrieved by drug dealers for illegal sale.

Doctor Shopping
Doctor shopping, an illegal activity, is the intentional use of multiple doctors to secure prescription narcotics or other controlled substances while withholding that the drug in question has already been prescribed by another doctor. The patient may have real, chronic pain that is being undertreated, or may be faking or exaggerating illness or injury to satisfy an addiction or to obtain medication to sell illegally.

Patients seek prescription drugs from emergency rooms, walk-in clinics, physicians, specialists, and dentists. They also may buy them on the street; may steal prescription pads; may alter prescriptions to get additional refills; might steal drugs from a pharmacy, friends, and family members (especially the elderly); might obtain drugs from disreputable Web-based pharmacies; or might visit physicians in states that have weak doctor-shopping laws.

Abuse of Prescription (Rx) Drugs
Affects Young Adults Most

Young adults (age 18 to 25) are the biggest abusers of prescription (Rx) opioid pain relievers, ADHD stimulants, and anti-anxiety drugs. They do it for all kinds of reasons, including to get high or because they think Rx stimulants will help them study better. But Rx abuse is dangerous. In 2014, more than 1,700 young adults died from prescription drug (mainly opioid) overdoses—more than died from overdoses of any other drug, including heroin and cocaine combined— and many more needed emergency treatment.[1]

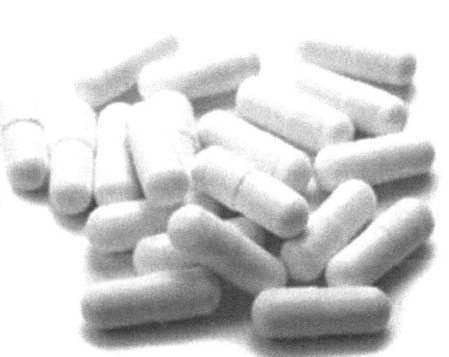

PAST-YEAR USE

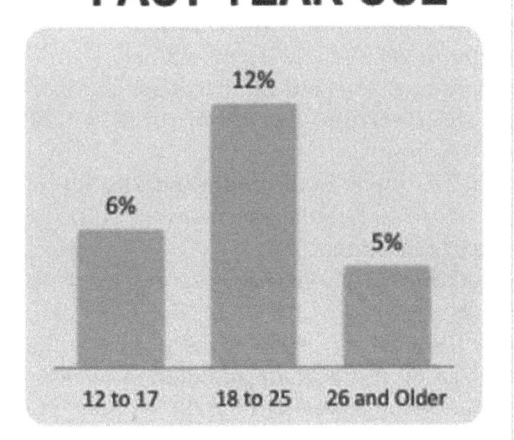

- 12 to 17: 6%
- 18 to 25: 12%
- 26 and Older: 5%

In 2014, the nonmedical use of prescription drugs was highest among young adults.[2]

MOTIVATIONS FOR USE
Most young adults say they use Rx drugs to[3,4,5]

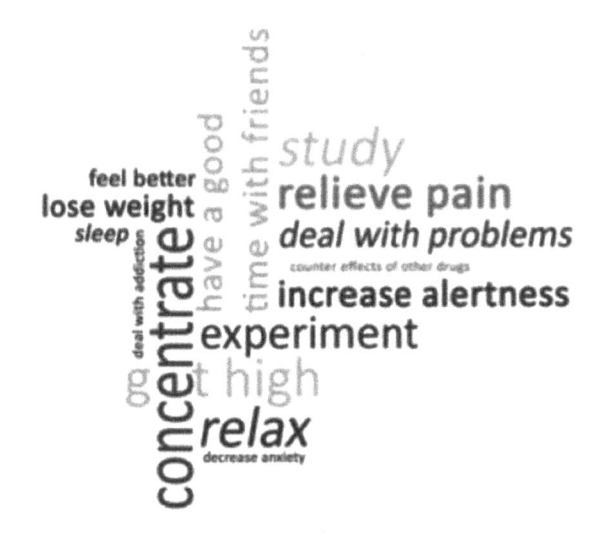

study, relieve pain, deal with problems, increase alertness, experiment, get high, relax, concentrate, feel better, lose weight, sleep, have a good time with friends, counter effects of other drugs, deal with addiction, decrease anxiety

Source: National Institute on Drug Abuse

The controlled substances most often sought are narcotics such as Vicodin (hydrocodone), OxyContin (oxycodone), Darvocet, Demerol (meperidine), Percocet (oxycodone with acetaminophen), and morphine. Addicts also seek stimulants (amphetamines) and sleeping pills (benzodiazepines).

Symptoms of Withdrawal
The problem of prescription drug dependence becomes evident when the person stops taking the addictive drug, whether voluntarily or because the person cannot obtain the drug. The addict will undergo withdrawal symptoms, which may be severe. Symptoms include such reactions as headache, tremors, vomiting, seizures, and even death.

Psychological symptoms too are common with a sudden withdrawal from prescription drugs of abuse; the person may experience severe anxiety, hallucinations, and delusions. To limit the withdrawal symptoms, persons who stop taking addictive prescription drugs should be under the care of a physician.

Treatment and Therapy
Prescription drug addiction is a treatable condition. The type of treatment will depend on the type of drug to which the person is addicted and on the needs of the individual. Successful treatment programs are usually a combination of detoxification, counseling, and, in some cases, medications. Many people go through more than one round of treatment before they are able to fully recover from their addiction.

Opioids. Initial treatment for opioid addiction may include medications to help alleviate the symptoms of withdrawal. Methadone and buprenorphine, both synthetic opioids, are the most commonly used drugs to treat symptoms of opioid withdrawal. Both are highly regulated drugs that are usually prescribed to people who are enrolled in a treatment program for opioid addiction.

Methadone and buprenorphine ease withdrawal symptoms and relieve cravings. Methadone has been used for decades to treat opioid addiction. Buprenorphine was approved by the US Food and Drug Administration for the treatment of opioid dependence in 2002. Patients will need medical supervision during treatment for opioid withdrawal.

Counseling following treatment for opioid withdrawal symptoms can help patients learn to function without drugs, handle drug cravings, cope with negative emotions without drug use, and avoid people and situations that could lead to relapse. Support groups and twelve-step programs such as Narcotics Anonymous can help with the treatment of opioid addiction and with the adjustment to a new, drug-free lifestyle. Some patients may choose in-patient treatment at a recovery center.

Stimulants. There are no medications to help alleviate withdrawal symptoms in patients who are addicted to prescription stimulants. One approach is to slowly decrease the dosage until the patient has been weaned. Patients will need medical supervision during treatment for withdrawal from stimulant medications. Once the patient has stopped taking the medication, behavioral therapy is often used to help patients recognize risky situations, avoid drug use, and more effectively cope with problems.

Another treatment that has been proven effective for stimulant addiction is contingency management. During contingency management, patients are given vouchers for drug-free urine tests. The vouchers can be exchanged for rewards that promote healthy living. Support groups and twelve-step programs such as Narcotics Anonymous also can help with the treatment of prescription stimulant addiction.

Prevention
Most people who take prescription medications as prescribed do not become addicted. There are some steps that people can take to decrease their risk of addiction, including the following:

Ask if the medication being prescribed is addictive and if there are any alternative medications.

Follow the directions on the medication label without exception.

Avoid increasing a medication dose without discussing it with the health care provider who prescribed the medication.

Never take medication that was prescribed for someone else.

Parents too can take steps to help ensure that their children do not become addicted to prescription drugs. Preventive steps include keeping prescription medications in a locked cabinet; discussing with children the dangers of prescription medications, including the dangers of sharing medications with others; and properly disposing of prescription medications.

Pharmacists can help prevent prescription drug addiction by giving patients clear information about how medications should be taken and by providing information about potential side effects or drug interactions. Prescribers can help to prevent prescription drug addiction by noting increases in the amount of drug a patient needs to get the same therapeutic effect, by tracking frequent requests for refills, and discussing the risks of addiction with patients.

—*Christine Adamec, BA, MBA*

For Further Information

Davis, W. Rees, and Bruce D. Johnson. "Prescription Opioid Use, Misuse, and Diversion among Street Drug Users in New York City." *Drug and Alcohol Dependence* vol. 92, 2008, pp. 267–76.

Gwinnell, Esther, and Christine Adamec. *The Encyclopedia of Drug Abuse*. Facts On File, 2008.

Inciardi, James A., et al. "Mechanisms of Prescription Drug Diversion among Drug-Involved Cluband Street-Based Populations." *Pain Medicine* vol. 8. no. 2, 2007, pp. 171–83.

McCabe, Sean E., et al. "Does Early Onset of Non-Medical Use of Prescription Drugs Predict Subsequent Prescription Drug Abuse and Dependence?" *Addiction* vol. 102 no. 12, 2007, pp. 1920–30.

■ Sedative-hypnotic misuse

CATEGORY: Addiction
ALSO KNOWN AS: Depressant misuse

History of Use

Bromide, the first sedative-hypnotic, originated in 1838 and was followed by chloral hydrate, paraldehyde, and barbiturates. Bromide compounds were frequently used as sedatives and anticonvulsants in the nineteenth and early twentieth century.

Barbiturates were first introduced for medical use in the early twentieth century. Since then, approximately fifty barbiturates were marketed but less than fifteen remain in medical use. Barbiturates became popular in the 1960s as treatment for anxiety, insomnia, and seizure disorders, but the dependence-producing potential and the dangers of overdose restricted their use significantly. Since the 1970s, barbiturates were largely replaced by the safer BDZ group.

The first BDZs, chlordiazepoxide and diazepam, were introduced in clinical practice in the early 1960s. Although more than two thousand different BDZs have been synthesized, less than twenty are currently approved in the United States. BDZ usage increased dramatically in the 1970s, with total sales accounting for about 10 percent of all prescriptions in many Western countries. The perceived desirable properties of anxiety alleviation, euphoria, disinhibition, and sleep promotion have led to the compulsive misuse of virtually all of the drugs classed as sedative-hypnotics.

Causes

Depressant misuse is on the rise because of the wide availability of drugs by prescription or through the illicit marketplace. Examples of illegal depressants of misuse include the date rape drugs flunitrazepam (Rohypnol) and gamma-hydroxybutyric acid (GHB, a natural depressant).

Overall, short-acting agents are more likely to be used nonmedically than those with long-lasting effects. Because of their wider margin of safety, benzodiazepines have largely replaced barbiturates. They now constitute the most prescribed central nervous system (CNS) depressants—and the most frequently misused, usually to achieve a general feeling of relaxation. However, barbiturates and barbiturate-like drugs still pose clinical problems, as many young people underestimate the risks these drugs carry. Non-benzodiazepine sedatives, such as zolpidem (Ambien), also can generate misuse and dependence.

Most sedative-hypnotic drugs work by enhancing the inhibitory activity of the neurotransmitter gamma-aminobutyric acid, thus reducing CNS activity and promoting relaxation and sleep. They are usually prescribed to treat sleep disorders, anxiety, acute stress reactions, panic attacks, and seizures. In higher doses, some agents become general anesthetics. Chronic use results in tolerance and dependence (both psychological and physical).

Risk Factors

Barbiturate misuse occurs most commonly in mature adults with a long history of use, while benzodiazepines are favored by younger persons (those younger than forty years of age). Two main categories of people misuse depressant drugs. The first category comprises people who receive depressant prescriptions for psychiatric disorders or who obtain them illicitly to cope with stressful life situations. These persons have a high risk of becoming dependent, especially if they receive high doses, take the drug for longer than one month, and have a history of substance misuse or a family history of alcoholism. However, if dose escalation is not evident and drugs are not used to achieve a state of intoxication, chronic benzodiazepine users should not be considered misusers.

A second important category comprises people who use sedative drugs in the context of alcohol or multiple-drug misuse. These people may take

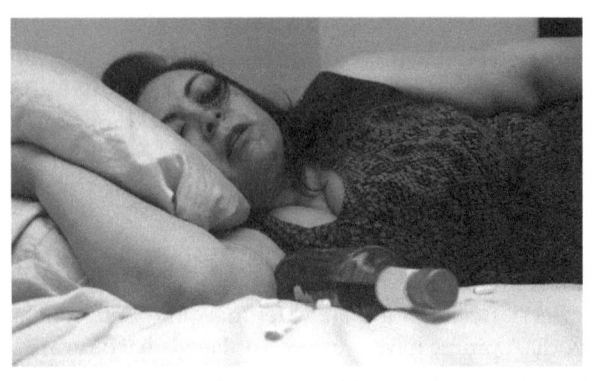

Abuse of hypnotics or sleeping pills often corresponds to misuse of alcohol, which is also a depressant. (rustycanuck via iStock)

benzodiazepines to alleviate insomnia and anxiety (sometimes induced by stimulants), to increase the euphoric effects of opioids, and to diminish cocaine (or alcohol) withdrawal symptoms.

Other Uses of Sedative-Hypnotics

Some of the sedative-hypnotics are used to commit sexual assaults. Because these drugs are sedating and induce a temporary amnesia, they are sometimes added to alcoholic beverages and soft drinks to incapacitate the intended victim of a rape. Flunitrazepam (Rohypnol), also known with the street names rophies, roofies, and roach, is a long-acting BDZ used as a favored sedative of misuse among adolescents and adults, and it is typically used in combination with alcohol as a party drug and a date rape drug.

Flunitrazepam has never been approved for medical use in the United States. Gamma-hydroxy butyrate (GHB), a natural CNS depressant resulting from the metabolism of the inhibitory neurotransmitter GABA, has emerged as a significant drug of misuse. It gained popularity for recreational use because of its pleasant, alcohol-like, hangover-free high with aphrodisiac properties.

Body-builders misuse GHB for its alleged utility as an anabolic agent. GHB is often taken by young polydrug misusers (who are called clubbers and ravers) in combination with amphetamines to produce euphoria and a hallucinatory state. Because of concerns about GHB misuse and date rape usage, in 2000 this drug was made a schedule I controlled substance. Because flunitrazepam and GHB are illegal in the United States, they are available only through the underground market.

Those who chronically misuse sedative-hypnotics prefer the short-acting barbiturates, the barbiturate-like depressants glutethimide and methaqualone, and the faster-acting BDZs diazepam, alprazolam, and lorazepam. Persons who misuse sedative-hypnotics are most likely to be those who use drugs to relieve stress; who use drugs to counteract unpleasant effects of other drugs of misuse; and who combine CNS depressants with alcohol or opiates to potentiate their effects.

Significant safety concerns with sedative-hypnotics include important drug interactions (for example, the inhibitors of drug metabolism such as antifungals, erythromycin, clarithromycin, or cimetidine significantly prolong their effect and increase their toxicity) and their appropriate use in special populations (elderly people, pregnant women, and persons with a history of substance misuse). Overdosing on sedative-hypnotics is among the most common methods for attempting suicide.

Symptoms

People who misuse depressants often engage in drug-seeking behaviors that include frequently requesting, borrowing, stealing, or forging prescriptions; ordering and purchasing medication online; and visiting several doctors to obtain prescriptions. These behaviors often accompany changes in sleep patterns and irritable mood and increased alcohol consumption. Recreational use and self-medication with depressants may lead to accidental overdoses and suicide attempts. Many persons use a "cocktail" of alcohol and depressant medications for enhanced relaxation and euphoria. This practice is dangerous, as it carries a high risk of overdose.

Sedative-hypnotic drug intoxication resembles alcohol, painkillers, and antihistamine intoxication. It presents with impaired judgment, confusion, drowsiness, dizziness, unsteady movements, slurred speech, and visual disturbances. Young adults attempting to get high may show excitement, loss of inhibition, and even aggressive behavior. Acute GHB intoxication leads to sleep and memory loss. These manifestations occur without alcohol odor on the breath, unless the misuser combined the drug with alcohol. In the case of barbiturates, the behavioral effects of intoxication can vary depending on the time of day, the surroundings, and even the user's expectations.

Tolerance to barbiturates is not accompanied by an increase in lethal dose, as it is with opiates. For this reason, an overdose can be fatal. Signs and symptoms of barbiturate overdose vary, and they include lethargy, decreased heart rate, diminished reflexes, respiratory depression, and cardiovascular collapse.

All sedative-hypnotics can induce physical dependence if taken in sufficient dosage over a long time. Withdrawal from depressant medication results in a "rebound" of nervous system activity. In a mild form, this leads to anxiety and insomnia. In cases of more severe dependence, withdrawal manifests with nausea, vomiting, tremors, seizures, delirium, and ultimately, death. Therefore, discontinuation of prescription drugs necessitates close medical supervision.

Screening and Diagnosis

To evaluate a person who might misuse depressant medication, a doctor will obtain a thorough medical history, ask questions about current and previous drug and alcohol use, and perform a physical examination. A psychiatric evaluation may also be required. The diagnosis of depressant drug misuse relies on evidence of dose escalation, on obtaining multiple prescriptions, and on taking the drug for purposes other than those stated in the prescription.

Multiple tests detect the presence of drugs and also potential medical complications. These include drug screening (urine and blood), electrolyte and liver profiles, an electrocardiogram, and X-ray and magnetic resonance imaging.

Treatment and Therapy

Therapeutic strategies for depressants misuse vary according to the drug used, the severity of the manifestations, and the duration of drug action. Common therapies include detoxification, which involves the use of agents that reverse the effects of the drug (for example, using Flumazenil for benzodiazepine misuse and using Naloxone for narcotics misuse). Other common therapies include the use of medications that mitigate withdrawal symptoms, counseling in inpatient or outpatient settings, support groups, and relaxation training. When a person receiving treatment has combined a CNS depressant with alcohol or other drugs, all aspects of this addiction have to be addressed and treated.

Prevention

Sedative-hypnotic medication should be used only as prescribed. Combinations of CNS depressants (such as alcohol/drug or over-the-counter drug/prescription medication) pose high risks and should be avoided.

People who are unsure of a drug's effects, or who suspect dependence, should consult a pharmacist or a doctor. Those people who are contemplating the discontinuation of a CNS depressant or who are experiencing withdrawal symptoms should seek medical care immediately.

A careful assessment is necessary before prescribing depressant medication in persons with a history of drug misuse. These individuals require close monitoring. Also, caregivers and health care providers should verify that there are no alternative sources for obtaining the drug of misuse.

—*Katia Marazova, MD, PhD,*
Mihaela Avramut, MD, PhD

References

Cooper, Jeffrey S. "Sedative-Hypnotic Toxicity." *Medscape*, 9 Nov. 2019, emedicine.medscape.com/article/818430-overview.

Erlach, Stephen P. "Sedative, Hypnotic, Anxiolytic Use Disorders Treatment & Management." *Medscape*, 9 Nov. 2019, emedicine.medscape.com/article/290585-treatment.

Ford, Jason A. "The Prescription Drug Problem We Are Missing: Risks Associated with the Misuse of Tranquilizers and Sedatives." *Journal of Adolescent Health*, vol. 63, no. 6, 2018, pp. 665–666., doi:10.1016/j.jadohealth.2018.09.007.

Hanson, Glen R., Peter J. Venturelli, and Annette E. Fleckenstein. *Drugs and Society*. 11th ed. Sudbury, MA: Jones, 2012.

Hasan, Aliya, and Valmiki Sharma. "Substance Abuse and Conscious Sedation: Theoretical and Practical Considerations." *British Dental Journal*, vol. 227, no. 10, 2019, pp. 923–927., doi:10.1038/s41415-019-0897-z.

Heller, Jacob L. "Barbiturate Intoxication and Overdose." *MedlinePlus*. National Library of Medicine, 15 Jan. 2014.

"Sedative, Hypnotic or Anxiolytic Drug Use Disorder." *Harvard Health Publishing*, Harvard Medical School, Dec. 2018, www.health.harvard.edu/a_to_z/sedative-hypnotic-or-anxiolytic-drug-use-disorder-a-to-z.

Weaver, Michael F. "Prescription Sedative Misuse and Abuse." *The Yale Journal of Biology and Medicine*, vol. 88, no. 3, Sept. 2015, pp. 247–256.

Common Ailments

■ Conditions InDepth: Carpal tunnel syndrome

Carpal tunnel syndrome is caused by a compressed nerve in the wrist that causes symptoms in the hand. Pressure on the median nerve, which is inside a narrow passage in the wrist called the carpal tunnel, causes the nerve to malfunction. This nerve provides feeling to the thumb, index and middle fingers, and half the ring finger. It also controls several muscles in the hand, including the muscle that allows the thumb to touch the little finger. Compression occurs when the tissues in the carpal tunnel swell up.

Carpal tunnel syndrome is a repetitive strain injury. Although there are many causes for carpal tunnel syndrome, by far the most common is doing repetitive motions as part of your job. Many experts believe that the increased incidence of carpal tunnel syndrome is due to changes in workplace responsibilities in which one person commonly does a single task over and over again. There are approximately 1 million new cases every year.

References

"Carpal Tunnel Syndrome." DynaMed, EBSCO Information Services, 30 Nov. 2018, www.dynamed.com/condition/carpal-tunnel-syndrome.

Katz, R. T. "Carpal Tunnel Syndrome: a Practical Review." *American Family Physician*, vol. 49, no. 6, 1 May 1994, pp. 1385–1386.

Viera, A, J. "Management of Carpal Tunnel Syndrome." *American Family Physician*, vol. 68, no. 2, 15 July 2003, pp. 265–272.

—James P. Cornell, MD
EBSCO Medical Review Board

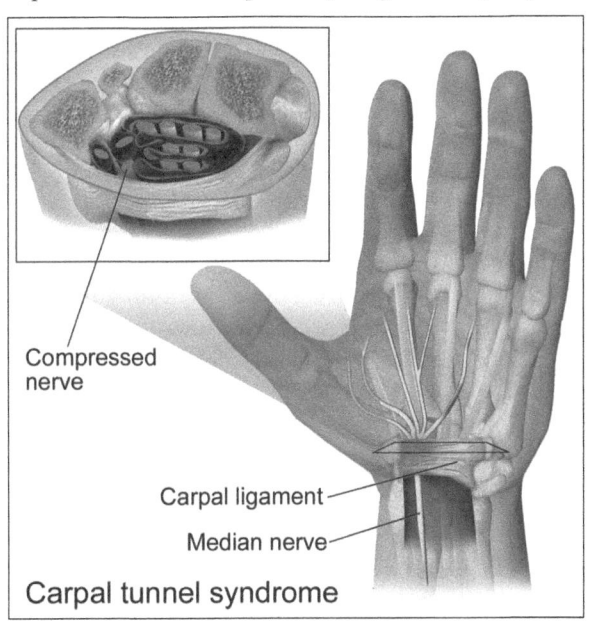

Anatomy of the carpal tunnel, showing the median nerve passing through the tight space it shares with the finger tendons. (Bruce-Blaus via Wikimedia Commons)

■ Medications for carpal tunnel syndrome

CATEGORY: Class of Drug

The information provided here is meant to give you a general idea about each of the medications listed below. Only the most general side effects are included. Ask your doctor if you need to take any special precautions. Use each of these medications as recommended by your doctor, or according to the instructions provided. If you have further questions about usage or side effects, contact your doctor.

Medications for carpal tunnel syndrome are prescribed to reduce swelling in the carpal tunnel. Two different kinds of medication may be effective. Both medications are aimed at reducing inflammation, a primary cause of swelling in this area.

Prescription Medications

Glucocorticoids

These cortisone-like drugs are given in short, sometimes tapering, bursts lasting a week or two. Glucocorticoids can produce a number of negative side effects, particularly when taken for prolonged periods. For this reason, your healthcare provider will prescribe them only for a short time. You will be monitored while taking them. These medications are often quite effective in reducing inflammation.

Common names include:
Prednisone
Prednisolone
Dexamethasone
Triamcinolone

Nonsteroidal Anti-inflammatory Drugs (NSAIDs)

There are currently twenty prescription NSAIDs on the market. Each medicine has a slightly different chemistry and side effect profile. NSAIDs can be as effective as cortisone and are safer over the long run. However, they do have side effects.

Take special care with NSAIDs if you have had an ulcer or gastritis. They can irritate these conditions. Tell your doctor if you have a stomach condition before you start taking any of these medications.

Common names include:
Indomethacin
Naproxen
Celecoxib

"Cortisone" Injection

An injection of synthetic glucocorticoids, commonly referred to as "cortisone." It is injected directly into the carpal tunnel. It may be used to treat carpal tunnel syndrome if rest, medications, and lifestyle changes are not working. This is a simple office procedure that is quite safe if done infrequently. It reduces inflammation and the swelling and pressure inside the carpal tunnel.

Injections rarely cause excessive bleeding and even more rarely cause infection. If there is excessive pain or swelling, contact your healthcare provider.

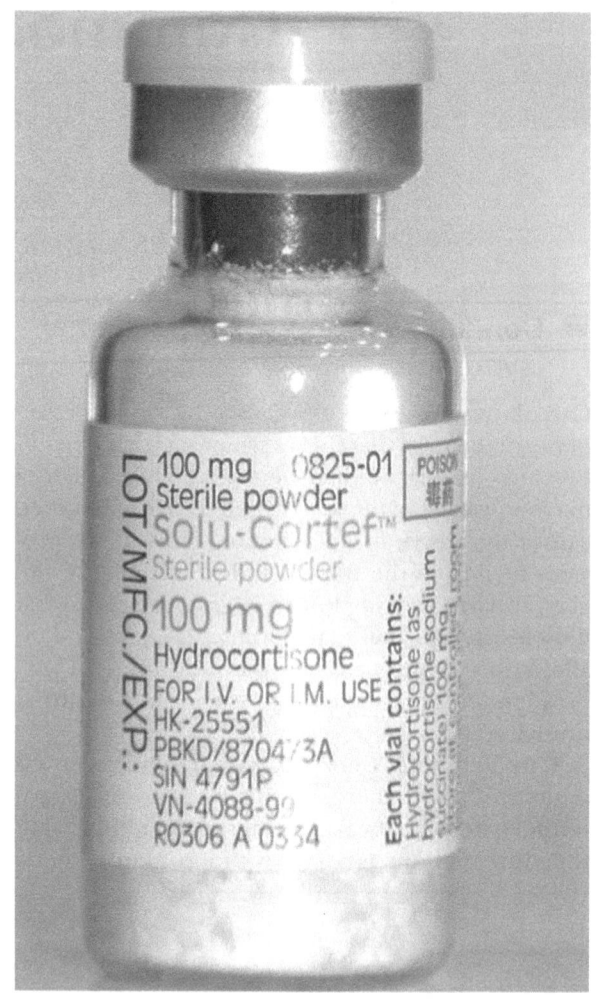

Corticosteroid injections can be effective for temporary relief from symptoms while a person develops a long-term strategy that fits their lifestyle. (LHcheM via Wikimedia Commons)

Over-the-Counter Medications

Lower doses of nonsteroidal anti-inflammatory drugs (NSAIDs) are sold over the counter and include:

- Aspirin
- Ibuprofen
- Naproxen
- Piroxicam

Take special care with NSAIDs if you have had an ulcer or gastritis, as they can irritate these conditions. Tell your doctor if you have a stomach condition before you start taking any of these medications.

Special Considerations

If you are taking medications, follow these general guidelines:

- Take your medication as directed. Do not change the amount or schedule.
- Ask what side effects could occur. Report them to your doctor.
- Talk to your doctor before you stop taking any prescription medication.
- Do not share your prescription medication.
- Medications can be dangerous when mixed. Talk to your doctor or pharmacist if you are taking more than one medication, including over-the-counter products and supplements.
- Plan ahead for refills as needed.

—*James P. Cornell, MD*
EBSCO Medical Review Board

References

"Carpal Tunnel Syndrome." DynaMed, EBSCO Information Services, 30 Nov. 2018, www.dynamed.com/condition/carpal-tunnel-syndrome.

Erickson, Mia, et al. "Hand Pain and Sensory Deficits: Carpal Tunnel Syndrome." *Journal of Orthopaedic & Sports Physical Therapy*, vol. 49, no. 5, 2019, doi:10.2519/jospt.2019.0301.

Saint-Lary, Olivier, et al. "Carpal Tunnel Syndrome: Primary Care and Occupational Factors." *Frontiers in Medicine*, vol. 2, 5 May 2015, doi:10.3389/fmed.2015.00028.

Thomson, J Grant. "Diagnosis and Treatment of Carpal Tunnel Syndrome." *The Lancet Neurology*, vol. 16, no. 4, 2017, p. 263., doi:10.1016/s1474-4422(17)30059-5.

Wipperman, Jennifer, and Kyle Goerl. "Carpal Tunnel Syndrome: Diagnosis and Management." *American Family Physician*, vol. 94, no. 12, 15 Dec. 2016, pp. 993–999.

■ Lifestyle changes to manage carpal tunnel syndrome

CATEGORY: Physiotherapy

If your carpal tunnel syndrome is caused by repetitive strain, then you'll need to make some lifestyle changes.

Check your Sleeping Position

A simple change in how your wrists are positioned during sleep may solve early symptoms. Sleep with your wrists cocked upward instead of bent downward to minimize pressure in the carpal tunnel. You can find carpel tunnel splint braces in the pharmacy. They can position your wrists correctly during sleep.

Check the Ergonomics of Your Workplace

Your workplace should be comfortable and your work activity should conform to the way your body works. To reduce the chance of discomfort or reduced performance:

- Minimize repetitive hand movements when possible.
- Alternate between activities or tasks to reduce the strain on your body.
- When using your wrists, keep them straight and let your arms and shoulders share the stress.
- Use your whole hand or both hands to pick up an item.
- Avoid holding an object the same way for a long time.

Check the Tools You Use at Work.

If you work in an office, adjust your desk, chair, and keyboard so you are in the best possible position:

- Back straight
- Feet flat on the floor or resting on a footrest
- Knees level with or slightly lower than your hips
- Shoulders in a neutral position, not forward or back
- Elbows bent at a 90 degree angle
- Forearms parallel to the floor and wrists straight

Warm Up Before and During Work

Take breaks at least once an hour to:

- Rest or shake your hands.
- Massage the palms and backs of your hands.
- Do a few stretches and loosening movements of the shoulders and arms before beginning work. Do them often during the day.
- Keep hands warm, with gloves if necessary.

- Avoid holding an object or tool the same way for a long time.
- Minimize time using vibrating tools. If this is not possible, then take frequent breaks and do the warm-up program listed below.
- Use gloves that dampen vibration

According to a report published by the American Academy of Orthopaedic Surgeons, a simple warm-up routine may reduce the incidence of carpal tunnel syndrome. This routine, combined with medication and rest, may prove to be better at treating symptoms than rest and medication.

- The warm-up routine is as follows:
- Hold your hands in front of you as if pushing on a wall. Count to 5.
- Relax your wrists and fingers.
- Make tight fists with both hands.
- Bend both fists downward. Count to 5.
- Repeat each step 10 times.
- Shake your arms loosely while hanging at your side.

Avoid Caffeine and Tobacco
Both caffeine and tobacco reduce blood flow to your hands. Nerve tissue is the most sensitive to reduced blood flow. Avoid caffeine and tobacco so that you don't decrease blood flow to these areas.

Contact your doctor when your symptoms begin to interfere with your activities.

—*James P. Cornell, MD*
EBSCO Medical Review Board

References
"Carpal Tunnel Syndrome Fact Sheet." *National Institute of Neurological Disorders and Stroke*, U.S. Department of Health and Human Services, 13 Aug. 2019, www.ninds.nih.gov/Disorders/ Patient-Caregiver-Education/Fact-Sheets/ Carpal-Tunnel-Syndrome-Fact-sheet.

"Carpal Tunnel Syndrome." *American Society for Surgery of the Hand*, 2015, handcare.assh.org/ Anatomy/Details-Page/ArticleID/27950/ Carpal-Tunnel-Syndrome.

Healthwise Staff. "Wrist Care: Preventing Carpal Tunnel Syndrome." *Penn Medicine Lancaster General Health*, 26 June 2019, www.lancastergeneralhealth.org/healthwise-library/healthwise-article?documentId=tn9041.

Rae-Grant, Alexander. "Carpal Tunnel Syndrome." DynaMed, EBSCO Information Services, 30 Nov. 2018, www.dynamed.com/condition/carpal-tunnel-syndrome.

Žídková, Věra, et al. "Effects of Exercise and Enzyme Therapy in Early Occupational Carpal Tunnel Syndrome: A Preliminary Study." *BioMed Research International*, vol. 2019, 23 Jan. 2019, pp. 1–7., doi:10.1155/2019/8720493.

■ Surgical procedures for carpal tunnel syndrome

CATEGORY: Procedure

When more conservative treatments fail, surgery is a successful option. Only 5% of patients experience symptoms after surgical treatment.

Carpal Tunnel Release
This simple procedure can be done in several ways, depending upon your particular case and the surgeon's experience and preference.

The thick ligament on the palm side of your carpal tunnel is cut, allowing the contents of the tunnel to expand and the pressure to be reduced. The procedure is ordinarily done in an outpatient setting under local anesthesia, some circumstances may recommend that a nerve block be used to interrupt pain signals. General anesthesia—where you're unconscious—is rarely necessary.

You'll be put into a hospital gown and taken to a surgical suite (operating room). After you lie down on an operating table, at least 1 IV line will be attached to a needle in your vein, and monitors may

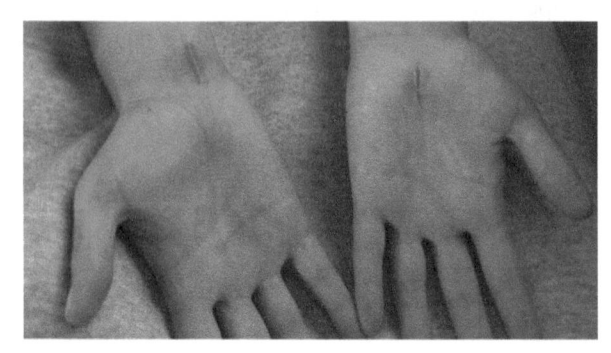

Scars from carpal tunnel release surgery. Two different techniques were used. The left scar is 6 weeks old, the right scar is 2 weeks old. (HenrykGerlach via Wikimedia Commons)

be attached to you to keep track of your heartbeat, blood pressure, and oxygen levels. If you've requested it, you may be sedated for additional comfort.

Approaches to carpal tunnel release include:

- The open approach, which cuts through the skin to expose the ligament, then cuts across the ligament with scissors
- A smaller incision that accommodates only the scissors
- An arthroscope to see the carpal tunnel in greater detail. This procedure will take slightly longer, mostly to set up the equipment. During the arthroscopy, the surgeon can put small instruments into the carpal tunnel to cut the ligament.

Each of these procedures takes only a few minutes. Afterward, your incision will be closed, and you will be taken briefly to a recovery room where the effects of the sedation or anesthesia can wear off and you can be monitored.

—*James P. Cornell, MD*
EBSCO Medical Review Board

References

"Carpal Tunnel Release." *Johns Hopkins Medicine*, 2019, www.hopkinsmedicine.org/health/treatment-tests-and-therapies/carpal-tunnel-release.

Ma, C. Benjamin, et al. "Carpal Tunnel Release." *MedlinePlus*, U.S. National Library of Medicine, 21 Apr. 2019, medlineplus.gov/ency/article/002976.htm.

Rae-Grant, Alexander. "Carpal Tunnel Syndrome." DynaMed, EBSCO Information Services, 30 Nov. 2018, www.dynamed.com/condition/carpal-tunnel-syndrome.

■ Other treatments for carpal tunnel syndrome

CATEGORY: Therapy or Technique; Physiotherapy

Rest, Ice, Elevation

Aside from surgery, medication and lifestyle changes, several other treatments can help ease the symptoms of carpal tunnel syndrome.

Along with taking anti-inflammatory medication, you will need to rest your hands and wrists for

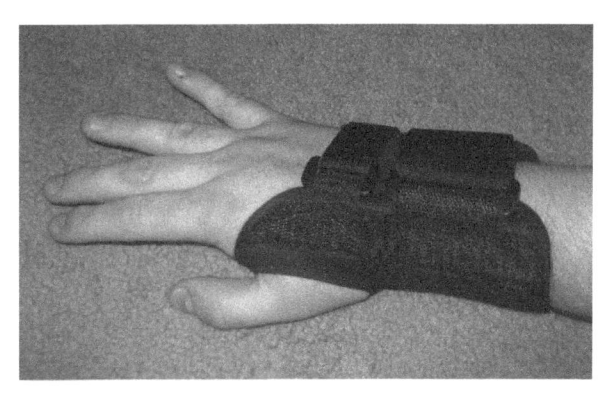

A carpal tunnel splint to keep the wrist straight. (SPUI via Wikimedia Commons)

a short time. In addition to rest and medications, ice and elevation can provide temporary relief from carpal tunnel syndrome while you are modifying your lifestyle to prevent recurrence.

Splinting

To assure that your wrist is rested, your doctor may choose to put your wrist in a splint. The splint holds the wrist in a cocked-up position. It may be worn only at night, when symptoms are usually at their worst, or throughout the day and night. Since any motion raises the pressure in the carpal tunnel and counteracts the effects of the splint, many doctors recommend the splint be worn continuously for the first week to 10 days.

Exercises

According to a report published by the American Academy of Orthopedic Surgeons, a simple warm-up routine may greatly reduce the incidence of carpal tunnel syndrome. This routine, combined with medication and rest, may prove to be better at treating symptoms than simple rest and medication.

The warm-up routine is as follows:
- Hold your hands in front of you as if pushing on a wall. Count to 5.
- Relax your wrists and fingers.
- Make tight fists with both hands.
- Bend both fists downward. Count to 5.
- Repeat each step 10 times.
- Then shake arms loosely while hanging at your side.

—*James P. Cornell, MD*
EBSCO Medical Review Board

References

Atroshi, Isam, et al. "Treatment of Carpal Tunnel Syndrome with Wrist Splinting: Study Protocol for a Randomized Placebo-Controlled Trial." *Trials*, vol. 20, no. 1, 27 Aug. 2019, doi:10.1186/s13063-019-3635-6.

Burg, Scott. "3 Steps to Fight Your Carpal Tunnel Syndrome." *Health Essentials*, Cleveland Clinic, 20 Sept. 2019, health.clevelandclinic.org/3-steps-to-fight-your-carpal-tunnel-syndrome/.

Faust, Katherine, and Charles D. Jennings. "Carpal Tunnel Syndrome." *OrthoInfo*, American Academy of Orthopaedic Surgeons, July 2016, orthoinfo.aaos.org/topic.cfm?topic=a00005.

Rae-Grant, Alexander. "Carpal Tunnel Syndrome." DynaMed, EBSCO Information Services, 30 Nov. 2018, www.dynamed.com/condition/carpal-tunnel-syndrome.

"Therapeutic Exercise Program for Carpal Tunnel Syndrome." *OrthoInfo*, Academy of Orthopaedic Surgeons, Dec. 2018, orthoinfo.aaos.org/en/recovery/carpal-tunnel-syndrome-therapeutic-exercise-program/.

■ Conditions InDepth: Foot pain

The foot is a complex structure of 26 bones, 33 joints, and many muscles, ligaments, and nerves. Only a small number of Americans are born with foot problems. Most problems develop due to neglect and poor care, including ill-fitting shoes. Some disorders begin early in life and are affected by heredity, walking patterns, and geography. However, most foot pain occurs as feet change with age or diseases develop over time. Most Americans will have foot pain at some point in their lives.

Common causes of foot pain include:

- Poor-fitting shoes
- High-heeled shoes
- Poor posture
- High impact exercise, such as running

Foot pain may also be caused by systemic diseases. Examples include:

- **Arthritis (osteoarthritis and rheumatoid arthritis)**—Arthritis can cause stiffness and reduced range of motion.
- **Peripheral arterial disease (PAD)**—This condition affects the legs and feet by causing reduced blood flow, swelling, and increased risk of infection.
- **Diabetes**—A common complication of diabetes is reduced blood flow, which causes a number of problems in the legs and feet, including abnormal sensation, swelling, and increased risk of infection.
- **Gout**—Gout is a buildup of uric acid crystals in one or several joints that causes pain and inflammation. The most common joint affected is the big toe.

—*Warren A. Bodine, DO, CAQSM*
EBSCO Medical Review Board

References

"Foot Complications." *American Diabetes Association*, 2019, www.diabetes.org/diabetes/complications/foot-complications.

"Foot Health." *American Podiatric Medical Association*, 2019, www.apma.org/Patients/FootHealthList.cfm?navItemNumber=25223.

"Healthy Feet: Preventing and Treating Common Foot Problems." *Harvard Health Publishing*, Harvard Medical School, 2019, www.health.harvard.edu/special-health-reports/Foot_Care_Basics.

Hospital for Special Surgery. "Foot Pain? New Study Says Look at Hip and Knee for Complete Diagnosis." *ScienceDaily*, 19 Sept. 2017, www.sciencedaily.com/releases/2017/09/170919181533.htm.

Ma, C. Benjamin, et al. "Foot Pain." *MedlinePlus*, U.S. National Library of Medicine, 20 Mar. 2018, medlineplus.gov/ency/article/003183.htm.

■ Medications for foot pain

CATEGORY: Class of Drug

The information provided here is meant to give you a general idea about each of the medications listed below. Only the most general side effects are included. Ask your doctor if you need to take any special care. Use each of these medications only as advised by your doctor, and according to the instructions provided. If you have further questions about usage or side effects, contact your doctor.

Prescription Medications
Glucocorticoids

You may be given glucocorticoids (cortisone-like drugs) to reduce inflammation. Sometimes these are given by mouth for a short period of time. This helps you avoid the side effects of a lengthy treatment. These medications should not be used when the body is fighting off an infection. More often, certain glucocorticoids are given by an injection into the affected area. This is done to try to avoid the whole-body side effects that occur more often when taking glucocorticoids by mouth.

There are many complications associated with this class of drugs. Even repeated doses separated by long periods of time may cause major damage. But a few sessions of glucocorticoids should not cause serious problems in most people.

Common names include:	*Possible side effects include:*
Prednisone	Puffy face
Prednisolone	Weight gain
Dexamethasone	High blood pressure
Triamcinolone	Increased risk of infection
	Bruising
	Acne
	Abnormal hair growth
	Osteoporosis
	Bone death (ischemic necrosis)
	Cataracts in the eyes
	Glaucoma
	Diabetes
	Muscle disease
	Blood chemistry abnormalities
	Menstrual disturbances
	Irritability
	Insomnia
	Psychosis

Nonsteroidal Anti-inflammatory Drugs (NSAIDs)

The standard nonsteroidal anti-inflammatory drugs (NSAIDs) can be as effective as glucocorticoids. These drugs reduce inflammation by other pathways than the glucocorticoid class of drugs. They are safer to use in the presence of infection. But they may have other harmful side effects.

Common names include:	*Possible side effects include:*
Ibuprofen	Stomach irritation, ulceration, and bleeding
Naproxen	Allergic reactions
Celecoxib	Kidney damage
Meloxicam	Possible increased risk of events such as heart attacks and strokes
Sulindac	
Diclofenac	
Piroxicam	
Ketoprofen	
Diflunisal	
Nabumetone	
Etodolac	
Oxaprozin	
Indomethacin	

Over-the-Counter Medications
Nonsteroidal Anti-inflammatory Drugs (NSAIDs)

Aspirin, which reduces inflammation, is really the first of the NSAIDs. There are minor differences among the available anti-inflammatory agents. These differences include dosing intervals, frequency of certain side effects, and other characteristics.

Common names include:	*Possible side effects include:*
Aspirin	Stomach irritation, ulceration, and bleeding
Ibuprofen	Allergic reactions
Naproxen	Kidney damage
	Possible increased risk of events such as heart attacks and strokes

Acetaminophen

Acetaminophen can help relieve mild aches and pains. Side effects such as allergic reactions can occur in some people. Symptoms can include:

- Rash
- Hives
- Itching
- Swelling of the face, throat, tongue, lips, eyes, hands, feet, ankles, or lower legs
- Hoarseness
- Difficulty breathing or swallowing

Be careful not to exceed overall dosing instructions with all medications containing acetaminophen. Liver damage can occur at high doses.

When to Contact Your Doctor

Contact your doctor if:

- The desired effect is not achieved
- An undesired effect appears
- You develop stomach problems

Special Considerations

If you are taking medications, follow these general guidelines:

- Take your medication as directed. Do not change the amount or schedule.
- Ask what side effects could occur. Report them to your doctor.
- Talk to your doctor before you stop taking any prescription medication.
- Do not share your prescription medication.
- Medications can be dangerous when mixed. Talk to your doctor or pharmacist if you are taking more than one medication, including over-the-counter products and supplements.
- Plan ahead for refills as needed.

—*Warren A. Bodine, DO, CAQSM*
EBSCO Medical Review Board

References

"Acetaminophen." *DynaMed*, EBSCO Information Services, 6 Feb. 2018, www.dynamed.com/topics/dmp~AN~T233023/Acetaminophen.

"Foot Complications." *American Diabetes Association*, 2019, www.diabetes.org/diabetes/complications/foot-complications.

"Foot Health." *American Podiatric Medical Association*, 2019, www.apma.org/Patients/FootHealthList.cfm?navItemNumber=25223.

"Healthy Feet: Preventing and Treating Common Foot Problems." *Harvard Health Publishing*, Harvard Medical School, 2019, www.health.harvard.edu/special-health-reports/Foot_Care_Basics.

Whittaker, Glen A., et al. "Corticosteroid Injection for Plantar Heel Pain: a Systematic Review and Meta-Analysis." *BMC Musculoskeletal Disorders*, vol. 20, no. 1, 17 Aug. 2019, doi:10.1186/s12891-019-2749-z.

■ Lifestyle changes to manage foot pain

CATEGORY: Physiotherapy

A number of lifestyle changes and self-care measures will help you relieve foot pain and prevent further damage to your feet. If you have trouble seeing and reaching your feet because of vision problems, paralysis, arthritis, or obesity, ask a friend, family member, or a professional to help you take care of your feet.

Wear Comfortable Shoes

In general, the best shoes are well cushioned and have a leather upper, stiff heel counter, and flexible area at the ball of the foot. The heel area should be strong and supportive, but not too stiff. The front of the shoe should be flexible. New shoes should feel comfortable right away, without a breaking in period. There should be plenty of room for all 5 toes.

Getting the Correct Fit

The best way to prevent nearly all foot problems is to choose well-fitted shoes with a firm sole and soft upper. You should purchase them in the afternoon or after a long walk, when your feet are at their largest size. There should be a ½ inch of space between your longest toe and the tip of the shoe, and the toes should be able to wiggle upward. You should stand when being measured, and both feet should be sized, with shoes bought for the larger foot. It is important to wear the same socks as you would regularly wear with the new shoes.

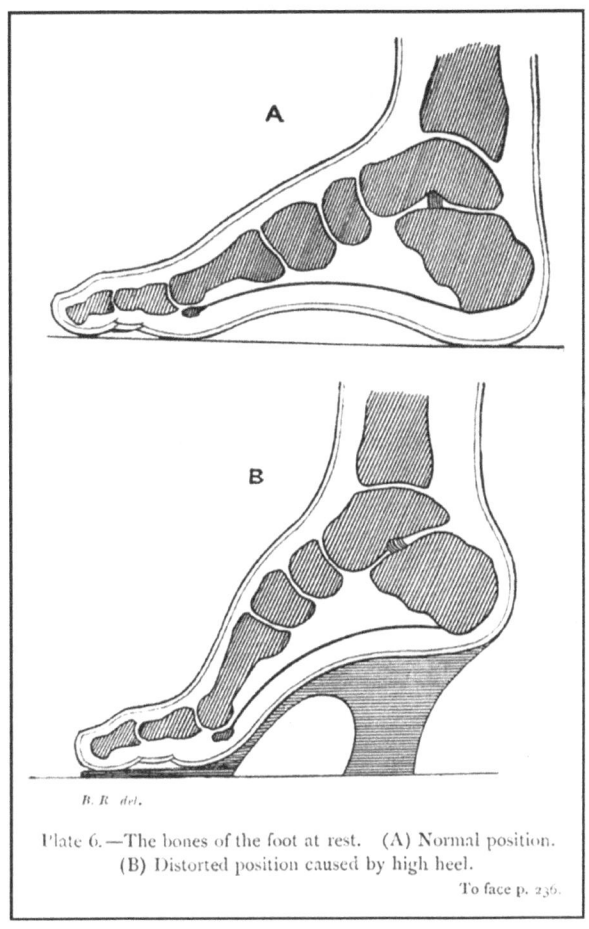

Plate 6.—The bones of the foot at rest. (A) Normal position. (B) Distorted position caused by high heel.

Wearing high heels is associated with musculoskeletal pain, specifically pain in the paraspinal muscles (muscles running up the back along the spine) and specifically with heel pain and plantar calluses. (Ada S. Ballin via Wikimedia Commons)

The Sole

Ideally, your shoes should have removable insoles (more information below). If you are an older person, thin hard soles may be the best choice. Elderly people wearing shoes with thick, inflexible soles may be unable to sense the position of their feet relative to the ground, which increases the risk of falling.

The Heel

High heels are a major cause of foot problems in women. If you insist on wearing high heels, look for shoes with a wide toe box (the part of the shoe that surrounds the toes), reinforced heels that are relatively wide, and cushioned insoles. You should also keep the amount of time you spend wearing high heels to a minimum.

Laces

The way shoes are laced can be important for preventing specific problems. Laces should always be loosened before putting shoes on. If you have narrow feet, you should buy shoes with eyelets more separated over the tongue than people with wider feet. This makes for a tighter fit for narrower feet and a looser fit for wider feet. If, after tying the shoe, less than an inch of tongue shows, then the shoes are probably too wide for you. Tightness should be adjusted both at the top of the laces and at the bottom. When high arches cause pain, eyelets should be skipped to relieve pressure.

Breaking In and Wearing Shoes

If your shoes require breaking in, place moleskin pads on areas of your skin where friction is likely to occur. Once a blister occurs, moleskin is not as effective. Change shoes during the day. As soon as the heels show noticeable wear, you should replace the shoes or heels.

Insoles

An insole is a flat cushioned insert that is placed inside the shoe. They are designed to reduce shock, provide support for your heels and arches, and absorb moisture and odor. People respond differently to specific insoles. What works for one person may not work for you. The thickness of your socks must be considered when purchasing insoles. You do not want insoles to squeeze your toes up against your shoes.

Exercise and Sports

The shoes you wear for exercise should be specifically designed for your preferred sport. For instance, a running shoe should cushion your forefoot, while tennis shoes should emphasize ankle support. Buy your shoes at a store with knowledgeable sales people.

Occupational Footwear

A number of occupations put the feet in danger. If you are in a high-risk job, you should be sure your footwear is protective. For example, nonelectric workers at risk for falling or rolling objects or punctures should wear shoes with steel toes and possibly other metal foot guards. Electric workers should wear footgear with no metal parts (or insulated steel toes) and rubber soles and heels. Chemical workers should wear shoes made of synthetics or rubber, not leather.

Insoles can be purchased in athletic and drug stores. Shoe stores that specialize in foot problems often make and sell customized insoles that are more expensive. In general, over-the-counter insoles offer enough support for most people's foot problems. Most well-known brands of athletic shoes have built-in insoles.

Care for Your Toenails

Toenails should be trimmed short and straight across. Filing should also be straight across using a single movement, lifting the file before the next stroke. The file should not saw back and forth. A cuticle stick can be used to clean under the nail.

Corns and Calluses

To prevent corns and calluses, and relieve discomfort:
- Do not wear shoes that are too tight or too loose. Wear well-padded shoes with open toes or a deep toe box. If necessary, have a cobbler stretch the shoes in the area where a corn or callus is located.
- Wear thick socks to absorb pressure, but do not wear tight socks or stockings.
- Apply petroleum jelly or lanolin hand cream to corns or calluses to soften them.
- Use doughnut-shaped pads that fit over a corn to decrease pressure and friction. They are available at most drug stores.
- Place cotton, lamb's wool, or moleskin between the toes to cushion any corns in these areas.

Walk and Exercise Correctly

In addition to wearing proper shoes and socks, you should also walk correctly to prevent foot injury and pain. Your head should be erect, your back straight, and your arms relaxed and swinging freely at your sides. You should step out on your heel, move forward with the weight on the outside of your foot, and complete the step by pushing off the big toe.

Report Injuries to Your Doctor

Do not take any foot injury lightly. If it is not healing at a reasonable speed, see your doctor or podiatrist.

—*Warren A. Bodine, DO, CAQSM*
EBSCO Medical Review Board

References

"10 Tips for Finding the Right Shoes." *Harvard Health Publishing*, Harvard Medical School, 2019, www.health.harvard.edu/staying-healthy/10-tips-for-finding-the-right-shoes.

AOFAS. "Five Tips for Healthy Feet." *American Orthopaedic Foot & Ankle Society*, 16 Apr. 2019, www.aofas.org/news/press-releases/2019/04/16/five-tips-for-healthy-feet.

Armstrong, David. "Diabetes and Foot Problems." *National Institute of Diabetes and Digestive and Kidney Diseases*, U.S. Department of Health and Human Services, 1 Jan. 2017, www.niddk.nih.gov/health-information/health-topics/Diabetes/prevent-diabetes-problems/Pages/keep-feet-healthy.aspx.

"Foot Complications." *American Diabetes Association*, 2019, www.diabetes.org/diabetes/complications/foot-complications.

■ Surgical procedures for foot pain

CATEGORY: Procedure

Surgery is always saved for conditions that haven't responded to medical treatment. This is particularly true with feet. Healing can be a problem, especially if you have diabetes. If you have diabetes and are thinking about surgery, check with the doctor who is handling your diabetes first. Consider the risks and benefits. Surgical procedures are available for the following foot problems.

Ingrown Toenails

In severe cases, treatments that are more intensive are needed. Surgery may involve cutting away the sharp portion of the ingrown nail. It may also involve removing part of the nail bed to stop the nail from growing.

Bunions

If discomfort persists after treatment, surgery may be necessary. Bunion surgery may include the following.

Bunionectomy

This procedure involves shaving down the large bone of your big toe joint. In a different method of this procedure, a very small incision is made. The bone-shaving drill is inserted through it. The doctor shaves off the bone, guided by feel or x-ray. Bunionectomy is not a cure.

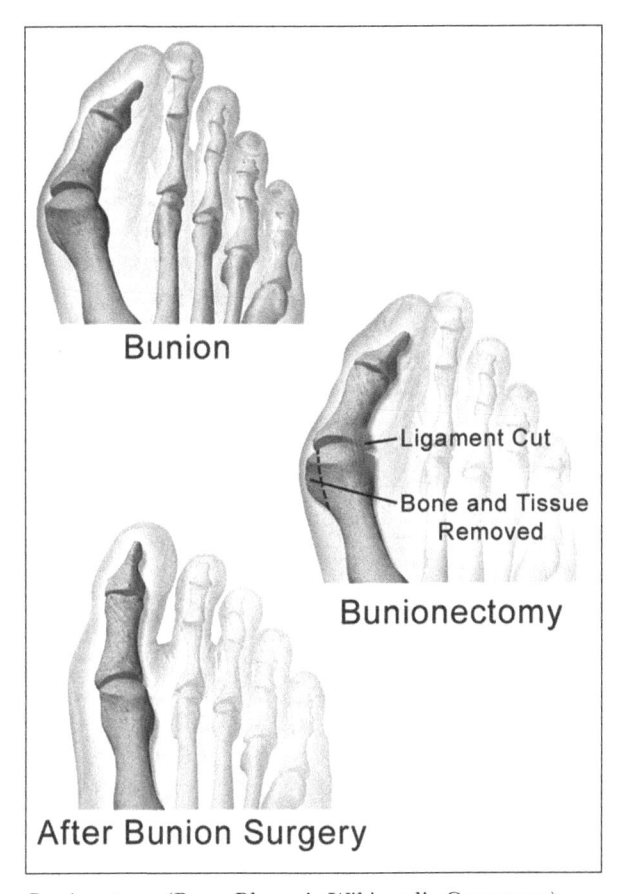

Bunionectomy. (BruceBlaus via Wikimedia Commons)

Bunion Surgery
Bunion surgery involves realigning your big toe joint and bone along with tendons and ligaments. For some people, a procedure that corrects the deformity without cutting or fusing the bone may be better. In severe cases, the metatarsal bone must be repositioned. Recovery takes 6-8 weeks. You will need to wear a cast or use crutches.

Hammertoes
Surgery may be needed in some severe cases. If your toe is still flexible, only the tendon or soft tissue may be involved. If your toe has become rigid, surgery on the bone may be needed. A procedure called PIP arthroplasty involves releasing the ligaments at the joint and removing a small piece of toe bone. This creates a new joint. It restores your toe to its normal position. Your toe is held in position with a rigid wire for about 3 weeks. Then, the wire is removed.

Neuromas
Neuroma surgery to remove the interdigital (between the toes) neuroma is usually successful. You will be able to walk immediately after the surgery. You may need a cane. Sometimes, the nerve tissue regrows and forms another neuroma.

Heel Pain
Heel surgery to relieve pain may be done for heel spurs, plantar fasciitis, and bursitis. Surgery is not advised until nonsurgical methods have failed for 6–12 months. Nonsurgical treatments for heel pain are useful in most people.

Plantar Fasciotomy for Plantar Fasciitis
This procedure releases the plantar fascia from the heel bone. The cause of the pain is the deteriorating fascia where it attaches to the heel bone. The procedure uses an incision. It takes about 2 months to resume normal activity.

Surgery for Heel Spurs
Surgery for heel spurs involves cutting and releasing the plantar fascia and removing the spurs. The heel spurs are usually caused by plantar fasciitis, and so the 2 problems are associated. This surgery is not always successful. In some cases, it is the only option. Recovery usually requires preventing the foot from moving and using crutches for about 2 weeks. Surgery should be a last resort.

Haglund's Deformity (Pump Bump)
In severe cases, surgery may be necessary to remove or reduce the bony growth. The growth is on the posterior part of the heel bone.

Tarsal Tunnel Syndrome
Surgery is sometimes performed to relieve pressure on the nerve.

Achilles Tendonitis
If your pain persists after other treatments, surgery is possible. The tendon is explored and the areas of degenerated tendon are removed.

Flat Feet
Children with flat feet often outgrow them, particularly tall, slender children with flexible joints. Many children and adults with flat feet have no symptoms at all.

In general, conservative treatment is advised for flat feet that begins in adulthood. Treatment includes pain relief and insoles or orthotics to support the foot and prevent the condition from getting worse. In very severe cases, a surgical procedure called arthrodesis is used to correct misalignment of the joints. Most adults with flat feet can be managed well with shoes and insoles.

—*Warren A. Bodine, DO, CAQSM*
EBSCO Medical Review Board

References

"Achilles Tendinopathy." *DynaMed*, EBSCO Information Services, 22 Jan. 2018, www.dynamed.com/condition/achilles-tendinopathy.

"Anterior Tarsal Tunnel Syndrome." *DynaMed*, EBSCO Information Services, 21 Dec. 2015, www.dynamed.com/condition/anterior-tarsal-tunnel-syndrome.

"Hallux Valgus and Bunion." *DynaMed*, EBSCO Information Services, 22 Nov. 2017, www.dynamed.com/condition/hallux-valgus-and-bunion.

"Hammer Toe." *DynaMed*, EBSCO Information Services, 30 Mar. 2015, www.dynamed.com/condition/hammer-toe.

"Morton Neuroma." *DynaMed*, EBSCO Information Services, 8 June 2016, www.dynamed.com/condition/morton-neuroma.

"Pes Planus (Flatfoot)." *DynaMed*, EBSCO Information Services, 26 Sept. 2017, www.dynamed.com/condition/pes-planus-flatfoot.

"Plantar Fasciitis." *DynaMed*, EBSCO Information Services, 12 July 2017, www.dynamed.com/condition/plantar-fasciitis.

■ Other treatments for foot pain

CATEGORY: Physiotherapy

Aside from medication and surgery, there are other treatments for foot pain. These treatments can help the following types of foot pain:

- Foot injuries
- Toe pain
- Forefoot pain
- Heel pain
- Arch and bottom-of-the-foot pain

Foot Injuries
RICE
RICE stands for rest, ice, compression, and elevation. These are the 4 basic elements of immediate treatment for injuries to the feet.

- **Rest**—Rest your foot as soon as possible.
- **Ice**—Ice is important to reduce swelling and promote recovery during the first 48 hours. A bag or towel that contains ice should be wrapped around the injured area. This should be done on a repetitive cycle of 20 minutes on, 40 minutes off. Do not put ice directly on the skin.
- **Compression**—An elastic bandage should be lightly wrapped around the area.
- **Elevation**—Use pillows to raise your foot above heart level.

Toe Pain
Removing Corns and Calluses
To remove a corn or callus, soak it in very warm water for 5 minutes or more to soften the hardened tissue. Then, gently sand it with a pumice stone. Several such treatments may be necessary. Do not trim corns or calluses with a razor blade or other sharp tool. If the cutting instrument is not sterile, infection can result. It is also easy to slip and cut too deeply, causing injury and bleeding.

Medicated Solutions and Pads
There are a number of over-the-counter pads, plasters, and medications to remove corns and calluses. These treatments commonly contain salicylic acid. This is a chemical that causes surface layers to peel off. It is possible for salicylic acid to cause irritation, burns, or infections that are more serious than the corn or callus.

Use caution with these medications and self-treatment. You should see your doctor for treatment if you have:

- Diabetes
- Reduced feeling in your feet due to blood flow problems or nerve damage
- Reduced flexibility or poor eyesight, which could impair your ability to use them properly

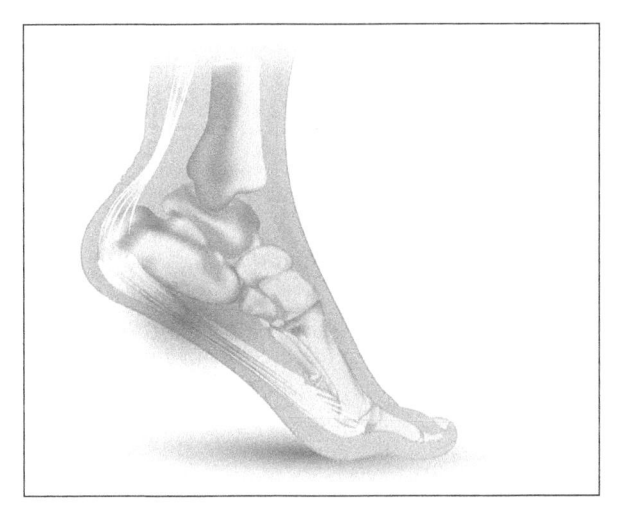

Plantar fasciitis is a disorder of the connective tissue which supports the arch of the foot. It results in pain in the heel and bottom of the foot that is usually most severe with the first steps of the day or following a period of rest. (Injury Map via Wikimedia Commons)

Ingrown Toenails

To relieve pain from ingrown toenails, try wearing sandals or open-toed shoes. Soak your toe for 5 minutes, twice a day. The water should be warm, but not hot. Seek professional treatment if you have diabetes or another condition that increases your risk of infection.

You can also apply antiseptic to a piece of cotton. Work the small wad of cotton under the nail. Get the cotton under the corner if possible, to lift the nail up. The cotton will also help force the toenail to grow out correctly. Change the cotton daily

Bunions and Bursitis

You can relieve pressure and pain from bunions, bunionettes (involving the little toe), and bursitis by wearing appropriate shoes:

- Soft, wide, low-heeled leather shoes that lace up
- Athletic shoes with soft toe boxes
- Open shoes or sandals with straps that don't touch the irritated area

A thick doughnut-shaped, moleskin pad can protect the area. In some cases, an orthotic can help take pressure off the bunion.

Hammertoes

At first, a hammertoe is flexible. You can usually relieve the pain by putting a toe pad into your shoe. Your shoes should have a deep, wide toe box. As the tendon becomes tighter and the toe stiffens, other treatments may be needed. These include exercises, splints, and custom-made shoe inserts called orthotics. Shoe inserts may help redistribute weight and ease the position of the toe.

Forefoot Pain

Neuromas

Roomier toe box shoes and metatarsal pads may be helpful.

Stress Fracture

In most cases, stress fractures heal by themselves if difficult physical activities are avoided.

Sesamoiditis

Rest and reducing stress on the ball of the foot are the first lines of treatment for sesamoiditis.

Heel Pain

It is important to have a correct diagnosis as to the exact cause of heel pain.

The American Orthopaedic Foot and Ankle Society (AOFAS) suggests shoe inserts, medications, and stretching of the Achilles tendon and calf muscles as the first line of therapy for heel pain. If these treatments fail, you may need prescription heel orthotics and extended physical therapy.

Surgery is not recommended until nonsurgical methods have failed for at least 6months and preferably up to 12 months

Plantar Fasciitis

There are many different methods to help treat plantar fasciitis. Some treatment methods include:

- Wearing proper shoes with a stiff heel and good arch support
- Stretching exercises
- Shoe inserts that slightly elevate the heel
- Night splints
- Taping the affected area
- Nonsteroidal anti-inflammatory drugs (NSAIDs) to relieve pain
- Massage
- Acupuncture
- Corticosteroid injection

Surgery is not recommended until nonsurgical methods have failed for at least 6 months and preferably up to 12 months.

Haglund's Deformity (Pump Bump)
A pump bump is an inflammation of the bursa due to bony enlargement at the back of the heel. Treatment is aimed at reducing inflammation of the bursa. Treatment methods include:

- NSAIDs
- Apply ice to reduce swelling
- Stretching exercises
- Shoe inserts such as heel lifts and heel pads
- Wearing shoes with a soft back or shoes that do not have a back
- Orthotics, such as custom arch supports
- Physical therapy
- A cast

If these treatments are not effective, then surgery may be needed. Talk to your doctor about whether it is an option for you.

Tarsal Tunnel Syndrome
Pain from tarsal tunnel syndrome may sometimes be relieved with orthotics. Orthotics are specially designed shoe inserts that help redistribute weight to try to take pressure off the nerve.

Achilles Tendinopathy
Like most athletic injuries, Achilles tendinopathy should be treated as early as possible. A tendinopathy may be a tendonitis or tendinosis. A tendonitis involves inflammation of the tendon and a tendinosis does not. Although the term tendonitis is used most often, most tendonopathies do not have inflammation and are tendinosis.

Rest is considered the first line treatment for achilles tendinopathy. Stretching and strengthening exercise are added after a period of rest.

If pain continues, surgery may be necessary.

Heel Spurs
Most heel spurs do not cause pain. They often show up when x-rays are taken. If there is pain, it is caused by the attachment of the plantar fascia to the heel bone causing the heel spur and the pain. With pain, insoles and NSAIDs may be helpful.

If the pain continues, surgery that involves cutting and releasing the plantar fascia and removing the spurs may be recommended. It is only used when other methods have failed.

Arch and Bottom-of-the-Foot Pain
Flat Foot
Treatment for flat feet (often due to posterior tibial tendon dysfunction) involves pain relief and insoles or custom-made orthotics. Insoles and orthotics support the foot and prevent flat feet from getting worse.

In severe cases, surgery may be needed to provide long-term arch support, particularly if people want to be active. Because of possible long-term problems, you should have flattened arches examined by a specialist.

Orthotics
A specialist may be needed for severe conditions, such as fallen arches or structural problems that cause imbalance. Podiatrists or physicians may need to fit and prescribe orthotics, or orthoses. These are insoles molded from a plaster cast of the patient's foot. Orthotics are usually categorized as rigid, soft, or semi-rigid.

When to Contact Your Doctor
Depending on your symptoms and your general health, experiment with shoe changes and over-the-counter products as long as you are making progress.

You should contact you doctor if you have persistent or progressive pain, or signs of an infection or arthritis.

—*Warren A. Bodine, DO, CAQSM*
EBSCO Medical Review Board

References
"Corns." *OrthoInfo*, American Academy of Orthopaedic Surgeons, Sept. 2012, orthoinfo.aaos.org/en/diseases–conditions/corns/.

"Heel Pain." *FootCareMD*, American Orthopaedic Foot & Ankle Society, 2019, www.footcaremd.org/conditions-treatments/heel/heel-pain.

"Onychomycosis." *DynaMed*, EBSCO Information Services, 15 Jan. 2018, www.dynamed.com/condition/onychomycosis.

"Orthotics." *FootCareMD*, American Orthopaedic Foot & Ankle Society, 2019, www.footcaremd.org/conditions-treatments/injections-and-other-treatments/orthotics.

"Plantar Fasciitis." *DynaMed*, EBSCO Information Services, 12 July 2017, www.dynamed.com/condition/plantar-fasciitis.

"Stress Fractures." *OrthoInfo*, American Academy of Orthopaedic Surgeons, Oct. 2007, orthoinfo.aaos.org/en/diseases--conditions/stress-fractures.

■ Conditions InDepth: Headache

Headache is pain in the head. There are many types, such as:

- Tension
- Migraine
- Cluster
- Sinus

They may be from:
- Taking medicine
- Using too much medicine to treat them
- Infections
- Bleeding
- Head injury
- Too much pressure in the head from a growth or other problem

The cause of many headaches is not known. It depends on the type of headache.

Tension Headache
This pain is from stress and muscle tightness. They may only happen once and a while because of a stressful event. They may also happen often. Some can be daily and differ in how painful they are. These headaches are when muscles in the neck, face, and scalp get tight and cause pain. The cause is not known. Stress, anxiety, depression, eyestrain, and other things may lead it.

Migraine
This headache involves blood vessels, nerves, and chemicals in the brain. Eyesight problems, called auras, may come before them. You can get these headaches many times a week or once every couple of years. They may be so strong that they get in the way of normal tasks.

A trigger sets off a process that causes headaches. The exact one is often not known. The nervous system may react to the it by making electrical activity that spreads across the brain. It may cause the brain to release chemicals that help regulate pain.

Cluster Headache
This is strong pain on one side of the head that keeps coming back. It follows a cluster or pattern. There are 2 types. Either type may change to the other.

- Episodic—(most common) one or more times each day for many months. Then they go away and come back months or years later.
- Chronic—(less common) almost each day with, at most, one headache-free month a year.

The cause is not known.

Sinus Headaches
Sinus headaches are from swelling of the sinuses. This is sinusitis. The sinuses are hollow parts of the skull. Colds and allergies cause swelling of the passages in the nose and can lead this. Allergies and viral infections cause mucus and cause tissue in the

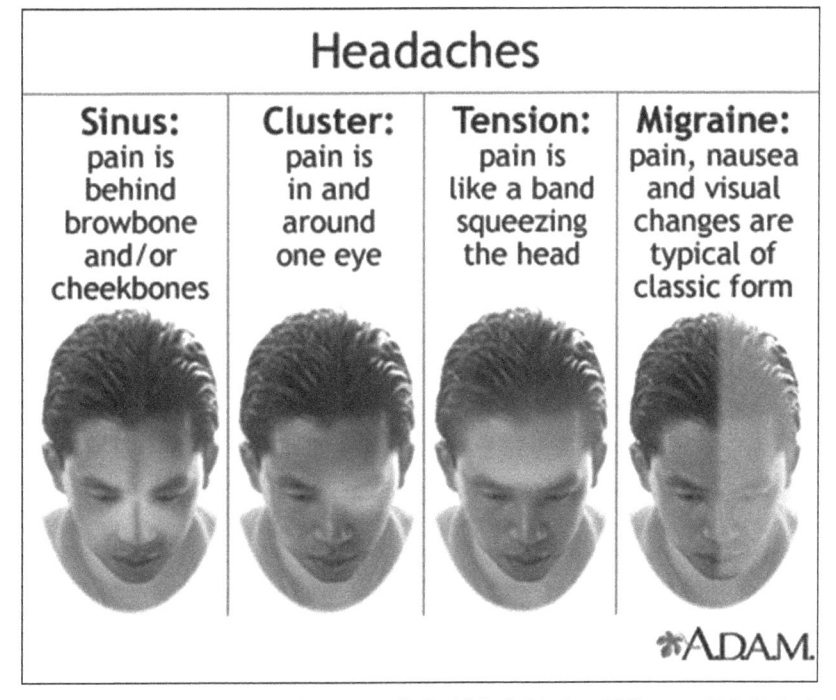

Where pain is felt in four types of headache. (A.D.A.M. via National Library of Medicine)

passages to swell. The passages become blocked and can't drain. Mucus that is trapped may get infected with bacteria or, rarely, fungus. The swollen tissues or infection may cause pain and pressure.

—*Rimas, Lukas, MD*
EBSCO Medical Review Board

References

"Cluster Headache." *DynaMed*, EBSCO Information Services, 20 Mar. 2018, www.dynamed.com/condition/cluster-headache.

"Frequently Asked Questions." *National Headache Foundation*, 2019, headaches.org/about/frequently-asked-questions/.

"Headache Information Page." *National Institute of Neurological Disorders and Stroke*, U.S. Department of Health and Human Services, 11 Oct. 2019, www.ninds.nih.gov/Disorders/All-Disorders/Headache-Information-Page.

International Headache Society. "The International Classification of Headache Disorders, 3rd Edition." *Cephalalgia*, vol. 38, no. 1, 2018, pp. 1–211., doi:10.1177/0333102417738202.

"Migraine in Adults." *DynaMed*, EBSCO Information Services, 8 Nov. 2018, www.dynamed.com/topics/dmp~AN~T114718/Migraine-in-adults.

"Tension-Type Headache." *DynaMed*, EBSCO Information Services, 20 Mar. 2018, www.dynamed.com/condition/tension-type-headache.

■ Medications for headache

CATEGORY: Class of Drug

Only the basic side effects are listed for each of the medicines below. Ask your doctor if you need to take any special steps. Use each of these medicines as advised by your doctor, or based on the instructions you were given. All medicines can cause or worsen some headaches. If you have questions about usage or side effects, call your doctor.

Prescription Medicine to Treat Migraines
Triptans (Serotonin Agonists)
Triptans are drugs that act like a chemical in the brain called serotonin. It tightens blood vessels in the brain. These drugs should be taken at the first signs of migraine or cluster headache. Some are injectable and others are taken by mouth or by nose spray. Don't use them within 24 hours of taking ergotamine tartrate or similar medicine. Do not take with monoamine oxidase (MAO) inhibitors.

Triptans shouldn't be used if you have uncontrolled high blood pressure, coronary artery disease, angina, liver disease, or neurovascular disease.

Common names are:	*Some side effects are:*
Sumatriptan	Dry mouth
Almotriptan	Headache
Naratriptan	Nausea
Rizatriptan	Tiredness
Zolmitriptan	A feeling of burning or tingling
Frovatriptan	

Ergot-based Preparations (Ergotamine Tartrate)
Ergotamine tartrate tightens blood vessels. It helps offset blood vessel widening during a migraine. Don't use within 24 hours of taking triptan drugs or serotonin agonists. Ergot preparations shouldn't be used if you have coronary artery disease, uncontrolled high blood pressure, kidney or liver disease, peripheral artery disease, or systemic infections.

Common names are:	*Some side effects are:*
Ergomar	Nausea and vomiting
Cafergot	Feelings of coldness in hands and feet
Migergot	Weakness and pain in the leg muscles

Dihydroergotamine
Dihydroergotamine tightens dilated blood vessels. It is injected to prevent or stop a migraine. Don't take this drug long-term. Tell your doctor right away if you have side effects.

Common names are:	*Some side effects are:*
DHE 45	Nausea and vomiting
Migranal	Feelings of coldness in hands and feet
	Weakness and pain in the leg muscles
	Chest pain
	Risk of heart attack and stroke

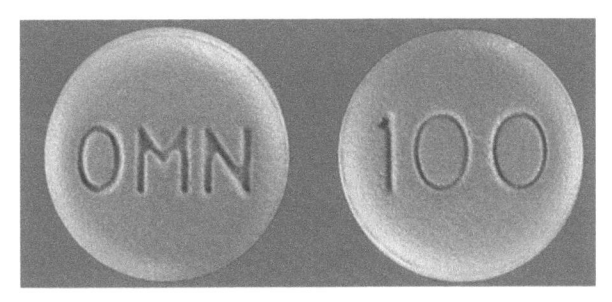

100mg of topiramate, sold as Topamax. (National Institutes of Health)

Phenothiazines
Certain phenothiazines have been FDA-approved to treat nausea and vomiting from migraines.

Common names are:	Some side effects are:
Prochlorperazine	Drowsiness
Metoclopramide	Lightheadedness
	Dry mouth
	Constipation
	Nausea

Over the Counter Medicine to Treat Migraines
Nonsteroidal Anti-inflammatory Drugs (NSAIDs)
These drugs shouldn't be used if you have peptic ulcer disease, recent bleeding from the digestive tract, kidney disease, or heart disease. These drugs work to control pain and swelling.

Common names are:	Some side effects are:
Naproxen sodium Ibuprofen	Rebound headache if the pain reliever is taken on a routine basis
Aspirin	Gastrointestinal bleeding
	Stomach upset

Analgesic Combinations
These drugs also work to control pain and swelling.

Common names are:	Some side effects are:
Excedrin Migraine—aspirin, acetaminophen, and caffeine	Rebound headache if the pain reliever is taken on a routine basis
Advil Migraine—has ibuprofen	Gastrointestinal bleeding
Motrin Migraine—has ibuprofen	Stomach upset

Acetaminophen can cause liver problems if taken with alcohol. Don't take more than the advised dose.

Medicine to Prevent Migraines
Beta-Blockers
Beta-blockers are used to treat high blood pressure, but are also used to prevent migraines. They work by swaying the response to some nerves in parts of the body. They also lower the heart's need for blood and oxygen by reducing its workload.

Common names are:	Some side effects are:
Propranolol	Lightheadedness
Metoprolol	Drowsiness
Timolol	Nausea
	Vomiting
	Upset stomach

Anti-Seizure Medicine
Valproic acid may be used to prevent migraines. Your doctor will order periodic blood tests to check drug levels and liver function. This drug shouldn't be used if you have liver disease. It shouldn't be used by women who are pregnant.

Common name:	Some side effects are:
Valproic acid	Sleepiness
	Nausea and vomiting
	Liver problems
	Blood problems
	Pancreatitis
	Hyperammonemia
	A risk of suicidal thinking and behavior

Topiramate
Topiramate may be used to treat migraines. Don't stop taking this drug without talking to your doctor first.

Common name:	Some side effects are:
Topiramate	Lightheadedness
	Problems with coordination and focus

(Continue)

Tiredness

Tingling in the fingertips and toes

Kidney stones

Glaucoma

Calcitonin Gene-Related Peptide Agonists (CGRP)
CGRP agonists are once monthly self-given injections.

Common names:	Some side effects are:
Erenumab-aooe	Tingling
Freemanezumab	Nausea
	Headaches
	Problems seeing

Other Medicine to Treat Migraines

Tricyclic Antidepressants
Antidepressants are given for their pain-relieving abilities. Don't stop taking antidepressants without first checking with your doctor. These drugs shouldn't be used if you have glaucoma, are healing from a recent heart attack, or have used MAO inhibitors within 2 weeks.

Common names:	Some side effects are:
Amitriptyline	Blurred eyesight
Nortiptyline	Dry mouth
	Lightheadedness when standing up
	Constipation
	Lack of strength

Botulinum Toxin Injections
Botulinum toxin is made from a type of bacteria. It blocks the chemical signals from the nerves to muscles. This will lower the muscle contraction. Botulinum toxin injections can be used to prevent migraines. This may also help to lessen the length and strength of migraines if they do happen.

Medicine to Treat Cluster Headaches
Many medicines may be given to treat cluster headaches. Examples are:
- Oxygen therapy
- Sumatriptan or other triptans
- Octreotide given as an injection

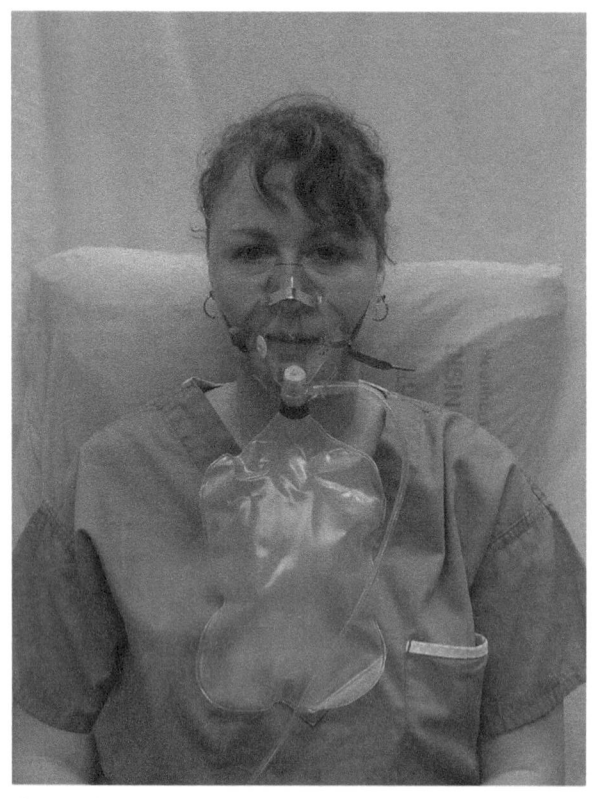

Oxygen therapy may help people with CH, but it does not help prevent future episodes. Typically it is given via a non-rebreather mask at 12–15 liters per minute for 15–20 minutes. (James Heilman, MD via Wikimedia Commons)

Medicine to Prevent Cluster Headache
Other medicines may be given to prevent or lower how often you have headaches. Examples are:

- Intranasal civamide and capsaicin cream
- Steroid injections
- Verapamil
- Lithium
- Melatonin
- Valproate or gabapentin
- Topiramate
- Baclofen
- Prednisone
- Clonidine

Medicine to Treat Sinus Headache

Antibiotics
Antibiotics may be needed to treat a sinus infection caused by bacteria. Take with food to decrease stomach upset. Take all pills as advised. Do not stop taking the antibiotics even if you feel better.

Common name:	Some side effects are:
Amoxicillin	Upset stomach
	Diarrhea
	Vaginal yeast infections

Decongestants

Decongestants may be given to treat sinusitis. They open clogged nasal passages, letting the sinuses drain. Don't use these drugs longer or more often than advised. Overuse of decongestant nose sprays may increase swelling and make your symptoms worse.

Common names are:	Some side effects are:
Pseudoephedrine hydrochloride	Higher blood pressure and pulse
Phenylephrine	Anxiety
	Rapid heartbeat

Special Considerations

If you are taking medicine:

- Take your medicine as advised. Don't change the amount or schedule.
- Ask what side effects could happen. Tell your doctor if you have any.
- Talk to your doctor before you stop taking any prescription medicine.
- Do not share your prescription medicine.
- Medicine can be harmful when mixed. Talk to your doctor or pharmacist if you are taking more than one, including over the counter products and supplements.
- Plan for refills.

—*Rimas Lukas, MD*
EBSCO Medical Review Board

References

Brandes, Jan Lewis, et al. "Sumatriptan-Naproxen for Acute Treatment of Migraine." *Jama*, vol. 297, no. 13, 2007, pp. 1443–1456., doi:10.1001/jama.297.13.1443.

Center for Drug Evaluation and Research. "Valproate Anti-Seizure Products Contraindicated for Migraine Preven…" *U.S. Food and Drug Administration*, 26 Feb. 2016, www.fda.gov/drugs/drug-safety-and-availability/fda-drug-safety-communication-valproate-anti-seizure-products-contraindicated-migraine-prevention.

Chankrachang, Siwaporn, et al. "Prophylactic Botulinum Type A Toxin Complex (Dysport®) for Migraine Without Aura." *Headache: The Journal of Head and Face Pain*, vol. 51, no. 1, 16 Nov. 2010, pp. 52–63., doi:10.1111/j.1526-4610.2010.01807.x.

"Cluster Headache." *DynaMed*, EBSCO Information Services, 20 Mar. 2018, www.dynamed.com/condition/cluster-headache.

"Dihydroergotamine." *DynaMed*, EBSCO Information Services, www.dynamed.com/drug-monograph/dihydroergotamine.

Francis, G. J., et al. "Acute and Preventive Pharmacologic Treatment of Cluster Headache." *Neurology*, vol. 75, no. 5, 2 Aug. 2010, pp. 463–473., doi:10.1212/wnl.0b013e3181eb58c8.

"Headache Information Page." *National Institute of Neurological Disorders and Stroke*, U.S. Department of Health and Human Services, 11 Oct. 2019, www.ninds.nih.gov/Disorders/All-Disorders/Headache-Information-Page.

Mannix, L. K, et al. "Rizatriptan for the Acute Treatment of ICHD-II Proposed Menstrual Migraine: Two Prospective, Randomized, Placebo-Controlled, Double-Blind Studies." *Cephalalgia*, vol. 27, no. 5, 2007, pp. 414–421., doi:10.1111/j.1468-2982.2007.01313.x.

"Migraine in Adults." *DynaMed*, EBSCO Information Services, 8 Nov. 2018, www.dynamed.com/topics/dmp~AN~T114718/Migraine-in-adults.

Serretti, Alessandro, and Laura Mandelli. "Antidepressants and Body Weight." *The Journal of Clinical Psychiatry*, vol. 71, no. 10, Oct. 2010, pp. 1259–1272., doi:10.4088/jcp.09r05346blu.

"Sumatriptan." *DynaMed*, EBSCO Information Services, 6 Nov. 2018, www.dynamed.com/drug-monograph/sumatriptan.

"Tension-Type Headache." *DynaMed*, EBSCO Information Services, 20 Mar. 2018, www.dynamed.com/condition/tension-type-headache.

Vikelis, Michail, et al. "A New Era in Headache Treatment." *Neurological Sciences*, vol. 39, no. S1, 2018, pp. 47–58., doi:10.1007/s10072-018-3337-y.

Lifestyle changes to manage headache

CATEGORY: Physiotherapy

Lifestyle changes can help ease headaches. Some changes can limit the number or strength of each type of headache.

- Tension headache
- Migraine headache
- Cluster headache
- Sinus headache

Managing Tension Headaches

Workout Often

Physical activity can help control stress. Aim for 30 minutes at time on most days of the week. Start out slowly and add to your routine over time. Talk to your doctor before you start any workout program.

Fix Your Posture

Poor posture leads to tension headaches. Don't slouch. Hold the phone or use a headset. Don't cradle it on your shoulder. Think about seeing a physical or occupational therapist for posture tips that may help you.

Ease Stress

Stress can lead to a headache. A therapist can work with you to find ways to manage stress and relax. You can also get help finding out which events start your headaches and how to resolve them.

Get Enough of Sleep

Normal sleep routines will help you fall asleep. Sleep helps ease tension and irritability.

Take Breaks From Tasks

Taking breaks helps stop your muscles from tightening up and can ease stress

Limit Stimuli During a Headache

Put an ice pack or heat pack on your head or neck to ease pain.
- Lie in a dark, quiet room.
- Massage your temples and neck.
- Use relaxation methods.

Managing Migraines

Keep a Headache Diary

Write down what starts your migraines and what eases them. This will help you and your doctor craft a plan to treat them.

Don't Overuse Pain Medicine

Overuse of pain medicine can make your headaches worse.

Ease Stress

Stress can lead to a headache. A therapist can work with you to find ways to manage stress and relax.

Workout Often

Working out helps control stress and ease depression. Swimming and walking can lower the number and strength of migraine headaches. However, working out can start a migraine attack in some people. Talk to your doctor about the activities you can do.

Don't Eat Foods That Start Your Migraines

Some foods bring on migraines. Don't eat foods that cause your headaches. These may be:

- Chocolate
- Any foods with monosodium glutamate (MSG), tyramine, or nitrates
- Alcohol, mainly red wine
- Aspartame

Eat Small Meals More Often

If low blood sugar happens before your migraines, eating small amounts of food more often may help keep your blood sugar from dropping.

Don't Change Your Sleep Pattern on the Weekend or During Vacation

Sleeping and waking at the same times may help prevent headaches.

Limit Stimuli During an Attack

Use cold packs on painful places on your head.
- Lie in a dark, quiet room.
- Apply gentle pressure to your temples.

Managing Cluster Headaches

Find a doctor who is a headache expert. Work with your doctor to craft a plan to treat and prevent your headaches.

Don't Drink Alcohol

Even a small amount of alcohol can start a headache during a cluster period.

Ease Stress

Stress can lead to a headache. A therapist can work with you to find ways to manage stress and relax.

Don't Smoke
Tobacco use has been linked to cluster headaches. If you smoke, talk to your doctor about the best ways you can quit

Don't Overuse Pain Medicine
Overuse of pain medicine can make your headaches worse.

Managing Sinus Headaches
Keep Nasal Passages Moist
This can be done by:

- Drinking plenty of fluids to keep hydrated
- Breathing in warm, moist air
- Using a mist of salt water nasal spray up to 6 times a day
- Nasal irrigation—ask your doctor how to do this at home

Avoid Exposure to Things that Trigger Allergy or Sinus Symptoms
Allergic reactions raise the amount of mucus in and swelling of the nasal passages. This can lead to sinusitis.

Get Help for Allergies or a Lasting Cold
Getting help for allergies and colds helps prevent sinusitis. If you are prone to sinus problems, ask your doctor about using a decongestant before air travel. This will help keep nasal passages open.

Wash Your Hands Often to Avoid Colds
Hand washing helps prevent colds and other infections passed from the hand to the nose, mouth, or eyes. Colds raise the amount of mucus in and swelling of the nasal passages, which can lead to sinusitis.

Don't Drink Alcohol
Alcohol can cause swelling of nasal and sinus tissues.

Don't Smoke
Don't smoke. Also, avoid second-hand smoke and polluted air. If you smoke, talk to your doctor about the best ways you can quit.

Don't Overuse Pain Medicine
Overuse of pain medicine can make your headaches worse.

When to Contact Your Doctor
Call your doctor if your headaches don't get better with lifestyle changes and prescribed medicine.

—Rimas, Lukas, MD
EBSCO Medical Review Board

References
"Cluster Headache." *DynaMed*, EBSCO Information Services, 20 Mar. 2018, www.dynamed.com/condition/cluster-headache.

"Dihydroergotamine." *DynaMed*, EBSCO Information Services, www.dynamed.com/drug-monograph/dihydroergotamine.

"Headache Information Page." *National Institute of Neurological Disorders and Stroke*, U.S. Department of Health and Human Services, 11 Oct. 2019, www.ninds.nih.gov/Disorders/All-Disorders/Headache-Information-Page.

"Migraine in Adults." *DynaMed*, EBSCO Information Services, 8 Nov. 2018, www.dynamed.com/topics/dmp~AN~T114718/Migraine-in-adults.

"Sumatriptan." *DynaMed*, EBSCO Information Services, 6 Nov. 2018, www.dynamed.com/drug-monograph/sumatriptan.

"Tension-Type Headache." *DynaMed*, EBSCO Information Services, 20 Mar. 2018, www.dynamed.com/condition/tension-type-headache.

■ Surgical procedures for headache

CATEGORY: Procedure

Surgery may needed in people with sinus headache, such as when you have problems in the nose passages or growths that block them from draining. It is rare for other headaches.

If other steps don't help your cluster headaches, some doctors may suggest cutting or harming some nerves in the face. But, the nerve may grow back.

Surgeries for Sinus Headache
Septoplasty
Septoplasty fixes a deviated septum. This is the wall that sets apart the left and right sides of the nose. The septum will be taken out or put it in the proper place.

Functional Endoscopic Sinus Surgery (FESS)
FESS opens the passages of the nose to make them drain better and let the sinuses go back to normal.

A thin tube is put in the nose to look at the openings into the sinuses and to remove anything blocking them. This may be done with the help of a CT scan.

Surgery for Cluster Headache
There are many surgeries that could be done if you don't get better with other methods. Nerves may be stimulated or harmed to do this.

Surgery for Migraine Headache
In some people, migraines start when a nerve in the head is stimulated. This surgery finds the nerve and turns it off. This may make the headaches go away or make you have fewer headaches if you don't get better with other methods.

—*Rimas Lukas, MD*
EBSCO Medical Review Board

References
"Cluster Headache." *DynaMed*, EBSCO Information Services, 20 Mar. 2018, www.dynamed.com/condition/cluster-headache.

"Deviated Septum." *ENT Health*, American Academy of Otolaryngology, Aug. 2018, www.enthealth.org/conditions/deviated-septum/.

Guyuron, Bahman, et al. "A Placebo-Controlled Surgical Trial of the Treatment of Migraine Headaches." *Plastic and Reconstructive Surgery*, vol. 124, no. 2, 2009, pp. 461–468., doi:10.1097/prs.0b013e3181adcf6a.

"Headache Information Page." *National Institute of Neurological Disorders and Stroke*, U.S. Department of Health and Human Services, 11 Oct. 2019, www.ninds.nih.gov/Disorders/All-Disorders/Headache-Information-Page.

International Headache Society. "The International Classification of Headache Disorders, 3rd Edition." *Cephalalgia*, vol. 38, no. 1, 2018, pp. 1–211., doi:10.1177/0333102417738202.

"Migraine in Adults." *DynaMed*, EBSCO Information Services, 8 Nov. 2018, www.dynamed.com/topics/dmp~AN~T114718/Migraine-in-adults.

"Tension-Type Headache." *DynaMed*, EBSCO Information Services, 20 Mar. 2018, www.dynamed.com/condition/tension-type-headache.

■ Other treatments for headache

CATEGORY: Physiotherapy; Psychotherapy

There are ways to treat each type of headache. Talk with your doctor before you try one.

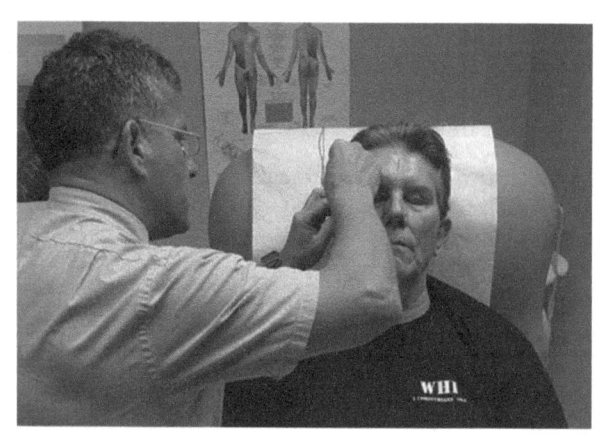

U.S. Navy Veteran Peter Johnson receives acupuncture to help relieve chronic headaches caused by massive head and eye injuries he received while serving in Vietnam. As a result of the acupuncture treatment offered at the Greenville Health Care Center, Johnson no longer has to rely on opioids to manage his pain. (Durham, Virginia Department of Veterans Affairs)

Other treatments are:

Biofeedback
Biofeedback teaches you how to control things the body does on its own. It may help you get fewer headaches and make them less painful. A therapist will guide you to relax certain muscles or control breathing. At the same time, an electronic device shows your body's response.

Relaxation
Relaxing the muscles can help you have fewer headaches from tension.

Relaxation methods are deep breathing, imagining being in a safe place, or clearing the mind of thoughts. A therapist can teach you how to do these methods.

Acupuncture
A trained specialist places small needles into the skin in specific places to ease pain.

Massage
Massage has been used to ease headaches.

Transcutaneous Electrical Nerve Stimulation (TENS)
TENS stimulates the nerves to put off migraines.

Oxygen
Breathing 100% oxygen for 10 to 15 minutes often helps ease cluster headache pain. It appears to lower blood flow to the part of the brain that is having problems.

Counseling

Counseling can help you learn new coping skills, ease stress, and change your thought pattern. This often means fewer tension headaches.

When to Call Your Doctor

Call your doctor if:
- Your headaches hurt more or happen more often
- You have a new type of headache
- You have new symptoms
- You have side effects

—*Rimas Lukas, MD*
EBSCO Medical Review Board

References

International Headache Society. "The International Classification of Headache Disorders, 3rd Edition." *Cephalalgia*, vol. 38, no. 1, 2018, pp. 1–211., doi:10.1177/0333102417738202.

"Frequently Asked Questions." *National Headache Foundation*, 2019, headaches.org/about/frequently-asked-questions/.

"Biofeedback." *National Headache Foundation*, 26 Oct. 2007, www.headaches.org/2007/10/25/biofeedback.

"Cluster Headache." *DynaMed*, EBSCO Information Services, 20 Mar. 2018, www.dynamed.com/condition/cluster-headache.

wwwwww*Neurological Disorders and Stroke*, U.S. Department of Health and Human Services, 11 Oct. 2019, www.ninds.nih.gov/Disorders/All-Disorders/Headache-Information-Page.

Jena, S, et al. "Acupuncture in Patients With Headache." *Cephalalgia*, vol. 28, no. 9, 2008, pp. 969–979., doi:10.1111/j.1468-2982.2008.01640.x.

"Migraine in Adults." *DynaMed*, EBSCO Information Services, 8 Nov. 2018, www.dynamed.com/topics/dmp~AN~T114718/Migraine-in-adults.

"Tension-Type Headache." *DynaMed*, EBSCO Information Services, 20 Mar. 2018, www.dynamed.com/condition/tension-type-headache.

■ Conditions InDepth: Low back pain and sciatica

Low back pain is an ache or discomfort in the lower part of the spinal column. It may radiate down into one or both legs. The lower spinal column consists of small, stacked bones (the vertebrae) that surround and protect the spinal cord and nerves. There are many possible causes for low back pain, including:

- Sprain or strain of muscles or ligaments in the area
- Herniated disc or ruptured disc—the cushions between the bones of the spine bulge out of place as a result of age-related changes or trauma.
- Disc degeneration—caused by arthritis or aging
- Scoliosis
- Lumbar spinal stenosis—bony narrowing of the spinal canal in the low back area
- Spondylolysis—fracture of part of the a bone in the back
- Spondylolisthesis—slippage of one bone over another, causing stretching or pinching of nerves
- Fractures due to trauma or osteoporosis
- Fibromyalgia—a condition that causes muscle aches and fatigue
- Ankylosing spondylitis—a disorder that causes spine stiffness and arthritis (believed to be hereditary)

In rare cases:
- Benign or malignant tumors
- Infections
- Arterial problems, such as hardening of the arteries

Sciatica is irritation of the sciatic nerve. It leads to pain that starts in the lower back and spreads to the buttocks and down the back of each thigh. The sciatic nerve is composed of several nerve roots that start from the lower part of the spinal cord. These nerves form a network that lead to individual nerves. These nerve bundles travel deep in the pelvis to the lower buttocks. From there, the nerve passes along the back of each upper leg and divides at the knee into branches that go to the feet.

Anything that causes irritation or puts pressure on the sciatic nerve can cause sciatica, including:

- Herniated disc (ruptured or slipped disc)
- Disc degeneration
- Spinal stenosis
- Spondylolisthesis
- Piriformis syndrome

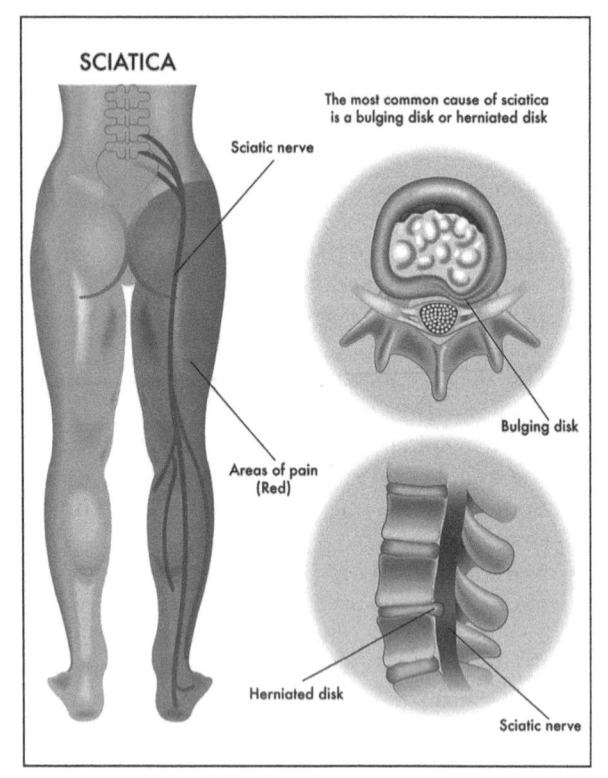

Bulging and herniated disks put pressure on the sciatic nerve, causing pain that can potentially reach the feet and toes. (Havard Health Publishing)

- In rare cases:
- Benign or malignant tumors
- Infections

Low back pain is very common. Over the course of a lifetime, almost 80% of Americans will suffer from at least one episode of back pain. Most back pain gets better with time. A small number of people will continue to have pain for longer than 3 months. About 5%-10% of people with low back pain will have sciatica

References

"Acute Low Back Pain." *DynaMed*, EBSCO Information Services, 25 Oct. 2017, www.dynamed.com/condition/acute-low-back-pain.

"Chronic Low Back Pain." *DynaMed*, EBSCO Information Services, 30 June 2017, www.dynamed.com/condition/chronic-low-back-pain.

Driscoll, T, et al. "The Global Burden of Occupationally Related Low Back Pain: Estimates from the Global Burden of Disease 2010 Study." *Annals of the Rheumatic Diseases*, vol. 73, no. 6, 24 Mar. 2014, pp. 975–981., doi:10.1136/annrheumdis-2013-204631.

"Low Back Pain." *OrthoInfo*, American Academy of Orthopaedic Surgeons, Dec. 2013, orthoinfo.aaos.org/en/diseases–conditions/low-back-pain.

"Sciatica." *Cleveland Clinic*, 11 Dec. 2017, my.clevelandclinic.org/health/diseases/12792-sciatica.

"Sciatica." *DynaMed*, EBSCO Information Services, 8 May 2017, www.dynamed.com/condition/sciatica.

—*Michael Woods, MD, FAAP*
EBSCO Medical Review Board

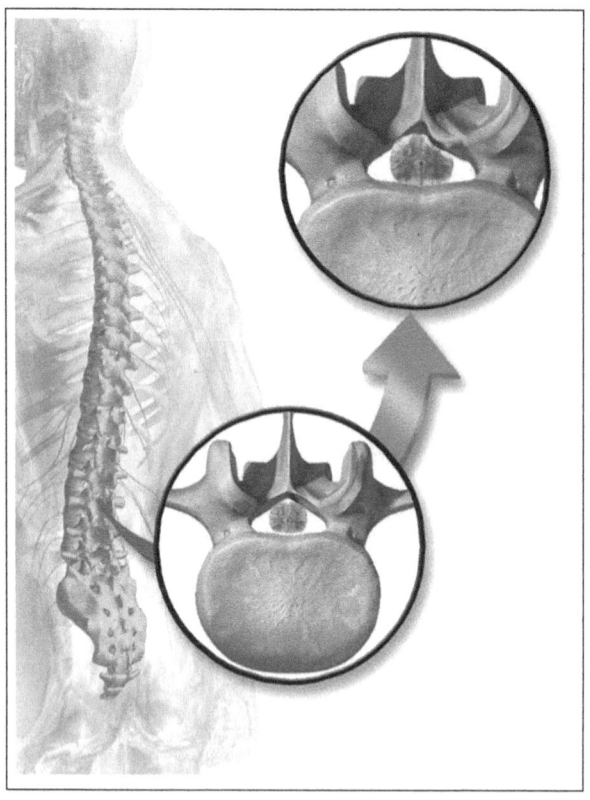

Drawing showing spinal stenosis with spinal cord compression. (BruceBlaus via Wikimedia Commons)

■ Medications for low back pain and sciatica

CATEGORY: Class of Drug

The information provided here is meant to give you a general idea about each of the medications listed below. Only the most general side effects are included. Ask your doctor if you need to take any special precautions. Use each of these medications as recommended by your doctor, or according to the instructions provided. If you have further questions about usage or side effects, contact your doctor.

Medications are used to control symptoms of low back pain and sciatica. The choice of medication depends on the nature and duration of the pain. The medications are listed by their generic name.

Prescription Medications

Nonsteroidal Anti-Inflammatory Drugs (NSAIDS)

These drugs work to control inflammation, which produces pain. They are used for acute and chronic low back pain, and sciatica.

Some prescription NSAIDs are higher doses of the same NSAIDs that are available without a prescription. Some NSAIDs come in topical forms.

Some prescription NSAIDs (such as celecoxib and meloxicam) have been associated with an increased risk of heart attack and stroke. Other studies show that some NSAIDs may cause complications in patients recovering from stroke, heart attacks, or open heart surgery. NSAIDs can also interfere with the actions of other drugs. Be certain your physician is aware of all drugs you take, including herbs and supplements even if you only take these occasionally.

Common names include:	Possible side effects include:
Naproxen	Gastrointestinal bleeding
Ibuprofen	Stomach upset
Diclofenac	Fluid retention
Celecoxib	Liver damage
Meloxicam	

Opioids

Prescription opioids may be prescribed short-term for severe acute low back pain and sciatica. Slow-release forms may be used in chronic low back pain.

Common names include:	Possible side effects include:
Codeine	Drowsiness
Oxycodone	Constipation
	Decreased breathing
	Longer use of opioids has a high risk of abuse or addiction

Antidepressants

Antidepressants may reduce pain in people with chronic low back pain.

Common names include:	Possible side effects include:
Fluoxetine	Risk of severe mood and behavior changes
Duloxetine	Stomach irritation
Amitriptyline	Nausea
	Diarrhea
	Lightheadedness
	Dry mouth
	Constipation
	Difficulty urinating

Muscle Relaxants

Muscle relaxants help calm muscle spasms. They may be ordered for short-term pain relief if spasm is present.

Common names include:	Possible side effects include:
Cyclobenzaprine	Drowsiness
Diazepam	Lightheadedness
	Addiction
	Allergic side-effects

Over-the-Counter Medications

Nonsteroidal Anti-Inflammatory Drugs (NSAIDS)

These drugs work to control inflammation, which produces pain. They are used for acute and chronic low back pain, and sciatica.

Common names include:	Possible side effects include:
Naproxen	Gastrointestinal bleeding
Ibuprofen	Stomach upset
	Liver damage
	Fluid retention
	Interaction with other drugs, including angiotensin-converting enzyme (ACE) inhibitors, blood thinners, and drugs to treat high blood pressure.

Acetaminophen

Acetaminophen relieves pain through different mechanisms than NSAIDs. It is used for acute and chronic low back pain, and sciatica.

- It can cause or exacerbate liver problems if recommended doses are exceeded.
- Do not drink alcohol while taking this drug.
- Do not take more than the recommended dose.
- Acetaminophen is unlikely to cause side effects associated with other pain medications such as gastrointestinal upset, fluid retention, and constipation.

When to Contact Your Doctor

Contact your doctor if you experience these symptoms:

- Pain that does not improve, or worsens, with rest
- Pain that is severe or that has gotten dramatically worse
- Progressive weakness in a leg or foot
- Difficulty walking, standing, or moving
- Numbness in the genital or rectal area
- Loss of bowel or bladder control
- Burning or difficulty with urination
- Fever, unexplained weight loss, or other signs of illness

Special Considerations

If you are taking medications, follow these general guidelines:

- Take the medication as directed. Do not change the amount or the schedule.
- Ask what side effects could occur. Report them to your doctor.
- Talk to your doctor before you stop taking any prescription medication.
- Do not share your prescription medication.
- Medications can be dangerous when mixed. Talk to your doctor or pharmacist if you are taking more than one medication, including over-the-counter products and supplements.
- Plan ahead for refills as needed.

—*Michael Woods, MD, FAAP*
EBSCO Medical Review Board

References

"Acute Low Back Pain." *DynaMed*, EBSCO Information Services, 25 Oct. 2017, www.dynamed.com/condition/acute-low-back-pain.

"Antidepressant Medication Overview." *DynaMed*, EBSCO Information Services, 18 Feb. 2011, www.dynamed.com/drug-review/antidepressant-medication-overview.

"Chronic Low Back Pain." *DynaMed*, EBSCO Information Services, 30 June 2017, www.dynamed.com/condition/chronic-low-back-pain.

"Low Back Pain." *OrthoInfo*, American Academy of Orthopaedic Surgeons, Dec. 2013, orthoinfo.aaos.org/en/diseases–conditions/low-back-pain.

National Guideline Centre. "Low Back Pain and Sciatica in over 16s: Assessment and Management: Guidance." *National Institute for Health and Care Excellence*, Nov. 2016, www.nice.org.uk/guidance/ng59.

"Sciatica." *Cleveland Clinic*, 11 Dec. 2017, my.clevelandclinic.org/health/diseases/12792-sciatica.

"Sciatica." *DynaMed*, EBSCO Information Services, 8 May 2017, www.dynamed.com/condition/sciatica.

Urquhart, Donna M, et al. "Antidepressants for Non-Specific Low Back Pain." *Cochrane Database of Systematic Reviews*, 2008, doi:10.1002/14651858.cd001703.pub3.

Serretti, Alessandro, and Laura Mandelli. "Antidepressants and Body Weight." *The Journal of Clinical Psychiatry*, vol. 71, no. 10, Oct. 2010, pp. 1259–1272., doi:10.4088/jcp.09r05346blu.

■ Lifestyle changes to manage low back pain and sciatica

CATEGORY: Physiotherapy, Psychotherapy

Modifying activities and learning techniques to decrease stress on the back are important to resolving or controlling low back pain and sciatica. Since back pain tends to recur, lifestyle changes should become a way of life if you hope to avoid future episodes.

Alter Your Activities

Prolonged bed rest is usually not advised. Bed rest can weaken muscles and slow recovery. In most cases, your doctor will recommend that you continue normal activities as much as is tolerated. Stay active within the limits of your pain and avoid activities that worsen the pain.

Guidelines for activity include:
- Avoid excessive, prolonged, or forceful bending or twisting of your back.
- Do not lift heavy objects.
- Learn the proper way to lift even light objects, using your knees rather than your back for leverage. If necessary, have a physical therapist or ergonomic specialist teach you proper body mechanics for daily activities.
- When lifting, squat down next to the object, hold the object close to your chest, maintain a straight back, and use your leg muscles to slowly rise.
- Plan ahead and ask for assistance with lifting or moving heavy objects.
- Avoid sitting for long periods. When you do sit, choose seats with good lumbar support. You may be able to use a standing desk at intervals to help avoid prolonged sitting.
- Avoid standing for long periods as well. If you need to stand, place a low footstool in front of you and alternate placing each foot on it for a period of time. This will take some of the load off your back.
- Consider job retraining if your work requires a lot of heavy lifting or sitting.
- Ask whether your company has someone who specializes in helping redesign the workplace for the restrictions an individual with back pain requires.

Practice Good Posture

Poor posture and slouching can put more pressure on your lower back. Stand and sit straight, and avoid sitting up in bed

Follow a Home Exercise Program

Exercises to stretch and strengthen the back and stomach muscles should be done regularly. You may also want to include balance exercises that work the trunk muscles.

A low-impact aerobic program will further improve your physical fitness and help you maintain a healthy weight. Choose exercises that you enjoy and that you can do on a routine basis. Activities that are back-friendly include walking, swimming, or biking. Exercise also can help you manage stress. Check with your doctor before starting any exercise program. The 2008 USDA Physical Activity Guidelines Advisory Committee Report recommends at minimum 2 hours and 30 minutes a week of moderate aerobic activity, and strengthening exercises at least 2 days a week.

Lose Weight If Needed

Maintenance of good weight is important for your overall health. While scientific evidence is inconclusive as to how much obesity contributes to back pain in general, extra pounds can increase pressure on the spinal muscles and discs. Follow the dietary and exercise plan recommended by your doctor. To lose weight, you have to consume fewer calories than you expend. To maintain a healthy weight, eat an equal number of calories to those you expend. Even more exercise than minimum recommendations may be required to lose weight.

If You Smoke, Quit

Smoking may contribute to degeneration of the discs in the spine. Also, smokers risk possible re-injury to the back during a coughing attack. Smoking can adversely affect healing if you are having back surgery. To heal properly, you should quit smoking at least 2 weeks before a spinal fusion procedure and stay tobacco-free for 6 months afterwards.

Manage Stress

Stress can increase muscle tension. Take time out to relax, exercise, and practice relaxation techniques. If you need support or assistance in reducing stress, you may want to try some of the following techniques:
- Cognitive-behavioral therapy
- Counseling
- Stress management classes
- Relaxation techniques
- Breathing exercises
- Meditation
- Yoga

Modify Your Environment

Certain changes to your workspace, attire, and home can reduce the stress on your back:
- Avoid wearing high-heeled shoes.
- If you sit for long periods of time, use a stool to bring your knees above your hips.
- Avoid having objects, such as a wallet, in your back pocket while sitting.
- Use a lumbar support pillow when sitting or driving.

- Sleep on a firm mattress.
- Avoid sleeping on your stomach.
- Sleep on your side or on your back with a wedge or pillow under the lower part of your legs.
- Find a mattress that suits your body and how you sleep. Everyone is different, so it may take time to find one that works for you.

While some people think that using shoe inserts will prevent back pain, so far there's not a lot of evidence to support this.

When to Contact Your Doctor

More serious symptoms associated with back pain that may require immediate medical attention include:
- Pain that does not subside, or worsens with rest
- Pain that is worse when you are reclining
- Pain that is severe or that has gotten dramatically worse
- Progressive weakness or numbness in a leg or foot
- Difficulty walking, standing, or moving
- Numbness in the genital or rectal area
- Loss of bowel or bladder control
- Burning or difficulty with urination
- Fever, unexplained weight loss, or other signs of illness
- If there has been any trauma, fall, or impact
- If you have a history of cancer, back pain should be evaluated

—*Michael Woods, MD, FAAP*
EBSCO Medical Review Board

References

"2008 Physical Activity Guidelines for Americans." *Health.gov*, Office of Disease Prevention and Health Promotion, 2008, health.gov/paguidelines/2008/chapter1.aspx.

"Acute Low Back Pain." *DynaMed*, EBSCO Information Services, 25 Oct. 2017, www.dynamed.com/condition/acute-low-back-pain.

"Chronic Low Back Pain." *DynaMed*, EBSCO Information Services, 30 June 2017, www.dynamed.com/condition/chronic-low-back-pain.

"Counseling and Education for Chronic Low Back Pain." *DynaMed*, EBSCO Information Services, 22 Dec. 2017, www.dynamed.com/topics/dmp~AN~T910282/Counseling-and-education-for-chronic-low-back-pain.

"Exercise Therapy for Chronic Low Back Pain." *DynaMed*, EBSCO Information Services, 27 Nov. 2017, www.dynamed.com/management/exercise-therapy-for-chronic-low-back-pain.

Gatti, Roberto, et al. "Efficacy of Trunk Balance Exercises for Individuals With Chronic Low Back Pain: A Randomized Clinical Trial." *Journal of Orthopaedic & Sports Physical Therapy*, vol. 41, no. 8, 2011, pp. 542–552., doi:10.2519/jospt.2011.3413.

Natour, Jamil, et al. "Pilates Improves Pain, Function and Quality of Life in Patients with Chronic Low Back Pain: a Randomized Controlled Trial." *Clinical Rehabilitation*, vol. 29, no. 1, 25 June 2014, pp. 59–68., doi:10.1177/0269215514538981.

Sahar, Tali, et al. "Insoles for Prevention and Treatment of Back Pain." *Cochrane Database of Systematic Reviews*, 2009, doi:10.1002/14651858.cd005275.pub2.

"Sciatica." *DynaMed*, EBSCO Information Services, 8 May 2017, www.dynamed.com/condition/sciatica.

Surgical procedures for low back pain and sciatica

CATEGORY: Procedure

Surgery may be necessary for persistent back pain that involves an anatomical problem such as a herniated disc, spinal stenosis, or spondylolisthesis.

Rarely, surgery may be performed on an emergency basis if there are severe symptoms, such as loss of bowel or bladder control, or if a tumor is present.

The 2 main surgical options to treat a herniated disc are laminectomy (with or without spinal fusion) and discectomy. Spinal decompression may be done to treat spinal stenosis. Spondylolisthesis is treated either with a fusion or with a fusion and a decompression.

Laminectomy (Spinal Decompression)

A laminectomy, also called spinal decompression, is an open surgical procedure. It involves removing a small portion of the lamina. The lamina is the small part of the vertebral bone over the area where the nerve is being pinched. It is removed to relieve pressure on spinal nerves. Along with bone, fragments of a ruptured disc also maybe removed.

Lumbar Laminectomy

Normal (Side View) — Spinal cord, Lamina, Intervertebral disc, Spinal nerve, Lumbar spine

Spinal Nerve Compression — Ruptured disc

Laminectomy — Portion of lamina removed

Normal (Top View) — Lamina, Spinal cord, Spinal nerve

Spinal Cord Compression — Bone spur

Laminectomy

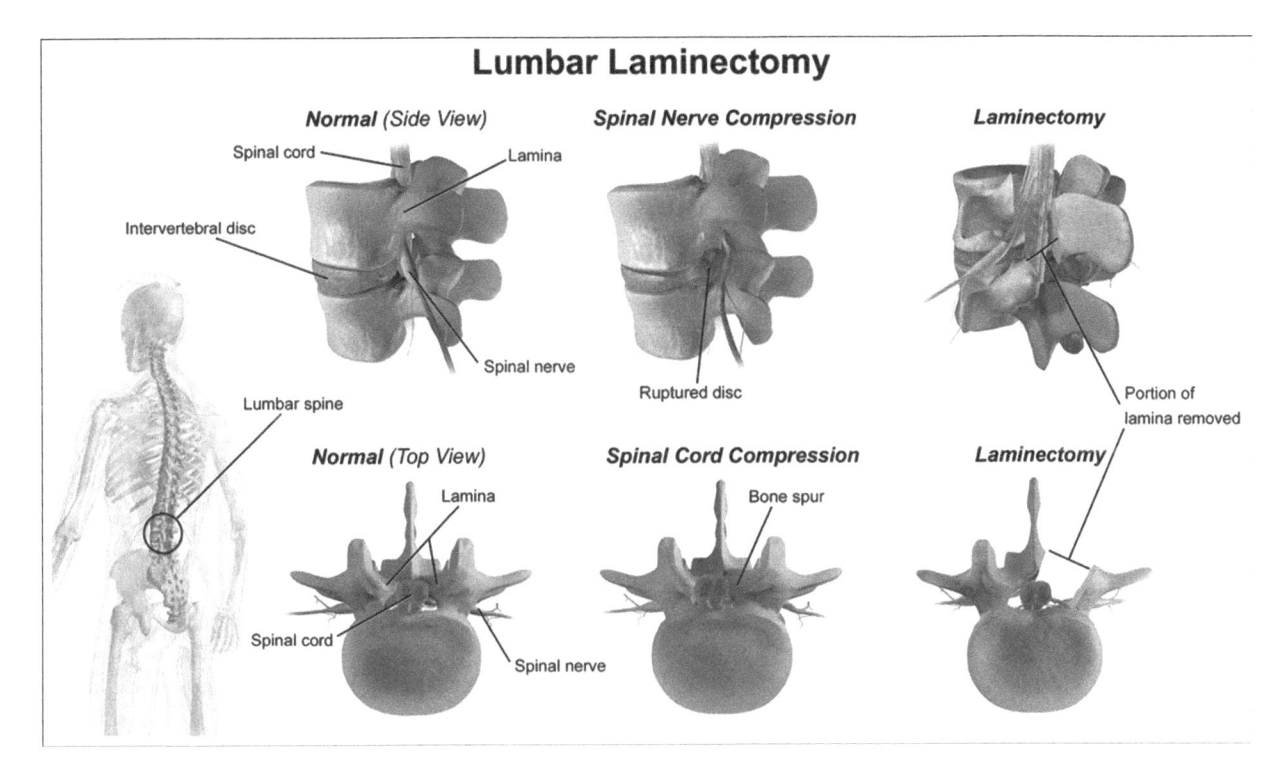

The surgeon makes an incision in the back, spreads the overlying muscles, and removes the lamina. After the bone is removed, the surgeon can see what is compressing the nerve and may remove the offending disc. The incision is closed with stitches or staples.

Spinal Fusion

Spinal fusion is a procedure that joins 2 bones (vertebrae) in the spinal column together to eliminate pain caused by movement.

Most of the time when a patient has a laminectomy and disc removal, a spinal fusion is *not* done. If a spinal fusion is to be performed, the adjacent vertebral bones are joined together with bone collected from the patient or a bone donor bank. Additional internal devices, such as metal rods and pins, may be used to provide added stability. The actual fusing of the vertebral segments occurs as the body stimulates new bone growth between the vertebrae over the course of the healing period. This process may take 3 to 6 months or longer.

Discectomy

Discectomy is the removal of the protruding disc and part of the backbone. The doctor makes an incision in the back. A small part of the bone is removed to obtain access to the disc. The disc is then removed to take pressure off the nerve.

In certain cases, the doctor can perform a microdiscectomy to remove a herniated disc. A microdiscectomy is a less invasive procedure. The doctor makes a smaller incision and uses a magnifying instrument to see the disc and nerves. It is not always possible to do a microdiscectomy.

Surgery is not always the better choice. People have been able to improve with nonoperative treatment options. Talk to your doctor about risks and benefits of surgery and other treatment options.

Disc Replacement

A relatively new procedure, total disc replacement, is now available as an alternative to fusion. It is chosen when the cause of the injury is a degenerated disc.

In the procedure, an artificial disc is used to replace the damaged disc. In theory, it offers the ability to repair the damaged portion of the spine while still maintaining the mobility of the spine. However, this new procedure remains controversial. It may be appropriate for only a limited group of patients.

Patients with multiple degenerating discs or those who have had multiple failed back surgeries

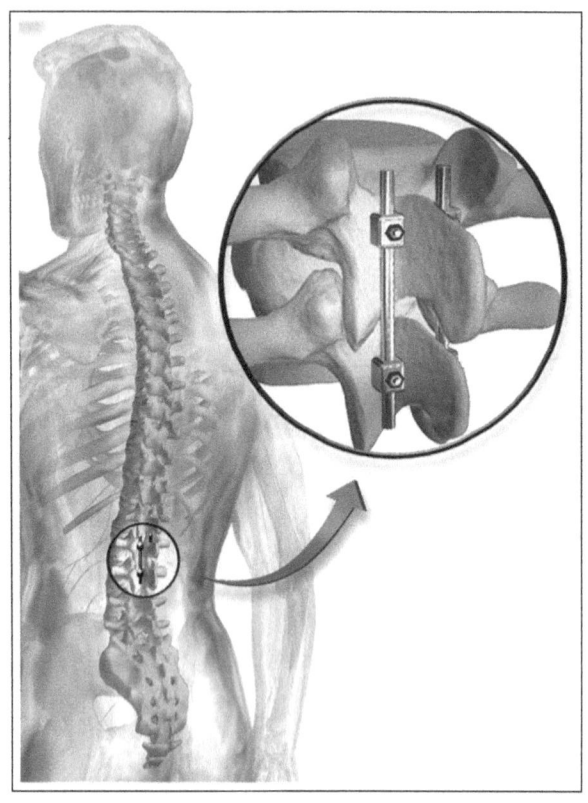

Stabilization rods used after spinal fusion surgery. (BruceBlaus via Wikimedia Commons)

may not be candidates for artificial disc replacement. There is also a device to replace only the nucleus pulposus. This is the soft inner part of the disc. The role of these new technologies is not yet established and long-term outcome data are lacking.

Radiofrequency Denervation
Radiofrequency denervation treats the nerves to stop them from sending pain messages to the body. During the procedure, a needle is placed in the nerve that is connected to the damaged joint. An anesthetic is injected. Then, the needle is heated to damage the nerve so it stops sending pain signals. The procedure is done on an outpatient basis.

Intra-articular Steroid Injections
An intra-articular steroid injection is a steroid medication that is injected into the joint space of a vertebrae to reduce pain.

—*Michael Woods, MD, FAAP*
EBSCO Medical Review Board

References
"Acute Low Back Pain." *DynaMed*, EBSCO Information Services, 25 Oct. 2017, www.dynamed.com/condition/acute-low-back-pain.

Bridwell, Keith H, et al. "What's New in Spine Surgery." *The Journal of Bone and Joint Surgery-American Volume*, vol. 97, no. 12, 2015, pp. 1022–1030., doi:10.2106/jbjs.o.00080.

"Chronic Low Back Pain." *DynaMed*, EBSCO Information Services, 30 June 2017, www.dynamed.com/condition/chronic-low-back-pain.

Lakemeier, Stefan, et al. "A Comparison of Intraarticular Lumbar Facet Joint Steroid Injections and Lumbar Facet Joint Radiofrequency Denervation in the Treatment of Low Back Pain." *Anesthesia & Analgesia*, vol. 117, no. 1, 2013, pp. 228–235., doi:10.1213/ane.0b013e3182910c4d.

"Radiofrequency Facet Denervation: Spine Center." *Oregon Health & Science University*, 2019, www.ohsu.edu/spine-center/radiofrequency-facet-denervation.

"Sciatica." *Cleveland Clinic*, 11 Dec. 2017, my.clevelandclinic.org/health/diseases/12792-sciatica.

"Sciatica." *DynaMed*, EBSCO Information Services, 8 May 2017, www.dynamed.com/condition/sciatica.

■ Other treatments for low back pain and sciatica

CATEGORY: Physiotherapy; Procedure; Psychotherapy; Therapy or Technique

Spinal manipulation is a therapy offered by chiropractors, osteopaths, and physical therapists. Physical leverage is combined with a series of exercises to adjust the spine and restore back mobility, while easing pain. Traditional massage is often used with spinal manipulation.

Physical Therapy
Physical therapy includes exercises, teaching back care principles, and using heat, ice, and other methods to relieve pain.

The purpose of physical therapy is to reduce the pain, strengthen the muscles, increase motion and function, and prevent future injury. Physical

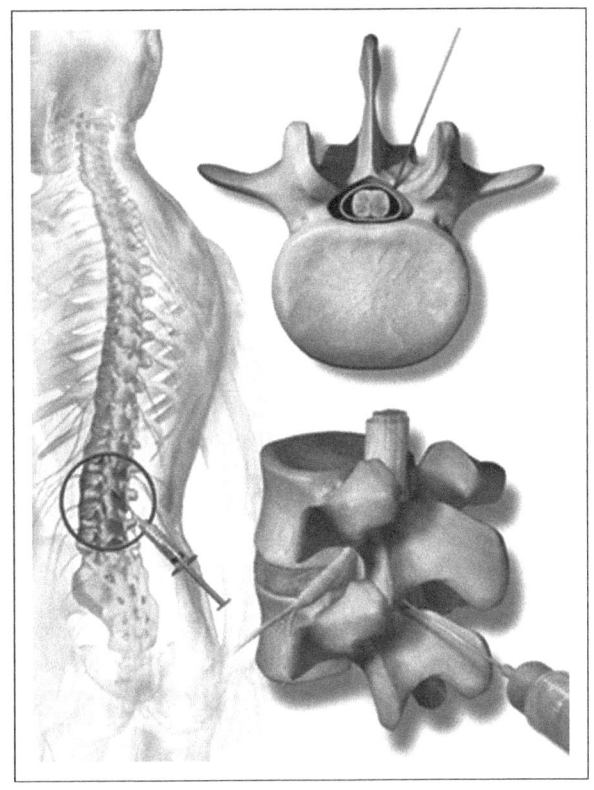

Steroids are injected into the cerebrospinal fluid in the canal surrounding the spine. Nerves branch out from the spine. The nerve roots, which may be compressed, are at the base of the nerves. (BruceBalus via Wikimedia Commons)

therapy should include a home exercise program. Treatments may include:

- Cold packs, which are usually used in the beginning to help reduce pain and muscle spasms
- Heat, which is used to relieve pain and muscle stiffness
- Aerobic exercises such as walking or swimming
- Stretching exercises
- Percutaneous nerve stimulation (PENS)
- Braces or other physical supports

Biofeedback

Biofeedback teaches people how to control body functions they normally do not think about. It may help you reduce the severity of the pain. A biofeedback therapist will guide you to relax certain muscles or control breathing. A device shows your body's response.

Relaxation Techniques

Relaxing the muscles can help prevent and reduce the severity of muscle tension and back pain.

Relaxation techniques may include conscious breathing, visualizing being in a relaxing place, or clearing the mind of any thoughts. A mental health professional can teach you how to perform different relaxation techniques.

Cognitive-Behavioral Therapy

Cognitive-behavioral therapy (CBT) is often used to help manage chronic pain and stress. It is a form of talk therapy that may be done individually or in a group. A therapist will help you identify negative thoughts and teach you to unlearn these thought patterns. You will also learn new, helpful habits to manage your pain with minimal disruption to your life.

Epidural Injections and Joint or Soft Tissue Injections

A steroid medication is injected into the epidural space in the spinal canal to decrease inflammation. Injections can be repeated if necessary. Other targets for injection include the facet and sacroiliac joints, as well as muscles and other soft tissues.

Exercise

Consult your physician about what exercises may be helpful for lower back pain. While there is mixed medical evidence about just which exercises will strengthen the back, specialists agree that it's important to keep moving. Low-impact activities like swimming, bicycling, and walking are especially recommended. Properly performed abdominal crunches and flexibility exercises are also important for strengthening the stomach muscles and relieving tight back muscles.

When to Contact Your Doctor

More serious symptoms associated with back pain that may require immediate medical attention include:

- Pain that does not subside or worsens with rest
- Pain that is worse when you are reclined
- Pain that is severe or that has gotten worse
- Progressive weakness or numbness in a leg or foot
- Difficulty walking, standing, or moving
- Numbness in the genital or rectal area

- Loss of bowel or bladder control
- Burning or difficulty with urination
- Fever, unexplained weight loss, or other signs of illness

—Michael Woods, MD, FAAP
EBSCO Medical Review Board

References

"2008 Physical Activity Guidelines for Americans." *Health.gov*, Office of Disease Prevention and Health Promotion, 2008, health.gov/paguidelines/2008/chapter1.aspx.

"Acupuncture and Related Therapies for Chronic Low Back Pain." *DynaMed*, EBSCO Information Services, 11 Aug. 2016, www.dynamed.com/management/acupuncture-and-related-therapies-for-chronic-low-back-pain.

"Acute Low Back Pain." *DynaMed*, EBSCO Information Services, 25 Oct. 2017, www.dynamed.com/condition/acute-low-back-pain.

Bronfort, Gert, et al. "Spinal Manipulation and Home Exercise With Advice for Subacute and Chronic Back-Related Leg Pain." *Annals of Internal Medicine*, vol. 161, no. 6, 16 Sept. 2014, pp. 381–391., doi:10.7326/m14-0006.

"Chronic Low Back Pain." *DynaMed*, EBSCO Information Services, 30 June 2017, www.dynamed.com/condition/chronic-low-back-pain.

"Counseling and Education for Chronic Low Back Pain." *DynaMed*, EBSCO Information Services, 22 Dec. 2017, www.dynamed.com/topics/dmp~AN~T910282/Counseling-and-education-for-chronic-low-back-pain.

Ebadi, Safoora, et al. "Therapeutic Ultrasound for Chronic Low-Back Pain." *Cochrane Database of Systematic Reviews*, 14 Mar. 2014, doi:10.1002/14651858.cd009169.pub2.

"Exercise Therapy for Chronic Low Back Pain." *DynaMed*, EBSCO Information Services, 27 Nov. 2017, www.dynamed.com/management/exercise-therapy-for-chronic-low-back-pain.

Gatti, Roberto, et al. "Efficacy of Trunk Balance Exercises for Individuals With Chronic Low Back Pain: A Randomized Clinical Trial." *Journal of Orthopaedic & Sports Physical Therapy*, vol. 41, no. 8, 2011, pp. 542–552., doi:10.2519/jospt.2011.3413.

"Manual Therapies for Chronic Low Back Pain." *DynaMed*, EBSCO Information Services, 30 June 2015, www.dynamed.com/management/manual-therapies-for-chronic-low-back-pain.

National Guideline Centre. "Low Back Pain and Sciatica in over 16s: Assessment and Management: Guidance." *National Institute for Health and Care Excellence*, Nov. 2016, www.nice.org.uk/guidance/ng59.

Natour, Jamil, et al. "Pilates Improves Pain, Function and Quality of Life in Patients with Chronic Low Back Pain: a Randomized Controlled Trial." *Clinical Rehabilitation*, vol. 29, no. 1, 25 June 2014, pp. 59–68., doi:10.1177/0269215514538981.

"Physical Supports for Chronic Low Back Pain." *DynaMed*, EBSCO Information Services, 30 June 2015, www.dynamed.com/management/physical-supports-for-chronic-low-back-pain.

Sahar, Tali, et al. "Insoles for Prevention and Treatment of Back Pain." *Cochrane Database of Systematic Reviews*, 2009, doi:10.1002/14651858.cd005275.pub2.

"Sciatica." *DynaMed*, EBSCO Information Services, 8 May 2017, www.dynamed.com/condition/sciatica.

"Thermal and Electromagnetic Therapies for Chronic Low Back Pain." *DynaMed*, EBSCO Information Services, 23 Mar. 2015, www.dynamed.com/management/thermal-and-electromagnetic-therapies-for-chronic-low-back-pain.

Wegner, Inge, et al. "Traction for Low-Back Pain with or without Sciatica." *Cochrane Database of Systematic Reviews*, 19 Aug. 2013, doi:10.1002/14651858.cd003010.pub5.

■ Conditions InDepth: Menopause

Stages of Menopause

Menopause is the natural end to menstruation. The average age of menopause in the US is 52 years old. However, it can start around age 40 and as late as around age 60. If menopause occurs prior to age 40, it is thought to be abnormal and is called premature menopause.

Menopause is the result of the depletion of egg cells from the ovaries and the reduction of female hormones. Menopause is considered complete when you have been without a menstrual period for a full year. Rather than a single point in time, menopause is a process or transitional period when women move away from the phase of life where reproduction is possible.

Symptoms of Menopause

Systemic
- Weight gain
- Heavy night sweats

Headache

Palpitations

Breasts
- Enlargement
- Pain

Skin
- Hot flashes
- Dryness
- Itching
- Thinning
- Tingling

Joints
- Soreness
- Stiffness

Back pain

Urinary
- Incontinence
- Urgency

Psychological
- Dizziness
- Interrupted sleeping patterns
- Anxiety
- Poor memory
- Inability to concentrate
- Depressive mood
- Irritability
- Mood swings
- Less interest in sexual activity

Transitional menstruations
- Shorter or longer cycles
- Bleeding between periods

Vaginal
- Dryness
- Painful intercourse

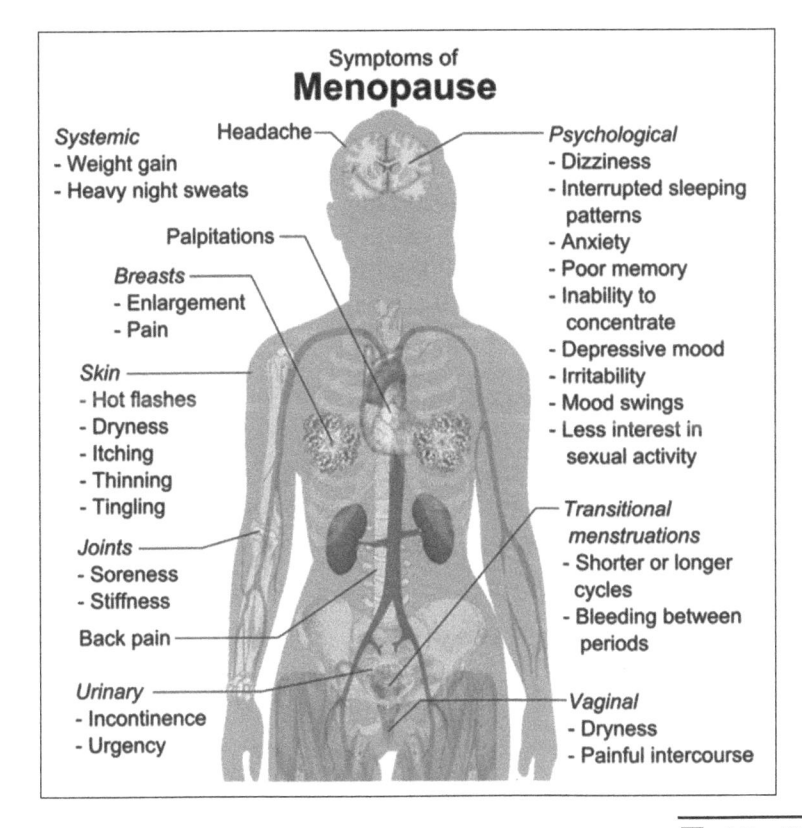

Postmenopause
- Begins after your last menstrual period
- You no longer menstruate
- The risk of certain health problems increases. These health problems include heart disease and osteoporosis

—*Marcie L. Sidman, MD*
EBSCO Medical Review Board

References

"Menopause." *DynaMed*, EBSCO Information Services, 15 Mar. 2018, www.dynamed.com/condition/menopause.

"Menopause Basics." *Office on Women's Health*, 18 Mar. 2019, www.womenshealth.gov/menopause/menopause-basics/.

"The Menopause Years." *American College of Obstetricians and Gynecologists*, Dec. 2018, www.acog.org/Patients/FAQs/The-Menopause-Years.

Menopause is a normal part of life. It marks the end of a long, slow process that begins when ovaries begin to produce less estrogen and progesterone. These female hormones are both important for normal menstrual cycles and successful pregnancy. An oophorectomy (removal of the ovaries) in women of reproductive age causes surgical menopause.

In addition to its role in reproduction, estrogen is an important hormone for maintaining bone health. It may also play important roles in heart health, skin elasticity, and brain function.

Perimenopause
- May begin 2-8 years before the last menstrual period
- Lasts about one year after the last menstrual period
- Signs and symptoms may appear during this phase

Menopause
- Complete cessation of menstrual periods
- You have had no menstrual periods for one year, undergo surgical menopause, or have a blood test confirmation of menopause
- Childbearing is no longer naturally possible

■ Medications for menopause

CATEGORY: Class of Drug

The information provided here is meant to give you a general idea about each of the medications listed below. Only the most general side effects are included. Ask your doctor if you need to take any special precautions. Use each of these medications as recommended by your doctor, or according to the instructions provided. If you have further questions about usage or side effects, contact your doctor.

There are a number of prescription therapies available to treat menopause-related symptoms. The most common drug used for menopause is estrogen. This hormone helps make up for the lower levels secreted by your ovaries at menopause.

Since each person is unique, a number of factors need to be considered before you make the decision to use hormone therapies, including your family and medical history. The results of recent studies on estrogen replacement therapy (ERT) and estrogen plus progestin (hormone replacement therapy or HRT) suggest that the risks of long-term hormone replacement therapy outweigh

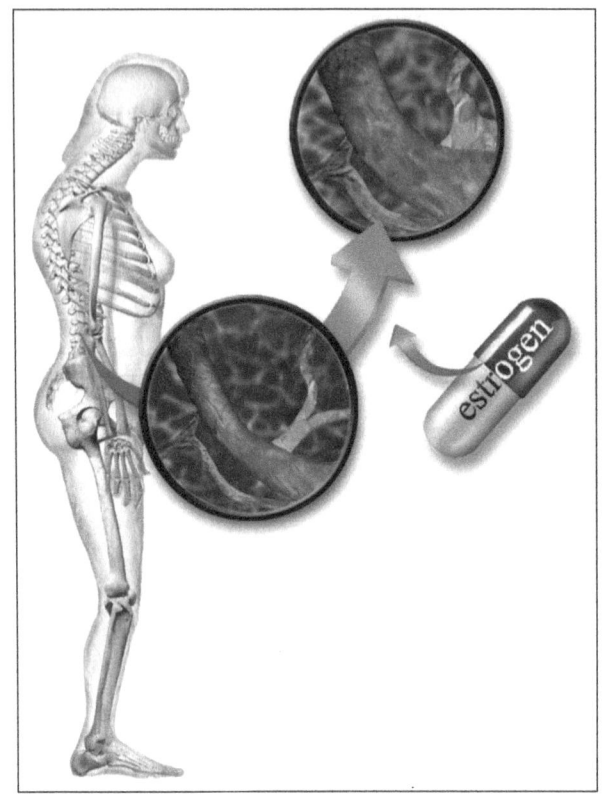

Hormone replacement therapy can reduce bone loss due to menopause. (BruceBlaus via Wikimeia Commons)

the benefits for many women. Therefore, you need to discuss the pros and cons of treatment with your doctor.

Prescription Medications

Estrogen Replacement Therapy (ERT)

ERT provides you with a fraction of the amount of estrogen that was produced by your ovaries before menopause. It helps reduce hot flashes, vaginal dryness, and may reduce the risk of urinary tract infections. Even low doses of estradiol (given as a skin patch) may help with vaginal dryness and pain during sexual activity. It may also reduce your risk of osteoporosis. Evamist, which is a spray, is another type of low-dose estradiol that may help reduce hot flashes.

Estrogen may be administered as an oral tablet, patch, injection, pellet placed under the skin, vaginal cream, ring, tablet, or spray.

Recent scientifically strong studies now show that ERT increases a woman's risk of heart disease, and uterine, ovarian, and breast cancers, blood clots, and stroke.

In general, you should NOT be using ERT if you have heart-related risk factors or known heart disease, are or may be pregnant, have a history of breast cancer or other hormone-sensitive cancer, have unexplained bleeding from your uterus, or a history of blood clotting disorders. You should also avoid long-term use of ERT. You should discuss the risks and benefits of ERT with your doctor.

Common names include:	*Possible side effects include:*
Conjugated equine estrogens	Uterine bleeding
Synthetic conjugated estrogens	Enlargement of benign uterine tumors
Esterified estrogens	Sore breasts
Estropipate	Abdominal bloating
Micronized 17-beta estradiol	Nausea
Estradiol hemihydrate	Fluid retention
Estradiol transdermal spray	Headache, including migraine
	Lightheadedness
	Corneal changes in the eye

Progestogen

If you choose ERT, the progesterone that your ovaries once produced must be replaced to reduce the increased risk of uterine cancer from taking ERT alone. Progesterone or progestin, a synthetic progesterone, is available as replacement therapy. If you had a hysterectomy, you are not at risk for uterine cancer and usually do not need to take progesterone with ERT.

Common names include:	*Possible side effects include:*
Progestin oral tablet:	Fluid retention
Medroxyprogesterone acetate	Weight gain
Norethindrone	Headache
Norethindrone acetate	Mood changes
Norgestrel	
Levonorgestrel	

(Continued)

Megestrol acetate

Progestin injectable:

Medroxyprogesterone acetate

Progestin IUD:

Levonorgestrel

Progesterone oral capsule:

Progesterone USP

Progesterone—vaginal gel:

Progesterone

Progesterone IUD:

Progesterone

Estrogen Plus Progestogen (Hormone Replacement Therapy–HRT)

When progesterone is taken with estrogen, it is called hormone replacement therapy (HRT). Options for HRT include cyclic, continuous-cyclic, continuous-combined, and intermittent-combined.

Long-term HRT increases the risk of strokes, blood clots, heart attacks, ovarian, uterine, and invasive breast cancers. Therefore, you and your doctor should carefully discuss the risks and benefits.

Common names include:	*Possible side effects include:*
Oral, continuous cycle	Uterine bleeding or spotting
Conjugated equine estrogens and medroxyprogesterone acetate	Fluid retention Sore breasts
	Headache
Oral, continuous-combined:	Mood changes
Conjugated equine estrogens and medroxyprogesterone acetate	Increased risk of gastroesophageal reflux disease (GERD)
Ethinyl estradiol and norethindrone acetate	
17-beta estradiol and norethindrone acetate	
Oral, intermittent-combined:	
17-beta estradiol and norgestimate	
Skin patch, continuous cycle:	
17-beta estradiol and norethindrone acetate	
Skin Patch, continuous combined:	
17-beta estradiol and norethindrone acetate	

Androgen

Androgen is a hormone produced by both males and females. In women, the ovaries secrete androgen as testosterone and androstenedione, which are then converted into estrogen and progesterone. As you get older, your ovaries produce less androgen and estrogen. As a result of less androgen, some women notice a decline in their sex drive. Androgen, which must be taken with estrogen, may help improve sex drive in some women.

Low dose androgen may be given through a patch or transdermal gel.

Common names include:	*Possible side effects* include:*
Androgen oral tablet:	Restlessness
Methyltestosterone and esterified estrogens	Depression
	Growth of facial and body hair
	Acne
	An enlarged clitoris
	Increased muscle mass
	A lowered voice
	Increased cardiovascular risks

*These side effects often occur as the result of improper dosages of androgen.

Bisphosphonates

These non-hormonal medications are used to prevent or treat osteoporosis. These agents effectively reduce both bone loss and your risk of fractures. Alendronate may cause gastrointestinal problems and irritation of your esophagus.

Common names include:
Alendronate
Risedronate
Pamidronate
Etidronate
Zoledronate

RANKL Inhibitor
Denosumab is used to prevent bone fractures in postmenopausal women with osteoporosis.

Common names include:	Side effects include:
Denosumab	Allergic reaction
	Low blood calcium
	Infection
	Skin problems
	Unusual fractures.

Selective Estrogen Receptor Modulators (SERMs)
SERMs are used to treat or prevent osteoporosis in postmenopausal women. They have some of the beneficial effects of estrogen, especially improved bone strength. They do not increase your risk of breast cancer or uterine bleeding. However, these medications tend to cause, rather than relieve, hot flashes. They also increase your risk of blood clots and gallstones.

Common names include:
Raloxifene

Nonhormonal Medications for Hot Flashes
Your doctor may prescribe other types of medication to relieve hot flashes. Examples include:
- Clonidine—medication that lowers blood pressure
- Gabapentin—an antiseizure medication
- Selective serotonin reuptake inhibitors (SSRIs) and serotonin and norepinephrine reuptake inhibitors (SNRIs)
- Note: SSRIs and SNRIs should not be used if you are taking tamoxifen, a medication to reduce the risk of breast cancer recurrence.

Common names include:
Fluoxetine
Paroxetine
Venlafaxine
Desvenlafaxine

Special Considerations
If you are taking medications, follow these general guidelines:
- Take the medication as directed. Do not change the amount or the schedule.
- Ask what side effects could occur. Report them to your doctor.
- Talk to your doctor before you stop taking any prescription medication.
- Do not share your prescription medication.
- Medications can be dangerous when mixed. Talk to your doctor or pharmacist if you are taking more than one medication, including over-the-counter products and supplements.
- Plan ahead for refills as needed.

—*Marcie L. Sidman, MD*
EBSCO Medical Review Board

References
Archer, David F., et al. "Desvenlafaxine for the Treatment of Vasomotor Symptoms Associated with Menopause: a Double-Blind, Randomized, Placebo-Controlled Trial of Efficacy and Safety." *American Journal of Obstetrics and Gynecology*, vol. 200, no. 3, 2009, doi:10.1016/j.ajog.2008.10.057.

Buster, John E., et al. "Low-Dose Estradiol Spray to Treat Vasomotor Symptoms." *Obstetrics & Gynecology*, vol. 111, no. 6, 2008, pp. 1343–1351., doi:10.1097/aog.0b013e318175d162.

Huang, Alison, et al. "The Effect of Ultralow-Dose Transdermal Estradiol on Sexual Function in Postmenopausal Women." *American Journal of Obstetrics and Gynecology*, vol. 198, no. 3, 2008, doi:10.1016/j.ajog.2007.09.039.

Jacobson, Brian C., et al. "Postmenopausal Hormone Use and Symptoms of Gastroesophageal Reflux." *Archives of Internal Medicine*, vol. 168, no. 16, 8 Sept. 2008, p. 1798., doi:10.1001/archinte.168.16.1798.

"Osteoporosis." *DynaMed*, EBSCO Information Services, 1 Feb. 2018, www.dynamed.com/condition/osteoporosis.

"Menopause." *DynaMed*, EBSCO Information Services, 15 Mar. 2018, www.dynamed.com/condition/menopause.

"The Menopause Years." *American College of Obstetricians and Gynecologists*, Dec. 2018, www.acog.org/Patients/FAQs/The-Menopause-Years.

"What Is Menopause?" *National Institute on Aging*, U.S. Department of Health and Human Services, 27 June 2017, www.nia.nih.gov/health/what-menopause.

■ Lifestyle changes to manage menopause

CATEGORY: Therapy or Technique; Physiotherapy

You may need to make some lifestyle changes that will help you maintain good health after menopause. Remember that the risk of heart disease and osteoporosis increases as you age. Some easy lifestyle changes may help reduce menopause symptoms and improve overall health.

Maintain Heart Health
You can reduce your risk of heart disease, stroke, and even some cancers by taking care of your heart.
- If you smoke, quit—Smoking is the number one preventable cause of premature death
- Eat a healthful diet—Increase intake of fruits, vegetables, and whole grains. Your diet should be low in saturated and transfats.
- Exercise regularly—Aim for 30-60 minutes of exercise every day. It releases chemicals in your brain, which make you feel better.
- Manage stress—Stress comes from every aspect of life. Learn to relax and find time for yourself. This includes exercise and other pleasurable activities. Some relaxation techniques include meditation, deep breathing, progressive relaxation, yoga, and biofeedback

Maintain Bone Health
Your body replaces bone tissue on a regular basis. With menopause and aging, bone loss speeds up which makes it harder to replace. This can lead to osteoporosis. You can reduce your risk of osteoporosis by getting 1,200-1,500 mg of calcium and 800 units of vitamin D each day.

Increase your dietary calcium intake by eating:
- Leafy green vegetables.
- Calcium-rich low-fat dairy foods, like yogurt or milk.
- Calcium-fortified fruits and juices.
- Vitamin D helps your body absorb calcium. Increase vitamin D intake by eating:
- Fortified milk or other low-fat dairy products
- Liver
- Tuna

You can also get vitamin D with sun exposure. Be sure to limit how much time you spend in the sun. You only need a few minutes at a time a few days a week.

Weight-bearing exercises like walking and strength exercises may also help keep bones healthy. A combination of exercises works best.

Talk to your doctor before you take any supplements with vitamin D or calcium.

Improve Sleep Patterns
If changes in sleeping patterns become bothersome:
- Get on a regular sleep schedule
- Reduce noise, temperature, and light in the bedroom
- Avoid caffeine, nicotine, and alcohol before bed
- Eat a light dinner and avoid heavy evening meals

Limit Caffeine and Alcohol
Cutting back on caffeine may reduce symptoms of anxiety and insomnia. It may also reduce the loss of calcium from your body and reduce your risk of other health problems. You can drink alcohol in moderation. Moderation is a maximum of one drink per day.

Stay Cool
If you are having hot flashes, try making a diary of when they happen and what seems to trigger them. This may help you find out what to avoid. Otherwise:
- When a hot flash starts, go somewhere that is cool.
- Sleeping in a cool room may keep hot flashes from waking you up during the night.
- Dress in layers that you can take off if you get warm.
- Use sheets and clothing that let your skin breathe.
- Carry a small, battery-operated fan in your briefcase or purse.
- Try having a cold drink like water or juice at the beginning of a hot flash.
- Avoid hot foods like soup or spicy foods.

—*Marcie L. Sidman, MD*
EBSCO Medical Review Board

References

Borrelli, Francesca, and Edzard Ernst. "Black Cohosh (Cimicifuga Racemosa): a Systematic Review of Adverse Events." *American Journal of Obstetrics and Gynecology*, vol. 199, no. 5, 2008, pp. 455–466., doi:10.1016/j.ajog.2008.05.007.

"Calcium and Vitamin D for Treatment and Prevention of Osteoporosis." *DynaMed*, EBSCO Information Services, 17 Jan. 2018, www.dynamed.com/management/calcium-and-vitamin-d-for-treatment-and-prevention-of-osteoporosis.

"Dietary Considerations for Cardiovascular Disease Risk Reduction." *DynaMed*, EBSCO Information Services, 22 Nov. 2017, www.dynamed.com/prevention/dietary-considerations-for-cardiovascular-disease-risk-reduction.

Kaszkin-Bettag, M., et al. "Confirmation Of The Efficacy Of Err 731® In Perimenopausal Women With Climacteric Symptoms." *Maturitas*, vol. 63, 2009, doi:10.1016/s0378-5122(09)70447-5.

"Menopause and Your Health." *Office on Women's Health*, 21 Sept. 2018, www.womenshealth.gov/menopause/menopause-and-your-health.

U.S. Department of Health and Human Services and U.S. Department of Agriculture. "Dietary Guidelines for Americans 2015–2020 8th Edition." *Health.gov*, Office of Disease Prevention and Health Promotion, health.gov/dietaryguidelines/2015/guidelines/.

"What Is Menopause?" *National Institute on Aging*, U.S. Department of Health and Human Services, 27 June 2017, www.nia.nih.gov/health/what-menopause.

Vitamin and Mineral Supplements

Many women can benefit from taking a multivitamin and mineral supplement. If your menstrual periods are very heavy during perimenopause, your doctor may recommend taking an iron supplement. If you do not get adequate calcium in your diet and your multivitamin and mineral supplement does not contain the daily requirement for calcium, you may need a separate calcium supplement. If you suffer from hot flashes, phytoestrogens or remifemin may be advised.

Vaginal Lubricants and Moisturizers

Water-soluble vaginal lubricants and moisturizers can help relieve problems due to vaginal dryness, such as painful intercourse. Unlike lubricants, moisturizers can work directly on the vaginal tissue to make it less dry. Do not use any products that are not designed for vaginal dryness. Though vaginal lubricants and moisturizers can help, they do not cure vaginal dryness and atrophy because the underlying cause is lack of estrogen. Prescription estrogen therapy can help treat vaginal atrophy.

—*Marcie L. Sidman, MD*
EBSCO Medical Review Board

References

"Menopause." *DynaMed*, EBSCO Information Services, 15 Mar. 2018, www.dynamed.com/condition/menopause.

"Menopause Basics." *Office on Women's Health*, 18 Mar. 2019, www.womenshealth.gov/menopause/menopause-basics/.

"The Menopause Years." *American College of Obstetricians and Gynecologists*, Dec. 2018, www.acog.org/Patients/FAQs/The-Menopause-Years.

■ Other treatments for menopause

CATEGORY: Herbs & Supplements

There are numerous over-the-counter products available that claim to relieve symptoms of menopause. The US Food and Drug Administration (FDA) has not approved the use of these nonprescription products for the treatment of menopause-related conditions. Since there may be potential risks involved in using any product, you should discuss these products with your doctor.

■ Conditions InDepth: Osteoarthritis

Osteoarthritis (OA) is the wearing down of structures in the joint. This leads to pain and stiffness. It can happen to any joint. It is most common in the knees, hip, spine, and hands.

Cartilage is a smooth tissue that covers bone surfaces inside the joint. It lets bones to move smoothly over each other. It is often the first part of the knee that wears down. The breakdown causes rough areas of the joint. This causes pain with movement.

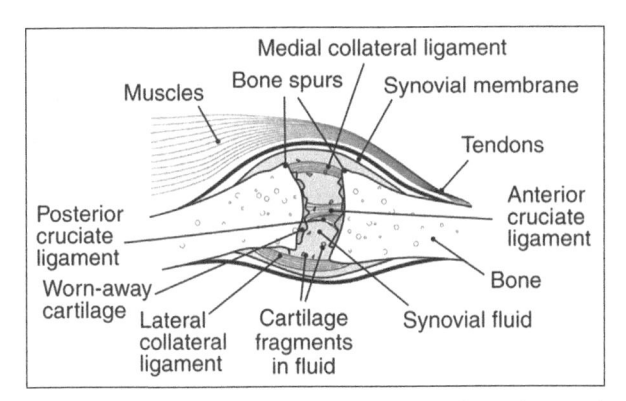

A joint with severe osteoarthritis. (National Institute of Arthritis and Musculoskeletal and Skin Diseases)

All the cartilage may wear away. This leaves the bone bare. It makes moving hard and painful. Over time, this can lead to extra stress and damage to other parts of the joint.

OA is a degenerative joint disease. This means it worsens over time. It is more common in women and older adults. OA is different from person to person. Some may have mild symptoms. Others may have symptoms that impact mobility and quality of life.

Causes

OA is often the result of wear and tear on joints over time. People may be more or less likely to have OA because of genetics and the environment. Things that can increase stress on joints and the amount of wear and tear include:

- Prior injury to the joint
- Bones that are not in line
- Certain sports, such as running
- Excess weight
- Repetitive movements over long periods of time
- Jobs with a lot of:
- Standing, lifting, and moving heavy objects (hip OA)
- Kneeling, squatting, walking, and moving heavy objects (knee OA

In some cases, the cause of OA may be unknown.
—*Warren A. Bodine, DO, CAQSM*
EBSCO Medical Review Board

References

"Osteoarthritis (OA) of the Hip." *DynaMed*, EBSCO Information Services, 15 Mar. 2018, www.dynamed.com/condition/osteoarthritis-oa-of-the-hip.

"Osteoarthritis (OA) of the Knee." *DynaMed*, EBSCO Information Services, 15 Mar. 2018, www.dynamed.com/condition/osteoarthritis-oa-of-the-knee.

"Osteoarthritis." *National Institute of Arthritis and Musculoskeletal and Skin Diseases*, U.S. Department of Health and Human Services, 30 May 2016, www.niams.nih.gov/health-topics/osteoarthritis.

Sinusas, Keith. "Osteoarthritis: Diagnosis and Treatment." *American Family Physician*, vol. 85, no. 1, 1 Jan. 2012, pp. 49–56.

■ Medications for osteoarthritis

CATEGORY: Class of Drug

This sheet gives you a basic idea about each of the medicines below. Only the most common side effects are listed. Ask your doctor if you need to take any special steps. Use each of these medicines the way your doctor tells you to. Follow the advice you are given. If you have questions, call your doctor.

There are many medicines to treat the pain and inflammation of osteoarthritis (OA). OA is not the same from one person to the next. It may take some time to find the right medicines that give you the least number of problems.

Prescription Medications

Nonsteroidal Anti-inflammatory Drugs (NSAIDs)
NSAIDs help to decrease inflammation, swelling, and joint pain. Many are available without a prescription. You may be given a prescription for a higher dose. Some may also be available as creams or patches. They can be placed on skin over the area.

Always take NSAIDs with food. This will decrease the risk of stomach upset. Do not drink alcohol while taking NSAIDs, it causes extra stress on the liver. If you are taking NSAIDs beware of any other medicine you are taking. Avoid taking other medicine that also has NSAIDs.

NSAIDs may cause an increased risk of serious problems. This includes a higher risk of a heart attack and stroke. This risk is important for those who already have heart disease or risk factors like high blood pressure.

Common names include:	Possible side effects include:
Naproxen	Stomach upset
Ketoprofen	Stomach ulcers and bleeding
Ibuprofen Indomethacin	Worsening of some health problems, such as high blood pressure heart failure, or kidney disease
Sulindac	Kidney damage
Meclofenamate	Liver inflammation
Ketorolac	Lightheadedness
Piroxicam Diclofenac	Severe allergic reaction, such as hives, problems breathing, or swelling around the eyes
	Risk of bleeding

Cyclooxygenase-2 or COX-2 Inhibitors

COX-2 inhibitors work like NSAIDs. They help with inflammation, swelling, and joint pain. They cause less stomach irritation than NSAIDs.

Drinking alcohol or taking NSAIDs while you are using a COX-2 inhibitor can raise your risk of side effects.

COX-2 inhibitors may cause a higher risk of heart problems. This can include a higher risk of heart attack or stroke. Talk to your doctor about medicine options if you already have heart disease or risk factors.

Common names include:	Possible side effects include:
Celecoxib	Stomach problems, such as stomach upset and ulcers
Meloxicam	Kidney damage
	Liver inflammation
	Severe allergic reaction, such as hives, problems breathing, or swelling around the eyes
	Worsening of chronic conditions, such as high blood pressure, heart failure, or kidney disease

Opioids

If you have severe pain from OA, your doctor may prescribe opioids to relieve pain. They work well, but may cause dependence. Your doctor will check in with you often while you are using them.

Some opioids may have acetaminophen. Acetaminophen is also a common ingredient in many over the counter medicines. You may be at risk for taking high doses of acetaminophen. High doses of it can harm your liver. Read the ingredient list on labels. Make sure you are not taking too much acetaminophen.

Common names include:	Some possible side effects include:
Hydrocodone Oxycodone	Feeling lightheaded, sleepy, having blurred vision, or a change in thinking clearly
Morphine	Nausea or vomiting
Hydromorphone	Constipation
Fentanyl	Itching
Methadone	Dry mouth

Antidepressants

Antidepressants may help decrease chronic pain. It may be prescribed for chronic pain caused by OA. This type of medicine can cause severe symptoms if it is stopped too fast. Do not stop taking this medicine without talking to your doctor first.

Common names include:	Possible side effects include:
Duloxetine	Lightheadedness
	Sleepiness
	Problems thinking clearly
	Feeling nervous or excited
	Blurred vision
	Dry mouth
	Headache
	Nausea and vomiting
	Diarrhea
	Insomnia
	Change in sexual ability or desire

Drug Facts

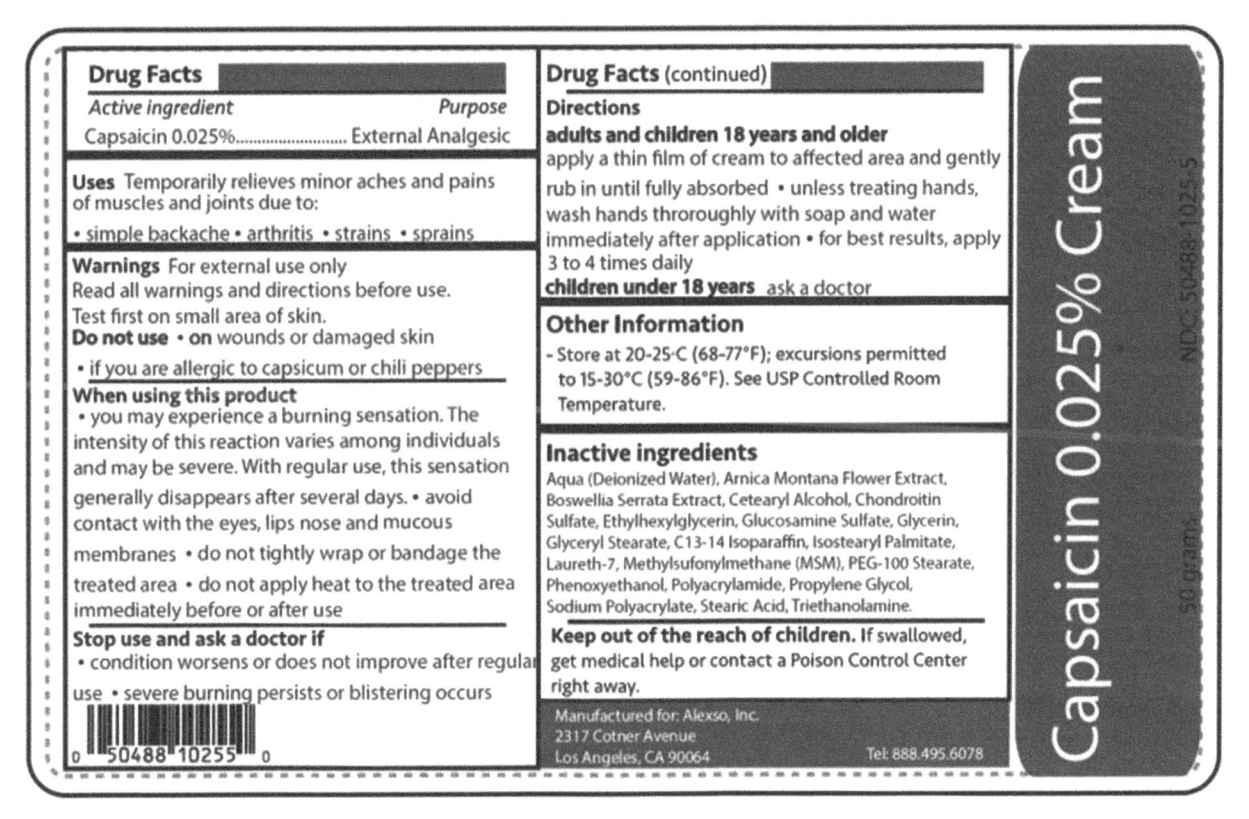

Active ingredient | Purpose
Capsaicin 0.025%.................. External Analgesic

Uses Temporarily relieves minor aches and pains of muscles and joints due to:
• simple backache • arthritis • strains • sprains

Warnings For external use only
Read all warnings and directions before use.
Test first on small area of skin.
Do not use • on wounds or damaged skin
• if you are allergic to capsicum or chili peppers
When using this product
• you may experience a burning sensation. The intensity of this reaction varies among individuals and may be severe. With regular use, this sensation generally disappears after several days. • avoid contact with the eyes, lips nose and mucous membranes • do not tightly wrap or bandage the treated area • do not apply heat to the treated area immediately before or after use
Stop use and ask a doctor if
• condition worsens or does not improve after regular use • severe burning persists or blistering occurs

0 50488 10255 0

Drug Facts (continued)
Directions
adults and children 18 years and older
apply a thin film of cream to affected area and gently rub in until fully absorbed • unless treating hands, wash hands throroughly with soap and water immediately after application • for best results, apply 3 to 4 times daily
children under 18 years ask a doctor

Other Information
- Store at 20-25°C (68-77°F); excursions permitted to 15-30°C (59-86°F). See USP Controlled Room Temperature.

Inactive ingredients
Aqua (Deionized Water), Arnica Montana Flower Extract, Boswellia Serrata Extract, Cetearyl Alcohol, Chondroitin Sulfate, Ethylhexylglycerin, Glucosamine Sulfate, Glycerin, Glyceryl Stearate, C13-14 Isoparaffin, Isostearyl Palmitate, Laureth-7, Methylsufonylmethane (MSM), PEG-100 Stearate, Phenoxyethanol, Polyacrylamide, Propylene Glycol, Sodium Polyacrylate, Stearic Acid, Triethanolamine.

Keep out of the reach of children. If swallowed, get medical help or contact a Poison Control Center right away.

Manufactured for: Alexso, Inc.
2317 Cotner Avenue
Los Angeles, CA 90064   Tel: 888.495.6078

NDC-50488-1025-5
Capsaicin 0.025% Cream
50 grams

Drug label for capsaicin cream. (National Library of Medicine)

Over-the-Counter Medications

Acetaminophen
Acetaminophen can help relieve pain from OA. Do not take a larger dose than your doctor tells you to. Do not drink alcohol if you take it every day. If you take it in high doses or with alcohol, it can harm your liver.

Side effects are rare. A few people may have an allergic reaction. If you get a rash, swelling, or have problems breathing, then stop taking it and get help.

Acetaminophen should be the first option in most people with OA.

Capsaicin Cream
Capsaicin cream is rubbed on the skin of a joint to relieve pain and inflammation.

It is made from the active part of hot chile peppers. Some people wear rubber gloves when they put it on. If you don't, be sure to wash your hands with soap and water after you use it. Do not get the cream near your eyes. It will burn and sting. If you do get some in your eyes, flush them well with cool water.

You may have burning, stinging, or a warm feeling when you first put it on

Common brand names include:
• Zostrix

Special Considerations
If you are taking medications, follow these steps:
- Take your medicine as directed. Do not change the amount or schedule.
- Ask what side effects could occur. Report them to your doctor.
- Talk to your doctor before you stop taking any prescription medicine.
- Do not share your prescription medicine.
- Medicine can be dangerous when mixed. Talk to your doctor or pharmacist if you are taking more than one medicine, including over-the-counter products and supplements.
- Plan ahead for refills as needed.

—*Warren A. Bodine, DO, CAQSM*
—*EBSCO Medical Review Board*

References

American College of Rheumatology. "ACR Issues Recommendations on Therapies for Osteoarthritis of the Hand, Hip, and Knee." *American Family Physician*, vol. 87, no. 7, 1 Apr. 2013, pp. 515–516.

Massey, Thomas, et al. "Topical NSAIDs for Acute Pain in Adults." *Cochrane Database of Systematic Reviews*, 16 June 2010, doi:10.1002/14651858.cd007402.pub2.

"Osteoarthritis (OA) of the Hip." *DynaMed*, EBSCO Information Services, 15 Mar. 2018, www.dynamed.com/condition/osteoarthritis-oa-of-the-hip.

"Osteoarthritis (OA) of the Knee." *DynaMed*, EBSCO Information Services, 15 Mar. 2018, www.dynamed.com/condition/osteoarthritis-oa-of-the-knee.

"Osteoarthritis." *National Institute of Arthritis and Musculoskeletal and Skin Diseases*, U.S. Department of Health and Human Services, 30 May 2016, www.niams.nih.gov/health-topics/osteoarthritis.

Sinusas, Keith. "Osteoarthritis: Diagnosis and Treatment." *American Family Physician*, vol. 85, no. 1, 1 Jan. 2012, pp. 49–56.

White, William B. "Cardiovascular Risk, Hypertension, and NSAIDs." *Current Rheumatology Reports*, vol. 9, no. 1, 2007, pp. 36–43., doi:10.1007/s11926-007-0020-3.

Wong, Melinda. "Cardiovascular Issues of COX-2 Inhibitors and NSAIDs." *Australian Family Physician*, vol. 34, no. 11, Dec. 2008, pp. 945–948.

■ Lifestyle changes to manage osteoarthritis

CATEGORY: Physiotherapy; Psychotherapy

Lifestyle changes can't cure OA. However, they can help to:
- Manage discomfort caused by OA
- Improve mobility and decrease disability
- Slow future damage to joints

Reach or Maintain a Healthy Weight

Maintaining a healthy weight can help:
- Improve symptoms caused by OA
- Slow OA from getting worse
- Reduce OA injury in other joints

Excess weight puts extra stress on your joints. If you are overweight, talk to your doctor or a dietitian. They can help find you find options that may work for you.

Exercise

Joint pain may make you less likely to be physically active. However, not moving can make the joints worse. Regular activity can help your joints move better and decrease stiffness. It can also decrease pain.

One important factor is strength. Strong muscles can decrease wear and tear on the joint. It also helps to absorb impact. This can protect the joint surfaces.

Exercise programs can be tailored to your needs. There are many options to work around sore joints. An exercise physiologist or physical therapist can help to design an effective program.

Reduce Stress

Stress can make pain worse. There are several ways to reduce stress, such as:
- Meditation
- Yoga
- Guided breathing and other relaxation techniques

Returning to Everyday Life

Chronic conditions like OA can be stressful. You may feel frustrated with changes in your lifestyle. Support groups or counseling can help you better meet these changes.

Talk to your care team if you are having trouble with pain. Other treatments options may be available to help better manage your OA.

Monitor Yourself for Depression

Mood changes can happen. It is most common within the first few months of a new diagnosis. It may also occur during periods of intense symptoms. Depression can make your symptoms worse. Call your doctor if you have more than 2 weeks of sadness, hopelessness, or have a loss of interest in your favorite things.

—*Warren A. Bodine, DO, CAQSM*
EBSCO Medical Review Board

References

American College of Rheumatology. "ACR Issues Recommendations on Therapies for Osteoarthritis of the Hand, Hip, and Knee." *American Family Physician*, vol. 87, no. 7, 1 Apr. 2013, pp. 515–516.

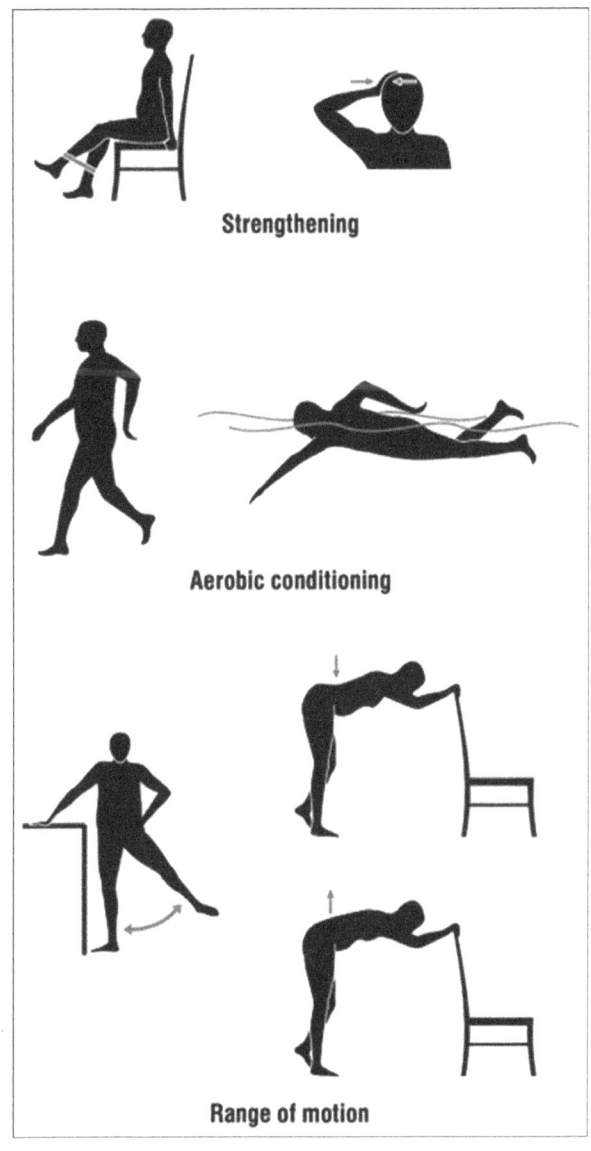

People with osteoarthritis should do different kinds of exercise for different benefits to the body. (National Library of Medicine)

Cadmus, Lisa, et al. "Community-Based Aquatic Exercise and Quality of Life in Persons with Osteoarthritis." *Medicine & Science in Sports & Exercise*, vol. 42, no. 1, 2010, pp. 8–15., doi:10.1249/mss.0b013e3181ae96a9.

Fransen, Marlene, and Sara Mcconnell. "Exercise for Osteoarthritis of the Knee." *Cochrane Database of Systematic Reviews*, 8 Oct. 2008, doi:10.1002/14651858.cd004376.pub2.

Mcalindon, Timothy, et al. "Effect of Vitamin D Supplementation on Progression of Knee Pain and Cartilage Volume Loss in Patients With Symptomatic Osteoarthritis." *Jama*, vol. 309, no. 2, 9 Jan. 2013, p. 155., doi:10.1001/jama.2012.164487.

"Osteoarthritis (OA) of the Hip." *DynaMed*, EBSCO Information Services, 15 Mar. 2018, www.dynamed.com/condition/osteoarthritis-oa-of-the-hip.

"Osteoarthritis (OA) of the Knee." *DynaMed*, EBSCO Information Services, 15 Mar. 2018, www.dynamed.com/condition/osteoarthritis-oa-of-the-knee.

"Osteoarthritis." *National Institute of Arthritis and Musculoskeletal and Skin Diseases*, U.S. Department of Health and Human Services, 30 May 2016, www.niams.nih.gov/health-topics/osteoarthritis.

Sinusas, Keith. "Osteoarthritis: Diagnosis and Treatment." *American Family Physician*, vol. 85, no. 1, 1 Jan. 2012, pp. 49–56.

■ Surgical and medical procedures for osteoarthritis

CATEGORY: Procedure

Medical Procedures

Injections may be recommended for severe joint pain. It may be needed if other care options are not able to relieve pain or mobility problems. These procedures can give temporary relief. They may need to be repeated to maintain benefits. Injections may not be advised for all types of osteoarthritis (OA).

Intra-articular Corticosteroid Injections

Corticosteroids (steroids) can decrease inflammation and pain. It can be injected directly injected into the joint.

Steroid injections may be repeated every several months. Frequent use of steroids can cause a breakdown of tissue in the joint. Because of this, they are often limited to 3-4 injections in a year.

Viscosupplementation Injections

This injection uses a substance called hyaluronic acid. It is a chemical found in normal cartilage and joint fluid. The injections are believed to help lubricate the joint. It allows better gliding of the joint and decreases pain and stiffness.

Surgical Procedures

Surgery can not treat OA itself. It may be needed to repair, rebuild, or replace damaged joints. Surgery is only recommended for those who don't have relief with other methods. Surgery may help to:

Reduce or eliminate pain
Correct joint deformities
Restore mobility

Arthroscopy

Several tiny incisions are made on or near the joint. A small lighted camera is inserted through one incision. Small surgical instruments are passed through a second incision. These instruments are used to clean out the joint. It may include removing shards of bone and cartilage that might be causing problems.

Osteotomy

This surgery helps to repair deformed joints. It is most often done for the knee, thigh bone, or leg bone. The joint will be realigned. It will change the balance of weight on the joint. The healthy areas of cartilage will then be able to bear more weight. This will put less pressure on the damaged tissue.

Arthroplasty

Arthroplasty replaces part or all of the damaged joint. It is more commonly referred to as a joint replacement. A synthetic joint or devices will be used. The replacement is often made of a chromium alloy and plastic. The replacement is done to decrease pain and improve function. The knee and hip are the most common joints replaced.

Arthrodesis

Arthrodesis may be considered for those who have not had good pain relief from other efforts. It is considered as a last resort. The two bones of the joint are permanently fused together. It can greatly improve pain. However, it also prevents normal movement of the joint.

—*Warren A. Bodine, DO, CAQSM*

References

American College of Rheumatology. "ACR Issues Recommendations on Therapies for Osteoarthritis of the Hand, Hip, and Knee." *American Family Physician*, vol. 87, no. 7, 1 Apr. 2013, pp. 515–516.

"Osteoarthritis (OA) of the Hip." *DynaMed*, EBSCO Information Services, 15 Mar. 2018, www.dynamed.com/condition/osteoarthritis-oa-of-the-hip.

"Osteoarthritis (OA) of the Knee." *DynaMed*, EBSCO Information Services, 15 Mar. 2018, www.dynamed.com/condition/osteoarthritis-oa-of-the-knee.

"Osteoarthritis." *National Institute of Arthritis and Musculoskeletal and Skin Diseases*, U.S. Department of Health and Human Services, 30 May 2016, www.niams.nih.gov/health-topics/osteoarthritis.

Sinusas, Keith. "Osteoarthritis: Diagnosis and Treatment." *American Family Physician*, vol. 85, no. 1, 1 Jan. 2012, pp. 49–56.

■ Other treatments for osteoarthritis

CATEGORY: Physiotherapy

Effects of osteoarthritis (OA) can vary from person to person. What works for one person may not work for someone else. Work with your doctor to find what works best for you. Some options that may help manage symptoms and improve function include:

Glucosamine and Chondroitin

Glucosamine and chondroitin are found naturally in the body. Glucosamine helps the body form and fix cartilage. Chondroitin sulfate stops certain enzymes from breaking down joint cartilage. It isVnot known if they are helpful as pills. If you are thinking of taking them, talk with your doctor first. They may cause problems with other medicines you are taking.

Transcutaneous Electrical Nerve Stimulation (TENS)

With TENS, a doctor or a physical therapist puts electrode patches on your skin. The patches connect you to a small machine. This machine sends painless electrical signals through the skin to the nerves. TENS may help with pain and improve function in people with knee OA.

Heat and Cold

Heat and cold may give you some relief. The one that works best for you may depend on your current activity and symptoms. Try one then the other to see which may work best for you.

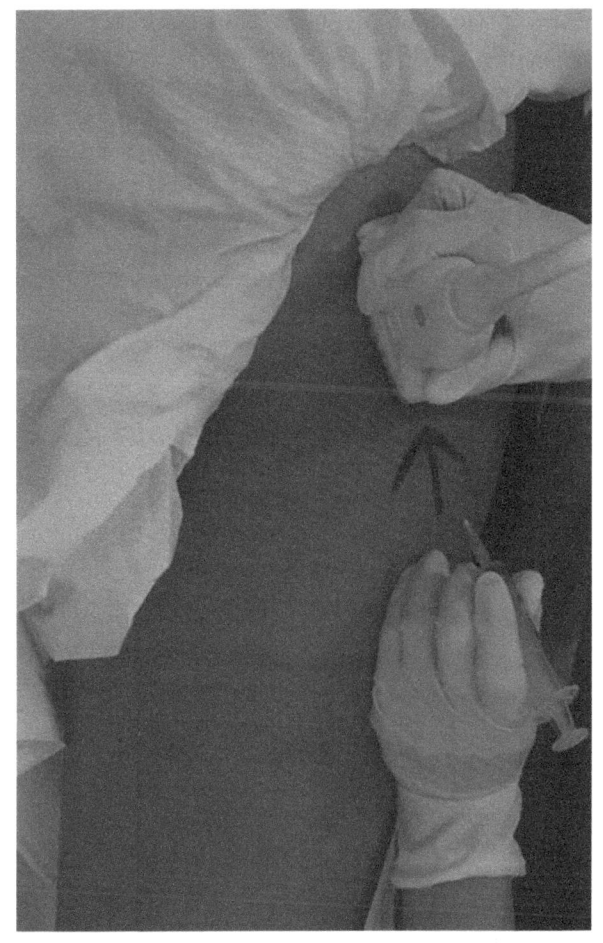

Ultrasound-guided hip joint injection: A skin mark is made to mark the optimal point of entry for the needle. (Phey Ming Yeap, Philip Robinson via Wikimedia Commons)

Heat helps blood and fluid circulate. This can make the site feel less stiff. Warm soaks, whirlpools, paraffin wax, or heating pads can be very soothing. Each method has its own safety steps. Talk to your doctor and try these methods to see what is best for you.

Cold can help decrease inflammation in a joint. You can put an ice pack on for 20-30 minutes at a time. You can do this for several times each day. Put a towel between the ice pack and your skin.

Assistive Devices and Splints

Using assisted devices may help you function. It may also decrease stress on joints. Options will depend on the joints that are affected. Here are some:

- A cane, walker, or crutches may help you move better if you have hip or knee OA. They spread body weight to the less affected joints.
- Splints or braces help align joints and spread body weight.
- Orthotic shoe inserts or special shoes may provide some relief while you are doing daily activities or exercising.

Certain daily activities can become challenging. Examples are buttoning or zipping your clothing, opening jars, or opening doors. Special tools can help you keep doing these tasks yourself. An occupational therapist can help you choose these tools and train you on how to use them to adapt.

Alternative Treatments

Some people have found success adding alternative therapies into their lives. They find they are helpful when used along with traditional therapies. Alternative therapies that have shown some benefit are:

- Acupuncture
- Balneotherapy—use of hot and cold baths
- Relaxation therapy—techniques used to lower stress
- Massage therapy—touch-based therapy to relax your mind and muscles
- Yoga—use of poses and breathing methods to increase flexibility and reduce stress
- Tai chi—martial art form that uses dance-like moves to increase physical endurance and promote emotional well-being

—*Warren A. Bodine, DO, CAQSM*
EBSCO Medical Review Board

References

American College of Rheumatology. "ACR Issues Recommendations on Therapies for Osteoarthritis of the Hand, Hip, and Knee." *American Family Physician*, vol. 87, no. 7, 1 Apr. 2013, pp. 515–516.

"Osteoarthritis (OA) of the Hip." *DynaMed*, EBSCO Information Services, 15 Mar. 2018, www.dynamed.com/condition/osteoarthritis-oa-of-the-hip.

"Osteoarthritis (OA) of the Knee." *DynaMed*, EBSCO Information Services, 15 Mar. 2018, www.dynamed.com/condition/osteoarthritis-oa-of-the-knee.

"Osteoarthritis." *National Institute of Arthritis and Musculoskeletal and Skin Diseases*, U.S. Department of Health and Human Services, 30 May 2016, www.niams.nih.gov/health-topics/osteoarthritis.

Sinusas, Keith. "Osteoarthritis: Diagnosis and Treatment." *American Family Physician*, vol. 85, no. 1, 1 Jan. 2012, pp. 49–56.

■ Conditions InDepth: Sinusitis

The sinuses are hollow areas in the skull that are arranged in pairs. Sinusitis occurs when the tissue lining the sinuses in the skull around the nose (the paranasal sinuses) becomes inflamed and infected. Sinusitis usually occurs with inflammation in the nasal passages (rhinitis). When they occur together, it is called rhinosinusitis. The infections are categorized by the length of time symptoms are present:

- Acute rhinosinusitis—duration less than 4 weeks
- Subacute rhinosinusitis—duration 4-12 weeks
- Recurrent acute rhinosinusitis—4 or more episodes per year with no symptoms between episodes
- Chronic rhinosinusitis—duration more than 12 weeks

Several viral, bacterial, or other causes are associated with acute sinusitis. All are bacteria that are often found in the nose and throat of healthy people, and which cause other common conditions, such as acute bronchitis and ear infections. Certain other bacteria and fungi can be a cause of chronic sinusitis.

A viral upper respiratory infection such as the common cold often occurs just before developing a bacterial infection.

Sinusitis starts with swelling of the nasal and sinus passages. Tiny hairs called cilia usually move constantly to help shift mucus out of the sinuses. With sinusitis, these hairs stop working as well as they should. Both the swelling and lack of movement from cilia make it difficult for mucus to move out of the sinuses. This buildup of mucus and air create the pressure and pain associated with sinusitis. It also creates a place for bacteria and viruses to grow.

Sinusitis is an extremely common problem. In a given year, about 37 million Americans suffer from sinusitis.

—*David L. Horn, MD, FACP*

References

"Acute Rhinosinusitis in Adults." *DynaMed*, EBSCO Information Services, 12 Sept. 2016, www.dynamed.com/condition/acute-rhinosinusitis-in-adults.

Alho, Olli-Pekka. "Viral Infections and Susceptibility to Recurrent Sinusitis." *Current Allergy and Asthma Reports*, vol. 5, no. 6, 2005, pp. 477–481., doi:10.1007/s11882-005-0029-5.

"Chronic Rhinosinusitis." *DynaMed*, EBSCO Information Services, 7 Apr. 2016, www.dynamed.com/condition/chronic-rhinosinusitis.

"Sinusitis." *American Academy of Allergy, Asthma & Immunology*, 2019, www.aaaai.org/conditions-and-treatments/allergies/sinusitis.

"Sinusitis." *ENT Health*, American Academy of Otolaryngology, Aug. 2018, www.enthealth.org/conditions/sinusitis/.

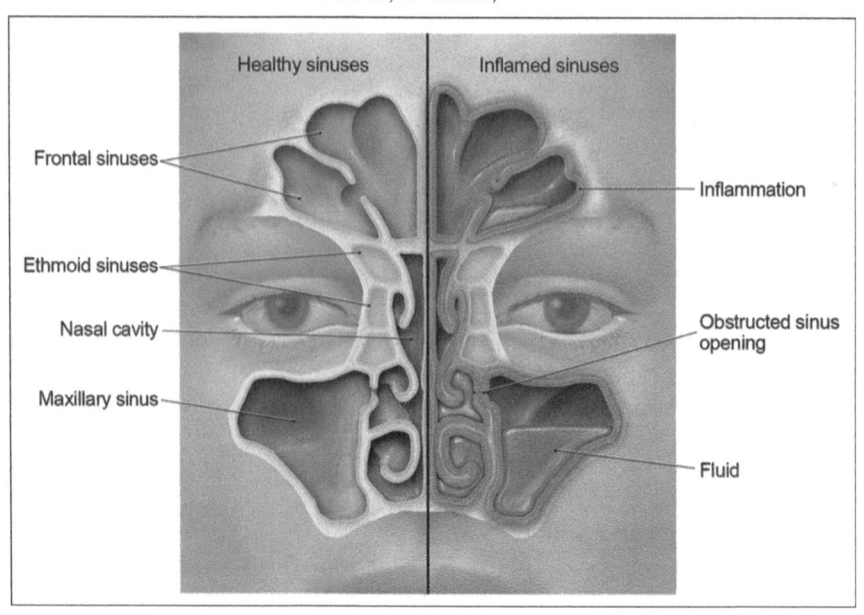

When you have a sinus infection, one or more of your sinuses becomes inflamed and fluid builds up, causing congestion and runny nose. (Centers of Disease Control and Prevention)

Medications for sinusitis

CATEGORY: Class of Drug

The information provided here is meant to give you a general idea about each of the medications listed below. Only the most general side effects are included, so ask your doctor if you need to take any special precautions. Use each of these medications as recommended by your doctor, or according to the instructions provided. If you have further questions about usage or side effects, contact your doctor.

Antibiotics

In most cases, acute sinusitis will get better without the use of antibiotics. Your doctor may prescribe an antibiotic if you have specific symptoms. It is important to take all antibiotics as prescribed, even when you are feeling better.

Beta-lactams

Common names include:	Possible side effects include:
Amoxicillin	Allergic reactions, such as rash, itchy skin, difficulty breathing
Amoxicillin-clavulanate	Diarrhea
Cefotaxime	Nausea, vomiting, stomach upset
Ceftriaxone	Decreased effectiveness of oral contraceptives—talk with your doctor about another form of contraception while you are taking these medications

Fluoroquinolones

If you are taking certain antacids or sucralfate, this may decrease the levels of antibiotic. Talk to your doctor about ways to avoid this interaction.

Common names include:	Possible side effects include:
Levofloxacin	Increased sensitivity to sunlight
Moxifloxacin	Lightheadedness
	Inflamed, torn tendons
	Nausea
	Diarrhea
	Allergic reactions, such as rash, itchy skin, difficulty breathing

Tetracyclines

Always take these medications with a full glass of water. The use of tetracyclines during pregnancy, and for children 8 years of age or less, are not recommended.

Common names include:	Possible side effects include:
Doxycycline	Stomach cramps, burning
	Diarrhea
	Nausea, vomiting
	Tooth discoloration in children, including those whose mothers took tetracycline while pregnant
	Increased sun sensitivity
	Lightheadedness
	Decreased effectiveness of oral contraceptives—talk with your doctor about another form of contraception while you are taking these medications

Other Prescription Medications

Nasal Corticosteroids

Nasal corticosteroids are inhaled directly into your nose through a special inhaler. These drugs may help relieve congestion by decreasing swelling in the lining of the nose. It will likely take a few days of using nasal corticosteroids before you notice an effect; they must be used daily to sustain this effect. These drugs are often used with antibiotics.

If any of the following occurs while you are taking a nasal corticosteroid, call your doctor:

- Severe coughing, wheezing, or trouble breathing
- Painful sores or white or red patches inside your mouth or nose

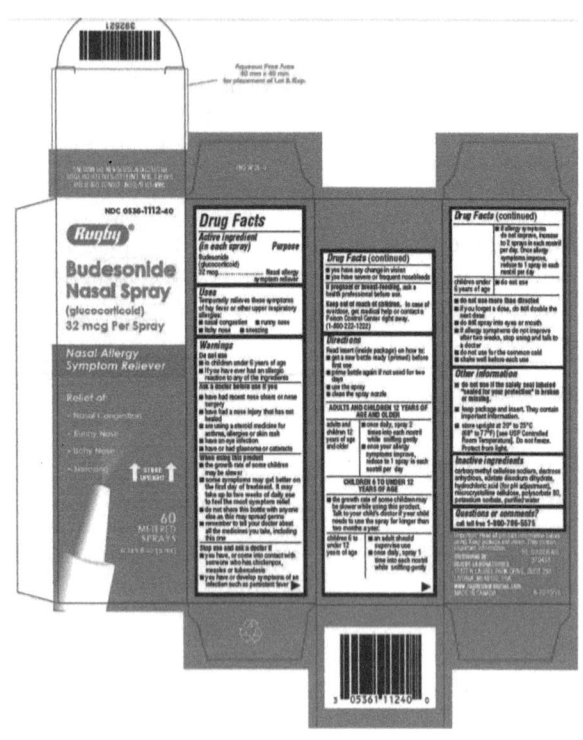

A nasal spray that contains the glucocorticoid Budesonide. (National Library of Medicine)

- Swelling of the tongue or throat
- Trouble swallowing
- Continuous stinging or burning feeling in your nose

Common names include:	Possible side effects include:
Beclomethasone	Dryness of irritation of your nose, including nosebleeds
Budesonide	Stuffy nose
Dexamethasone	Sneezing
Flunisolide	Changes in the sense of smell or taste
Fluticasone	
Mometasone	
Triamcinolone	

Over-the-Counter Medications

Acetaminophen

Acetaminophen can be helpful in relieving some of the pain and discomfort associated with sinusitis. It's also safe to give to children. Do not take a larger dose than is recommended by your

Common brand names include:

Tylenol

Ibuprofen

Ibuprofen can also help relieve some of the pain associated with sinusitis. Because some people find ibuprofen to be very hard on the stomach, you should take this medication with food. Drinking alcoholic beverages while you are taking ibuprofen can increase your risk of stomach irritation.

On rare occasions, people have allergic reactions to ibuprofen. If you notice a new skin rash, difficulty breathing, or puffiness or swelling in your face or around your eyes, stop taking ibuprofen and immediately contact your doctor.

Common brand names include:

Motrin

Advil

Decongestants

Decongestants have been popular choices in the past for acute sinusitis. However, certain professional medical groups such as the Infectious Disease Society of America (IDSA), no longer recommend these medications. These recommendations are based the lack of evidence that they are helpful. Talk to your doctor about medications that are safe for you.

Special Considerations

If you are taking medications, follow these general guidelines:

- Take the medication as directed. Do not change the amount or the schedule.
- Ask what side effects could occur. Report them to your doctor.
- Talk to your doctor before you stop taking any prescription medication.
- Do not share your prescription medication.
- Medications can be dangerous when mixed. Talk to your doctor or pharmacist if you are taking more than one medication, including over-the-counter products and supplements.
- Plan ahead for refills as needed.

—*David L. Horn, MD, FACP*

References

"Acute Rhinosinusitis in Adults." *DynaMed*, EBSCO Information Services, 12 Sept. 2016, www.dynamed.com/condition/acute-rhinosinusitis-in-adults.

De Sutter, An, et al. "Predicting Prognosis and Effect of Antibiotic Treatment in Rhinosinusitis." *The Annals of Family Medicine*, vol. 4, no. 6, 1 Nov. 2006, pp. 486–493., doi:10.1370/afm.600.

Gosepath, Jan, and Wolf J. Mann. "Current Concepts in Therapy of Chronic Rhinosinusitis and Nasal Polyposis." *Orl*, vol. 67, no. 3, 2005, pp. 125–136., doi:10.1159/000086075.

Pichichero, Michael E., and Diana I. Brixner. "A Review of Recommended Antibiotic Therapies with Impact on Outcomes in Acute Otitis Media and Acute Bacterial Sinusitis." *Search Results Web Result with Site Links American Journal of Managed Care*, vol. 12, no. 10, 1 Aug. 2006, pp. S292–S302.

"Sinusitis." *American Academy of Allergy, Asthma & Immunology*, 2019, www.aaaai.org/conditions-and-treatments/allergies/sinusitis.

"Sinusitis." *ENT Health*, American Academy of Otolaryngology, Aug. 2018, www.enthealth.org/conditions/sinusitis/.

Slavin, R, et al. "The Diagnosis and Management of Sinusitis: A Practice Parameter Update." *Journal of Allergy and Clinical Immunology*, vol. 116, no. 6, 2005, doi:10.1016/j.jaci.2005.09.048.

Vining, Eugenia M. "Evolution of Medical Management of Chronic Rhinosinusitis." *Annals of Otology, Rhinology & Laryngology*, vol. 115, no. 9_suppl, 2006, pp. 54–60., doi:10.1177/00034894061150s909.

Williamson, Ian G., et al. "Antibiotics and Topical Nasal Steroid for Treatment of Acute Maxillary Sinusitis." *Jama*, vol. 298, no. 21, 5 Dec. 2007, pp. 2487–2496., doi:10.1001/jama.298.21.2487.

■ Lifestyle changes to manage sinusitis

CATEGORY: Therapy or Technique

General Guidelines for Managing Sinusitis

Quit Smoking
Smoking increases your risk of sinusitis and may hamper your ability to heal from the infection. When you quit smoking, the benefits are immediate. Talk to your doctor about programs and medications that may help you quit.

Drink More Water
Drinking more water might help keep your nasal secretions thinner and easier to blow out. However, there is no evidence showing that fluid intake changes the outcome of sinus infections.

It is also reasonable to increase the consumption of fluids in hot weather or following intense exercise.

Avoid Flying
If possible, avoid flying when you are congested. Changes in air pressure may make your condition worse.

—David L. Horn, MD, FACP

References

"Acute Rhinosinusitis in Adults." *DynaMed*, EBSCO Information Services, 12 Sept. 2016, www.dynamed.com/condition/acute-rhinosinusitis-in-adults.

"Chronic Rhinosinusitis." *DynaMed*, EBSCO Information Services, 7 Apr. 2016, www.dynamed.com/condition/chronic-rhinosinusitis.

"Sinusitis." *American Academy of Allergy, Asthma & Immunology*, 2019, www.aaaai.org/conditions-and-treatments/allergies/sinusitis.

"Sinusitis." *ENT Health*, American Academy of Otolaryngology, Aug. 2018, www.enthealth.org/conditions/sinusitis/.

■ Surgical procedures for sinusitis

CATEGORY: Procedure

Your doctor may recommend that you undergo sinus surgery if you have:

- Chronic sinusitis
- Frequently recurring sinusitis
- Little or no relief from treatments
- Developed complications of sinusitis
- Obstruction of the sinuses by nasal polyps
- Fungal sinusitis

Surgical treatments include the following:

Functional Endoscopic Sinus Surgery (FESS)
This operation is performed using an endoscope, a rigid tube with a light on one end. The tube is threaded into your nose and up into the sinus openings. Using this technique, your sinuses can be drained and the sinus openings can be

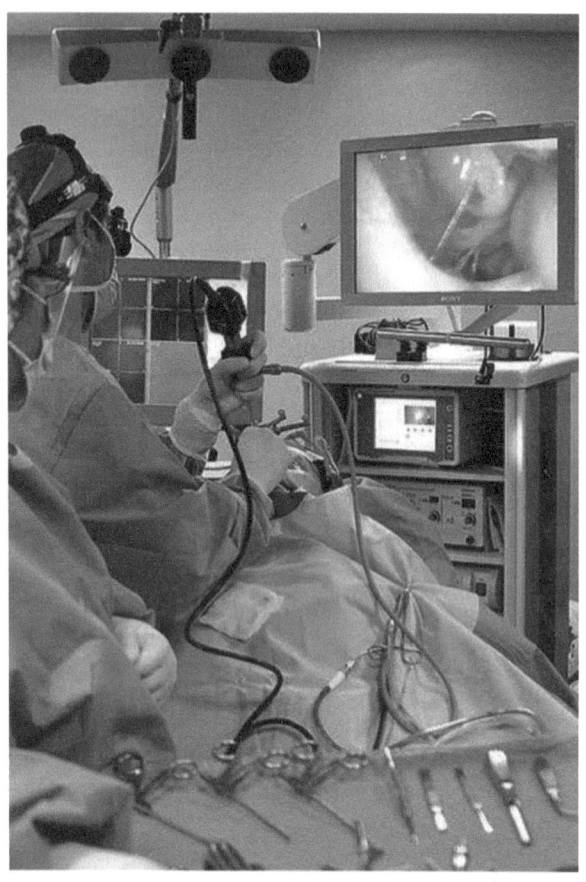

Functional endoscopic sinus surgery (FESS) is a minimally invasive surgical treatment which uses nasal endoscopes to enlarge the nasal drainage pathways of the paranasal sinuses to improve sinus ventilation. (James C. Mutter via Wikimedia Commons)

enlarged, allowing better drainage in the future. If polyps (benign growths) are discovered, they can be removed. This type of sinus surgery has a high rate of success and a low rate of complications. However if complications occur, they may be serious.

Conventional Open Sinus Surgery

Conventional open sinus surgery is also used to enlarge the sinuses for better drainage. Infected sinus linings may be removed during this procedure. Now that FESS is such a successful method, this type of surgery is rarely used. In general, if it is recommended that you have conventional sinus surgery, you should get a second opinion.

—*David L. Horn, MD, FACP*

References

"Acute Rhinosinusitis in Adults." *DynaMed*, EBSCO Information Services, 12 Sept. 2016, www.dynamed.com/condition/acute-rhinosinusitis-in-adults.

"Chronic Rhinosinusitis." *DynaMed*, EBSCO Information Services, 7 Apr. 2016, www.dynamed.com/condition/chronic-rhinosinusitis.

Djukic, Vojko, et al. "Clinical Outcomes and Quality of Life in Patients with Nasal Polyposis after Functional Endoscopic Sinus Surgery." *European Archives of Oto-Rhino-Laryngology*, vol. 272, no. 1, 24 Apr. 2014, pp. 83–89., doi:10.1007/s00405-014-3054-y.

Li, H, et al. "Effects of Functional Endoscopic Sinus Surgery on Chronic Rhinosinusitis Resistant to Medication." *The Journal of Laryngology & Otology*, vol. 128, no. 11, 17 Oct. 2014, pp. 976–980., doi:10.1017/s002221511400228x.

Luong, Amber, and Bradley F. Marple. "Sinus Surgery: Indications and Techniques." *Clinical Reviews in Allergy & Immunology*, vol. 30, no. 3, 2006, pp. 217–222., doi:10.1385/criai:30:3:217.

"Sinusitis." *American Academy of Allergy, Asthma & Immunology*, 2019, www.aaaai.org/conditions-and-treatments/allergies/sinusitis.

"Sinusitis." *ENT Health*, American Academy of Otolaryngology, Aug. 2018, www.enthealth.org/conditions/sinusitis/.

■ Other treatments for sinusitis

CATEGORY: Therapy or Technique

Inhale Steam

Even though studies have not been performed to evaluate its benefit, some people find that inhaling steam can be very soothing in the management of acute sinusitis. Studies do show a small benefit when steam is used in this way to treat symptoms of the common cold.

One way to use steam treatment is to fill a bowl with steamy hot water. Then lean over the bowl in a comfortable position, and drape a towel over the bowl and your head to keep the steam in. Relax and breathe in the steam for about 10 minutes at a time. You can repeat this several times a day. Be careful not to scald your face by touching the water.

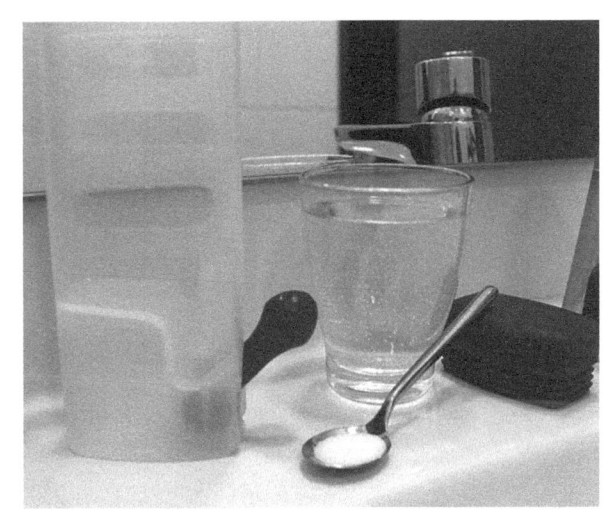

To prepare an isotonic saline solution for nasal rinsing, approx. 0.25 liter lukewarm drinking water and 2.5 ml of table salt (about half a level teaspoon) is required. (Rillke via Wikimedia Commons)

You can also find steam inhalers made for this purpose in stores. You can also try hot packs over your face several times a day.

Saline Nasal Sprays/Nasal Irrigation

Some doctors recommend a nasal irrigation device and warm salt solution to wash out your sinuses and nasal passages. Check with your doctor to see if they recommend a particular device.

Nasal irrigation is most often used in the management of chronic sinusitis. There is some evidence that it may be helpful and little to suggest that it is harmful. Be sure to use distilled water if advised.

—David L. Horn, MD, FACP

References

"Acute Rhinosinusitis in Adults." *DynaMed*, EBSCO Information Services, 12 Sept. 2016, www.dynamed.com/condition/acute-rhinosinusitis-in-adults.

Alho, Olli-Pekka. "Viral Infections and Susceptibility to Recurrent Sinusitis." *Current Allergy and Asthma Reports*, vol. 5, no. 6, 2005, pp. 477–481., doi:10.1007/s11882-005-0029-5.

"Chronic Rhinosinusitis." *DynaMed*, EBSCO Information Services, 7 Apr. 2016, www.dynamed.com/condition/chronic-rhinosinusitis.

"Sinusitis." *American Academy of Allergy, Asthma & Immunology*, 2019, www.aaaai.org/conditions-and-treatments/allergies/sinusitis.

"Sinusitis." *ENT Health*, American Academy of Otolaryngology, Aug. 2018, www.enthealth.org/conditions/sinusitis/.

APPENDICES

Bibliography

■ General Bibliography

"10 Tips for Finding the Right Shoes." *Harvard Health Publishing*, Harvard Medical School, 2019, www.health.harvard.edu/staying-healthy/10-tips-for-finding-the-right-shoes.

"2008 Physical Activity Guidelines for Americans." *Health.gov*, Office of Disease Prevention and Health Promotion, 2008, health.gov/paguidelines/2008/chapter1.aspx.

A.D.A.M. " Willow Bark." *Milton S. Hershey Medical Center*, Penn State Hershey, 5 Aug. 2015, pennstatehershey.adam.com/content.aspx?productId=107&pid=33&gid=000281.

——. "Rosemary." *Milton S. Hershey Medical Center*, Penn State Hershey , 20 Jan. 2017, pennstatehershey.adam.com/content.aspx?productId=107&pid=33&gid=000271.

Abbott, Ryan, and Helen Lavretsky. "Tai Chi and Qigong for the Treatment and Prevention of Mental Disorders." *Psychiatric Clinics of North America*, vol. 36, no. 1, 2013, pp. 109–119., doi:10.1016/j.psc.2013.01.011.

Abdulla, Fuad A., et al. "Effects of Pulsed Low-Frequency Magnetic Field Therapy on Pain Intensity in Patients with Musculoskeletal Chronic Low Back Pain: Study Protocol for a Randomised Double-Blind Placebo-Controlled Trial." *BMJ Open*, vol. 9, no. 6, 9 June 2019, doi:10.1136/bmjopen-2018-024650.

"About Psychoanalysis." *APsaA*, American Psychoanalytic Association, apsa.org/content/about-psychoanalysis.

"Acetaminophen Information." *U.S. Food and Drug Administration*, 14 Nov. 2017, www.fda.gov/drugs/information-drug-class/acetaminophen-information.

"Acetaminophen." *DynaMed*, EBSCO Information Services, 6 Feb. 2018, www.dynamed.com/topics/dmp~AN~T233023/Acetaminophen.

"Achilles Tendinopathy." *DynaMed*, EBSCO Information Services, 22 Jan. 2018, www.dynamed.com/condition/achilles-tendinopathy.

Ackerman, Courtney E. "Psychoanalysis: A Brief History of Freud's Psychoanalytic Theory [2019]." *PositivePsychology.com*, 27 Oct. 2019, positivepsychology.com/psychoanalysis/.

"Acupuncture and Related Therapies for Chronic Low Back Pain." *DynaMed*, EBSCO Information Services, 11 Aug. 2016, www.dynamed.com/management/acupuncture-and-related-therapies-for-chronic-low-back-pain.

"Acute Low Back Pain." *DynaMed*, EBSCO Information Services, 25 Oct. 2017, www.dynamed.com/condition/acute-low-back-pain.

"Acute Rhinosinusitis in Adults." *DynaMed*, EBSCO Information Services, 12 Sept. 2016, www.dynamed.com/condition/acute-rhinosinusitis-in-adults.

Adams, Angela, et al. "Acupressure for Chronic Low Back Pain: a Single System Study." *Journal of Physical Therapy Science*, vol. 29, no. 8, 2017, pp. 1416–1420., doi:10.1589/jpts.29.1416.

"Addiction to Muscle Relaxers: Carisoprodol (Soma)." *American Addiction Centers*, 17 Oct. 2019, americanaddictioncenters.org/prescription-drugs/soma-addiction.

Agarwal, Sumit D., and Bruce E. Landon. "Patterns in Outpatient Benzodiazepine Prescribing in the United States." *JAMA Network Open*, vol. 2, no. 1, 25 Jan. 2019, doi:10.1001/jamanetworkopen.2018.7399.

Ahmadi, Jamshid, et al. "A Randomized Clinical Trial on the Effects of Bupropion and Buprenorphine on the Reduction of Methamphetamine Craving." *Trials*, vol. 20, no. 1, 30 July 2019, doi:10.1186/s13063-019-3554-6.

Alammar, N., et al. "The Impact of Peppermint Oil on the Irritable Bowel Syndrome: a Meta-Analysis of the Pooled Clinical Data." *BMC Complementary and Alternative Medicine*, vol. 19, no. 1, 17 Jan. 2019, doi:10.1186/s12906-018-2409-0.

Alho, Olli-Pekka. "Viral Infections and Susceptibility to Recurrent Sinusitis." *Current Allergy and Asthma Reports*, vol. 5, no. 6, 2005, pp. 477–481., doi:10.1007/s11882-005-0029-5.

Ali, Babar, et al. "Essential Oils Used in Aromatherapy: A Systemic Review." *Asian Pacific Journal of Tropical Biomedicine*, vol. 5, no. 8, 2015, pp. 601–611., doi:10.1016/j.apjtb.2015.05.007.

Allen, Laura. "Case Study: The Use of Massage Therapy to Relieve Chronic Low-Back Pain." International Journal of Therapeutic Massage & Bodywork: Research, Education, & Practice, vol. 9, no. 3, Sept. 2016, doi:10.3822/ijtmb.v9i3.267.

"Alleviating Pain & Symptoms with Palliative Medicine." *JourneyCare*, 30 July 2019, journeycare.org/alleviating-pain-symptoms-palliative-medicine/.

Altug, Ziya. *Integrative Healing: Developing Wellness in the Mind and Body*. Plain Sight Publishing, An Imprint of Cedar Fort, Inc., 2018.

Ambrose, Kirsten R., and Yvonne M. Golightly. "Physical Exercise as Non-Pharmacological Treatment of Chronic Pain: Why and When." *Best Practice & Research Clinical Rheumatology*, vol. 29, no. 1, 2015, pp. 120–130., doi:10.1016/j.berh.2015.04.022.

Ameisen, Olivier, and Hilary Hinzmann. *The End of My Addiction: How One Man Cured Himself of Alcoholism*. Piatkus, 2010.

American Chemical Society. "Kratom's Reputed Pain-Relief Benefits Could Come from One of Its Metabolites." *ScienceDaily*, 29 May 2019, www.sciencedaily.com/releases/2019/05/190529113045.htm.

American College of Emergency Physicians. "Street 'Norco' Looks like the Real Thing but Really, Really Isn't." *ScienceDaily*, 28 July 2016, www.sciencedaily.com/releases/2016/07/160728110433.htm.

American College of Rheumatology. "ACR Issues Recommendations on Therapies for Osteoarthritis of the Hand, Hip, and Knee." *American Family Physician*, vol. 87, no. 7, 1 Apr. 2013, pp. 515–516.

American Pain Society. "Cognitive Behavioral Therapy Improves Functioning for People with Chronic Pain, Study Shows." *ScienceDaily*, 11 July 2017, www.sciencedaily.com/releases/2017/07/170711125851.htm.

American Physiological Society. "Flaxseed Fiber Ferments in Gut to Improve Health, Reduce Obesity." *ScienceDaily*, 5 Feb. 2019, www.sciencedaily.com/releases/2019/02/190205090541.htm.

"Analgesics." *Arthritis Foundation*, www.arthritis.org/living-with-arthritis/treatments/medication/drug-guide/drug-class/analgesics.php.

Ananth, Kartik, et al. "Managing Chronic Pain: Consider Psychotropics and Other Non-Opioids." *Current Psychiatry*, vol. 11, no. 2, Feb. 2012, pp. 38–43.

Anderson, William. *Deep Brain Stimulation Techniques and Practices*. Thieme Medical Publishers, 2019.

Ando, Hironori. *Handbook of Hormones: Comparative Endocrinology for Basic and Clinical Research*. Academic Press Inc, 2015.

Andrade, Chittaranjan, and Rajiv Radhakrishnan. "Prayer and Healing: A Medical and Scientific Perspective on Randomized Controlled Trials." *Indian Journal of Psychiatry*, vol. 51, no. 4, 2009, p. 247., doi:10.4103/0019-5545.58288.

Angoules, Antonios, et al. "A Review of Efficacy of Hippotherapy for the Treatment of Musculoskeletal Disorders." *British Journal of Medicine and Medical Research*, vol. 8, no. 4, Apr. 2015, pp. 289–297., doi:10.9734/bjmmr/2015/17023.

Anim-Somuah, Millicent, et al. "Epidural versus Non-Epidural or No Analgesia for Pain Management in Labour." *Cochrane Database of Systematic Reviews*, 21 May 2018, doi:10.1002/14651858.cd000331.pub4.

"Anterior Tarsal Tunnel Syndrome." *DynaMed*, EBSCO Information Services, 21 Dec. 2015, www.dynamed.com/condition/anterior-tarsal-tunnel-syndrome.

"Antidepressant Medication Overview." *DynaMed*, EBSCO Information Services, 18 Feb. 2011, www.dynamed.com/drug-review/antidepressant-medication-overview.

AOFAS. "Five Tips for Healthy Feet." *American Orthopaedic Foot & Ankle Society*, 16 Apr. 2019, www.aofas.org/news/press-releases/2019/04/16/five-tips-for-healthy-feet.

Aparna, L. Mercy et al. "Assessment of Sputum Quality and Its Importance in the Rapid Diagnosis of Pulmonary Tuberculosis." *Archives of Clinical Microbiology*, vol. 08, no. 04, 2017, doi:10.4172/1989-8436.100053.

Archer, David F., et al. "Desvenlafaxine for the Treatment of Vasomotor Symptoms Associated with Menopause: a Double-Blind, Randomized,

Placebo-Controlled Trial of Efficacy and Safety." *American Journal of Obstetrics and Gynecology*, vol. 200, no. 3, 2009, doi:10.1016/j.ajog.2008.10.057.

Armstrong, David. "Diabetes and Foot Problems." *National Institute of Diabetes and Digestive and Kidney Diseases*, U.S. Department of Health and Human Services, 1 Jan. 2017, www.niddk.nih.gov/health-information/health-topics/Diabetes/prevent-diabetes-problems/Pages/keep-feet-healthy.aspx.

Arreola, Rodrigo, et al. "Immunomodulation and Anti-Inflammatory Effects of Garlic Compounds." *Journal of Immunology Research*, 19 Apr. 2015, pp. 1–13., doi:10.1155/2015/401630.

Arrowhead Health. "Remedies for Muscle and Joint Pain." *Arrowhead Health Centers*, 7 Aug. 2015, arrowheadhealth.com/home-remedies-for-muscle-and-joint-pain/.

"Arthroplasty." *Johns Hopkins Medicine*, 2019, www.hopkinsmedicine.org/health/treatment-tests-and-therapies/arthroplasty.

"Aspirin and Your Heart: Many Questions, Some Answers." *Harvard Health*, 21 May 2018, www.health.harvard.edu/heart-health/aspirin-and-your-heart-many-questions-some-answers.

"Aspirin." *MedlinePlus*, U.S. National Library of Medicine, 15 Feb. 2018, medlineplus.gov/druginfo/meds/a682878.html.

Atroshi, Isam, et al. "Treatment of Carpal Tunnel Syndrome with Wrist Splinting: Study Protocol for a Randomized Placebo-Controlled Trial." *Trials*, vol. 20, no. 1, 27 Aug. 2019, doi:10.1186/s13063-019-3635-6.

Babb, Malaika, et al. "Treating Pain during Pregnancy." *Canadian Family Physician*, vol. 56, no. 1, Jan. 2010, pp. 25–27.

Babl, Anna, et al. "Psychotherapy Integration under Scrutiny: Investigating the Impact of Integrating Emotion-Focused Components into a CBT-Based Approach: a Study Protocol of a Randomized Controlled Trial." *BMC Psychiatry*, vol. 16, no. 1, 24 Nov. 2016, doi:10.1186/s12888-016-1136-7.

Backes, Michael. *Cannabis Pharmacy: the Practical Guide to Medical Marijuana*. Black Dog & Leventhal Publishers, 2017.

"Baclofen." *MedlinePlus*, U.S. National Library of Medicine, 15 July 2017, medlineplus.gov/druginfo/meds/a682530.html.

Bajwa, Sukhminder Jitsingh, and Rudrashish Haldar. "Pain Management Following Spinal Surgeries: An Appraisal of the Available Options." *Journal of Craniovertebral Junction and Spine*, vol. 6, no. 3, 2015, p. 105., doi:10.4103/0974-8237.161589.

Baltenberger, Elizabeth P., et al. "Review of Antidepressants in the Treatment of Neuropathic Pain." *Mental Health Clinician*, vol. 5, no. 3, 2015, pp. 123–133., doi:10.9740/mhc.2015.05.123.

Bandelow, Borwin, et al. "Treatment of Anxiety Disorders." *Dialogues in Clinical Neuroscience*, vol. 19, no. 2, June 2017, pp. 93–107.

Barton, Debra L., et al. "The Use of Valeriana Officinalis (Valerian) in Improving Sleep in Patients Who Are Undergoing Treatment for Cancer: A Phase III Randomized, Placebo-Controlled, Double-Blind Study (NCCTG Trial, N01C5)." *The Journal of Supportive Oncology*, vol. 9, no. 1, 2011, pp. 24–31., doi:10.1016/j.suponc.2010.12.008.

Batmanabane, Gitanjali. "Why Patients in Pain Cannot Get 'God's Own Medicine?'." *Journal of Pharmacology and Pharmacotherapeutics*, vol. 5, no. 2, 2014, p. 81., doi:10.4103/0976-500x.130040.

Bauer, Brent A. "Valerian: A Safe and Effective Herbal Sleep Aid?" *Mayo Clinic*, Mayo Foundation for Medical Education and Research, 15 Feb. 2018, www.mayoclinic.org/diseases-conditions/insomnia/expert-answers/valerian/faq-20057875.

Bauer, Brent A., et al. "Complementary and Alternative Medicine Therapies for Chronic Pain." *Chinese Journal of Integrative Medicine*, vol. 22, no. 6, 2016, pp. 403–411., doi:10.1007/s11655-016-2258-y.

Beliveau, Peter J. H., et al. "The Chiropractic Profession: a Scoping Review of Utilization Rates, Reasons for Seeking Care, Patient Profiles, and Care Provided." *Chiropractic & Manual Therapies*, vol. 25, no. 1, 22 Nov. 2017, doi:10.1186/s12998-017-0165-8.

Bell, Rae Frances, and Eija Anneli Kalso. "Ketamine for Pain Management." *PAIN Reports*, vol. 3, no. 5, 2018, doi:10.1097/pr9.0000000000000674.

Bellnier, Terrance, et al. "Preliminary Evaluation of the Efficacy, Safety, and Costs Associated with the Treatment of Chronic Pain with Medical

Cannabis." *Mental Health Clinician*, vol. 8, no. 3, 2018, pp. 110–115., doi:10.9740/mhc.2018.05.110.

Benini, Franca, and Egidio Barbi. "Doing without Codeine: Why and What Are the Alternatives?" *Italian Journal of Pediatrics*, vol. 40, no. 1, 11 Feb. 2014, doi:10.1186/1824-7288-40-16.

"Benzodiazepines (and the Alternatives)." *Harvard Health Publishing*, Harvard Medical School, 15 Mar. 2019, www.health.harvard.edu/mind-and-mood/benzodiazepines_and_the_alternatives.

Bergland, Christopher. "How Does Yoga Relieve Chronic Pain?" *Psychology Today*, Sussex Publishers, 27 May 2015, www.psychologytoday.com/us/blog/the-athletes-way/201505/how-does-yoga-relieve-chronic-pain.

Bermudes, Richard A., et al. *Transcranial Magnetic Stimulation: Clinical Applications for Psychiatric Practice*. American Psychiatric Association Publishing, 2018.

Berridge, Virginia. "Opium through History." *The Lancet*, vol. 379, no. 9834, 2012, p. 2332., doi:10.1016/s0140-6736(12)61005-8.

Bervoets, Diederik C, et al. "Massage Therapy Has Short-Term Benefits for People with Common Musculoskeletal Disorders Compared to No Treatment: a Systematic Review." Journal of Physiotherapy, vol. 61, no. 3, 2015, pp. 106–116., doi:10.1016/j.jphys.2015.05.018.

Bhandari, Monika, et al. "Recent Updates on Codeine." *Pharmaceutical Methods*, vol. 2, no. 1, 2011, pp. 3–8., doi:10.4103/2229-4708.81082.

Bhatia, ByJuhie, et al. "Herbal Remedies for Natural Pain Relief." *EverydayHealth.com*, 10 Feb. 2016, www.everydayhealth.com/pain-management/natural-pain-remedies.aspx.

Bhatnagar, Sushma, and Mayank Gupta. "Integrated Pain and Palliative Medicine Model." *Annals of Palliative Medicine*, vol. 5, no. 3, 2016, pp. 196–208., doi:10.21037/apm.2016.05.02.

"Biofeedback Glossary." *Association for Applied Psychophysiology and Biofeedback*, 2011, www.aapb.org/i4a/pages/index.cfm?pageid=3462.

Bisen, Prakash S., and Mila Emerald. "Nutritional and Therapeutic Potential of Garlic and Onion (Allium Sp.)." *Current Nutrition & Food Science*, vol. 12, no. 3, 2016, pp. 190–199., doi:10.2174/1573401312666160608121954.

Black, Christopher D., et al. "Ginger (Zingiber Officinale) Reduces Muscle Pain Caused by Eccentric Exercise." *The Journal of Pain*, vol. 11, no. 9, 2010, pp. 894–903., doi:10.1016/j.jpain.2009.12.013.

Blanchette, Marc-André, et al. "Effectiveness and Economic Evaluation of Chiropractic Care for the Treatment of Low Back Pain: A Systematic Review of Pragmatic Studies." *Plos One*, vol. 11, no. 8, 3 Aug. 2016, doi:10.1371/journal.pone.0160037.

Bleecker, Deborah. *Acupuncture Points Handbook: a Patient's Guide to the Locations and Functions of Over 400 Acupuncture Points*. Draycott Design Books, 2017.

Blistein, David, and John Halpern. *Opium: How an Ancient Flower Shaped and Poisoned Our World*. Hachette Books, 2019.

Blödt, Susanne, et al. "Effectiveness of App-Based Relaxation for Patients with Chronic Low Back Pain (Relaxback) and Chronic Neck Pain (Relaxneck): Study Protocol for Two Randomized Pragmatic Trials." *Trials*, vol. 15, no. 1, 2014, doi:10.1186/1745-6215-15-490.

Blokdijk, G. J. *Bupropion: 523 Questions to Ask That Matter to You*. CreateSpace Independent Publishing Platform, 2018.

BMJ. "Do Not Give Decongestants to Young Children for Common Cold Symptoms." *ScienceDaily*, 11 Oct. 2018, www.sciencedaily.com/releases/2018/10/181011103628.htm.

Boehnke, Kevin F., et al. "Pills to Pot: Observational Analyses of Cannabis Substitution Among Medical Cannabis Users With Chronic Pain." *The Journal of Pain*, vol. 20, no. 7, 2019, pp. 830–841., doi:10.1016/j.jpain.2019.01.010.

Bonnie, Richard J., et al. "Pain Management and Opioid Regulation: Continuing Public Health Challenges." *American Journal of Public Health*, vol. 109, no. 1, Jan. 2019, pp. 31–34., doi:10.2105/ajph.2018.304881.

Booth, Jessie W., and James T. Neill. "Coping Strategies and the Development of Psychological Resilience." *Journal of Outdoor and Environmental Education*, vol. 20, no. 1, 2017, pp. 47–54., doi:10.1007/bf03401002.

Borrelli, Francesca, and Edzard Ernst. "Black Cohosh (Cimicifuga Racemosa): a Systematic

Review of Adverse Events." *American Journal of Obstetrics and Gynecology*, vol. 199, no. 5, 2008, pp. 455–466., doi:10.1016/j.ajog.2008.05.007.

Bortolato, Beatrice, et al. "Cognitive Remission: a Novel Objective for the Treatment of Major Depression?" *BMC Medicine*, vol. 14, no. 1, 22 Jan. 2016, doi:10.1186/s12916-016-0560-3.

Bost, Jeffreyw, et al. "Natural Anti-Inflammatory Agents for Pain Relief." *Surgical Neurology International*, vol. 1, no. 1, 2010, p. 80., doi:10.4103/2152-7806.73804.

Brady, Kathleen T., et al. "Prescription Opioid Misuse, Abuse, and Treatment in the United States: An Update." *American Journal of Psychiatry*, vol. 173, no. 1, 2016, pp. 18–26., doi:10.1176/appi.ajp.2015.15020262.

Brämberg, Elisabeth Björk, et al. "Effects of Yoga, Strength Training and Advice on Back Pain: a Randomized Controlled Trial." *BMC Musculoskeletal Disorders*, vol. 18, no. 1, 29 Mar. 2017, doi:10.1186/s12891-017-1497-1.

Brandes, Jan Lewis, et al. "Sumatriptan-Naproxen for Acute Treatment of Migraine." *Jama*, vol. 297, no. 13, 2007, pp. 1443–1456., doi:10.1001/jama.297.13.1443.

Brazier, Yvette. "Drama Therapy: Unlocking the Door to Change." *Medical News Today*, MediLexicon International, 30 Mar. 2016, www.medicalnewstoday.com/articles/308452.php#1.

—. "Euthanasia and Assisted Suicide: What Are They and What Do They Mean?" *Medical News Today*, MediLexicon International, 17 Dec. 2018, www.medicalnewstoday.com/articles/182951.php.

Brazier, Yvette. "Peppermint: Health Benefits and Precautions." *Medical News Today*, MediLexicon International, 27 June 2017, www.medicalnewstoday.com/articles/265214.php.

Brazil, Rachel. "Pain Relief: Designing Better Opioids." *The Pharmaceutical Journal*, vol. 300, no. 7912, 19 Apr. 2018, doi:10.1211/pj.2018.20204708.

Brett, Jonathan, and Bridin Murnion. "Management of Benzodiazepine Misuse and Dependence." *Australian Prescriber*, vol. 38, no. 5, 1 Oct. 2015, pp. 152–155., doi:10.18773/austprescr.2015.055.

Bridgeman, Mary Barna, and Daniel T. Abazia. "Medicinal Cannabis: History, Pharmacology, And Implications for the Acute Care Setting." *Pharmacy & Therapeutics*, vol. 42, no. 3, Mar. 2017, pp. 180–188.

Bridwell, Keith H, et al. "What's New in Spine Surgery." *The Journal of Bone and Joint Surgery-American Volume*, vol. 97, no. 12, 2015, pp. 1022–1030., doi:10.2106/jbjs.o.00080.

Brien, Sarah. "Trial Evaluating Devil's Claw for the Treatment of Hip and Knee Osteoarthritis." *ClinicalTrials.gov*, U.S. National Library of Medicine, 12 Sept. 2011, clinicaltrials.gov/ct2/show/NCT00295490.

Brittain, Danielle R., et al. "Moving Forward with Physical Activity: Self-Management of Chronic Pain among Women." *Women's Health Issues*, vol. 28, no. 2, 2018, pp. 113–116., doi:10.1016/j.whi.2017.12.006.

Bronfort, Gert, et al. "Spinal Manipulation and Home Exercise With Advice for Subacute and Chronic Back-Related Leg Pain." *Annals of Internal Medicine*, vol. 161, no. 6, 16 Sept. 2014, pp. 381–391., doi:10.7326/m14-0006.

Brugnoli, Maria Paola, et al. "The Role of Clinical Hypnosis and Self-Hypnosis to Relief Pain and Anxiety in Severe Chronic Diseases in Palliative Care: a 2-Year Long-Term Follow-up of Treatment in a Nonrandomized Clinical Trial." *Annals of Palliative Medicine*, vol. 7, no. 1, 2018, pp. 17–31., doi:10.21037/apm.2017.10.03.

Bryson, Ethan O., and Jeffrey H. Silverstein. "Addiction and Substance Abuse in Anesthesiology." *Anesthesiology*, vol. 109, no. 5, 2008, pp. 905–917., doi:10.1097/aln.0b013e3181895bc1.

"Bupropion: MedlinePlus Drug Information." *MedlinePlus*, U.S. National Library of Medicine, 15 Feb. 2015, medlineplus.gov/druginfo/meds/a695033.html.

Burchiel, Kim J., and Ahmed M. Raslan. "Contemporary Concepts of Pain Surgery." *Journal of Neurosurgery*, vol. 130, no. 4, 2019, pp. 1039–1049., doi:10.3171/2019.1.jns181620.

Burg, Scott. "3 Steps to Fight Your Carpal Tunnel Syndrome." *Health Essentials*, Cleveland Clinic, 20 Sept. 2019, health.clevelandclinic.org/3-steps-to-fight-your-carpal-tunnel-syndrome/.

Buster, John E., et al. "Low-Dose Estradiol Spray to Treat Vasomotor Symptoms." *Obstetrics & Gynecology*, vol. 111, no. 6, 2008, pp. 1343–1351., doi:10.1097/aog.0b013e318175d162.

C, Griffith, and La France B. "The Benefits and Effects of Using Marijuana as a Pain Agent to Treat Opioid Addiction." *Journal of Hospital & Medical Management*, vol. 04, no. 02, 2018, doi:10.4172/2471-9781.100051.

Cadmus, Lisa, et al. "Community-Based Aquatic Exercise and Quality of Life in Persons with Osteoarthritis." *Medicine & Science in Sports & Exercise*, vol. 42, no. 1, 2010, pp. 8–15., doi:10.1249/mss.0b013e3181ae96a9.

Cafasso, Jacqueline, and Alan Carter. "Antiemetic Drugs." *Healthline*, 12 June 2017, www.healthline.com/health/antiemetic-drugs-list.

Cafasso, Jacqueline, and Cynthia Cobb. "Red Light Therapy Benefits." *Healthline*, 11 May 2018, www.healthline.com/health/red-light-therapy.

Çakici, Özer Ural, et al. "Open Stone Surgery: Still-in-Use Approach for Complex Stone Burden." *Central European Journal of Urology*, vol. 70, no. 2, 2017, doi:10.5173/ceju.2017.1205.

Calado, Ana, et al. "The Effect of Flaxseed in Breast Cancer: A Literature Review." *Frontiers in Nutrition*, vol. 5, 7 Feb. 2018, doi:10.3389/fnut.2018.00004.

Calcaterra, Nicholas E., and James C. Barrow. "Classics in Chemical Neuroscience: Diazepam (Valium)." *ACS Chemical Neuroscience*, vol. 5, no. 4, 2014, pp. 253–260., doi:10.1021/cn5000056.

"Calcium and Vitamin D for Treatment and Prevention of Osteoporosis." *DynaMed*, EBSCO Information Services, 17 Jan. 2018, www.dynamed.com/management/calcium-and-vitamin-d-for-treatment-and-prevention-of-osteoporosis.

Cano, Annmarie, et al. "A Couple-Based Psychological Treatment for Chronic Pain and Relationship Distress." *Cognitive and Behavioral Practice*, vol. 25, no. 1, 2018, pp. 119–134., doi:10.1016/j.cbpra.2017.02.003.

"Carbamazepine." *MedlinePlus*, U.S. National Library of Medicine, 15 Apr. 2019, medlineplus.gov/druginfo/meds/a682237.html.

Cardia, Luigi, et al. "Preclinical and Clinical Pharmacology of Hydrocodone for Chronic Pain: A Mini Review." *Frontiers in Pharmacology*, vol. 9, 1 Oct. 2018, p. 1122., doi:10.3389/fphar.2018.01122.

Carere, Amy, and Robin Orr. "The Impact of Hydrotherapy on a Patient's Perceived Well-Being: a Critical Review of the Literature." *Physical Therapy Reviews*, vol. 21, no. 2, 16 Sept. 2016, pp. 91–101., doi:10.1080/10833196.2016.1228510.

"Carisoprodol." *MedlinePlus*, U.S. National Library of Medicine, 15 Oct. 2018, medlineplus.gov/druginfo/meds/a682578.html.

Carney, Tara, et al. "A Comparative Analysis of Pharmacists' Perspectives on Codeine Use and Misuse – a Three Country Survey." *Substance Abuse Treatment, Prevention, and Policy*, vol. 13, no. 1, 27 Mar. 2018, doi:10.1186/s13011-018-0149-2.

"Carpal Tunnel Release." *Johns Hopkins Medicine*, 2019, www.hopkinsmedicine.org/health/treatment-tests-and-therapies/carpal-tunnel-release.

"Carpal Tunnel Syndrome Fact Sheet." *National Institute of Neurological Disorders and Stroke*, U.S. Department of Health and Human Services, 13 Aug. 2019, www.ninds.nih.gov/Disorders/Patient-Caregiver-Education/Fact-Sheets/Carpal-Tunnel-Syndrome-Fact-sheet.

"Carpal Tunnel Syndrome." *American Society for Surgery of the Hand*, 2015, handcare.assh.org/Anatomy/Details-Page/ArticleID/27950/Carpal-Tunnel-Syndrome.

"Carpal Tunnel Syndrome." DynaMed, EBSCO Information Services, 30 Nov. 2018, www.dynamed.com/condition/carpal-tunnel-syndrome.

Carter, Greg T. "The Argument for Medical Marijuana for the Treatment of Chronic Pain." *Pain Medicine*, vol. 14, no. 6, 2013, pp. 800–800., doi:10.1111/pme.12137_2.

Castro, Jessica, and Maureen F. Cooney. "Intravenous Magnesium in the Management of Postoperative Pain." *Journal of PeriAnesthesia Nursing*, vol. 32, no. 1, Feb. 2017, pp. 72–76., doi:10.1016/j.jopan.2016.11.007.

Castro-Sánchez, Adelaida María, et al. "Hydrotherapy for the Treatment of Pain in People with Multiple Sclerosis: A Randomized Controlled Trial." *Evidence-Based Complementary and Alternative Medicine*, 2012, pp. 1–8., doi:10.1155/2012/473963.

Cazacu, Irina, et al. "Safety Issues of Current Analgesics: an Update." *Medicine and Pharmacy Reports*, vol. 88, no. 2, 15 Apr. 2015, pp. 128–136., doi:10.15386/cjmed-413.

"CDC Guideline for Prescribing Opioids for Chronic Pain." *Centers for Disease Control and Prevention*, 28 Aug. 2019, www.cdc.gov/drugoverdose/prescribing/guideline.html.

Center for Drug Evaluation and Research. "Valproate Anti-Seizure Products Contraindicated for Migraine Preven..." *U.S. Food and Drug Administration*, 26 Feb. 2016, www.fda.gov/drugs/drug-safety-and-availability/fda-drug-safety-communication-valproate-anti-seizure-products-contraindicated-migraine-prevention.

Center for Substance Abuse Treatment. *Substance Abuse and Mental Health Services Administration*, 23 Aug. 2017, www.samhsa.gov/about-us/who-we-are/offices-centers/csat.

Centers of Disease Control and Prevention. "Counterfeit Norco Poses New Danger." *JAMA Network*, vol. 315, no. 22, 14 June 2016, p. 2390., doi:10.1001/jama.2016.6975.

"Cervical Epidural." *Department of Radiology*, University of Wisconsin School of Medicine and Public Health, 18 Dec. 2017, www.radiology.wisc.edu/documents/cervical-epidural/.

"Cervical Radicular Pain and Radiculopathy." Edited by Brian C. Callaghan et al., *DynaMed*, EBSCO Information Services, 18 Nov. 2018, www.dynamed.com/condition/cervical-radicular-pain-and-radiculopathy.

Chang, Jongwha, et al. "Prescription to over-the-Counter Switches in the United States." *Journal of Research in Pharmacy Practice*, vol. 5, no. 3, 2016, pp. 149–154., doi:10.4103/2279-042x.185706.

Chang, Victor T., et al. "Pain and Palliative Medicine." *The Journal of Rehabilitation Research and Development*, vol. 44, no. 2, 2007, p. 279., doi:10.1682/jrrd.2006.06.0067.

Chankrachang, Siwaporn, et al. "Prophylactic Botulinum Type A Toxin Complex (Dysport®) for Migraine Without Aura." *Headache: The Journal of Head and Face Pain*, vol. 51, no. 1, 16 Nov. 2010, pp. 52–63., doi:10.1111/j.1526-4610.2010.01807.x.

Cheatham SW, Lee M, Cain M, Baker R. "The Efficacy of Instrument Assisted Soft Tissue Mobilization: A Systematic Review." Journal of the Canadian Chiropractic Association 60, no. 3. Sept. 2016, pp. 200-211.

Cheatle, Martin D., and Rachel Shmuts. "The Risk and Benefit of Benzodiazepine Use in Patients with Chronic Pain." *Pain Medicine*, vol. 16, no. 2, 2015, pp. 219–221., doi:10.1111/pme.12674.

Check, Devon K., and Ethan M. Basch. "Appropriate Use of Antiemetics to Prevent Chemotherapy-Induced Nausea and Vomiting." *JAMA Oncology*, vol. 3, no. 3, 1 Mar. 2017, pp. 307–309., doi:10.1001/jamaoncol.2016.2616.

Chen, Chia-Hui, and Shih-Ku Lin. "Carbamazepine Treatment of Bipolar Disorder: a Retrospective Evaluation of Naturalistic Long-Term Outcomes." *BMC Psychiatry*, vol. 12, no. 1, 23 May 2012, doi:10.1186/1471-244x-12-47.

Chen, Lucy, and Andreas Michalsen. "Management of Chronic Pain Using Complementary and Integrative Medicine." *Bmj*, 24 Apr. 2017, doi:10.1136/bmj.j1284.

Chen, Yan-Jiao, et al. "What Is the Appropriate Acupuncture Treatment Schedule for Chronic Pain? Review and Analysis of Randomized Controlled Trials." *Evidence-Based Complementary and Alternative Medicine*, 18 June 2019, pp. 1–10., doi:10.1155/2019/5281039.

Cheng, Tianze, et al. "Valium without Dependence? Individual GABAA Receptor Subtype Contribution toward Benzodiazepine Addiction, Tolerance, and Therapeutic Effects." *Neuropsychiatric Disease and Treatment*, vol. 14, 2018, pp. 1351–1361., doi:10.2147/ndt.s164307.

Cherry, Kendra. "How Psychoanalysis Influenced the Field of Psychology." *Verywell Mind*, 13 Oct. 2019, www.verywellmind.com/what-is-psychoanalysis-2795246.

Cheungpasitporn, Wisit, et al. "White Willow Bark Induced Acute Respiratory Distress Syndrome." *North American Journal of Medical Sciences*, vol. 5, no. 5, 2013, p. 330., doi:10.4103/1947-2714.112483.

"Chiropractic Care for Pain Relief." *Harvard Health*, Harvard Medical School, 6 June 2016, www.health.harvard.edu/pain/chiropractic-care-for-pain-relief.

"Chiropractic." *MedlinePlus*, U.S. National Library of Medicine, 28 Jan. 2019, medlineplus.gov/chiropractic.html.

Choi, Jin Young, et al. "Factors That Affect Quality of Dying and Death in Terminal Cancer Patients on Inpatient Palliative Care Units: Perspectives of Bereaved Family Caregivers." *Journal of Pain and Symptom Management*, vol. 45, no. 4, 2013, pp. 735–745., doi:10.1016/j.jpainsymman.2012.04.010.

Chou, Roger, et al. "Comparative Efficacy and Safety of Skeletal Muscle Relaxants for Spasticity and Musculoskeletal Conditions: a Systematic Review." *Journal of Pain and Symptom Management*, vol. 28, no. 2, 2004, pp. 140–175., doi:10.1016/j.jpainsymman.2004.05.002.

———. "Methadone Safety: A Clinical Practice Guideline From the American Pain Society and College on Problems of Drug Dependence, in Collaboration With the Heart Rhythm Society." *The Journal of Pain*, vol. 15, no. 4, 2014, pp. 321–337., doi:10.1016/j.jpain.2014.01.494.

"Chronic Low Back Pain." *DynaMed*, EBSCO Information Services, 30 June 2017, www.dynamed.com/condition/chronic-low-back-pain.

"Chronic Pain and Mental Health: Mental Health America." *Mental Health America*, 2019, www.mhanational.org/chronic-pain-and-mental-health.

"Chronic Rhinosinusitis." *DynaMed*, EBSCO Information Services, 7 Apr. 2016, www.dynamed.com/condition/chronic-rhinosinusitis.

Chughtai, Morad, et al. "Astym® Therapy: a Systematic Review." *Annals of Translational Medicine*, vol. 7, no. 4, Feb. 2019, p. 70., doi:10.21037/atm.2018.11.49.

Cicero, Theodore J. "No End in Sight: The Abuse of Prescription Narcotics." *Cerebrum*, 1 Sept. 2015.

Clark, Stephanie D., et al. "Effect of Integrative Medicine Services on Pain for Hospitalized Patients at an Academic Health Center." *Explore*, vol. 15, no. 1, 2019, pp. 61–64., doi:10.1016/j.explore.2018.07.006.

"Cluster Headache." *DynaMed*, EBSCO Information Services, 20 Mar. 2018, www.dynamed.com/condition/cluster-headache.

"Codeine." *MedlinePlus*, U.S. National Library of Medicine, 15 Mar. 2018, medlineplus.gov/druginfo/meds/a682065.html.

"Cognitive-Behavioral Therapy Skills for Modern Pain Care Practitioners." *Integrative Pain Science Institute*, 31 Aug. 2019, www.integrativepainscienceinstitute.com/cognitive-behavioral-therapy/.

Cohen, N., and J. Cohen-Lévy. "Healing Processes Following Tooth Extraction in Orthodontic Cases." *Journal of Dentofacial Anomalies and Orthodontics*, vol. 17, no. 3, 2014, p. 304., doi:10.1051/odfen/2014006.

"Comfort Measures (Pharmacologic) During Labor." Edited by Allen Shaughnessy and Alan Ehrlich, *DynaMed*, EBSCO Information Services, 13 Aug. 2018, www.dynamed.com/topics/dmp~AN~T116857/Comfort-measures-pharmacologic-during-labor.

Cook, Gareth. "The Science of Healing Thoughts." *Scientific American*, 19 Jan. 2016, www.scientificamerican.com/article/the-science-of-healing-thoughts/.

Cooper, Jeffrey S. "Sedative-Hypnotic Toxicity." *Medscape*, 9 Nov. 2019, emedicine.medscape.com/article/818430-overview.

Corbett, Christina, et al. "A Randomised Comparison of Two 'Stress Control' Programmes: Progressive Muscle Relaxation versus Mindfulness Body Scan." *Mental Health & Prevention*, vol. 15, 2019, p. 200163., doi:10.1016/j.mph.2019.200163.

Cordovilla-Guardia, Sergio, et al. "The Effect of Central Nervous System Depressant, Stimulant and Hallucinogenic Drugs on Injury Severity in Patients Admitted for Trauma." *Gaceta Sanitaria*, vol. 33, no. 1, 2019, pp. 4–9., doi:10.1016/j.gaceta.2017.06.006.

"Corns." *OrthoInfo*, American Academy of Orthopaedic Surgeons, Sept. 2012, orthoinfo.aaos.org/en/diseases–conditions/corns/.

Corr, Charles A., Clyde M. Nabe, and Donna M. Corr. *Death and Dying, Life and Living*. 7th ed. Wadsworth/Cengage Learning, 2013.

"Corticosteroids." *Cleveland Clinic*, 16 Mar. 2015, my.clevelandclinic.org/health/drugs/4812-corticosteroids.

"Counseling and Education for Chronic Low Back Pain." *DynaMed*, EBSCO Information Services, 22 Dec. 2017, www.dynamed.com/topics/dmp~AN~T910282/Counseling-and-education-for-chronic-low-back-pain.

Cour, Peter La, and Marian Petersen. "Effects of Mindfulness Meditation on Chronic Pain: A

Randomized Controlled Trial." *Pain Medicine*, vol. 16, no. 4, 2015, pp. 641–652., doi:10.1111/pme.12605.

Court, C., et al. "Thoracic Disc Herniation: Surgical Treatment." *Orthopaedics & Traumatology: Surgery & Research*, vol. 104, no. 1, 2018, doi:10.1016/j.otsr.2017.04.022.

Courtney, Suzanne Whitney, et al. "Is Garlic Effective in Reducing Cardiovascular Risk Factors?" *Evidence-Based Practice*, 22 July 2019, doi:10.1097/EBP.0000000000000566.

Cousins, Michael J., P. O. Bridenbaugh, et al., eds. *Neural Blockade in Clinical Anesthesia and Management of Pain*. 4th ed. J. B. Lippincott, 2008.

Crisp, Bryan, and David Knox. *Behavioral Family Therapy: An Evidence Based Approach*. Carolina Academic Press, 2009.

Crofford, Leslie J. "Psychological Aspects of Chronic Musculoskeletal Pain." *Best Practice & Research Clinical Rheumatology*, vol. 29, no. 1, 2015, pp. 147–155., doi:10.1016/j.berh.2015.04.027.

Cronkleton, Emily, and Debra Rose Wilson. "Oregano Oil for Cold and Flu: Does It Work?" *Healthline*, 6 Mar. 2018, www.healthline.com/health/oregano-oil-for-cold.

Crosby, Vincent, et al. "Magnesium." *Journal of Pain and Symptom Management*, vol. 45, no. 1, 2013, pp. 137–144., doi:10.1016/j.jpainsymman.2012.10.005.

Cuncic, Arlin. "Chill Out: How to Use Progressive Muscle Relaxation to Quell Anxiety." *Verywell Mind*, 13 July 2019, www.verywellmind.com/how-do-i-practice-progressive-muscle-relaxation-3024400.

Cunningham, Julie, et al. "Benzodiazepine Use in Patients with Chronic Pain in an Interdisciplinary Pain Rehabilitation Program." *Journal of Pain Research*, vol. 10, 2017, pp. 311–317., doi:10.2147/jpr.s123487.

Dail, Clarence W., and Charles Thomas. *Hydrotherapy: Simple Treatments for Common Ailments*. Teach Services, Inc., 2013.

"Daily Aspirin Therapy: Understand the Benefits and Risks." *Mayo Clinic*, Mayo Foundation for Medical Education and Research, 9 Jan. 2019, www.mayoclinic.org/diseases-conditions/heart-disease/in-depth/daily-aspirin-therapy/art-20046797.

Daily, James W., et al. "Efficacy of Turmeric Extracts and Curcumin for Alleviating the Symptoms of Joint Arthritis: A Systematic Review and Meta-Analysis of Randomized Clinical Trials." *Journal of Medicinal Food*, vol. 19, no. 8, 2016, pp. 717–729., doi:10.1089/jmf.2016.3705.

Davies, Claire, et al. "Astym Therapy Improves Function and Range of Motion Following Mastectomy." *Breast Cancer: Targets and Therapy*, vol. 8, 8 Mar. 2016, pp. 39–45., doi:10.2147/bctt.s102598.

Davis, Abigail, and John Robson. "The Dangers of NSAIDs: Look Both Ways." *British Journal of General Practice*, vol. 66, no. 645, Apr. 2016, pp. 172–173., doi:10.3399/bjgp16x684433.

Davis, Jennifer S, et al. "Use of Non-Steroidal Anti-Inflammatory Drugs in US Adults: Changes over Time and by Demographic." *Open Heart*, vol. 4, no. 1, 2017, doi:10.1136/openhrt-2016-000550.

Davis, Kathleen. "Barbiturates: Uses, Side Effects, and Risks." *Medical News Today*, MediLexicon International, 25 June 2018, www.medicalnewstoday.com/articles/310066.php.

Davis, W. Rees, and Bruce D. Johnson. "Prescription Opioid Use, Misuse, and Diversion among Street Drug Users in New York City." *Drug and Alcohol Dependence* vol. 92, 2008, pp. 267–76.

De Cássia Da Silveira E Sá, Rita, et al. "Analgesic-Like Activity of Essential Oil Constituents: An Update." *International Journal of Molecular Sciences*, vol. 18, no. 12, 9 Dec. 2017, p. 2392., doi:10.3390/ijms18122392.

De Sutter, An, et al. "Predicting Prognosis and Effect of Antibiotic Treatment in Rhinosinusitis." *The Annals of Family Medicine*, vol. 4, no. 6, 1 Nov. 2006, pp. 486–493., doi:10.1370/afm.600.

Dean, Carolyn. *The Magnesium Miracle*. 2nd ed., Ballantine Books, 2017.

DeAngelo, Steve. *The Cannabis Manifesto: a New Paradigm for Wellness*. 2nd ed., North Atlantic Books, 2015.

Deckx, Laura, et al. "Nasal Decongestants in Monotherapy for the Common Cold." *Cochrane Database of Systematic Reviews*, vol. 2016, no. 10, 17 Oct. 2016, doi:10.1002/14651858.cd009612.pub2.

"Decongestants: OTC Relief for Congestion." *Familydoctor.org*, American Academy of Family

Physicians, 16 Nov. 2017, familydoctor.org/decongestants-otc-relief-for-congestion/.

Dedeli, Ozden, and Gulten Kaptan. "Spirituality and Religion in Pain and Pain Management." *Health Psychology Research*, vol. 1, no. 3, 23 Sept. 2013, p. 29., doi:10.4081/hpr.2013.e29.

"Deep Brain Stimulation." *American Association of Neurological Surgeons*, 2019, www.aans.org/en/Patients/Neurosurgical-Conditions-and-Treatments/Deep-Brain-Stimulation.

Del Pozo, Jessica. "Biofeedback." *Institute for Chronic Pain*, 2017, www.instituteforchronicpain.org/treating-common-pain/what-is-pain-management/biofeedback.

Desai, Rishi, et al. "Prescription Opioids in Pregnancy and Birth Outcomes: A Review of the Literature." *Journal of Pediatric Genetics*, vol. 4, no. 2, 2015, pp. 56–70., doi:10.1055/s-0035-1556740.

Desantana, Josimari M., et al. "Effectiveness of Transcutaneous Electrical Nerve Stimulation for Treatment of Hyperalgesia and Pain." *Current Rheumatology Reports*, vol. 10, no. 6, 2008, pp. 492–499., doi:10.1007/s11926-008-0080-z.

Deshpande, Amol, and Angela Mailis. "Medical Cannabis and Pain Management: How Might the Role of Cannabis Be Defined in Pain Medicine?" *The Journal of Applied Laboratory Medicine: An AACC Publication*, vol. 2, no. 4, Dec. 2017, pp. 485–488., doi:10.1373/jalm.2017.023184.

"Deviated Septum." *ENT Health*, American Academy of Otolaryngology, Aug. 2018, www.enthealth.org/conditions/deviated-septum/.

"Devil's Claw: MedlinePlus Supplements." *MedlinePlus*, U.S. National Library of Medicine, 22 Mar. 2018, medlineplus.gov/druginfo/natural/984.html.

Devitt, Michael. "Research Finds Acupuncture Effective for Chronic Pain." *American Academy of Family Physicians*, 21 May 2018, www.aafp.org/news/health-of-the-public/20180521acupuncture.html.

"Dextromethorphan." *MedlinePlus*, U.S. National Library of Medicine, 15 Feb. 2018, medlineplus.gov/druginfo/meds/a682492.html.

D'Hotman, Daniel, et al. "Methadone for Prisoners." *The Lancet*, vol. 387, no. 10015, 2016, p. 224., doi:10.1016/s0140-6736(16)00044-1.

"Diazepam." *MedlinePlus*, U.S. National Library of Medicine, 15 July 2019, medlineplus.gov/druginfo/meds/a682047.html.

"Dietary Considerations for Cardiovascular Disease Risk Reduction." *DynaMed*, EBSCO Information Services, 22 Nov. 2017, www.dynamed.com/prevention/dietary-considerations-for-cardiovascular-disease-risk-reduction.

"Dihydroergotamine." *DynaMed*, EBSCO Information Services, www.dynamed.com/drug-monograph/dihydroergotamine.

Dima, Delia, et al. "The Use of Rotation to Fentanyl in Cancer-Related Pain." *Journal of Pain Research*, vol. 10, 2017, pp. 341–348., doi:10.2147/jpr.s121920.

Dirks, April. "The Opioid Epidemic: Impact on Children and Families." *Journal of Psychiatry and Psychiatric Disorders*, vol. 02, no. 01, 2018, pp. 9–11., doi:10.26502/jppd.2572-519x0035.

Djukic, Vojko, et al. "Clinical Outcomes and Quality of Life in Patients with Nasal Polyposis after Functional Endoscopic Sinus Surgery." *European Archives of Oto-Rhino-Laryngology*, vol. 272, no. 1, 24 Apr. 2014, pp. 83–89., doi:10.1007/s00405-014-3054-y.

Donk, Tine Van De, et al. "An Experimental Randomized Study on the Analgesic Effects of Pharmaceutical-Grade Cannabis in Chronic Pain Patients with Fibromyalgia." *Pain*, vol. 160, no. 4, 2019, pp. 860–869., doi:10.1097/j.pain.0000000000001464.

"Don't Let Decongestants Squeeze Your Heart." *Harvard Health Publishing*, Harvard Medical School, 3 Apr. 2019, www.health.harvard.edu/heart-health/dont-let-decongestants-squeeze-your-heart.

Dowbiggin, Ian Robert. *A Merciful End: The Euthanasia Movement in Modern America*. Oxford University Press, 2003.

Dreher, Diane. "Why Do Horses Help Us Heal?" *Psychology Today*, 6 Jan. 2018, www.psychologytoday.com/us/blog/your-personal-renaissance/201801/why-do-horses-help-us-heal.

Driscoll, T, et al. "The Global Burden of Occupationally Related Low Back Pain: Estimates from the Global Burden of Disease 2010 Study." *Annals of the Rheumatic Diseases*, vol. 73, no. 6, 24 Mar. 2014, pp. 975–981., doi:10.1136/annrheumdis-2013-204631.

Du, Jerry, et al. "Microdiscectomy for the Treatment of Lumbar Disc Herniation: An Evaluation of Reoperations and Long-Term Outcomes." *Evidence-Based Spine-Care Journal*, vol. 05, no. 02, Oct. 2014, pp. 77–86., doi:10.1055/s-0034-1386750.

Duenas, María, et al. "A Review of Chronic Pain Impact on Patients, Their Social Environment and the Health Care System." *Journal of Pain Research*, vol. 9, 2016, pp. 457–467., doi:10.2147/jpr.s105892.

Dugdale, David C. "Over-the-Counter Pain Relievers." *MedlinePlus*, U.S. National Library of Medicine, 12 Oct. 2018, medlineplus.gov/ency/article/002123.htm.

Dunford, Emma, and Miles Thompson. "Relaxation and Mindfulness in Pain: A Review." *Reviews in Pain*, vol. 4, no. 1, 2010, pp. 18–22., doi:10.1177/204946371000400105.

Earley, Paul H., and Torin Finver. "Addiction to Propofol." *Journal of Addiction Medicine*, vol. 7, no. 3, 2013, pp. 169–176., doi:10.1097/adm.0b013e3182872901.

Eaves, Emery R. "'Just Advil': Harm Reduction and Identity Construction in the Consumption of over-the-Counter Medication for Chronic Pain." *Social Science & Medicine*, vol. 146, 19 Oct. 2015, pp. 147–154., doi:10.1016/j.socscimed.2015.10.033.

Ebadi, Safoora, et al. "Therapeutic Ultrasound for Chronic Low-Back Pain." *Cochrane Database of Systematic Reviews*, 14 Mar. 2014, doi:10.1002/14651858.cd009169.pub2.

Edens, Pat Stanfill, et al. "Developing and Financing a Palliative Care Program." *American Journal of Hospice and Palliative Medicine®*, vol. 25, no. 5, 2008, pp. 379–384., doi:10.1177/1049909108319269.

Ellis, Deborah. " Holistic Approaches to Chronic Pain." *U.S. Pain Foundation*, 6 Mar. 2019, uspainfoundation.org/blog/holistic-approaches-to-chronic-pain/.

Elmokhallalati, Yousuf, et al. "Specialist Palliative Care Support Is Associated with Improved Pain Relief at Home during the Last 3 Months of Life in Patients with Advanced Disease: Analysis of 5-Year Data from the National Survey of Bereaved People (VOICES)." *BMC Medicine*, vol. 17, no. 1, 22 Mar. 2019, doi:10.1186/s12916-019-1287-8.

Encinosa, William, and Amy J. Davidoff. "Changes in Antiemetic Overuse in Response to Choosing Wisely Recommendations." *JAMA Oncology*, vol. 3, no. 3, Mar. 2017, p. 320., doi:10.1001/jamaoncol.2016.2530.

"Epidural Injections." *RadiologyInfo.org*, Radiological Society of North America, Inc, 20 Mar. 2019, www.radiologyinfo.org/en/info.cfm?pg=epidural.

Erdek, Michael. "Pain Medicine and Palliative Care as an Alternative to Euthanasia in End-of-Life Cancer Care." *The Linacre Quarterly*, vol. 82, no. 2, 2015, pp. 128–134., doi:10.1179/2050854915y.0000000003.

Erickson, Mia, et al. "Hand Pain and Sensory Deficits: Carpal Tunnel Syndrome." *Journal of Orthopaedic & Sports Physical Therapy*, vol. 49, no. 5, 2019, doi:10.2519/jospt.2019.0301.

Erlach, Stephen P. "Sedative, Hypnotic, Anxiolytic Use Disorders Treatment & Management." *Medscape*, 9 Nov. 2019, emedicine.medscape.com/article/290585-treatment.

Eustice, Carol. "*Boswellia* Frankincense for Osteoarthritis." *Verywell Health*, 15 May 2019, www.verywellhealth.com/Boswellia-for-osteoarthritis-2551981.

Evans, Nicole. *Herbal Remedies: the Ultimate Guide to Herbal Remedies for Pain Relief, Stress Relief, Weight Loss, and Skin Conditions*. VDV Publishing, 2014.

"Exercise Therapy for Chronic Low Back Pain." *DynaMed*, EBSCO Information Services, 27 Nov. 2017, www.dynamed.com/management/exercise-therapy-for-chronic-low-back-pain.

Falowski, Steven M. "Deep Brain Stimulation for Chronic Pain." *Current Pain and Headache Reports*, vol. 19, no. 7, July 2015, doi:10.1007/s11916-015-0504-1.

Fanous, Summer, and Natalie Butler. "The Health Potential of Rosemary." *Healthline*, 27 May 2016, www.healthline.com/health/rosemary-health-potential.

Farrell, Sarah, et al. "The Current State of Deep Brain Stimulation for Chronic Pain and Its Context in Other Forms of Neuromodulation." *Brain Sciences*, vol. 8, no. 8, 20 Aug. 2018, p. 158., doi:10.3390/brainsci8080158.

Faust, Katherine, and Charles D. Jennings. "Carpal Tunnel Syndrome." *OrthoInfo*,

American Academy of Orthopaedic Surgeons, July 2016, orthoinfo.aaos.org/topic.cfm?topic=a00005.

"FDA and Marijuana." *U.S. Food and Drug Administration*, 19 June 2019, www.fda.gov/news-events/public-health-focus/fda-and-marijuana.

Fei, Joni Teoh Bing, et al. "Effectiveness of Methadone Maintenance Therapy and Improvement in Quality of Life Following a Decade of Implementation." *Journal of Substance Abuse Treatment*, vol. 69, 2016, pp. 50–56., doi:10.1016/j.jsat.2016.07.006.

Felson, David T. "Safety of Nonsteroidal Antiinflammatory Drugs." *New England Journal of Medicine*, vol. 375, no. 26, 29 Dec. 2016, pp. 2595–2596., doi:10.1056/nejme1614257.

Feng, James, et al. "Total Knee Arthroplasty: Improving Outcomes with a Multidisciplinary Approach." *Journal of Multidisciplinary Healthcare*, vol. 11, 2018, pp. 63–73., doi:10.2147/jmdh.s140550.

"Fentanyl." *MedlinePlus*, U.S. National Library of Medicine, 15 Oct. 2019, medlineplus.gov/druginfo/meds/a605043.html.

Filshie, Jacqueline, et al. *Medical Acupuncture: a Western Scientific Approach*. 2nd ed., Elsevier, 2016.

Fine, Perry G. "Long-Term Consequences of Chronic Pain: Mounting Evidence for Pain as a Neurological Disease and Parallels with Other Chronic Disease States." *Pain Medicine*, vol. 12, no. 7, 2011, pp. 996–1004., doi:10.1111/j.1526-4637.2011.01187.x.

——. "Bridging the Gap: Pain Medicine and Palliative Care: Table 1." *Pain Medicine*, vol. 14, no. 9, 2013, pp. 1277–1279., doi:10.1111/pme.12187.

Fishman, Loren. *Healing Yoga: Proven Postures to Treat Twenty Common Ailments – from Backache to Bone Loss, Shoulder Pain to Bunions, and More*. W.W. Norton & Company, 2015.

Flores, Diane. *Nonsteroidal Anti-Inflammatory Drugs (NSAIDs): Common Uses, Risks and Effectiveness*. Nova Biomedical, 2017.

Florida Atlantic University. "First Study to Show Chair Yoga as Effective Alternative Treatment for Osteoarthritis." *ScienceDaily*, 11 Jan. 2017, www.sciencedaily.com/releases/2017/01/170111091417.htm.

Fluyau, Dimy, et al. "Challenges of the Pharmacological Management of Benzodiazepine Withdrawal, Dependence, and Discontinuation." *Therapeutic Advances in Psychopharmacology*, vol. 8, no. 5, 9 Feb. 2018, pp. 147–168., doi:10.1177/2045125317753340.

Flynn, Daniel, et al. "Dialectical Behaviour Therapy for Treating Adults and Adolescents with Emotional and Behavioural Dysregulation: Study Protocol of a Coordinated Implementation in a Publicly Funded Health Service." *BMC Psychiatry*, vol. 18, no. 1, 26 Feb. 2018, doi:10.1186/s12888-018-1627-9.

Follett, Kenneth A. *Neurosurgical Pain Management*. W.B. Saunders, 2004.

Fookes, C. "Nonsteroidal Anti-Inflammatory Drugs." *Drugs.com*, 22 Mar. 2018, www.drugs.com/drug-class/nonsteroidal-anti-inflammatory-agents.html.

"Foot Complications." *American Diabetes Association*, 2019, www.diabetes.org/diabetes/complications/foot-complications.

"Foot Health." *American Podiatric Medical Association*, 2019, www.apma.org/Patients/FootHealthList.cfm?navItemNumber=25223.

Ford, Jason A. "The Prescription Drug Problem We Are Missing: Risks Associated with the Misuse of Tranquilizers and Sedatives." *Journal of Adolescent Health*, vol. 63, no. 6, 2018, pp. 665–666., doi:10.1016/j.jadohealth.2018.09.007.

Francis, G. J., et al. "Acute and Preventive Pharmacologic Treatment of Cluster Headache." *Neurology*, vol. 75, no. 5, 2 Aug. 2010, pp. 463–473., doi:10.1212/wnl.0b013e3181eb58c8.

Frank, Lone. *The Pleasure Shock: the Rise of Deep Brain Stimulation and Its Forgotten Inventor*. Dutton, 2018.

Fransen, Marlene, and Sara Mcconnell. "Exercise for Osteoarthritis of the Knee." *Cochrane Database of Systematic Reviews*, 8 Oct. 2008, doi:10.1002/14651858.cd004376.pub2.

"Frequently Asked Questions." *National Headache Foundation*, 2019, headaches.org/about/frequently-asked-questions/.

Friedberg, Robert D. "A Cognitive-Behavioral Approach to Family Therapy." *Journal of Contemporary Psychotherapy*, vol. 36, no. 4, 2006, pp. 159–165., doi:10.1007/s10879-006-9020-2.

Friedman, Robi. "Individual or Group Therapy? Indications for Optimal Therapy." *Group Analysis*, vol. 46, no. 2, 22 Apr. 2013, pp. 164–170., doi:10.1177/0533316413483691.

Frizon, Leonardo A, et al. "Deep Brain Stimulation for Pain in the Modern Era: A Systematic Review." *Neurosurgery*, 25 Feb. 2019, doi:10.1093/neuros/nyy552.

Fukuda, Ken-Ichi. "Diagnosis and Treatment of Abnormal Dental Pain." *Journal of Dental Anesthesia and Pain Medicine*, vol. 16, no. 1, 2016, p. 1., doi:10.17245/jdapm.2016.16.1.1.

Gaffey, Andrew, et al. "The Effects of Curcumin on Musculoskeletal Pain: a Systematic Review Protocol." *JBI Database of Systematic Reviews and Implementation Reports*, vol. 13, no. 2, 2015, pp. 59–73., doi:10.11124/jbisrir-2015-1684.

Gass, Natalia, et al. "Differences between Ketamine's Short-Term and Long-Term Effects on Brain Circuitry in Depression." *Translational Psychiatry*, vol. 9, no. 1, 28 June 2019, doi:10.1038/s41398-019-0506-6.

Gatti, Roberto, et al. "Efficacy of Trunk Balance Exercises for Individuals With Chronic Low Back Pain: A Randomized Clinical Trial." *Journal of Orthopaedic & Sports Physical Therapy*, vol. 41, no. 8, 2011, pp. 542–552., doi:10.2519/jospt.2011.3413.

Gauntlett-Gilbert, Jeremy, et al. "Benzodiazepines May Be Worse Than Opioids." *The Clinical Journal of Pain*, vol. 32, no. 4, 2016, pp. 285–291., doi:10.1097/ajp.0000000000000253.

Geneen, Louise J, et al. "Physical Activity and Exercise for Chronic Pain in Adults: an Overview of Cochrane Reviews." *Cochrane Database of Systematic Reviews*, 24 Apr. 2017, doi:10.1002/14651858.cd011279.pub3.

"General Anesthesia—Interactive Tutorial." Medline Plus, 2013. Katz, Jordan. *Atlas of Regional Anesthesia*. 4th ed. Appleton & Lange, 2010.

George, Renuka, et al. "'Oh Mg!' Magnesium: A Powerful Tool in the Perioperative Setting." *ASRA News*, American Society of Regional Anesthesia and Pain Medicine, Aug. 2018, www.asra.com/asra-news/article/105/oh-mg-magnesium-a-powerful-tool-in-the.

Ghanavatian, Shirin, and Armen Derian. "Baclofen." *StatPearls*, 1 Oct. 2019.

Giacolini, Teodosio, and Ugo Sabatello. "Psychoanalysis and Affective Neuroscience. The Motivational/Emotional System of Aggression in Human Relations." *Frontiers in Psychology*, vol. 9, 14 Jan. 2019, doi:10.3389/fpsyg.2018.02475.

Gibson, William, et al. "Transcutaneous Electrical Nerve Stimulation (TENS) for Chronic Pain an Overview of Cochrane Reviews." *Cochrane Database of Systematic Reviews*, vol. 4, Apr. 2019, doi:10.1002/14651858.CD011890.pub3.

Gierbolini, Jaime, et al. "Carbamazepine-Related Antiepileptic Drugs for the Treatment of Epilepsy - a Comparative Review." *Expert Opinion on Pharmacotherapy*, vol. 17, no. 7, 21 Mar. 2016, pp. 885–888., doi:10.1517/14656566.2016.1168399.

Giggins, Oonagh M, et al. "Biofeedback in Rehabilitation." *Journal of NeuroEngineering and Rehabilitation*, vol. 10, no. 60, 18 June 2013, doi:10.1186/1743-0003-10-60.

Giller, Cole A. "The Neurosurgical Treatment of Pain." *Archives of Neurology*, vol. 60, no. 11, Nov. 2003, pp. 1537–1540., doi:10.1001/archneur.60.11.1537.

Gillihan, Seth J. "What Happens When Partners Fight Chronic Pain Together?" *Psychology Today*, 19 June 2017, www.psychologytoday.com/us/blog/think-act-be/201706/what-happens-when-partners-fight-chronic-pain-together.

Gladding, Samuel T. *Family Therapy: History, Theory, and Practice*. 7th ed., Pearson, 2019.

Godman, Heidi, and Zara Risoldi Cochrane. "Understanding Hydrocodone Addiction." *Healthline*, 8 Jan. 2019, www.healthline.com/health/understanding-hydrocodone-addiction.

Gogineni, Hrishikesh C., et al. "Transition to Outpatient Total Hip and Knee Arthroplasty: Experience at an Academic Tertiary Care Center." *Arthroplasty Today*, vol. 5, no. 1, Mar. 2019, pp. 100–105., doi:10.1016/j.artd.2018.10.008.

Gokhale, Sankalp, and Ciro Ramos-Estebanez. "An Interesting Case of Barbiturate Automatism and Review of Literature." *Case Reports in Neurological Medicine*, vol. 2013, 2013, pp. 1–2., doi:10.1155/2013/713065.

Goldenberg, Irene, et al. *Family Therapy: An Overview*. 9th ed., Cengage Learning, 2017.

Goldman, Rena, and Debra Rose Wilson. "What Is Comfrey?" *Healthline*, 18 July 2016, www.healthline.com/health/what-is-comfrey.

Goldstein, Leonard, and Scott Falkowitz. "Pain Management in a Palliative Care Setting." *Practical Pain Management*, 20 Dec. 2011, www.practicalpainmanagement.com/resources/hospice/pain-management-palliative-care-setting.

Gosepath, Jan, and Wolf J. Mann. "Current Concepts in Therapy of Chronic Rhinosinusitis and Nasal Polyposis." *Orl*, vol. 67, no. 3, 2005, pp. 125–136., doi:10.1159/000086075.

Gotter, Ana, and Christine Frank. "What to Expect During a Tooth Extraction." *Healthline*, 9 Feb. 2018, www.healthline.com/health/tooth-extraction.

Goyal, Ankit, et al. "Flax and Flaxseed Oil: an Ancient Medicine & Modern Functional Food." *Journal of Food Science and Technology*, vol. 51, no. 9, 10 Jan. 2014, pp. 1633–1653., doi:10.1007/s13197-013-1247-9.

Grady, Sarah E., et al. "Ketamine for the Treatment of Major Depressive Disorder and Bipolar Depression: A Review of the Literature." *Mental Health Clinician*, vol. 7, no. 1, 2017, pp. 16–23., doi:10.9740/mhc.2017.01.016.

Greive, Kerryn, et al. "Evaluation of a Topical Treatment for the Relief of Sensitive Skin." *Clinical, Cosmetic and Investigational Dermatology*, vol. 8, 2015, p. 405., doi:10.2147/ccid.s87509.

Grinspoon, Peter. "Kratom: Fear-Worthy Foliage or Beneficial Botanical?" *Harvard Health Publishing*, Harvard Medical School, 26 Sept. 2019, www.health.harvard.edu/blog/kratom-fear-worthy-foliage-or-beneficial-botanical-2019080717466.

—. "Medical Marijuana." *Harvard Health Blog*, Harvard Medical School, 25 June 2019, www.health.harvard.edu/blog/medical-marijuana-2018011513085.

Groninger, Hunter, and Jaya Vijayan. "Pharmacologic Management of Pain at the End of Life." *American Family Physician*, vol. 90, no. 1, July 2014, pp. 26–32.

Grover, Casey, et al. "Transcutaneous Electrical Nerve Stimulation (TENS) in the ED for Pain Relief: A Preliminary Study of Feasibility and Efficacy." *Western Journal of Emergency Medicine*, vol. 19, no. 5, 9 Aug. 2018, pp. 872–876., doi:10.5811/westjem.2018.7.38447.

Gugliotta, Marinella, et al. "Surgical versus Conservative Treatment for Lumbar Disc Herniation: a Prospective Cohort Study." *BMJ Open*, vol. 6, no. 12, 2016, doi:10.1136/bmjopen-2016-012938.

Gulur, Padma, et al. "Morphine versus Hydromorphone: Does Choice of Opioid Influence Outcomes?" *Pain Research and Treatment*, 1 Nov. 2015, pp. 1–6., doi:10.1155/2015/482081.

Guyuron, Bahman, et al. "A Placebo-Controlled Surgical Trial of the Treatment of Migraine Headaches." *Plastic and Reconstructive Surgery*, vol. 124, no. 2, 2009, pp. 461–468., doi:10.1097/prs.0b013e3181adcf6a.

Gwinnell, Esther, and Christine Adamec. *The Encyclopedia of Drug Abuse*. Facts On File, 2008.

Haber, Stacy L., and Shareen Y. El-Ibiary. "Peppermint Oil for Treatment of Irritable Bowel Syndrome." *American Journal of Health-System Pharmacy*, vol. 73, no. 2, 15 Jan. 2016, pp. 22–31., doi:10.2146/ajhp140801.

Håkanson, Margareta, et al. "The Horse as the Healer—A Study of Riding in Patients with Back Pain." *Journal of Bodywork and Movement Therapies*, vol. 13, no. 1, 2009, pp. 43–52., doi:10.1016/j.jbmt.2007.06.002.

Hall, Kevin P., et al. "Cannabis and Pain: A Clinical Review." *Cannabis and Cannabinoid Research*, vol. 2, no. 1, 1 May 2017, pp. 96–104., doi:10.1089/can.2017.0017.

"Hallux Valgus and Bunion." *DynaMed*, EBSCO Information Services, 22 Nov. 2017, www.dynamed.com/condition/hallux-valgus-and-bunion.

"Hammer Toe." *DynaMed*, EBSCO Information Services, 30 Mar. 2015, www.dynamed.com/condition/hammer-toe.

Han, Xuesheng, and Tory L. Parker. "Anti-Inflammatory, Tissue Remodeling, Immunomodulatory, and Anticancer Activities of Oregano (Origanum Vulgare) Essential Oil in a Human Skin Disease Model." *Biochimie Open*, vol. 4, 2017, pp. 73–77., doi:10.1016/j.biopen.2017.02.005.

Hanson, Glen R., Peter J. Venturelli, and Annette E. Fleckenstein. *Drugs and Society*. 11th ed. Sudbury, MA: Jones, 2012.

Harari, Michal Doron. "'To Be On Stage Means To Be Alive' Theatre Work with Education Undergraduates as a Promoter of Students' Mental Resilience." *Procedia - Social and Behavioral Sciences*, vol. 209, 2015, pp. 161–166., doi:10.1016/j.sbspro.2015.11.272.

Hardy, Sheila, et al. "Transcranial Magnetic Stimulation in Clinical Practice." *BJPsych Advances*, vol. 22, no. 6, 2016, pp. 373–379., doi:10.1192/apt.bp.115.015206.

Harris, Leah S., et al. "Astym® Therapy Improves FOTO® Outcomes for Patients with Musculoskeletal Disorders: an Observational Study." *Annals of Translational Medicine*, vol. 7, no. S7, 2019, doi:10.21037/atm.2019.04.09.

Hasan, Aliya, and Valmiki Sharma. "Substance Abuse and Conscious Sedation: Theoretical and Practical Considerations." *British Dental Journal*, vol. 227, no. 10, 2019, pp. 923–927., doi:10.1038/s41415-019-0897-z.

Hassamal, Sameer, et al. "Tramadol: Understanding the Risk of Serotonin Syndrome and Seizures." *The American Journal of Medicine*, vol. 131, no. 11, 2018, doi:10.1016/j.amjmed.2018.04.025.

He, Hong-Gu, et al. "The Effectiveness of Therapeutic Play Intervention in Reducing Perioperative Anxiety, Negative Behaviors, and Postoperative Pain in Children Undergoing Elective Surgery: A Systematic Review." *Pain Management Nursing*, vol. 16, no. 3, 2015, pp. 425–439., doi:10.1016/j.pmn.2014.08.011.

"Headache Information Page." *National Institute of Neurological Disorders and Stroke*, U.S. Department of Health and Human Services, 11 Oct. 2019, www.ninds.nih.gov/Disorders/All-Disorders/Headache-Information-Page.

Health.com. "Real Life Strategies for Coping with Chronic Pain." *Health.com*, 29 Feb. 2016, www.health.com/health/condition-article/0,20189626,00.html.

Healthwise Staff. "Wrist Care: Preventing Carpal Tunnel Syndrome." *Penn Medicine Lancaster General Health*, 26 June 2019, www.lancastergeneralhealth.org/healthwise-library/healthwise-article?documentId=tn9041.

"Healthy Feet: Preventing and Treating Common Foot Problems." *Harvard Health Publishing*, Harvard Medical School, 2019, www.health.harvard.edu/special-health-reports/Foot_Care_Basics.

"Heel Pain." *FootCareMD*, American Orthopaedic Foot & Ankle Society, 2019, www.footcaremd.org/conditions-treatments/heel/heel-pain.

Heffer, Taylor, and Teena Willoughby. "A Count of Coping Strategies: A Longitudinal Study Investigating an Alternative Method to Understanding Coping and Adjustment." *Plos One*, vol. 12, no. 10, 5 Oct. 2017, doi:10.1371/journal.pone.0186057.

Heitler, Susan. "Anxiety Treatment: Should You Be Wary of Anxiety Medication?" *Psychology Today*, Sussex Publishers, 20 Jan. 2017, www.psychologytoday.com/us/blog/resolution-not-conflict/201701/anxiety-treatment-should-you-be-wary-anxiety-medication.

Heller, Jacob L. "Barbiturate Intoxication and Overdose." *MedlinePlus*. National Library of Medicine, 15 Jan. 2014.

Herrera-Gómez, Antonio, et al. "Risk Assessments of Epidural Analgesia During Labor and Delivery." *Clinical Nursing Research*, vol. 27, no. 7, 28 July 2017, pp. 841–852., doi:10.1177/1054773817722689.

Hertz, Sharon. "The Benefits and Risks of Pain Relievers: Q & A on NSAIDs." *U.S. Food and Drug Administration*, 24 Sept. 2015, www.fda.gov/consumers/consumer-updates/benefits-and-risks-pain-relievers-q-nsaids-sharon-hertz-md.

Hewlings, Susan, and Douglas Kalman. "Curcumin: A Review of Its' Effects on Human Health." *Foods*, vol. 6, no. 10, 22 Oct. 2017, p. 92., doi:10.3390/foods6100092.

Hill, John. *Valerian. or, the Virtues of That Root in Nervous Disorders*. 2nd ed., Gale Ecco, 2018.

Hillier, Susan, and Anthea Worley. "The Effectiveness of the Feldenkrais Method: A Systematic Review of the Evidence." *Evidence-Based Complementary and Alternative Medicine*, 8 Apr. 2015, pp. 1–12., doi:10.1155/2015/752160.

Hilton, Lara, et al. "Mindfulness Meditation for Chronic Pain: Systematic Review and Meta-Analysis." *Annals of Behavioral Medicine*, vol. 51, no. 2, 22 Sept. 2016, pp. 199–213., doi:10.1007/s12160-016-9844-2.

Hines, Roberta L., and Katherine Marschall. *Stoelting's Anesthesia and Co-Existing Disease*, 7th ed. Elsevier, 2017.

Ho, Kok Yuen, et al. "Nonsteroidal Anti-Inflammatory Drugs in Chronic Pain: Implications of New Data for Clinical Practice." *Journal of Pain Research*, vol. 11, 2018, pp. 1937–1948., doi:10.2147/jpr.s168188.

Ho, Rainbow T H, et al. "Psychophysiological Effects of Dance Movement Therapy and Physical Exercise on Older Adults With Mild Dementia: A Randomized Controlled Trial." *The Journals of Gerontology: Series B*, 2018, doi:10.1093/geronb/gby145.

Holland, Kimberly, and Alyson Lozicki. "Vicodin vs. Percocet for Pain Reduction." *Healthline*, 30 Nov. 2017, www.healthline.com/health/pain-relief/vicodin-vs-percocet.

Hong, Bosun, et al. "Minimally Invasive Vertical versus Conventional Tooth Extraction." *The Journal of the American Dental Association*, vol. 149, no. 8, 2018, pp. 688–695., doi:10.1016/j.adaj.2018.03.022.

Hongratanaworakit, Tapanee, et al. "Development of Aroma Massage Oil for Relieving Muscle Pain and Satisfaction Evaluation in Humans." *Journal of Applied Pharmaceutical Science*, vol. 8, no. 4, 2018, pp. 126–130., doi:10.7324/japs.2018.8418.

Hooten, W. Michael. "Chronic Pain and Mental Health Disorders." *Mayo Clinic Proceedings*, vol. 91, no. 7, 2016, pp. 955–970., doi:10.1016/j.mayocp.2016.04.029.

Horsfall, Joseph T., and Jon E. Sprague. "The Pharmacology and Toxicology of the 'Holy Trinity.'" *Basic & Clinical Pharmacology & Toxicology*, vol. 120, no. 2, 2016, pp. 115–119., doi:10.1111/bcpt.12655.

"Hospice Care." *National Hospice and Palliative Care Organization*, 20 Feb. 2019, www.nhpco.org/about/hospice-care.

Hospital for Special Surgery. "Foot Pain? New Study Says Look at Hip and Knee for Complete Diagnosis." *ScienceDaily*, 19 Sept. 2017, www.sciencedaily.com/releases/2017/09/170919181533.htm.

Hou, Wen-Hsuan, et al. "Treatment Effects of Massage Therapy in Depressed People." The Journal of Clinical Psychiatry, vol. 71, no. 07, 2010, pp. 894–901., doi:10.4088/jcp.09r05009blu.

"How to Spell Pain Relief in the Wake of COX-2 Problems." *Harvard Health*, Harvard Medical School, Mar. 2014, www.health.harvard.edu/newsletter_article/How_to_spell_pain_relief_in_the_wake_of_COX-2_problems.

Huang, Alison, et al. "The Effect of Ultralow-Dose Transdermal Estradiol on Sexual Function in Postmenopausal Women." *American Journal of Obstetrics and Gynecology*, vol. 198, no. 3, 2008, doi:10.1016/j.ajog.2007.09.039.

Huang, Hui-Chuan, et al. "Reminiscence Therapy Improves Cognitive Functions and Reduces Depressive Symptoms in Elderly People With Dementia: A Meta-Analysis of Randomized Controlled Trials." *Journal of the American Medical Directors Association*, vol. 16, no. 12, 2015, pp. 1087–1094., doi:10.1016/j.jamda.2015.07.010.

Huang, S., et al. "The Effectiveness of Bright Light Therapy on Depressive Symptoms in Older Adults with Nonseasonal Depression." *International Journal of Evidence-Based Healthcare*, vol. 14, 2016, doi:10.1097/01.xeb.0000511626.75195.51.

"Hydrocodone Combination Products." *MedlinePlus*, U.S. National Library of Medicine, 15 Oct. 2019, medlineplus.gov/druginfo/meds/a601006.html.

"Hydrocodone." *MedlinePlus*, U.S. National Library of Medicine, 15 March 2018. https://medlineplus.gov/druginfo/meds/a614045.html

Inaba, Darryl S., William E. Cohen, and Michael E. Holstein. Uppers, Downers, All Arounders: Physical and Mental Effects of Psychoactive Drugs. 8th ed. CNS, 2014.

Inciardi, James A., et al. "Mechanisms of Prescription Drug Diversion among Drug-Involved Cluband Street-Based Populations." *Pain Medicine* vol. 8.no. 2, 2007, pp. 171–83.

Ingraham, Paul. "Hydrotherapy: Water Powered Rehab." *PainScience.com*, 1 Aug. 2016, www.painscience.com/articles/hydrotherapy.php.

——. "Massage Therapy: Does It Work?" PainScience.com, 18 July 2018, www.painscience.com/articles/does-massage-work.php.

International Headache Society. "The International Classification of Headache Disorders, 3rd

Edition." *Cephalalgia*, vol. 38, no. 1, 2018, pp. 1–211., doi:10.1177/0333102417738202.

Interrante, Julia D., et al. "Risk Comparison for Prenatal Use of Analgesics and Selected Birth Defects, National Birth Defects Prevention Study 1997–2011." *Annals of Epidemiology*, vol. 27, no. 10, 2017, pp. 645–653., doi:10.1016/j.annepidem.2017.09.003.

Iram, Farah, et al. "Phytochemistry and Potential Therapeutic Actions of Boswellic Acids: A Mini-Review." *Asian Pacific Journal of Tropical Biomedicine*, vol. 7, no. 6, 2017, pp. 513–523., doi:10.1016/j.apjtb.2017.05.001.

Iverach, Lisa, et al. "Death Anxiety and Its Role in Psychopathology: Reviewing the Status of a Transdiagnostic Construct." *Clinical Psychology Review*, vol. 34, no. 7, 2014, pp. 580–593., doi:10.1016/j.cpr.2014.09.002.

Ivker, Rav. *Cannabis for Chronic Pain: a Proven Prescription for Using Marijuana to Relieve Your Pain and Heal Your Life*. Touchstone, 2017.

Jacob, Julie A. "As Opioid Prescribing Guidelines Tighten, Mindfulness Meditation Holds Promise for Pain Relief." *Jama*, vol. 315, no. 22, 14 June 2016, p. 2385., doi:10.1001/jama.2016.4875.

Jacobson, Brian C., et al. "Postmenopausal Hormone Use and Symptoms of Gastroesophageal Reflux." *Archives of Internal Medicine*, vol. 168, no. 16, 8 Sept. 2008, p. 1798., doi:10.1001/archinte.168.16.1798.

Janicak, Philip, and Mehmet E. Dokucu. "Transcranial Magnetic Stimulation for the Treatment of Major Depression." *Neuropsychiatric Disease and Treatment*, 2015, p. 1549., doi:10.2147/ndt.s67477.

Jantos, Marek, and Hosen Kiat. "Prayer as Medicine: How Much Have We Learned?" *Medical Journal of Australia*, vol. 186, no. S10, 2007, doi:10.5694/j.1326-5377.2007.tb01041.x.

Javaherian, Atash, and Pasha Latifpour. *Acetaminophen: Properties, Clinical Uses and Adverse Effects*. Nova Science, 2012.

Jermakowicz, Walter J., et al. "Deep Brain Stimulation Improves the Symptoms and Sensory Signs of Persistent Central Neuropathic Pain from Spinal Cord Injury: A Case Report." *Frontiers in Human Neuroscience*, vol. 11, 6 Apr. 2017, doi:10.3389/fnhum.2017.00177.

Jeurgens, Jeffrey, and Theresa Parisi. "Morphine Addiction and Abuse." *AddictionCenter*, 12 Sept. 2019, www.addictioncenter.com/opiates/morphine/.

——. "Oxycodone Addiction and Abuse." *AddictionCenter*, 16 July 2019, www.addictioncenter.com/opiates/oxycodone/.

——. "Tramadol Addiction and Abuse." *AddictionCenter*, 16 July 2019, www.addictioncenter.com/opiates/tramadol/.

Jimenez, Xavier F., et al. "A Systematic Review of Atypical Antipsychotics in Chronic Pain Management." *The Clinical Journal of Pain*, vol. 34, no. 6, 2018, pp. 585–591., doi:10.1097/ajp.0000000000000567.

Johannes, Laura. "A Plant to Ease Muscle and Joint Pain." *The Wall Street Journal*, Dow Jones & Company, 20 Apr. 2015, www.wsj.com/articles/a-plant-to-ease-muscle-and-joint-pain-1429568686.

——. "Can Mint Make Migraines Less Miserable?" *The Wall Street Journal*, Dow Jones & Company, 19 Oct. 2015, www.wsj.com/articles/can-mint-make-migraines-less-miserable-1445271218.

Johnson, Brian, and Daniela Flores Mosri. "The Neuropsychoanalytic Approach: Using Neuroscience as the Basic Science of Psychoanalysis." *Frontiers in Psychology*, vol. 7, 13 Oct. 2016, doi:10.3389/fpsyg.2016.01459.

Johnson, Jon. "Turmeric for Rheumatoid Arthritis: Does It Work?" *Medical News Today*, MediLexicon International, 19 June 2019, www.medicalnewstoday.com/articles/325508.php.

Jones, Mark R., et al. "A Brief History of the Opioid Epidemic and Strategies for Pain Medicine." *Pain and Therapy*, vol. 7, no. 1, 24 Apr. 2018, pp. 13–21., doi:10.1007/s40122-018-0097-6.

Jonkman, Kelly, et al. "Ketamine for Pain." *F1000Research*, vol. 6, 20 Sept. 2017, p. 1711., doi:10.12688/f1000research.11372.1.

Joseph, Andrew. "New Details Revealed about Purdue's Marketing of OxyContin." *STAT*, 18 Jan. 2019, www.statnews.com/2019/01/15/massachusetts-purdue-lawsuit-new-details/.

Jun, Yang Suk, et al. "Effect of Eucalyptus Oil Inhalation on Pain and Inflammatory Responses after Total Knee Replacement: A Randomized Clinical Trial." *Evidence-Based Complementary and Alternative Medicine*, 2013, pp. 1–7., doi:10.1155/2013/502727.

Kaklauskas, Francis J., and Les R. Greene. *Core Principles of Group Psychotherapy: a Training Manual for Theory, Research, and Practice*. Routledge, 2019.

Kamangar, Farin, et al. "Opium Use: an Emerging Risk Factor for Cancer?" *The Lancet Oncology*, vol. 15, no. 2, 2014, doi:10.1016/s1470-2045(13)70550-3.

Kaplan, Gary, and Donna Beech. *Total Recovery: Solving the Mystery of Chronic Pain and Depression: How We Get Sick, Why We Stay Sick, How We Can Recover*. Rodale Books, 2015.

Kar, Sujita Kumar. "Predictors of Response to Repetitive Transcranial Magnetic Stimulation in Depression: A Review of Recent Updates." *Clinical Psychopharmacology and Neuroscience*, vol. 17, no. 1, 28 Feb. 2019, pp. 25–33., doi:10.9758/cpn.2019.17.1.25.

Karachalios, Theofilos, et al. "Total Hip Arthroplasty." *EFORT Open Reviews*, vol. 3, no. 5, 2018, pp. 232–239., doi:10.1302/2058-5241.3.170068.

Karkou, Vicky, et al. "Effectiveness of Dance Movement Therapy in the Treatment of Adults With Depression: A Systematic Review With Meta-Analyses." *Frontiers in Psychology*, vol. 10, 3 May 2019, doi:10.3389/fpsyg.2019.00936.

Kastenbaum, Robert J. *Death, Society, and Human Experience*. 11th ed. Pearson, 2014.

Kaszkin-Bettag, M., et al. "Confirmation Of The Efficacy Of Err 731® In Perimenopausal Women With Climacteric Symptoms." *Maturitas*, vol. 63, 2009, doi:10.1016/s0378-5122(09)70447-5.

Katz, Jeffrey A. "COX-2 Inhibition: What We Learned—A Controversial Update on Safety Data." *Pain Medicine*, vol. 14, no. suppl 1, 23 Dec. 2013, doi:10.1111/pme.12252.

Katz, R. T. "Carpal Tunnel Syndrome: a Practical Review." American Family Physician, vol. 49, no. 6, 1 May 1994, pp. 1385–1386.

Keefe, Francis J., et al. "Group Therapy for Patients with Chronic Pain." *Psychological Approaches to Pain Management: a Practitioner's Handbook*, edited by Dennis C. Turk and Robert J. Gatchel, 3rd ed., The Guilford Press, 2018, pp. 205–229.

Kellicker, Patricia. "General Anesthesia." *Health Library*, 10 Sept. 2012.

Kelsey, Amber. "The Healing Properties of Oregano Oil." *Livestrong.com*, Leaf Group, 20 Jan. 2019, www.livestrong.com/article/153766-the-healing-properties-of-oregano-oil/.

Kenny, Kathleen. "OTC Pain Medications: The Pros and Cons." *Pharmacy Times*, 30 Apr. 2017, www.pharmacytimes.com/publications/issue/2017/august2017/otc-pain-medications-the-pros-and-cons.

Kerner, Nancy, and Joan Prudic. "Current Electroconvulsive Therapy Practice and Research in the Geriatric Population." *Neuropsychiatry*, vol. 4, no. 1, 2014, pp. 33–54., doi:10.2217/npy.14.3.

Kessler, David. *The Needs of the Dying: A Guide for Bringing Hope, Comfort, and Love to Life's Final Chapter*. New York: Harper, 2007.

Khouzam, Hani Raoul. "Psychopharmacology of Chronic Pain: a Focus on Antidepressants and Atypical Antipsychotics." *Postgraduate Medicine*, vol. 128, no. 3, 16 Feb. 2016, pp. 323–330., doi:10.1080/00325481.2016.1147925.

Kiefer, Dale, et al. "Decongestants to Treat Allergy Symptoms." *Healthline*, 11 Mar. 2016, www.healthline.com/health/allergies/decongestants#1.

Kim, Jooyoung, et al. "Therapeutic Effectiveness of Instrument-Assisted Soft Tissue Mobilization for Soft Tissue Injury: Mechanisms and Practical Application." *Journal of Exercise Rehabilitation*, vol. 13, no. 1, 28 Feb. 2017, pp. 12–22., doi:10.12965/jer.1732824.412.

Kim, Young Hoon. "The Role and Position of Antipsychotics in Managing Chronic Pain." *The Korean Journal of Pain*, vol. 32, no. 1, 2019, p. 1., doi:10.3344/kjp.2019.32.1.1.

Kimmel, Ryan J., et al. "Pharmacological Treatments for Panic Disorder, Generalized Anxiety Disorder, Specific Phobia, and Social Anxiety Disorder." *Oxford Clinical Psychology*, 2015, doi:10.1093/med:psych/9780199342211.003.0015.

Kindt, Sara, et al. "Helping Motivation and Well-Being of Chronic Pain Couples." *Pain*, vol. 157, no. 7, 2016, pp. 1551–1562., doi:10.1097/j.pain.0000000000000550.

——. "Helping Your Partner with Chronic Pain: The Importance of Helping Motivation, Received Social Support, and Its Timeliness." *Pain Medicine*, vol. 20, no. 1, Jan. 2019, pp. 77–89., doi:10.1093/pm/pny006.

King, Kristi Mcclary, and Olivia Estill. "Exercise as a Treatment for Chronic Pain." *ACSM s Health & Fitness Journal*, vol. 23, no. 2, 2019, pp. 36–40., doi:10.1249/fit.0000000000000461.

Kingston University. "Age-Old Remedies Using White Tea, Witch Hazel and Rose May Be Beneficial, Study Suggests." *ScienceDaily*, 2 Dec. 2011, www.sciencedaily.com/releases/2011/12/111201132501.htm.

Kinney, Adam R., et al. "Equine-Assisted Interventions for Veterans with Service-Related Health Conditions: a Systematic Mapping Review." *Military Medical Research*, vol. 6, no. 1, 29 Aug. 2019, doi:10.1186/s40779-019-0217-6.

Kivlan, Benjamin R., et al. "The Effect of Astym® Therapy on Muscle Strength: a Blinded, Randomized, Clinically Controlled Trial." *BMC Musculoskeletal Disorders*, vol. 16, 29 Oct. 2015, doi:10.1186/s12891-015-0778-9.

Klein, Penelope, et al. "Meditative Movement, Energetic, and Physical Analyses of Three Qigong Exercises: Unification of Eastern and Western Mechanistic Exercise Theory." *Medicines*, vol. 4, no. 4, 23 Sept. 2017, p. 69., doi:10.3390/medicines4040069.

Klever, Sandy. "Reminiscence Therapy." *Nursing*, vol. 43, no. 4, 2013, pp. 36–37., doi:10.1097/01.nurse.0000427988.23941.51.

Klimas, Jan, et al. "Strategies to Identify Patient Risks of Prescription Opioid Addiction When Initiating Opioids for Pain." *JAMA Network Open*, vol. 2, no. 5, 3 May 2019, doi:10.1001/jamanetworkopen.2019.3365.

Knaul, Felicia M, et al. "The Lancet Commission on Palliative Care and Pain Relief—Findings, Recommendations, and Future Directions." *The Lancet Global Health*, vol. 6, 1 Mar. 2018, doi:10.1016/s2214-109x(18)30082-2.

Koch, Sabine C., et al. "Effects of Dance Movement Therapy and Dance on Health-Related Psychological Outcomes. A Meta-Analysis Update." *Frontiers in Psychology*, vol. 10, 20 Aug. 2019, doi:10.3389/fpsyg.2019.01806.

Koliqi, Rozafa, et al. "Prevalence of Side Effects Treatment with Carbamazepine and Other Antiepileptics in Patients with Epilepsy." *Materia Socio Medica*, vol. 27, no. 3, 2015, p. 167., doi:10.5455/msm.2015.27.167-171.

Koulivand, Peir Hossein, et al. "Lavender and the Nervous System." *Evidence-Based Complementary and Alternative Medicine*, 2013, pp. 1–10., doi:10.1155/2013/681304.

Kramer, Peter D. *Ordinarily Well: the Case for Antidepressants*. Farrar, Straus & Giroux, 2017.

Kress, Hans-Georg, et al. "A Holistic Approach to Chronic Pain Management That Involves All Stakeholders: Change Is Needed." *Current Medical Research and Opinion*, vol. 31, no. 9, 20 Aug. 2015, pp. 1743–1754., doi:10.1185/03007995.2015.1072088.

Kübler-Ross, Elisabeth. *On Death and Dying*. Reprint ed. Routledge, 2009.

Kucera, Alexander, et al. "Tolerability and Effectiveness of an Antitrauma Cream with Comfrey Herb Extract in Pediatric Use with Application on Intact and on Broken Skin." *International Journal of Pediatrics and Adolescent Medicine*, vol. 5, no. 4, 2018, pp. 135–141., doi:10.1016/j.ijpam.2018.11.002.

Kuebler, Karen M. "Using Morphine in End-of-Life Care." *Nursing*, vol. 44, no. 4, 2014, p. 69., doi:10.1097/01.nurse.0000444548.72595.ac.

Kulish, Peter. *Conquering Pain: the Art of Healing with BioMagnetism*. 6th ed., BioMag Science, 2016.

Kumarswamy, A. "Multimodal Management of Dental Pain with Focus on Alternative Medicine: A Novel Herbal Dental Gel." *Contemporary Clinical Dentistry*, vol. 7, no. 2, 2016, p. 131., doi:10.4103/0976-237x.183066.

Kuroda, Shinnosuke, et al. "A New Prediction Model for Operative Time of Flexible Ureteroscopy with Lithotripsy for the Treatment of Renal Stones." *Plos One*, vol. 13, no. 2, 13 Feb. 2018, doi:10.1371/journal.pone.0192597.

Kyota, Ayumi, and Kiyoko Kanda. "How to Come to Terms with Facing Death: a Qualitative Study Examining the Experiences of Patients with Terminal Cancer." *BMC Palliative Care*, vol. 18, no. 1, 4 Apr. 2019, doi:10.1186/s12904-019-0417-6.

Lafferty, Keith A., et al. "Barbiturate Toxicity." *Medscape*, 14 Jan. 2017, emedicine.medscape.com/article/813155-overview.

Lakemeier, Stefan, et al. "A Comparison of Intraarticular Lumbar Facet Joint Steroid Injections and Lumbar Facet Joint Radiofrequency Denervation in the Treatment of Low Back Pain." *Anesthesia & Analgesia*, vol. 117, no. 1, 2013, pp. 228–235., doi:10.1213/ane.0b013e3182910c4d.

Lakhan, Shaheen E., et al. "The Effectiveness of Aromatherapy in Reducing Pain: A Systematic Review and Meta-Analysis." *Pain Research and Treatment*, 2016, pp. 1–13., doi:10.1155/2016/8158693.

Lakhan, Shaheen E., et al. "Zingiberaceae Extracts for Pain: a Systematic Review and Meta-Analysis." *Nutrition Journal*, vol. 14, no. 1, 14 May 2015, doi:10.1186/s12937-015-0038-8.

Lambert, Jonathan. "Antidepressants Can Interfere With Pain Relief Of Common Opioids." *National Public Radio*, 6 Feb. 2019, www.npr.org/sections/health-shots/2019/02/06/691998300/antidepressants-can-interfere-with-pain-relief-of-common-opioids.

Lane, Trevor, et al. "Public Awareness and Perceptions of Palliative and Comfort Care." *The American Journal of Medicine*, vol. 132, no. 2, 2019, pp. 129–131., doi:10.1016/j.amjmed.2018.07.032.

Lee, Chun-Hsien, et al. "Inappropriate Self-Medication among Adolescents and Its Association with Lower Medication Literacy and Substance Use." *Plos One*, vol. 12, no. 12, 14 Dec. 2017, doi:10.1371/journal.pone.0189199.

Lee, Courtney, et al. "Mind–Body Therapies for the Self-Management of Chronic Pain Symptoms." *Pain Medicine*, vol. 15, no. S1, Apr. 2014, pp. S21–S39., doi:10.1111/pme.12383.

Lee, Jin-Seong, and Young Don Pyun. "Use of Hypnosis in the Treatment of Pain." *The Korean Journal of Pain*, vol. 25, no. 2, 2012, p. 75., doi:10.3344/kjp.2012.25.2.75.

Lee, Sangseok. "Guilty, or Not Guilty?: a Short Story of Propofol Abuse." *Korean Journal of Anesthesiology*, vol. 65, no. 5, 2013, p. 377., doi:10.4097/kjae.2013.65.5.377.

Lee, Yong Seuk. "Comprehensive Analysis of Pain Management after Total Knee Arthroplasty." *Knee Surgery & Related Research*, vol. 29, no. 2, 1 June 2017, pp. 80–86., doi:10.5792/ksrr.16.024.

LeFebvre, Ron, et al. "Evidence-Based Practice and Chiropractic Care." *Journal of Evidence-Based Complementary & Alternative Medicine*, vol. 18, no. 1, 28 Dec. 2012, pp. 75–79., doi:10.1177/2156587212458435.

Leggieri, Melissa, et al. "Music Intervention Approaches for Alzheimer's Disease: A Review of the Literature." *Frontiers in Neuroscience*, vol. 13, 12 Mar. 2019, doi:10.3389/fnins.2019.00132.

Lemerond, Terry. "Reduce Inflammation from Respiratory Diseases with *Boswellia*." *Chiropractic Economics*, 4 June 2018, www.chiroeco.com/breathing-easier-Boswellia/.

Leonard, Jayne. "Anxiety Medication: List, Types, and Side Effects." *Medical News Today*, MediLexicon International, 13 Nov. 2018, www.medicalnewstoday.com/articles/323666.php.

Leubner, Daniel, and Thilo Hinterberger. "Reviewing the Effectiveness of Music Interventions in Treating Depression." *Frontiers in Psychology*, vol. 8, 7 July 2017, doi:10.3389/fpsyg.2017.01109.

Leyva-López, Nayely, et al. "Essential Oils of Oregano: Biological Activity beyond Their Antimicrobial Properties." *Molecules*, vol. 22, no. 6, 14 June 2017, p. 989., doi:10.3390/molecules22060989.

Li, Dian-Jeng, et al. "Significant Treatment Effect of Bupropion in Patients With Bipolar Disorder but Similar Phase-Shifting Rate as Other Antidepressants." *Medicine*, vol. 95, no. 13, Mar. 2016, doi:10.1097/md.0000000000003165.

Li, H, et al. "Effects of Functional Endoscopic Sinus Surgery on Chronic Rhinosinusitis Resistant to Medication." *The Journal of Laryngology & Otology*, vol. 128, no. 11, 17 Oct. 2014, pp. 976–980., doi:10.1017/s002221511400228x.

Li, Mo, et al. "The Clinical Efficacy of Reminiscence Therapy in Patients with Mild-to-Moderate Alzheimer Disease." *Medicine*, vol. 96, no. 51, 2017, doi:10.1097/md.0000000000009381.

Li, William H. C., et al. "Play Interventions to Reduce Anxiety and Negative Emotions in Hospitalized Children." *BMC Pediatrics*, vol. 16, no. 1, 11 Mar. 2016, doi:10.1186/s12887-016-0570-5.

Lieber, Mark. "Equine Therapy May Help Autism, PTSD and Pain." *CNN*, Cable News Network, 10 July 2018, www.cnn.com/2018/06/18/health/equine-assisted-therapy-cfc/index.html.

Liebrenz, Michael, et al. "High-Dose Benzodiazepine Dependence: A Qualitative Study of Patients' Perceptions on Initiation, Reasons for Use, and

Obtainment." *Plos One*, vol. 10, no. 11, 10 Nov. 2015, doi:10.1371/journal.pone.0142057.

Liew, Zeyan, et al. "Acetaminophen Use During Pregnancy, Behavioral Problems, and Hyperkinetic Disorders." *JAMA Pediatrics*, vol. 168, no. 4, Apr. 2014, pp. 313–320., doi:10.1001/jamapediatrics.2013.4914.

Lilienfeld, Scott O. "The Truth about Shock Therapy." *Scientific American*, 1 May 2014, www.scientificamerican.com/article/the-truth-about-shock-therapy/.

Lima, Liliana De, and Lukas Radbruch. "The International Association for Hospice and Palliative Care: Advancing Hospice and Palliative Care Worldwide." *Journal of Pain and Symptom Management*, vol. 55, no. 2, 8 Aug. 2017, doi:10.1016/j.jpainsymman.2017.03.023.

Linton, Steven J. "Applying Dialectical Behavior Therapy to Chronic Pain: A Case Study." *Scandinavian Journal of Pain*, vol. 1, no. 1, 2010, pp. 50–54., doi:10.1016/j.sjpain.2009.09.005.

Liska, Ken. Drugs and the Human Body, with Implications for Society. 8th ed. Pearson/Prentice Hall, 2009.

Litt, Mark D., and Howard Tennen. "What Are the Most Effective Coping Strategies for Managing Chronic Pain?" *Pain Management*, vol. 5, no. 6, 2015, pp. 403–406., doi:10.2217/pmt.15.45.

Liu, Dora, et al. "A Practical Guide to the Monitoring and Management of the Complications of Systemic Corticosteroid Therapy." *Allergy, Asthma & Clinical Immunology*, vol. 9, no. 1, 2013, p. 30., doi:10.1186/1710-1492-9-30.

Locke, Amy B., et al. "Diagnosis and Management of Generalized Anxiety Disorder and Panic Disorder in Adults." *American Family Physician*, vol. 91, no. 9, May 2015, pp. 617–624.

Lök, Neslihan, et al. "The Effect of Reminiscence Therapy on Cognitive Functions, Depression, and Quality of Life in Alzheimer Patients: Randomized Controlled Trial." *International Journal of Geriatric Psychiatry*, vol. 34, no. 1, 2018, pp. 47–53., doi:10.1002/gps.4980.

López-Muñoz, Francisco, et al. "The History of Barbiturates a Century after Their Clinical Introduction." *Neuropsychiatric Disease and Treatment*, vol. 1, no. 4, Dec. 2005, pp. 329–343.

"Low Back Pain." *OrthoInfo*, American Academy of Orthopaedic Surgeons, Dec. 2013, orthoinfo.aaos.org/en/diseases--conditions/low-back-pain.

Lozano, Andres M., et al. "Deep Brain Stimulation: Current Challenges and Future Directions." *Nature Reviews Neurology*, vol. 15, no. 3, Mar. 2019, pp. 148–160., doi:10.1038/s41582-018-0128-2.

Lucille, Holly. *The Healing Power of Trauma Comfrey*. Take Charge Books, 2013.

Luo, Ailin, et al. "Sevoflurane Addiction Due to Workplace Exposure." *Medicine*, vol. 97, no. 38, 2018, doi:10.1097/md.0000000000012454.

Luong, Amber, and Bradley F. Marple. "Sinus Surgery: Indications and Techniques." *Clinical Reviews in Allergy & Immunology*, vol. 30, no. 3, 2006, pp. 217–222., doi:10.1385/criai:30:3:217.

Lyapustina, Tatyana, and G. Caleb Alexander. "The Prescription Opioid Addiction and Abuse Epidemic: How It Happened and What We Can Do about It." *The Pharmaceutical Journal*, vol. 294, no. 7866, 11 June 2015, doi:10.1211/pj.2015.20068579.

Ma, C. Benjamin, et al. "Carpal Tunnel Release." *MedlinePlus*, U.S. National Library of Medicine, 21 Apr. 2019, medlineplus.gov/ency/article/002976.htm.

——. "Foot Pain." *MedlinePlus*, U.S. National Library of Medicine, 20 Mar. 2018, medlineplus.gov/ency/article/003183.htm.

Macguire, Eoghan. "Equine-Assisted psychotherapy: Horses as healers." CNN, Cable News Network, 30 Nov. 2015, www.cnn.com/2015/11/30/sport/horse-psychotherapy-otra-mas/index.html.

Mackeen, Dawn. "What Are the Benefits of Turmeric?" *The New York Times*, 16 Oct. 2019, www.nytimes.com/2019/10/16/style/self-care/turmeric-benefits.html.

Maeng, S., et al. "Changes In Coping Strategy With Age." *Innovation in Aging*, vol. 1, no. suppl_1, 30 July 2017, pp. 897–897., doi:10.1093/geroni/igx004.3218.

Mafetoni, Reginaldo Roque, and Antonieta Keiko Kakuda Shimo. "The Effects of Acupressure on Labor Pains during Child Birth: Randomized Clinical Trial." *Revista Latino-Americana De Enfermagem*, vol. 24, 8 Aug. 2016, doi:10.1590/1518-8345.0739.2738.

"Magnets for Pain." *National Center for Complementary and Integrative Health*, U.S. Department of Health and Human Services, 27 Dec. 2017, nccih.nih.gov/Health/magnets-for-pain.

Mahdi, Jassem G. "Medicinal Potential of Willow: A Chemical Perspective of Aspirin Discovery." *Journal of Saudi Chemical Society*, vol. 14, no. 3, 2010, pp. 317–322., doi:10.1016/j.jscs.2010.04.010.

Mannix, L. K, et al. "Rizatriptan for the Acute Treatment of ICHD-II Proposed Menstrual Migraine: Two Prospective, Randomized, Placebo-Controlled, Double-Blind Studies." *Cephalalgia*, vol. 27, no. 5, 2007, pp. 414–421., doi:10.1111/j.1468-2982.2007.01313.x.

"Manual Therapies for Chronic Low Back Pain." *DynaMed*, EBSCO Information Services, 30 June 2015, www.dynamed.com/management/manual-therapies-for-chronic-low-back-pain.

Mao, Jun J., and Jeffery A. Dusek. "Integrative Medicine as Standard Care for Pain Management: The Need for Rigorous Research." *Pain Medicine*, vol. 17, no. 6, 26 May 2016, pp. 1181–1182., doi:10.1093/pm/pnw102.

Marrelli, Tina M. *Hospice & Palliative Care Handbook: Quality, Compliance, and Reimbursement.* 3rd ed., Sigma Theta Tau International, 2018.

Martin, Laura J., et al. "Palliative Care - Managing Pain." *MedlinePlus*, U.S. National Library of Medicine, 18 Feb. 2018, medlineplus.gov/ency/patientinstructions/000532.htm.

Martinak, Bridgette, et al. "Dextromethorphan in Cough Syrup: The Poor Man's Psychosis." *Psychopharmacology Bulletin*, vol. 47, no. 4, Sept. 2017, pp. 47–51.

Mathew, Sam T., et al. "Efficacy and Safety of COX-2 Inhibitors in the Clinical Management of Arthritis: Mini Review." *ISRN Pharmacology*, 2011, pp. 1–4., doi:10.5402/2011/480291.

Matyjaszczyk, Ewa, and Regina Schumann. "Risk Assessment of White Willow (Salix Alba) in Food." *EFSA Journal*, vol. 16, no. S1, 28 Aug. 2018, doi:10.2903/j.efsa.2018.e16081.

May, Jennifer M, et al. "Dialectical Behavior Therapy as Treatment for Borderline Personality Disorder." *Mental Health Clinician*, vol. 6, no. 2, 2016, pp. 62–67., doi:10.9740/mhc.2016.03.62.

Mayo Clinic Staff. "Bladder Stones." *Mayo Clinic*, Mayo Foundation for Medical Education and Research, 16 Aug. 2019, www.mayoclinic.org/diseases-conditions/bladder-stones/diagnosis-treatment/drc-20354345.

—. "Cognitive Behavioral Therapy." *Mayo Clinic*, Mayo Foundation for Medical Education and Research, 16 Mar. 2019, www.mayoclinic.org/tests-procedures/cognitive-behavioral-therapy/about/pac-20384610.

—. "Electroconvulsive Therapy (ECT)." *Mayo Clinic*, Mayo Foundation for Medical Education and Research, 12 Oct. 2018, www.mayoclinic.org/tests-procedures/electroconvulsive-therapy/about/pac-20393894.

—. "Gallstones." *Mayo Clinic*, Mayo Foundation for Medical Education and Research, 8 Aug. 2019, www.mayoclinic.org/diseases-conditions/gallstones/diagnosis-treatment/drc-20354220.

—. "Kidney Stones." *Mayo Clinic*, Mayo Foundation for Medical Education and Research, 8 Feb. 2019, www.mayoclinic.org/diseases-conditions/kidney-stones/diagnosis-treatment/drc-20355759.

—. "Light Therapy." *Mayo Clinic*, Mayo Foundation for Medical Education and Research, 8 Feb. 2017, www.mayoclinic.org/tests-procedures/light-therapy/about/pac-20384604.

—. "Transcranial Magnetic Stimulation." *Mayo Clinic*, Mayo Foundation for Medical Education and Research, 27 Nov. 2018, www.mayoclinic.org/tests-procedures/transcranial-magnetic-stimulation/about/pac-20384625.

—. "Yoga: Fight Stress and Find Serenity." *Mayo Clinic*, Mayo Foundation for Medical Education and Research, 19 Sept. 2019, www.mayoclinic.org/healthy-lifestyle/stress-management/in-depth/yoga/art-20044733.

—. "Historically 'Safer' Tramadol More Likely than Other Opioids to Result in Prolonged Use." *ScienceDaily*, 14 May 2019, www.sciencedaily.com/releases/2019/05/190514090953.htm.

McAlindon, Timothy, et al. "Effect of Vitamin D Supplementation on Progression of Knee Pain and Cartilage Volume Loss in Patients With Symptomatic Osteoarthritis." *Jama*, vol. 309, no. 2, 9 Jan. 2013, p. 155., doi:10.1001/jama.2012.164487.

McCabe, Sean E., et al. "Does Early Onset of Non-Medical Use of Prescription Drugs Predict Subsequent Prescription Drug Abuse and Dependence?" *Addiction* vol. 102 no. 12, 2007, pp. 1920–30.

McGregor, Gerard, et al. "Devil's Claw (Harpagophytum Procumbens): An Anti-Inflammatory Herb with Therapeutic Potential." *Phytochemistry Reviews*, vol. 4, no. 1, 2005, pp. 47–53., doi:10.1007/s11101-004-2374-8.

McGregor, Jennifer. "How Holistic Methods May Help Your Chronic Pain." *Pain Connection*, 1 Sept. 2016, www.painconnection.org/blog/how-holistic-methods-may-help-your-chronic-pain/.

McHugh, R. Kathryn, et al. "Prescription Drug Abuse: from Epidemiology to Public Policy." *Journal of Substance Abuse Treatment*, vol. 48, no. 1, 2015, pp. 1–7., doi:10.1016/j.jsat.2014.08.004.

Mehta, Piyush, et al. "Contemporary Acupressure Therapy: Adroit Cure for Painless Recovery of Therapeutic Ailments." *Journal of Traditional and Complementary Medicine*, vol. 7, no. 2, 2017, pp. 251–263., doi:10.1016/j.jtcme.2016.06.004.

Meisner, Robert C. "Ketamine for Major Depression: New Tool, New Questions." *Harvard Health Blog*, Harvard Medical School, 20 May 2019, www.health.harvard.edu/blog/ketamine-for-major-depression-new-tool-new-questions-2019052216673.

"Menopause and Your Health." *Office on Women's Health*, 21 Sept. 2018, www.womenshealth.gov/menopause/menopause-and-your-health.

"Menopause Basics." *Office on Women's Health*, 18 Mar. 2019, www.womenshealth.gov/menopause/menopause-basics/.

"Menopause." *DynaMed*, EBSCO Information Services, 15 Mar. 2018, www.dynamed.com/condition/menopause.

Menzies, Rachel E., et al. "The Effects of Psychosocial Interventions on Death Anxiety: A Meta-Analysis and Systematic Review of Randomised Controlled Trials." *Journal of Anxiety Disorders*, vol. 59, 2018, pp. 64–73., doi:10.1016/j.janxdis.2018.09.004.

Messer, Stanley D. "Assimilative Psychotherapy Integration." *The SAGE Encyclopedia of Theory in Counseling and Psychotherapy*, 27 Sept. 2017, doi:10.4135/9781483346502.n29.

"Methadone." *MedlinePlus*, U.S. National Library of Medicine, 15 Oct. 2019, medlineplus.gov/druginfo/meds/a682134.html.

"Methadone." *Substance Abuse and Mental Health Services Administration*, 30 Sept. 2019, www.samhsa.gov/medication-assisted-treatment/treatment/methadone.

"Migraine in Adults." *DynaMed*, EBSCO Information Services, 8 Nov. 2018, www.dynamed.com/topics/dmp~AN~T114718/Migraine-in-adults.

Millard, Michael A., and Eduardo A. Hernandez-Vila. "What Do the Guidelines Really Say About Aspirin?" *Texas Heart Institute Journal*, vol. 45, no. 4, 2018, pp. 228–230., doi:10.14503/thij-18-6673.

Miller, Glen E. *Living Thoughtfully, Dying Well: A Doctor Explains How to Make Death a Natural Part of Life*. Herald, 2014.

Miller, Scott, and David Zieve. "Spinal and Epidural Anesthesia." *Medline Plus*, 28 Mar. 2011.

Mirsadraei, Majid, et al. "Effects of Rosemary and Platanus Extracts on Asthmatic Subjects Resistant to Traditional Treatments." *European Respiratory Journal*, vol. 42, 2013.

Mncwangi, Nontobeko, et al. "Devil's Claw—A Review of the Ethnobotany, Phytochemistry and Biological Activity of Harpagophytum Procumbens." *Journal of Ethnopharmacology*, vol. 143, no. 3, 2012, pp. 755–771., doi:10.1016/j.jep.2012.08.013.

Moccia, Lorenzo, et al. "The Experience of Pleasure: A Perspective Between Neuroscience and Psychoanalysis." *Frontiers in Human Neuroscience*, vol. 12, 2018, doi:10.3389/fnhum.2018.00359.

Moghadam, Zahra Behboodi, et al. "The Effect of Valerian Root Extract on the Severity of Pre Menstrual Syndrome Symptoms." *Journal of Traditional and Complementary Medicine*, vol. 6, no. 3, 2016, pp. 309–315., doi:10.1016/j.jtcme.2015.09.001.

Moments of Life: Made Possible by Hospice, National Hospice and Palliative Care Organization, moments.nhpco.org/.

Moncivaiz, Aaron, and Debra Rose Wilson. "*Boswellia* (Indian Frankincense)." *Healthline*, 9 Nov. 2017, www.healthline.com/health/*Boswellia*.

Montánchez Torres, M.I. et al. "Benefits of Using Music Therapy in Mental Disorders." *Journal of

Biomusical Engineering, vol. 04, no. 02, 2016, doi:10.4172/2090-2719.1000116.

Moore, Paul A., et al. "Why Do We Prescribe Vicodin?" *The Journal of the American Dental Association*, vol. 147, no. 7, 2016, pp. 530–533., doi:10.1016/j.adaj.2016.05.005.

Moradi, Mohammad, et al. "Use of Oxycodone in Pain Management." *Anesthesiology and Pain Medicine*, vol. 1, no. 4, 2012, pp. 262–264., doi:10.5812/aapm.4529.

Morales-Rodríguez, Francisco Manuel, and José Manuel Pérez-Mármol. "The Role of Anxiety, Coping Strategies, and Emotional Intelligence on General Perceived Self-Efficacy in University Students." *Frontiers in Psychology*, vol. 10, 7 Aug. 2019, doi:10.3389/fpsyg.2019.01689.

"Morphine." *MedlinePlus*, U.S. National Library of Medicine, 15 Oct. 2019, medlineplus.gov/druginfo/meds/a682133.html.

Morrow, Angela. "Pain Management in Palliative Care." *Verywell Health*, 22 July 2016, www.verywellhealth.com/pain-management-in-palliative-care-1132349.

"Morton Neuroma." *DynaMed*, EBSCO Information Services, 8 June 2016, www.dynamed.com/condition/morton-neuroma.

Moscano, Filomena, et al. "An Observational Study of Fixed-Dose Tanacetum Parthenium Nutraceutical Preparation for Prophylaxis of Pediatric Headache." *Italian Journal of Pediatrics*, vol. 45, no. 1, 12 Mar. 2019, doi:10.1186/s13052-019-0624-z.

Moss, Mark, et al. "Acute Ingestion of Rosemary Water: Evidence of Cognitive and Cerebrovascular Effects in Healthy Adults." *Journal of Psychopharmacology*, vol. 32, no. 12, 15 Oct. 2018, pp. 1319–1329., doi:10.1177/0269881118798339.

Mountain, Vivienne. "Play Therapy – Respecting the Spirit of the Child." *International Journal of Children's Spirituality*, vol. 21, no. 3-4, 30 Sept. 2016, pp. 191–200., doi:10.1080/1364436x.2016.1228616.

Moyle, Sally. "The Emotional and Psychological Impacts of Chronic Pain." *Ausmed*, 2 Feb. 2016, www.ausmed.com/cpd/articles/chronic-pain-emotional-psychological-impacts.

Murina, Filippo, and Stefania Di Francesco. "Transcutaneous Electrical Nerve Stimulation." *Electrical Stimulation for Pelvic Floor Disorders*, by Jacopo Martellucci, Springer International Publishing, 2015, pp. 105–117.

Muzyk, Andrew, et al. "Clinical Effectiveness of Baclofen for the Treatment of Alcohol Dependence: a Review." *Clinical Pharmacology: Advances and Applications*, vol. 5, 2013, p. 99., doi:10.2147/cpaa.s32434.

"Narcotics (Opioids)." *United States Drug Enforcement Administration*, U.S. Department of Justice, 16 Sept. 2019, www.dea.gov/taxonomy/term/331.

Naste, Tiffany M., et al. "Equine Facilitated Therapy for Complex Trauma (EFT-CT)." *Journal of Child & Adolescent Trauma*, vol. 11, no. 3, 17 Aug. 2017, pp. 289–303., doi:10.1007/s40653-017-0187-3.

National Guideline Centre. "Low Back Pain and Sciatica in over 16s: Assessment and Management: Guidance." *National Institute for Health and Care Excellence*, Nov. 2016, www.nice.org.uk/guidance/ng59.

Natour, Jamil, et al. "Pilates Improves Pain, Function and Quality of Life in Patients with Chronic Low Back Pain: a Randomized Controlled Trial." *Clinical Rehabilitation*, vol. 29, no. 1, 25 June 2014, pp. 59–68., doi:10.1177/0269215514538981.

Nekovarova, Tereza, et al. "Common Mechanisms of Pain and Depression: Are Antidepressants Also Analgesics?" *Frontiers in Behavioral Neuroscience*, vol. 8, 25 Mar. 2014, doi:10.3389/fnbeh.2014.00099.

Nelson, Harry. *The United States of Opioids: a Prescription for Liberating a Nation in Pain*. Ingram Pub Services, 2019.

Nelson, Nicole L., and James R. Churilla. "Massage Therapy for Pain and Function in Patients With Arthritis." American Journal of Physical Medicine & Rehabilitation, vol. 96, no. 9, 2017, pp. 665–672., doi:10.1097/phm.0000000000000712.

Newman, Tim. "Garlic: Proven Health Benefits and Uses." *Medical News Today*, MediLexicon International, 18 Aug. 2017, www.medicalnewstoday.com/articles/265853.php.

——. "Just How Effective Is Hypnosis at Relieving Pain?" *Medical News Today*, MediLexicon International, 28 Apr. 2019, www.medicalnewstoday.com/articles/325041.php#1.

Nichols, Hannah. "The Research-Backed Benefits of Yoga." *Medical News Today*, MediLexicon International, 23 Sept. 2019, www.medicalnewstoday.com/articles/326414.php.

NIDA. "Fentanyl." *National Institute on Drug Abuse*, 6 June 2016, www.drugabuse.gov/drugs-abuse/fentanyl.

——. "Kratom." *National Institute on Drug Abuse*, National Institutes of Health, Apr. 2019, www.drugabuse.gov/publications/drugfacts/kratom.

——. "Misuse of Prescription Drugs." *National Institute on Drug Abuse*, Dec. 2018, www.drugabuse.gov/publications/misuse-prescription-drugs/overview.

Ning, Zhipeng, and Lixing Lao. "Acupuncture for Pain Management in Evidence-Based Medicine." *Journal of Acupuncture and Meridian Studies*, vol. 8, no. 5, 2015, pp. 270–273., doi:10.1016/j.jams.2015.07.012.

Nita, Maria. "'Spirituality' in Health Studies: Competing Spiritualities and the Elevated Status of Mindfulness." *Journal of Religion and Health*, vol. 58, no. 5, 26 Feb. 2019, pp. 1605–1618., doi:10.1007/s10943-019-00773-2.

Noll, Eric, et al. "Randomized Trial of Acupressure to Improve Patient Satisfaction and Quality of Recovery in Hospitalized Patients: Study Protocol for a Randomized Controlled Trial." *Trials*, vol. 18, no. 1, 7 Mar. 2017, doi:10.1186/s13063-017-1839-1.

Nordqvist, Christian. "All about Antidepressants." *Medical News Today*, MediLexicon International, 16 Feb. 2018, www.medicalnewstoday.com/kc/antidepressants-work-248320.

Nordqvist, Joseph, and Debra Rose Wilson. "Flaxseed: Health Benefits, Nutritional Content, and Risks." *Medical News Today*, MediLexicon International, 20 Nov. 2017, www.medicalnewstoday.com/articles/263405.php.

——. "Benzodiazepines: Uses, Types, Side Effects, and Risks." *Medical News Today*, MediLexicon International, 7 Mar. 2019, www.medicalnewstoday.com/articles/262809.php.

——. "Lavender: Health Benefits and Uses." *Medical News Today*, MediLexicon International, 4 Mar. 2019, www.medicalnewstoday.com/articles/265922.php.

Norton, Amy. "Could Hypnotherapy Be Alternative to Opioids for Pain?" *U.S. News & World Report*, 17 May 2019, www.usnews.com/news/health-news/articles/2019-05-17/could-hypnotherapy-be-alternative-to-opioids-for-pain.

Novotney, Amy. "Not Your Great-Grandfather's Psychoanalysis." *Monitor on Psychology*, American Psychological Association, Dec. 2017, www.apa.org/monitor/2017/12/psychoanalysis.

O'Rourke, Mark A., et al. "Reasons to Reject Physician Assisted Suicide/Physician Aid in Dying." *Journal of Oncology Practice*, vol. 13, no. 10, 2017, pp. 683–686., doi:10.1200/jop.2017.021840.

Oakes, Kari. "Green Light Therapy: A Stop Sign for Pain?" *MDedge Neurology*, 15 May 2019, www.mdedge.com/neurology/article/200743/pain/green-light-therapy-stop-sign-pain.

Oakley, Simon, et al. "Recognition of Anesthetic Barbiturates by a Protein Binding Site: A High Resolution Structural Analysis." *PLoS ONE*, vol. 7, no. 2, 16 Feb. 2012, doi:10.1371/journal.pone.0032070.

Ogal, Hans P., and Wolfram Stor. *Pictorial Atlas of Acupuncture: an Illustrated Manual of Acupuncture Points*. H.F. Ullman Publishing, 2012.

Ogbru, Omudhome, and Jay W. Marks. "Acetaminophen Uses, Side Effects, and Dosage." *MedicineNet*, 19 June 2018, www.medicinenet.com/acetaminophen/article.htm.

——. "Cox-2 Inhibitors Side Effects, List, Uses & Dosage." *MedicineNet*, 28 Feb. 2019, www.medicinenet.com/cox-2_inhibitors/article.htm.

Oliveira, Jonatas Rafael De, et al. "Rosmarinus Officinalis L. (Rosemary) as Therapeutic and Prophylactic Agent." *Journal of Biomedical Science*, vol. 26, no. 1, 9 Jan. 2019, doi:10.1186/s12929-019-0499-8.

O'Malley, Patricia Anne. "Lavender for Sleep, Rest, and Pain." *Clinical Nurse Specialist*, vol. 31, no. 2, 2017, pp. 74–76., doi:10.1097/NUR.0000000000000273.

"Onychomycosis." *DynaMed*, EBSCO Information Services, 15 Jan. 2018, www.dynamed.com/condition/onychomycosis.

"Opioid Overdose Crisis." *National Institute on Drug Abuse*, National Institutes of Health, 22 Jan. 2019, www.drugabuse.gov/drugs-abuse/opioids/opioid-overdose-crisis.

Orhurhu, Vwaire, et al. "Ketamine Infusions for Chronic Pain." *Anesthesia & Analgesia*, vol. 129, no. 1, 2019, pp. 241–254., doi:10.1213/ane.0000000000004185.

"Orthotics." *FootCareMD*, American Orthopaedic Foot & Ankle Society, 2019, www.footcaremd.org/conditions-treatments/injections-and-other-treatments/orthotics.

Osafo, Newman, et al. "Mechanism of Action of Nonsteroidal Anti-Inflammatory Drugs." *Nonsteroidal Anti-Inflammatory Drugs*, 23 Aug. 2017, doi:10.5772/68090.

"Osteoarthritis (OA) of the Hip." *DynaMed*, EBSCO Information Services, 15 Mar. 2018, www.dynamed.com/condition/osteoarthritis-oa-of-the-hip.

"Osteoarthritis." *National Institute of Arthritis and Musculoskeletal and Skin Diseases*, U.S. Department of Health and Human Services, 30 May 2016, www.niams.nih.gov/health-topics/osteoarthritis.

"Osteoporosis." *DynaMed*, EBSCO Information Services, 1 Feb. 2018, www.dynamed.com/condition/osteoporosis.

"OTC Drug Facts Label." *U.S. Food and Drug Administration*, 5 June 2015, www.fda.gov/drugs/drug-information-consumers/otc-drug-facts-label.

"OTC Medicines: Know Your Risks and Reduce Them." *Familydoctor.org*, 23 May 2018, familydoctor.org/otc-medicines-know-your-risks-and-reduce-them/.

"Over-the-Counter Medicines." *MedlinePlus*, U.S. National Library of Medicine, 23 Oct. 2019, medlineplus.gov/overthecountermedicines.html.

"Over-the-Counter Pain Relievers." *MedlinePlus*, U.S. National Library of Medicine, 12 Oct. 2018, medlineplus.gov/ency/article/002123.htm.

"Oxycodone." *MedlinePlus*, U.S. National Library of Medicine, 15 Oct. 2019, medlineplus.gov/druginfo/meds/a682132.html.

"Pain, Anxiety, and Depression." *Harvard Health Publishing*, Harvard Medical School, 5 June 2019, www.health.harvard.edu/mind-and-mood/pain-anxiety-and-depression.

Palermo, Elizabeth. "Does Magnetic Therapy Work?" *LiveScience*, Future US, Inc., 12 Feb. 2015, www.livescience.com/40174-magnetic-therapy.html.

Pangotra, Aditi, et al. "Effectiveness of Progressive Muscle Relaxation, Biofeedback and L-Theanine in Patients Suffering from Anxiety Disorder." *Journal Of Psychosocial Research*, vol. 13, no. 1, 2018, pp. 219–228., doi:10.32381/jpr.2018.13.01.21.

Pareek, Anil, et al. "Feverfew (Tanacetum Parthenium L.): A Systematic Review." *Pharmacognosy Reviews*, vol. 5, no. 9, 2011, pp. 103–110., doi:10.4103/0973-7847.79105.

Paris, Joel. "Is Psychoanalysis Still Relevant to Psychiatry?" *The Canadian Journal of Psychiatry*, vol. 62, no. 5, 31 Jan. 2017, pp. 308–312., doi:10.1177/0706743717692306.

Park, Kyoung Sik. "A Systematic Review on Anti-Inflammatory Activity of Harpagoside." *Journal of Biochemistry and Molecular Biology Research*, vol. 2, no. 3, 2016, pp. 166–169., doi:10.17554/j.issn.2313-7177.2016.02.27.

Park, Kyung Moo, and Ji Hwan Kim. "Herbal Medicine for the Management of Postoperative Pain." *Medicine*, vol. 98, no. 1, 2019, doi:10.1097/md.0000000000014016.

Park, Rex, et al. "Magnesium for the Management of Chronic Noncancer Pain in Adults: Protocol for a Systematic Review." *JMIR Research Protocols*, vol. 8, no. 1, 11 Jan. 2019, doi:10.2196/11654.

Parker, Linda A, et al. "Regulation of Nausea and Vomiting by Cannabinoids." *British Journal of Pharmacology*, vol. 163, no. 7, 2011, pp. 1411–1422., doi:10.1111/j.1476-5381.2010.01176.x.

Parks, Troy. "Neurosurgery Makes Pain Management Curricular Breakthroughs." *American Medical Association*, 2 Aug. 2016, www.ama-assn.org/delivering-care/opioids/neurosurgery-makes-pain-management-curricular-breakthroughs.

——. "Using Neurosurgical Solutions to Manage Chronic Back Pain." *American Medical Association*, 23 Aug. 2016, www.ama-assn.org/delivering-care/opioids/using-neurosurgical-solutions-manage-chronic-back-pain.

Parsaik, Ajay K., et al. "Efficacy of Ketamine in Bipolar Depression." *Journal of Psychiatric Practice*, vol. 21, no. 6, 2015, pp. 427–435., doi:10.1097/pra.0000000000000106.

Patel, Krisna, et al. "Bupropion: a Systematic Review and Meta-Analysis of Effectiveness as an Antidepressant." *Therapeutic Advances in Psychopharmacology*, vol. 6, no. 2, 2016, pp. 99–144., doi:10.1177/2045125316629071.

Patterson, Terence. "A Cognitive Behavioral Systems Approach to Family Therapy." *Journal of Family Psychotherapy*, vol. 25, no. 2, 2014, pp. 132–144., doi:10.1080/08975353.2014.910023.

Paul, Gunchan, et al. "Carisoprodol Withdrawal Syndrome Resembling Neuroleptic Malignant Syndrome: Diagnostic Dilemma." *Journal of Anaesthesiology Clinical Pharmacology*, vol. 32, no. 3, 2016, p. 387., doi:10.4103/0970-9185.173346.

Pavan, Rajendra, et al. "Properties and Therapeutic Application of Bromelain: A Review." *Biotechnology Research International*, 2012, pp. 1–6., doi:10.1155/2012/976203.

Pearson, Neil, et al. *Yoga and Science in Pain Care: Treating the Person in Pain.* Singing Dragon, 2019.

Peck, Sheldon. "Extractions, Retention and Stability: the Search for Orthodontic Truth." *European Journal of Orthodontics*, vol. 39, no. 2, 23 Feb. 2017, pp. 109–115., doi:10.1093/ejo/cjx004.

Penman, Danny. "Can Mindfulness Meditation Really Reduce Pain and Suffering?" *Psychology Today*, 9 Jan. 2015, www.psychologytoday.com/us/blog/mindfulness-in-frantic-world/201501/can-mindfulness-meditation-really-reduce-pain-and-suffering.

"Peppermint Oil." *National Center for Complementary and Integrative Health*, U.S. Department of Health and Human Services, 1 Dec. 2016, nccih.nih.gov/health/peppermintoil.

Perkins, Kimberly, et al. "Efficacy of Curcuma for Treatment of Osteoarthritis." *Journal of Evidence-Based Complementary & Alternative Medicine*, vol. 22, no. 1, 23 Mar. 2016, pp. 156–165., doi:10.1177/2156587216636747.

"Pes Planus (Flatfoot)." *DynaMed*, EBSCO Information Services, 26 Sept. 2017, www.dynamed.com/condition/pes-planus-flatfoot.

Peterson, Stacy M. "Why Aromatherapy Is Showing up in Hospital Surgical Units." *Mayo Clinic*, Mayo Foundation for Medical Education and Research, 27 Oct. 2017, www.mayoclinic.org/healthy-lifestyle/stress-management/in-depth/why-aromatherapy-is-showing-up-in-hospital-surgical-units/art-20342126.

Phd, Nebojsa Nick Knezevic Md, et al. "Treatment of Chronic Low Back Pain – New Approaches on the Horizon." *Journal of Pain Research*, vol. 10, 2017, pp. 1111–1123., doi:10.2147/jpr.s132769.

Phend, Crystal. "FDA Advisors Weigh COX-2 Inhibitor Safety." *MedPage Today*, Everyday Health Group, 25 Apr. 2018, www.medpagetoday.com/painmanagement/painmanagement/72522.

"Physical Supports for Chronic Low Back Pain." *DynaMed*, EBSCO Information Services, 30 June 2015, www.dynamed.com/management/physical-supports-for-chronic-low-back-pain.

Pichichero, Michael E., and Diana I. Brixner. "A Review of Recommended Antibiotic Therapies with Impact on Outcomes in Acute Otitis Media and Acute Bacterial Sinusitis." *Search Results Web Result with Site Links American Journal of Managed Care*, vol. 12, no. 10, 1 Aug. 2006, pp. S292–S302.

Piotrowski, Monica. "Frequently Asked Questions About Hospice and Palliative Care." *Palliative Doctors*, palliativedoctors.org/faq.

Pitta, Patricia J. *Solving Modern Family Dilemmas Assimilative Therapy.* Routledge, 2015.

"Plantar Fasciitis." *DynaMed*, EBSCO Information Services, 12 July 2017, www.dynamed.com/condition/plantar-fasciitis.

Pourianezhad, Farzaneh, et al. "Review on Feverfew, a Valuable Medicinal Plant." *Journal of Herbmed Pharmacology*, vol. 5, no. 2, 2016, pp. 45–49.

Prabhavathi, K, et al. "A Randomized, Double Blind, Placebo Controlled, Cross over Study to Evaluate the Analgesic Activity of *Boswellia* Serrata in Healthy Volunteers Using Mechanical Pain Model." *Indian Journal of Pharmacology*, vol. 46, no. 5, 2014, p. 475., doi:10.4103/0253-7613.140570.

Pringle, A, et al. "Cognitive Mechanisms of Diazepam Administration: a Healthy Volunteer Model of Emotional Processing." *Psychopharmacology*, vol. 233, no. 12, 6 May 2016, pp. 2221–2228., doi:10.1007/s00213-016-4269-y.

Prozialeck, Walter C., et al. "Kratom Policy: The Challenge of Balancing Therapeutic Potential with Public Safety." *International Journal of Drug Policy*, vol. 70, 2019, pp. 70–77., doi:10.1016/j.drugpo.2019.05.003.

Qidwai, Waris, and Tabinda Ashfaq. "Role of Garlic Usage in Cardiovascular Disease Prevention: An Evidence-Based Approach." *Evidence-Based Complementary and Alternative Medicine*, 2013, pp. 1–9., doi:10.1155/2013/125649.

"Radiofrequency Facet Denervation: Spine Center." *Oregon Health & Science University*, 2019, www.ohsu.edu/spine-center/radiofrequency-facet-denervation.

Rae-Grant, Alexander C. "Epidural Steroid Injection." *DynaMed*, EBSCO Information Services, 5 Sept. 2016, www.dynamed.com/topics/dmp~AN~T901362/Epidural-steroid-injection.

——. "Carpal Tunnel Syndrome." DynaMed, EBSCO Information Services, 30 Nov. 2018, www.dynamed.com/condition/carpal-tunnel-syndrome.

Raffa, R.B., et al. "Oxycodone Combinations for Pain Relief." *Drugs of Today*, vol. 46, no. 6, 2010, p. 379., doi:10.1358/dot.2010.46.6.1470106.

Rahnama, Parvin, et al. "Effect of Zingiber Officinale R. Rhizomes (Ginger) on Pain Relief in Primary Dysmenorrhea: a Placebo Randomized Trial." *BMC Complementary and Alternative Medicine*, vol. 12, no. 1, 2012, doi:10.1186/1472-6882-12-92.

Rajan, J, and J Scott-Warren. "The Clinical Use of Methadone in Cancer and Chronic Pain Medicine." *BJA Education*, vol. 16, no. 3, 2016, pp. 102–106., doi:10.1093/bjaceaccp/mkv023.

Raleigh, M. D., et al. "Safety and Efficacy of an Oxycodone Vaccine: Addressing Some of the Unique Considerations Posed by Opioid Abuse." *Plos One*, vol. 12, no. 12, 2017, doi:10.1371/journal.pone.0184876.

Ramamoorthy, Sivapriya, and John A. Cidlowski. "Corticosteroids." *Rheumatic Disease Clinics of North America*, vol. 42, no. 1, 2016, pp. 15–31., doi:10.1016/j.rdc.2015.08.002.

Ramli, Aizi Nor Mazila, et al. "Bromelain: from Production to Commercialisation." *Journal of the Science of Food and Agriculture*, vol. 97, no. 5, 28 Oct. 2016, pp. 1386–1395., doi:10.1002/jsfa.8122.

Ramos-Matos, Carlos F., and Wilfredo Lopez-Ojeda. "Fentanyl." *StatPearls*, 3 Oct. 2019.

Ramsahai, J Michael, and Peter Ab Wark. "Appropriate Use of Oral Corticosteroids for Severe Asthma." *Medical Journal of Australia*, vol. 209, no. S2, 17 July 2018, doi:10.5694/mja18.00134.

Rapaport, Lisa. "Use of Benzodiazepines for Pain Rising in US." *Psychiatry & Behavioral Health Learning Network*, 1 Feb. 2019, www.psychcongress.com/news/use-benzodiazepines-pain-rising-us.

Rathnavelu, Vidhya, et al. "Potential Role of Bromelain in Clinical and Therapeutic Applications." *Biomedical Reports*, vol. 5, no. 3, 18 July 2016, pp. 283–288., doi:10.3892/br.2016.720.

Rayati, Farshid, et al. "Comparison of Anti-Inflammatory and Analgesic Effects of Ginger Powder and Ibuprofen in Postsurgical Pain Model: A Randomized, Double-Blind, Case–Control Clinical Trial." *Dental Research Journal*, vol. 14, no. 1, 2017, p. 1., doi:10.4103/1735-3327.201135.

Ray-Griffith, Shona, et al. "Chronic Pain during Pregnancy: a Review of the Literature." *International Journal of Women's Health*, vol. 10, 2018, pp. 153–164., doi:10.2147/ijwh.s151845.

Read, John, et al. "Should We Stop Using Electroconvulsive Therapy?" *BMJ*, 30 Jan. 2019, doi:10.1136/bmj.k5233.

Reddy, M. S., and M. Starlin Vijay. "Empirical Reality of Dialectical Behavioral Therapy in Borderline Personality." *Indian Journal of Psychological Medicine*, vol. 39, no. 2, 2017, p. 105., doi:10.4103/ijpsym.ijpsym_132_17.

Reeves, Gloria M., et al. "Improvement in Depression Scores After 1 Hour of Light Therapy Treatment in Patients With Seasonal Affective Disorder." *The Journal of Nervous and Mental Disease*, vol. 200, no. 1, 2012, pp. 51–55., doi:10.1097/nmd.0b013e31823e56ca.

Reeves, Roy R., et al. "Carisoprodol." *Southern Medical Journal*, vol. 105, no. 11, 2012, pp. 619–623., doi:10.1097/smj.0b013e31826f5310.

Reichel, Chloe. "Benzodiazepines: Another Prescription Drug Problem." *Journalist's Resource*, 30 May 2019, journalistsresource.org/studies/society/public-health/benzodiazepines-what-journalists-should-know/.

Reissig, Chad J., et al. "High Doses of Dextromethorphan, an NMDA Antagonist, Produce Effects Similar to Classic Hallucinogens." *Psychopharmacology*, vol. 223, no. 1, 2012, pp. 1–15., doi:10.1007/s00213-012-2680-6.

Ricciotti, Hope. "Contrary to Popular Belief, Epidurals Don't Prolong Labor. Phew." *Harvard*

Richeimer, Steven. "Couples-Based Therapy May Help with Chronic Pain." *Medium*, 25 May 2018, medium.com/@stevenricheimer/couples-based-therapy-may-help-with-chronic-pain-138d1cafa681.

Riediger, Carina, et al. "Adverse Effects of Antidepressants for Chronic Pain: A Systematic Review and Meta-Analysis." *Frontiers in Neurology*, vol. 8, 14 July 2017, doi:10.3389/fneur.2017.00307.

Rietjens, Judith A. C., et al. "Terminal Sedation and Euthanasia." *Archives of Internal Medicine*, vol. 166, no. 7, 10 Apr. 2006, p. 749., doi:10.1001/archinte.166.7.749.

Rismanchi, Mojtaba. "Chronic Pain and Voluntary Euthanasia." *Journal of Medical Ethics and History of Medicine*, vol. 2, no. 1, 19 Oct. 2008.

Roberts, R Lynae, et al. "Hypnosis for Burn-Related Pain: Case Studies and a Review of the Literature." *World Journal of Anesthesiology*, vol. 6, no. 1, 2017, pp. 1–13., doi:10.5313/wja.v6.i1.1.

Rodriguez-Garcia, I., et al. "Oregano Essential Oil as an Antimicrobial and Antioxidant Additive in Food Products." *Critical Reviews in Food Science and Nutrition*, vol. 56, no. 10, 2015, pp. 1717–1727., doi:10.1080/10408398.2013.800832.

Rodriguez-Merchan, E. Carlos, et al. "The Current Role of Astym Therapy in the Treatment of Musculoskeletal Disorders." *Postgraduate Medicine*, 28 Aug. 2019, pp. 1–6., doi:10.1080/00325481.2019.1654836.

Rojas, Katia M., and Huiyang Li. "Adverse Events and Over-the-Counter (OTC) Drugs: Is Inappropriate Labeling the Problem? - The Case of Acetaminophen." *Proceedings of the Human Factors and Ergonomics Society Annual Meeting*, vol. 61, no. 1, 2017, pp. 676–680., doi:10.1177/1541931213601656.

Romaniuk, Madeline, et al. "Evaluation of an Equine-Assisted Therapy Program for Veterans Who Identify as 'Wounded, Injured or Ill' and Their Partners." *Plos One*, vol. 13, no. 9, 27 Sept. 2018, doi:10.1371/journal.pone.0203943.

Rooney, Steven M., and J.N Campbell. *How Aspirin Entered Our Medicine Cabinet*. Springer, 2017.

Roth, Christine. "Study Pokes Holes in Kratom's 'Bad Rap'." *University of Rochester Medical Center*, 14 Dec. 2017, www.urmc.rochester.edu/news/story/5202/study-pokes-holes-in-kratoms-bad-rap.aspx.

Roy-Byrne, Peter. "What Medications Are Used to Treat Anxiety Disorders?" *Anxiety and Depression Association of America*, Feb. 2019, adaa.org/learn-from-us/from-the-experts/blog-posts/what-medications-are-used-treat-anxiety-disorders.

Ruijs, Cees Dm, et al. "Unbearable Suffering and Requests for Euthanasia Prospectively Studied in End-of-Life Cancer Patients in Primary Care." *BMC Palliative Care*, vol. 13, no. 1, 2014, doi:10.1186/1472-684x-13-62.

Russo, Emilio, et al. "Corticosteroid-Related Central Nervous System Side Effects." *Journal of Pharmacology and Pharmacotherapeutics*, vol. 4, no. 5, 2013, pp. 94–98., doi:10.4103/0976-500x.120975.

Rzepa, Ewelina, et al. "Bupropion Administration Increases Resting-State Functional Connectivity in Dorso-Medial Prefrontal Cortex." *International Journal of Neuropsychopharmacology*, vol. 20, no. 6, 11 Mar. 2017, pp. 455–462., doi:10.1093/ijnp/pyx016.

Sackeim, Harold A. "Modern Electroconvulsive Therapy." *JAMA Psychiatry*, vol. 74, no. 8, 1 Aug. 2017, p. 779., doi:10.1001/jamapsychiatry.2017.1670.

Saha, Felix J., et al. "Integrative Medicine for Chronic Pain." *Medicine*, vol. 95, no. 27, 2016, doi:10.1097/md.0000000000004152.

Sahar, Tali, et al. "Insoles for Prevention and Treatment of Back Pain." *Cochrane Database of Systematic Reviews*, 2009, doi:10.1002/14651858.cd005275.pub2.

Sahebkar, Amirhossein, and Yves Henrotin. "Analgesic Efficacy and Safety of Curcuminoids in Clinical Practice: A Systematic Review and Meta-Analysis of Randomized Controlled Trials." *Pain Medicine*, vol. 17, no. 6, June 2016, pp. 1192–1202., doi:10.1093/pm/pnv024.

Saini, Rajivkumar, et al. "Transcranial Magnetic Stimulation: A Review of Its Evolution and Current Applications." *Industrial Psychiatry Journal*, vol. 27, no. 2, 2018, p. 172., doi:10.4103/ipj.ipj_88_18.

Saint-Lary, Olivier, et al. "Carpal Tunnel Syndrome: Primary Care and Occupational Factors." *Frontiers in Medicine*, vol. 2, 5 May 2015, doi:10.3389/fmed.2015.00028.

Salehi, Alireza, et al. "Chiropractic: Is It Efficient in Treatment of Diseases? Review of Systematic Reviews." *International Journal of Community Based Nursing and Midwifery*, vol. 3, Oct. 2015, pp. 244–254.

Salottolo, Kristin, et al. "The Grass Is Not Always Greener: a Multi-Institutional Pilot Study of Marijuana Use and Acute Pain Management Following Traumatic Injury." *Patient Safety in Surgery*, vol. 12, no. 16, 19 June 2018, doi:10.1186/s13037-018-0163-3.

Sandoiu, Ana. "Treating Pain with Magnetic Fields." *Medical News Today*, MediLexicon International, 9 Aug. 2018, www.medicalnewstoday.com/articles/322718.php#1.

Sanger, Gareth J., and Paul L. R. Andrews. "A History of Drug Discovery for Treatment of Nausea and Vomiting and the Implications for Future Research." *Frontiers in Pharmacology*, vol. 9, 4 Sept. 2018, p. 913., doi:10.3389/fphar.2018.00913.

Sansgiry, Sujit, et al. "Abuse of over-the-Counter Medicines: a Pharmacist's Perspective." *Integrated Pharmacy Research and Practice*, vol. 6, 2016, pp. 1–6., doi:10.2147/iprp.s103494.

Scarponi, Dorella, and Andrea Pession. "Play Therapy to Control Pain and Suffering in Pediatric Oncology." *Frontiers in Pediatrics*, vol. 4, 8 Dec. 2016, doi:10.3389/fped.2016.00132.

Scheer, Nicole A., et al. "Astym Therapy Improves Bilateral Hamstring Flexibility and Achilles Tendinopathy in a Child with Cerebral Palsy: A Retrospective Case Report." *Clinical Medicine Insights: Case Reports*, vol. 9, Oct. 2016, pp. 95–98., doi:10.4137/ccrep.s40623.

Schmidt-Hansen, Mia, et al. "Oxycodone for Cancer-Related Pain." *Cochrane Database of Systematic Reviews*, 2017, doi:10.1002/14651858.cd003870.pub6.

Schmitz, Allison. "Benzodiazepine Use, Misuse, and Abuse: A Review." *Mental Health Clinician*, vol. 6, no. 3, 2016, pp. 120–126., doi:10.9740/mhc.2016.05.120.

Schottelkorb, April A., et al. "Effectiveness of Play Therapy on Problematic Behaviors of Preschool Children With Somatization." *Journal of Child and Adolescent Counseling*, vol. 1, no. 1, 2 May 2015, pp. 3–16., doi:10.1080/23727810.2015.1015905.

Schubiner, Howard. "Mindfulness, CBT and ACT for Chronic Pain." *Psychology Today*, 8 Dec. 2014, www.psychologytoday.com/us/blog/unlearn-your-pain/201412/mindfulness-cbt-and-act-chronic-pain.

Schwartz, Mark S., and Frank Andrasik. *Biofeedback: a Practitioner's Guide*. 4th ed., The Guilford Press, 2017.

"Sciatica." *Cleveland Clinic*, 11 Dec. 2017, my.clevelandclinic.org/health/diseases/12792-sciatica.

"Sciatica." *DynaMed*, EBSCO Information Services, 8 May 2017, www.dynamed.com/condition/sciatica.

"Sedative, Hypnotic or Anxiolytic Drug Use Disorder." *Harvard Health Publishing*, Harvard Medical School, Dec. 2018, www.health.harvard.edu/a_to_z/sedative-hypnotic-or-anxiolytic-drug-use-disorder-a-to-z.

Seidel, Stefan, et al. "Antipsychotics for Acute and Chronic Pain in Adults." *Cochrane Database of Systematic Reviews*, 2013, doi:10.1002/14651858.cd004844.pub3.

Seigner, Jacqueline, et al. "A Symphytum Officinale Root Extract Exerts Anti-Inflammatory Properties by Affecting Two Distinct Steps of NF- B Signaling." *Frontiers in Pharmacology*, vol. 10, 26 Apr. 2019, doi:10.3389/fphar.2019.00289.

Seladi-Schulman, Jill. "About Peppermint Oil Uses and Benefits." *Healthline*, 25 Apr. 2019, www.healthline.com/health/benefits-of-peppermint-oil.

Selhub, Eva. "The Alexander Technique Can Help You (Literally) Unwind." *Harvard Health*, Harvard Medical School, 19 Nov. 2015, www.health.harvard.edu/blog/the-alexander-technique-can-help-you-literally-unwind-201511238652.

Seliger, Corinna, et al. "Use of Selective Cyclooxygenase-2 Inhibitors, Other Analgesics, and Risk of Glioma." *Plos One*, vol. 11, no. 2, 12 Feb. 2016, doi:10.1371/journal.pone.0149293.

Selva, Joaquin. "Progressive Muscle Relaxation (PMR): A Positive Psychology Guide."

PositivePsychology.com, 4 July 2019, positivepsychology.com/progressive-muscle-relaxation-pmr/.

Sen, Ingrid. *Lavender Essential Oil: Your Complete Guide to Lavender Essential Oil Uses, Benefits, Applications and Natural Remedies*. CreateSpace Independent Publishing Platform, 2016.

Serafini, Gianluca, et al. "The Role of Ketamine in Treatment-Resistant Depression: A Systematic Review." *Current Neuropharmacology*, vol. 12, no. 5, 12 Sept. 2014, pp. 444–461., doi:10.2174/1570159x12666140619204251.

Serretti, Alessandro, and Laura Mandelli. "Antidepressants and Body Weight." *The Journal of Clinical Psychiatry*, vol. 71, no. 10, Oct. 2010, pp. 1259–1272., doi:10.4088/jcp.09r05346blu.

Setayesh, Mohammad, et al. "A Topical Gel From Flax Seed Oil Compared With Hand Splint in Carpal Tunnel Syndrome: A Randomized Clinical Trial." *Journal of Evidence-Based Complementary & Alternative Medicine*, vol. 22, no. 3, 2016, pp. 462–467., doi:10.1177/2156587216677822.

Sevier, Thomas L., and Caroline W. Stegink-Jansen. "Astym Treatmentvs.eccentric Exercise for Lateral Elbow Tendinopathy: a Randomized Controlled Clinical Trial." *PeerJ*, vol. 3, May 2015, doi:10.7717/peerj.967.

Shad, Bijan, et al. "Does Opium Have Benefit for Coronary Artery Disease? A Systematic Review." *Research in Cardiovascular Medicine*, vol. 7, no. 2, 2018, p. 51., doi:10.4103/rcm.rcm_12_17.

Shader, Richard I. "An Anecdote About Arthritis and *Boswellia* Serrata." *Clinical Therapeutics*, vol. 40, no. 5, 2018, pp. 669–671., doi:10.1016/j.clinthera.2018.04.008.

Shah, Shalini, et al. "Pain Management in Pregnancy: Multimodal Approaches." *Pain Research and Treatment*, 2015, pp. 1–15., doi:10.1155/2015/987483.

Shahgholian, Nahid, and Sekine Keshavarzian. "Comparison of the Effect of Topical Application of Rosemary and Menthol for Musculoskeletal Pain in Hemodialysis Patients." *Iranian Journal of Nursing and Midwifery Research*, vol. 22, no. 6, 2017, p. 436., doi:10.4103/ijnmr.ijnmr_163_16.

Shamji, Mohammed F., et al. "The Advancing Role of Neuromodulation for the Management of Chronic Treatment-Refractory Pain." *Neurosurgery*, vol. 80, no. 3S, 21 Feb. 2017, doi:10.1093/neuros/nyw047.

Shara, Mohd, and Sidney J. Stohs. "Efficacy and Safety of White Willow Bark (Salix Alba) Extracts." *Phytotherapy Research*, vol. 29, no. 8, 22 May 2015, pp. 1112–1116., doi:10.1002/ptr.5377.

Sharbaugh, Adam, et al. "Contemporary Best Practice in the Management of Staghorn Calculi." *Therapeutic Advances in Urology*, vol. 11, 2019, p. 175628721984709., doi:10.1177/1756287219847099.

Sharma, Muktika, et al. "A Comprehensive Pharmacognostic Report on Valerian." *International Journal of Pharmaceutical Sciences and Research*, vol. 1, no. 7, 1 July 2010, pp. 6–40., doi:10.13040/ijpsr.0975-8232.1(7).6-40.

Sheng, Jiyao, et al. "The Link between Depression and Chronic Pain: Neural Mechanisms in the Brain." *Neural Plasticity*, 2017, pp. 1–10., doi:10.1155/2017/9724371.

Shepard, Nicholas, and Woojin Cho. "Recurrent Lumbar Disc Herniation: A Review." *Global Spine Journal*, vol. 9, no. 2, 18 Dec. 2017, pp. 202–209., doi:10.1177/2192568217745063.

Sherman, Karen J., et al. "Effectiveness of Therapeutic Massage for Generalized Anxiety Disorder: a Randomized Controlled Trial." *Depression and Anxiety*, vol. 27, no. 5, 2010, pp. 441–450., doi:10.1002/da.20671.

Shirvalkar, Prasad, et al. "Closed-Loop Deep Brain Stimulation for Refractory Chronic Pain." *Frontiers in Computational Neuroscience*, vol. 12, 26 Mar. 2018, p. 18., doi:10.3389/fncom.2018.00018.

Shmerling, Robert H. "Are You Taking Too Much Anti-Inflammatory Medication?" *Harvard Health Blog*, 23 Mar. 2018, www.health.harvard.edu/blog/are-you-taking-too-much-anti-inflammatory-medication-2018040213540.

———. "Is Tramadol a Risky Pain Medication?" *Harvard Health Blog*, Harvard Medical School, 16 Aug. 2019, www.health.harvard.edu/blog/is-tramadol-a-risky-pain-medication-2019061416844.

Sholjakova, Marija, et al. "Pain Relief as an Integral Part of the Palliative Care." *Open Access Macedonian Journal of Medical Sciences*, vol. 6, no. 4, 6 Apr. 2018, pp. 739–741., doi:10.3889/oamjms.2018.163.

Shuchang, He, et al. "Emotional and Neurobehavioural Status in Chronic Pain Patients." *Pain*

Research and Management, vol. 16, no. 1, 2011, pp. 41–43., doi:10.1155/2011/825636.

Siddall, Philip J., et al. "Spirituality: What Is Its Role in Pain Medicine?" *Pain Medicine*, vol. 16, no. 1, 2015, pp. 51–60., doi:10.1111/pme.12511.

Siddiqui, Mahtab Z. "*Boswellia* Serrata, A Potential Antiinflammatory Agent: An Overview." *Indian Journal of Pharmaceutical Sciences*, vol. 73, no. 3, May 2011, pp. 255–261., doi:10.4103/0250-474X.93507.

Sielski, Robert, et al. "Efficacy of Biofeedback in Chronic Back Pain: a Meta-Analysis." *International Journal of Behavioral Medicine*, vol. 24, no. 1, Feb. 2017, pp. 25–41., doi:10.1007/s12529-016-9572-9.

Silva, Jeane, et al. "Analgesic and Anti-Inflammatory Effects of Essential Oils of Eucalyptus." *Journal of Ethnopharmacology*, vol. 89, no. 2-3, 2003, pp. 277–283., doi:10.1016/j.jep.2003.09.007.

Simotas, Alexander C. "Cervical Radiculopathy: Nonsurgical Treatment Options." *Hospital for Special Surgery*, 1 May 2009, www.hss.edu/conditions_cervical-radiculopathy-nonoperative-treatments-epidural.asp#.VJMhbtLF-So.

Singh, Aditya, et al. "Personalized Repetitive Transcranial Magnetic Stimulation Temporarily Alters Default Mode Network in Healthy Subjects." *Scientific Reports*, vol. 9, no. 1, 4 Apr. 2019, doi:10.1038/s41598-019-42067-3.

Singh, Amit, and Sujita Kumar Kar. "How Electroconvulsive Therapy Works?: Understanding the Neurobiological Mechanisms." *Clinical Psychopharmacology and Neuroscience*, vol. 15, no. 3, 31 Aug. 2017, pp. 210–221., doi:10.9758/cpn.2017.15.3.210.

Sinusas, Keith. "Osteoarthritis: Diagnosis and Treatment." *American Family Physician*, vol. 85, no. 1, 1 Jan. 2012, pp. 49–56.

"Sinusitis." *American Academy of Allergy, Asthma & Immunology*, 2019, www.aaaai.org/conditions-and-treatments/allergies/sinusitis.

"Sinusitis." *ENT Health*, American Academy of Otolaryngology, Aug. 2018, www.enthealth.org/conditions/sinusitis/.

Sirois, Jay, and Stefanie P. Ferreri. "OTC Combination Products in Pharmacistassisted Self-Care." *Pharmacy Today*, vol. 19, no. 6, June 2013, pp. 49–53., doi:10.1016/s1042-0991(15)31306-2.

Slavin, R, et al. "The Diagnosis and Management of Sinusitis: A Practice Parameter Update." *Journal of Allergy and Clinical Immunology*, vol. 116, no. 6, 2005, doi:10.1016/j.jaci.2005.09.048.

Smith, Benjamin E, et al. "Musculoskeletal Pain and Exercise—Challenging Existing Paradigms and Introducing New." *British Journal of Sports Medicine*, vol. 53, no. 14, 20 June 2018, pp. 907–912., doi:10.1136/bjsports-2017-098983.

Smith, Cooper. "Codeine: Drug Effects, Addiction, Abuse and Treatment - Rehab Spot." *RehabSpot*, 9 July 2019, www.rehabspot.com/opioids/codeine/.

Smith, Karen E., and Greg J. Norman. "Brief Relaxation Training Is Not Sufficient to Alter Tolerance to Experimental Pain in Novices." *Plos One*, vol. 12, no. 5, 11 Mar. 2017, doi:10.1371/journal.pone.0177228.

Smith, Karmen R., and Kevin P. Lyness. "Solving Modern Family Dilemmas: An Assimilative Therapy Model." *Journal of Marital and Family Therapy*, vol. 42, no. 2, Apr. 2016.

Smith, Shannon M., et al. "Couple Interventions for Chronic Pain." *The Clinical Journal of Pain*, vol. 35, no. 11, 2019, pp. 916–922., doi:10.1097/ajp.0000000000000752.

Solloway, Michele R., et al. "An Evidence Map of the Effect of Tai Chi on Health Outcomes." *Systematic Reviews*, vol. 5, no. 1, 27 July 2016, doi:10.1186/s13643-016-0300-y.

Solomon, Daniel H. "Overview of COX-2 Selective NSAIDs." *UpToDate*, 30 Mar. 2019, www.uptodate.com/contents/overview-of-cox-2-selective-nsaids?topicRef=35&source=see_link.

——. "Patient Education: Nonsteroidal Antiinflammatory Drugs (NSAIDs) (Beyond the Basics)." *UpToDate*, 21 Feb. 2019, www.uptodate.com/contents/nonsteroidal-antiinflammatory-drugs-nsaids-beyond-the-basics.

Song, Man-Kyu, et al. "Effects of Cognitive-Behavioral Therapy on Empathy in Patients with Chronic Pain." *Psychiatry Investigation*, vol. 15, no. 3, 2018, pp. 285–291., doi:10.30773/pi.2017.07.03.

Soyka, Michael. "Treatment of Benzodiazepine Dependence." *New England Journal of Medicine*, vol. 376, no. 12, 23 Mar. 2017, pp. 1147–1157., doi:10.1056/nejmra1611832.

St. Michael's Hospital. "Dangerous Increases in Patients Mixing Opioids, Benzodiazepines or Z-Drugs." *ScienceDaily*, 17 Jan. 2019, www.sciencedaily.com/releases/2019/01/190117090455.htm.

Staiger, Christiane. "Comfrey Root: from Tradition to Modern Clinical Trials." *Wiener Medizinische Wochenschrift*, vol. 163, no. 3-4, Feb. 2013, pp. 58–64., doi:10.1007/s10354-012-0162-4.

——. "Comfrey: A Clinical Overview." *Phytotherapy Research*, vol. 26, no. 10, 23 Feb. 2012, pp. 1441–1448., doi:10.1002/ptr.4612.

Stanley, Theodore H. "The Fentanyl Story." *The Journal of Pain*, vol. 15, no. 12, 2014, pp. 1215–1226., doi:10.1016/j.jpain.2014.08.010.

"Stress Fractures." *OrthoInfo*, American Academy of Orthopaedic Surgeons, Oct. 2007, orthoinfo.aaos.org/en/diseases--conditions/stress-fractures.

Sturgeon, John. "Psychological Therapies for the Management of Chronic Pain." *Psychology Research and Behavior Management*, vol. 7, 2014, pp. 115–124., doi:10.2147/prbm.s44762.

Subedi, Muna, et al. "An Overview of Tramadol and Its Usage in Pain Management and Future Perspective." *Biomedicine & Pharmacotherapy*, vol. 111, 2019, pp. 443–451., doi:10.1016/j.biopha.2018.12.085.

Sulmasy, Lois Snyder, and Paul S. Mueller. "Ethics and the Legalization of Physician-Assisted Suicide: An American College of Physicians Position Paper." *Annals of Internal Medicine*, vol. 167, no. 8, 2017, p. 576., doi:10.7326/m17-0938.

"Sumatriptan." *DynaMed*, EBSCO Information Services, 6 Nov. 2018, www.dynamed.com/drug-monograph/sumatriptan.

Sun, Jia, et al. "Role of Curcumin in the Management of Pathological Pain." *Phytomedicine*, vol. 48, 2018, pp. 129–140., doi:10.1016/j.phymed.2018.04.045.

Suso-Ribera, Carlos, et al. "Empathic Accuracy in Chronic Pain: Exploring Patient and Informal Caregiver Differences and Their Personality Correlates." *Medicina*, vol. 55, no. 9, 27 Aug. 2019, p. 539, doi:10.3390/medicina55090539.

Swan, Karrie L., and Dee C. Ray. "Effects of Child-Centered Play Therapy on Irritability and Hyperactivity Behaviors of Children With Intellectual Disabilities." *The Journal of Humanistic Counseling*, vol. 53, no. 2, 2014, pp. 120–133., doi:10.1002/j.2161-1939.2014.00053.x.

Swanberg, Sarah. *A Patient's Guide to Acupuncture: Everything You Need to Know*. Althea Press, 2019.

Sweeney, Frank. *The Anesthesia Fact Book: Everything You Need to Know Before Surgery*. Perseus, 2003.

Sysko, Helen, et al. "Dialectical Behavior Therapy for Chronic Pain in Gastrointestinal Disorders." *Inflammatory Bowel Diseases*, vol. 22, Mar. 2016, doi:10.1097/01.mib.0000480106.40651.21.

Szalay, Jessie. "What Is Inflammation?" *LiveScience*, 19 Oct. 2018, www.livescience.com/52344-inflammation.html.

Tayabali, Khadija, et al. "Kratom: a Dangerous Player in the Opioid Crisis." *Journal of Community Hospital Internal Medicine Perspectives*, vol. 8, no. 3, 4 June 2018, pp. 107–110., doi:10.1080/20009666.2018.1468693.

Taylor & Francis Group. "Could Marijuana Be an Effective Pain Alternative to Prescription Medications?" *ScienceDaily*, 1 July 2019, www.sciencedaily.com/releases/2019/07/190701224523.htm.

Taylor, Charles P., et al. "Pharmacology of Dextromethorphan: Relevance to Dextromethorphan/Quinidine (Nuedexta®) Clinical Use." *Pharmacology & Therapeutics*, vol. 164, 2016, pp. 170–182., doi:10.1016/j.pharmthera.2016.04.010.

Teitelbaum, Jacob. "Magnesium for Pain Relief." *Psychology Today*, Sussex Publishers, 16 Sept. 2010, www.psychologytoday.com/us/blog/complementary-medicine/201009/magnesium-pain-relief.

"Tension-Type Headache." *DynaMed*, EBSCO Information Services, 20 Mar. 2018, www.dynamed.com/condition/tension-type-headache.

Terrie, Yvette C. "A Guide to the Proper Use of Nonprescription Decongestant Products." *Pharmacy Times*, 17 Nov. 2018, www.pharmacytimes.com/publications/issue/2018/november2018/a-guide-to-the-proper-use-of-nonprescription-decongestant-products.

Terry, Rohini, et al. "The Use of Ginger (Zingiber Officinale) for the Treatment of Pain: A Systematic Review of Clinical Trials." *Pain Medicine*, vol. 12, no. 12, 2011, pp. 1808–1818., doi:10.1111/j.1526-4637.2011.01261.x.

Teut, Michael, et al. "Qigong or Yoga Versus No Intervention in Older Adults With Chronic Low Back Pain—A Randomized Controlled Trial." *The Journal of Pain*, vol. 17, no. 7, 2016, pp. 796–805., doi:10.1016/j.jpain.2016.03.003.

"The Menopause Years." *American College of Obstetricians and Gynecologists*, Dec. 2018, www.acog.org/Patients/FAQs/The-Menopause-Years.

"The Secret to Joint Pain Relief - Exercise." *Harvard Health*, Harvard Medical School, www.health.harvard.edu/healthbeat/the-secret-to-joint-pain-relief-exercise.

"Therapeutic Exercise Program for Carpal Tunnel Syndrome." *OrthoInfo*, Academy of Orthopaedic Surgeons, Dec. 2018, orthoinfo.aaos.org/en/recovery/carpal-tunnel-syndrome-therapeutic-exercise-program/.

"Therapeutic Massage for Pain Relief." Harvard Health, Harvard Medical School, July 2016, www.health.harvard.edu/alternative-and-complementary-medicine/therapeutic-massage-for-pain-relief.

Therkleson, Tessa. "Topical Ginger Treatment With a Compress or Patch for Osteoarthritis Symptoms." *Journal of Holistic Nursing*, vol. 32, no. 3, Sept. 2013, pp. 173–182., doi:10.1177/0898010113512182.

"Thermal and Electromagnetic Therapies for Chronic Low Back Pain." *DynaMed*, EBSCO Information Services, 23 Mar. 2015, www.dynamed.com/management/thermal-and-electromagnetic-therapies-for-chronic-low-back-pain.

Thiele, Rainer. *Chiropractic Treatment for Headache and Lower Back Pain Systematic Review of Randomised Controlled Trials*. Springer Fachmedien Wiesbaden GmbH, 2019.

Thiels, Cornelius A, et al. "Chronic Use of Tramadol after Acute Pain Episode: Cohort Study." *Bmj*, 14 May 2019, doi:10.1136/bmj.l1849.

Thimm, Jens C, and Liss Antonsen. "Effectiveness of Cognitive Behavioral Group Therapy for Depression in Routine Practice." *BMC Psychiatry*, vol. 14, no. 1, 21 Oct. 2014, doi:10.1186/s12888-014-0292-x.

Thomson, Gill, et al. "Women's Experiences of Pharmacological and Non-Pharmacological Pain Relief Methods for Labour and Childbirth: a Qualitative Systematic Review." *Reproductive Health*, vol. 16, no. 1, 30 May 2019, doi:10.1186/s12978-019-0735-4.

Thomson, J Grant. "Diagnosis and Treatment of Carpal Tunnel Syndrome." *The Lancet Neurology*, vol. 16, no. 4, 2017, p. 263., doi:10.1016/s1474-4422(17)30059-5.

Thring, Tamsyn Sa, et al. "Antioxidant and Potential Anti-Inflammatory Activity of Extracts and Formulations of White Tea, Rose, and Witch Hazel on Primary Human Dermal Fibroblast Cells." *Journal of Inflammation*, vol. 8, no. 1, 2011, p. 27., doi:10.1186/1476-9255-8-27.

Tolou-Ghamari, Zahra, et al. "A Quick Review of Carbamazepine Pharmacokinetics in Epilepsy from 1953 to 2012." *Journal of Research in Medical Studies*, vol. 18, no. Suppl1, Mar. 2013, pp. S81–S85.

Tort, Sera, and Adrian Preda. "How Does Bupropion Compare with Placebo for Preventing Seasonal Affective Disorder (SAD)?" *Cochrane Clinical Answers*, 2019, doi:10.1002/cca.2226.

"Tramadol." *MedlinePlus*, U.S. National Library of Medicine, 15 Jan. 2019, medlineplus.gov/druginfo/meds/a695011.html.

"Treating Generalized Anxiety Disorder in the Elderly." *Harvard Health Publishing*, Harvard Medical School, 29 May 2019, www.health.harvard.edu/mind-and-mood/treating-generalized-anxiety-disorder-in-the-elderly.

Trescot, Andrea, et al. "Extended-Release Hydrocodone – Gift or Curse?" *Journal of Pain Research*, vol. 6, 2013, p. 53., doi:10.2147/jpr.s33062.

Trice-Black, Shannon, et al. "Play Therapy in School Counseling." *Professional School Counseling*, vol. 16, no. 5, 2013, doi:10.1177/2156759x1201600503.

Trüeb, Ralphm. "North American Virginian Witch Hazel (Hamamelis Virginiana): Based Scalp Care and Protection for Sensitive Scalp, Red Scalp, and Scalp Burn-Out." *International Journal of Trichology*, vol. 6, no. 3, 2014, pp. 100–103., doi:10.4103/0974-7753.139079.

Tsu, Peter Shiu Hwa. "Pain Control and Euthanasia." *Journal of Palliative Care & Medicine*, vol. 02, no. 01, 2012, doi:10.4172/2165-7386.1000e109.

Tuerk, Elena Hontoria, et al. "Collaboration in Family Therapy." *Journal of Clinical Psychology*, vol. 68, no. 2, 2012, pp. 168–178., doi:10.1002/jclp.21833.

Turk, Dennis C., et al. "Assessment of Psychosocial and Functional Impact of Chronic Pain." *The Journal of Pain*, vol. 17, no. 9, 2016, doi:10.1016/j.jpain.2016.02.006.

U.S. Department of Health and Human Services and U.S. Department of Agriculture. "Dietary Guidelines for Americans 2015–2020 8th Edition." *Health.gov*, Office of Disease Prevention and Health Promotion, health.gov/dietaryguidelines/2015/guidelines/.

"Understanding Over-the-Counter Medicines." *U.S. Food and Drug Administration*, 16 May 2018, www.fda.gov/drugs/buying-using-medicine-safely/understanding-over-counter-medicines.

University of Arizona. "Promise in Light Therapy to Treat Chronic Pain." *ScienceDaily*, 28 Feb. 2017, www.sciencedaily.com/releases/2017/02/170228185325.htm.

University of Georgia. "Daily Ginger Consumption Eases Muscle Pain by 25 Percent, Study Suggests." *ScienceDaily*, 20 May 2010, www.sciencedaily.com/releases/2010/05/100519131130.htm.

Urquhart, Donna M, et al. "Antidepressants for Non-Specific Low Back Pain." *Cochrane Database of Systematic Reviews*, 2008, doi:10.1002/14651858.cd001703.pub3.

"Use Only as Directed." *ProPublica*, 20 Sept. 2013, www.propublica.org/article/tylenol-mcneil-fda-use-only-as-directed.

Vadalà, Maria, et al. "Mechanisms and Therapeutic Effectiveness of Pulsed Electromagnetic Field Therapy in Oncology." *Cancer Medicine*, vol. 5, no. 11, 17 Oct. 2016, pp. 3128–3139., doi:10.1002/cam4.861.

Vadivelu, Nalini, et al. "Options for Perioperative Pain Management in Neurosurgery." *Journal of Pain Research*, vol. 9, 2016, p. 37., doi:10.2147/jpr.s85782.

"Valium: Side Effects, Addiction, Symptoms & Treatment: What Is Valium?" *American Addiction Centers*, 14 Nov. 2019, americanaddictioncenters.org/valium-treatment.

Vallath, Nandini. "Perspectives On Yoga inputs in the Management of Chronic Pain." *Indian Journal of Palliative Care*, vol. 16, no. 1, 2010, pp. 1–7., doi:10.4103/0973-1075.63127.

Van Den Bosch, A. A. S., et al. "Maternal Quality of Life in Routine Labor Epidural Analgesia versus Labor Analgesia on Request: Results of a Randomized Trial." *Quality of Life Research*, vol. 27, no. 8, 30 Mar. 2018, pp. 2027–2033., doi:10.1007/s11136-018-1838-z.

Vance, Carol Gt, et al. "Using TENS for Pain Control: the State of the Evidence." *Pain Management*, vol. 4, no. 3, 2014, pp. 197–209., doi:10.2217/pmt.14.13.

Vanderlaan, Jennifer. "Retrospective Cohort Study of Hydrotherapy in Labor." *Journal of Obstetric, Gynecologic & Neonatal Nursing*, vol. 46, no. 3, 2017, pp. 403–410., doi:10.1016/j.jogn.2016.11.018.

Veltri, Charles, and Oliver Grundmann. "Current Perspectives on the Impact of Kratom Use." *Substance Abuse and Rehabilitation*, vol. 10, 2019, pp. 23–31., doi:10.2147/sar.s164261.

Viera, A, J. "Management of Carpal Tunnel Syndrome." American Family Physician, vol. 68, no. 2, 15 July 2003, pp. 265–272.

Vikelis, Michail, et al. "A New Era in Headache Treatment." *Neurological Sciences*, vol. 39, no. S1, 2018, pp. 47–58., doi:10.1007/s10072-018-3337-y.

Villines, Zawn. "10 Natural Remedies for Reducing Anxiety and Stress." *Medical News Today*, MediLexicon International, 9 July 2018, www.medicalnewstoday.com/articles/322396.php.

Vining, Eugenia M. "Evolution of Medical Management of Chronic Rhinosinusitis." *Annals of Otology, Rhinology & Laryngology*, vol. 115, no. 9_suppl, 2006, pp. 54–60., doi:10.1177/00034894061150s909.

Vlachojannis, J. E., et al. "A Systematic Review on the Effectiveness of Willow Bark for Musculoskeletal Pain." *Phytotherapy Research*, vol. 23, no. 7, 2009, pp. 897–900., doi:10.1002/ptr.2747.

Voigt, Jeffrey, et al. "A Systematic Literature Review of the Clinical Efficacy of Repetitive Transcranial Magnetic Stimulation (RTMS) in Non-Treatment Resistant Patients with Major

Depressive Disorder." *BMC Psychiatry*, vol. 19, no. 1, 8 Jan. 2019, doi:10.1186/s12888-018-1989-z.

Vučković, Sonja, et al. "Cannabinoids and Pain: New Insights From Old Molecules." *Frontiers in Pharmacology*, vol. 9, 13 Nov. 2018, doi:10.3389/fphar.2018.01259.

Wachter, Kerri. "Navigating Cannabis Options for Chronic Pain." *Practical Pain Management*, 24 June 2019, www.practicalpainmanagement.com/patient/treatments/marijuana-cannabis/navigating-cannabis-options-chronic-pain.

Wadehra, Sunali, and Charles F. van Gunten. "Ketamine for Chronic Pain Management." *Practical Pain Management*, 4 Dec. 2018, www.practicalpainmanagement.com/patient/treatments/medications/ketamine-chronic-pain-management-current-role-future-directions.

Waljee, Akbar K, et al. "Short Term Use of Oral Corticosteroids and Related Harms among Adults in the United States: Population Based Cohort Study." *Bmj*, 12 Apr. 2017, doi:10.1136/bmj.j1415.

Walker, Bruce F. "The New Chiropractic." *Chiropractic & Manual Therapies*, vol. 24, no. 1, 30 June 2016, doi:10.1186/s12998-016-0108-9.

Wang, Sicong, and Qing Quan Lian. "Addictions and Stress: Implications for Propofol Abuse." *Neuropsychiatry*, vol. 07, no. 05, 2017, doi:10.4172/neuropsychiatry.1000260.

Ware, Megan. "Ginger: Health Benefits and Dietary Tips." *Medical News Today*, MediLexicon International, 11 Sept. 2017, www.medicalnewstoday.com/articles/265990.php.

Warwick, Hunter, et al. "Immediate Physical Therapy Following Total Joint Arthroplasty: Barriers and Impact on Short-Term Outcomes." *Advances in Orthopedics*, vol. 2019, 8 Apr. 2019, pp. 1–7., doi:10.1155/2019/6051476.

Weant, Kyle A., et al. "Antiemetic Use in the Emergency Department." *Advanced Emergency Nursing Journal*, vol. 39, no. 2, 2017, pp. 97–105., doi:10.1097/tme.0000000000000141.

Weaver, Michael F. "Prescription Sedative Misuse and Abuse." *The Yale Journal of Biology and Medicine*, vol. 88, no. 3, Sept. 2015, pp. 247–256.

Weber, Jim M. *Bringing It All Together: The Chiropractic Perspective for Better Structural and Functional Health.* Babypie, 2019.

Weber, Markus, et al. "Predicting Outcome after Total Hip Arthroplasty: The Role of Preoperative Patient-Reported Measures." *BioMed Research International*, vol. 2019, 29 Jan. 2019, pp. 1–9., doi:10.1155/2019/4909561.

Wegner, Inge, et al. "Traction for Low-Back Pain with or without Sciatica." *Cochrane Database of Systematic Reviews*, 19 Aug. 2013, doi:10.1002/14651858.cd003010.pub5.

Weinbroum, Avi A., et al. "The Role of Dextromethorphan in Pain Control." *Canadian Journal of Anesthesia/Journal Canadien D'anesthésie*, vol. 47, no. 6, 2000, pp. 585–596., doi:10.1007/bf03018952.

Wells, Cherie, et al. "The Effectiveness of Pilates Exercise in People with Chronic Low Back Pain: A Systematic Review." *PLoS ONE*, vol. 9, no. 7, 1 July 2014, doi:10.1371/journal.pone.0100402.

Wells, Karen, et al. "Decision Making and Support Available to Individuals Considering and Undertaking Electroconvulsive Therapy (ECT): a Qualitative, Consumer-Led Study." *BMC Psychiatry*, vol. 18, no. 1, 24 July 2018, doi:10.1186/s12888-018-1813-9.

Westhoff, Ben. *Fentanyl, Inc.: How Rogue Chemists Are Creating the Deadliest Wave of the Opioid Epidemic.* Atlantic Monthly Press, 2019.

Wexler, Alyse. "Valerian Root for Insomnia and Anxiety: Benefits, Dosage, and More." *Medical News Today*, MediLexicon International, 25 June 2017, www.medicalnewstoday.com/articles/318088.php.

"What Is a Methadone Clinic? MedMark's Guide to Methadone Clinics." *MedMark Treatment Centers*, medmark.com/resources/comprehensive-guide-to-methadone-clinics/.

"What Is Menopause?" National Institute on Aging, U.S. Department of Health and Human Services, 27 June 2017, www.nia.nih.gov/health/what-menopause.

Whelan, Corey, and Debra Rose Wilson. "Bromelain." *Healthline*, 22 Dec. 2017, www.healthline.com/health/bromelain.

Whitley, Nancy. *A Manual of Clinical Obstetrics.* Lippincott, 1985.

Whitman, Sarah M. "Group Psychotherapy for Chronic Pain Patients." *Practical Pain Management*, 16 May 2011, www.practicalpainmanagement.com/treatments/psychological/group-psychotherapy-chronic-pain-patients.

Whittaker, Glen A., et al. "Corticosteroid Injection for Plantar Heel Pain: a Systematic Review and Meta-Analysis." *BMC Musculoskeletal Disorders*, vol. 20, no. 1, 17 Aug. 2019, doi:10.1186/s12891-019-2749-z.

Wider, Barbara, et al. "Feverfew for Preventing Migraine." *Cochrane Database of Systematic Reviews*, 20 Apr. 2015, doi:10.1002/14651858.cd002286.pub3.

Wilkie, Diana J., and Miriam O. Ezenwa. "Pain and Symptom Management in Palliative Care and at End of Life." *Nursing Outlook*, vol. 60, no. 6, 2012, pp. 357–364., doi:10.1016/j.outlook.2012.08.002.

Williams, Amy M., and Annmarie Cano. "Spousal Mindfulness and Social Support in Couples With Chronic Pain." *The Clinical Journal of Pain*, vol. 30, no. 6, 2014, pp. 528–535., doi:10.1097/ajp.0000000000000009.

Williams, Craig D., et al. "Aspirin Use Among Adults in the U.S." *American Journal of Preventive Medicine*, vol. 48, no. 5, 2015, pp. 501–508., doi:10.1016/j.amepre.2014.11.005.

Williams, Sarah C.P. "Study Identifies Brain Areas Altered during Hypnotic Trances." *Stanford Medicine*, 28 July 2016, med.stanford.edu/news/all-news/2016/07/study-identifies-brain-areas-altered-during-hypnotic-trances.html.

Williamson, Ian G., et al. "Antibiotics and Topical Nasal Steroid for Treatment of Acute Maxillary Sinusitis." *Jama*, vol. 298, no. 21, 5 Dec. 2007, pp. 2487–2496., doi:10.1001/jama.298.21.2487.

Wipperman, Jennifer, and Kyle Goerl. "Carpal Tunnel Syndrome: Diagnosis and Management." *American Family Physician*, vol. 94, no. 12, 15 Dec. 2016, pp. 993–999.

Wise, Jacqui. "Yoga Is Reasonable Alternative to Physical Therapy for Lower Back Pain, Say Researchers." *Bmj*, 20 June 2017, doi:10.1136/bmj.j2964.

Wolf, Laurie Goldrich, and Mary Wolf. *The Medical Marijuana Dispensary: Understanding, Medicating, and Cooking with Cannabis.* Althea Press, 2016.

Wollenweber, Vanessa, et al. "Study of the Effectiveness of Hippotherapy on the Symptoms of Multiple Sclerosis – Outline of a Randomised Controlled Multicentre Study (MS-HIPPO)." *Contemporary Clinical Trials Communications*, vol. 3, 2016, pp. 6–11., doi:10.1016/j.conctc.2016.02.001.

Wong, Cathy. "Can Willow Bark Relieve Pain?" *Verywell Health*, 17 July 2019, www.verywellhealth.com/white-willow-bark-89085.

—. "The Benefits and Uses of Valerian Root." *Verywell Health*, 17 July 2019, www.verywellhealth.com/what-you-need-to-know-about-valerian-88336.

—. "The Health Benefits of Eucalyptus Oil." *Verywell Health*, 24 June 2019, www.verywellhealth.com/steam-inhalation-with-eucalyptus-essential-oil-88169.

—. "The Health Benefits of Turmeric." *Verywell Health*, 16 Sept. 2019, www.verywellhealth.com/turmeric-for-pain-relief-can-it-help-4173236.

—. "The Health Benefits of Witch Hazel." *Verywell Health*, 17 July 2019, www.verywellhealth.com/the-benefits-of-witch-hazel-90061.

—. "What Is Feverfew and What Does It Do?" *Verywell Health*, 17 July 2019, www.verywellhealth.com/the-health-benefits-of-feverfew-89562.

Wong, Rebecca S. Y. "Role of Nonsteroidal Anti-Inflammatory Drugs (NSAIDs) in Cancer Prevention and Cancer Promotion." *Advances in Pharmacological Sciences*, vol. 2019, 31 Jan. 2019, pp. 1–10., doi:10.1155/2019/3418975.

Wood, Evan, et al. "Pain Management With Opioids in 2019-2020." *Jama*, 10 Oct. 2019, doi:10.1001/jama.2019.15802.

Woods, Bernadette A. *Carbamazepine: Indications, Contraindications and Adverse Effects.* Nova Science Publishers, 2017.

Woods, Bob, et al. "Reminiscence Therapy for Dementia." *Cochrane Database of Systematic Reviews*, 1 Mar. 2018, doi:10.1002/14651858.cd001120.pub3.

Woolston, Chris. "Massage for Pain Relief." Consumer HealthDay, 1 Jan. 2019, consumer.healthday.com/encyclopedia/holistic-medicine-25/mis-alternative-medicine-news-19/massage-for-pain-relief-645793.html.

Wrenn, Paula, and Jo Gustely. *Dying Well with Hospice: a Compassionate Guide to End of Life Care*. Amans Vitae Press, 2017.

Wu, Song, et al. "Effect of Low-Level Laser Therapy on Tooth-Related Pain and Somatosensory Function Evoked by Orthodontic Treatment." *International Journal of Oral Science*, vol. 10, no. 3, 2 July 2018, doi:10.1038/s41368-018-0023-0.

Xiang, Anfeng, et al. "The Immediate Analgesic Effect of Acupuncture for Pain: A Systematic Review and Meta-Analysis." *Evidence-Based Complementary and Alternative Medicine*, 25 Oct. 2017, pp. 1–13., doi:10.1155/2017/3837194.

Xiong, Ming, et al. "Neurobiology of Propofol Addiction and Supportive Evidence: What Is the New Development?" *Brain Sciences*, vol. 8, no. 2, 22 Feb. 2018, p. 36., doi:10.3390/brainsci8020036.

Yaksh, Tony L., et al. "Development of New Analgesics: An Answer to Opioid Epidemic." *Trends in Pharmacological Sciences*, vol. 39, no. 12, 1 Dec. 2018, pp. 1000–1002., doi:10.1016/j.tips.2018.10.003.

Yang, Ziyi, et al. "The Effectiveness of Acupuncture for Chronic Pain with Depression." *Medicine*, vol. 96, no. 47, 27 Nov. 2017, doi:10.1097/md.0000000000008800.

Yasin, Waqas, et al. "Does Bupropion Impact More than Mood? A Case Report and Review of the Literature." *Cureus*, vol. 11, no. 3, 19 Mar. 2019, doi:10.7759/cureus.4277.

"Yoga for Pain Relief." *Harvard Health Publishing*, Harvard Medical School, Apr. 2015, www.health.harvard.edu/alternative-and-complementary-medicine/yoga-for-pain-relief.

"Yoga for Pain." *National Center for Complementary and Integrative Health*, U.S. Department of Health and Human Services, 21 Sept. 2018, nccih.nih.gov/health/providers/digest/yoga-pain.

Yuhas, Daisy. "Forget Pills and Surgery for Back Pain." *Scientific American*, 1 Oct. 2017, www.scientificamerican.com/article/forget-pills-and-surgery-for-back-pain/.

Zamunér, Antonio Roberto, et al. "Impact of Water Therapy on Pain Management in Patients with Fibromyalgia: Current Perspectives." *Journal of Pain Research*, vol. 12, 2019, pp. 1971–2007., doi:10.2147/jpr.s161494.

Zarbo, Cristina, et al. "Integrative Psychotherapy Works." *Frontiers in Psychology*

Zare, Afshin, et al. "Analgesic Effect of Valerian Root and Turnip Extracts." *World Journal Of Plastic Surgery*, vol. 7, no. 3, Sept. 2018, pp. 345–350., doi:10.29252/wjps.7.3.345.

Zarnaghash, Maryam, et al. "The Influence of Family Therapy on Marital Conflicts." *Procedia - Social and Behavioral Sciences*, vol. 84, 2013, pp. 1838–1844., doi:10.1016/j.sbspro.2013.07.044.

Zeidan, Fadel, and David R. Vago. "Mindfulness Meditation-Based Pain Relief: a Mechanistic Account." *Annals of the New York Academy of Sciences*, vol. 1373, no. 1, 2016, pp. 114–127., doi:10.1111/nyas.13153.

Zeratsky, Katherine. "Why Buy Ground Flaxseed?" *Mayo Clinic*, Mayo Foundation for Medical Education and Research, 18 Jan. 2019, www.mayoclinic.org/healthy-lifestyle/nutrition-and-healthy-eating/expert-answers/flaxseed/faq-20058354.

Žídková, Vĕra, et al. "Effects of Exercise and Enzyme Therapy in Early Occupational Carpal Tunnel Syndrome: A Preliminary Study." *BioMed Research International*, vol. 2019, 23 Jan. 2019, pp. 1–7., doi:10.1155/2019/8720493.

Zilles, David. "Beneficial Effects of Electroconvulsive Therapy in Elderly People." *The Lancet Psychiatry*, vol. 5, no. 9, 2018, pp. 697–698., doi:10.1016/s2215-0366(18)30264-5.

Zisman, Anna L. "Effectiveness of Treatment Modalities on Kidney Stone Recurrence." *Clinical Journal of the American Society of Nephrology*, vol. 12, no. 10, 22 Oct. 2017, pp. 1699–1708., doi:10.2215/cjn.11201016.

Journals

Anaesthesia
Editor: A. A. Klein
Publisher: Wiley-Blackwell
ISSN: 0003-2409 (print)
1365-2044 (web)
https://onlinelibrary.wiley.com/journal/13652044
anaesthesia@aagbi.org

Anesthesia & Analgesia
Editor: Jean-Francois Pittet
Publisher: Lippincott Williams & Wilkins
ISSN: 0003-2999 (print)
1526-7598 (web)
https://journals.lww.com/anesthesia-analgesia/pages/default.aspx
(240) 646-7089
info@iars.org

Anesthesiology
Editor: Evan Kharasch
Publisher: Lippincott Williams & Wilkins
ISSN: 0003-3022 (print)
1528-1175 (web)
https://anesthesiology.pubs.asahq.org/journal.aspx
managing-editor@anesthesiology.org

The Clinical Journal of Pain
Editor: Dennis C. Yurk, PhD
Publisher: Lippincott Williams & Wilkins
ISSN: 0749-8047 (print)
1536-5409 (web)
https://journals.lww.com/clinicalpain/pages/default.aspx
(215) -521-8300

Current Pain and Headache Reports
Editor: Stephen D. Silberstein
Lawrence C. Newman
Publisher: Springer Science+Business Media
ISSN: 1531-3433 (print)
1534-3081 (web)
https://www.springer.com/journal/11916

Headache
Editor: Thomas N. Ward
Publisher: Wiley-Blackwell
ISSN: 0017-8748 (print)
1526-4610 (web)
https://headachejournal.onlinelibrary.wiley.com/

International Journal of Palliative Nursing
Editor: Brian Nyatanga
Publisher: Mark Allen Group
ISSN: 1357-6321 (print)
2052-286X (web)
https://www.magonlinelibrary.com/journal/ijpn
+44 (0)20 3874 9213
laura.glenny@markallengroup.com

The Journal of Headache and Pain
Editor: Paolo Martelletti
Publisher: BioMed Central
ISSN: 1129-2369 (print)
1129-2377 (web)
https://thejournalofheadacheandpain.biomed-central.com/
+39-06-33775111
paolo.martelletti@uniroma1.it

The Journal of Pain
Editor: Mark Jensen
Publisher: Elsevier
ISSN: 1526-5900
https://www.journals.elsevier.com/the-journal-of-pain

Journal of Pain & Palliative Care Pharmacotherapy
Editor: Arthur G. Lipman
Publisher: Taylor & Francis
ISSN: 1536-0288 (print)
1536-0239 (web)
https://www.tandfonline.com/toc/ippc20/current

Journal of Pain and Symptom Management
Editor: Russell K. Portenoy
Publisher: Elsevier
ISSN: 0885-3924 (print)
1873-6513 (web)
https://www.jpsmjournal.com/
(508) 732-6767 x11
jpsm@stellarmed.com

Journal of Pain Research
Editor: Michael Schataman, MD
Publisher: Dove Medical Press
ISSN: 1178-7090
https://www.dovepress.com/journal-of-pain-research-journal

Journal of Palliative Medicine
Editor: Charles F. von Gunten
Publisher: Mary Ann Liebert
ISSN: 1096-6218 (print)
1557-7740 (web)
https://home.liebertpub.com/publications/journal-of-palliative-medicine/41

Molecular Pain
Editor: Jianguo Gu
Min Zhuo
Publisher: BioMed Central
ISSN: 1744-8069
https://journals.sagepub.com/home/mpx

Pain
Editor: Francis J. Keefe
Publisher: Lippincott Williams & Wilkins
ISSN: 0304-3959 (print)
1872-6623 (web)
https://journals.lww.com/pain/pages/default.aspx

Pain Medicine
Editor: Rollin Gallagher
Publisher: Wiley-Blackwell
ISSN: 1526-2375 (print)
1526-4637 (web)
https://academic.oup.com/painmedicine

Pain Physician
Editor: Alan David Kaye, MD, PhD
Publisher: American Society of Interventional Pain Physicians
ISSN: 1533-3159 (print)
2150-1149 (web)
https://www.painphysicianjournal.com/
(270) 554-9412
editor@painphysicianjournal.com

Pain Practice
Editor: Craig T. Hartrick
Publisher: John Wiley & Sons
ISSN: 1530-7085 (print)
1533-2500 (web)
https://onlinelibrary.wiley.com/journal/15332500
papr@wiley.com

Pain Research & Management
Editor: Kenneth D. Craig
Publisher: Hindawi Publishing Corp.
ISSN: 1203-6765 (print)
1918-1523 (web)
https://www.hindawi.com/journals/prm/

Glossary

5-Hydroxytryptamine: also known as 5-HT; another name for the neurotransmitter serotonin.

acathisia: a condition of severe restlessness, in which the very thought of sitting still causes strong feelings of anxiety.

acetabulum: the portion of the pelvic bone joining the femoral head to create the hip joint.

action potential: a fast, sudden, transient, and propagating change of the resting membrane potential of excitable cells.

activator: a small handheld spring-loaded instrument which delivers a controlled and reproducible impulse to the spine.

active euthanasia: administration of a drug or some other means that directly causes death; the motivation is to relieve patient suffering.

adjunctive: referring to the treatment of symptoms associated with a condition, not the condition itself.

adjuvant analgesic: drugs with a primary indication other than pain that have analgesic properties in some painful conditions and are usually given in combination with other analgesics.

aerobic exercise: brisk exercise that promotes the circulation of oxygen through the blood and is associated with an increased rate of breathing.

agonist: a drug that mimics the effects of a hormone or neurotransmitter normally found in the body.

Alexander technique: a process that teaches how to properly coordinate body and mind to release harmful tension and to improve posture, coordination and general health.

alternating pole devices: magnets that expose the skin to both north and south magnetic fields .

AMPA receptor: a subtype of ionotropic glutamate receptor that modulates the glutamate-mediated stimulation of neurons by allowing the influx of calcium and sodium ions.

analgesia: relief of pain; analgesics are compounds that stop the neurotransmission of pain messages.

analgesic: a substance that reduces pain.

anesthetic: any of a variety of drugs used to cause a patient to become unconscious and amnesiac for a brief period of time; very short-acting anesthetics, such as methohexital, thiamylal sodium, thiopental sodium, and etomidate, are often used in conjunction with electroconvulsive therapy.

aneurysm: the swelling of a blood vessel, which occurs with the stretching of a weak place in the vessel wall.

angina pectoris: chest pain caused by partial blockages of the arteries that feed blood to the heart.

antagonist: a drug that acts to block the effects of a hormone or neurotransmitter normally found in the body.

anticonvulsant: a medication that prevents or relieves the spontaneous movements of convulsions.

antipyretic: a substance that lowers body temperature.

arachidonic acid: an omega-6 unsaturated fatty acid the body requires to function properly; when broken down in the body, prostaglandins are produced.

arthritis: a painful condition that involves inflammation of one or more joints.

asana: (in Sanskrit seat or posture); a yogic posture or position; the ability to sit unmoving with a straight spine for long periods of time.

ataxia: a neurological sign characterized by a lack of voluntary coordination of muscle movements that may include gait abnormality, speech changes, and abnormalities in eye movement.

autonomic nervous system: the part of the nervous system responsible for control of the bodily functions not consciously directed, such as breathing, the heartbeat, and digestive processes.

Ayurveda: the traditional Hindu system of medicine, which is based on the idea of balance in bodily systems and uses diet, herbal treatment, and yogic breathing.

behavioral medicine: an interdisciplinary field of research and practice that focuses on how people's thoughts and behavior affect their health.

biodisplay: audio or visual information about the physiological activity within an organism displayed by various instruments and processes.

biofeedback instrument: a device (usually electronic) that is capable of measuring and displaying information about a physiologic process in a way that allows an individual to monitor the physiologic activity through his or her own senses.

biofeedback: the provision of information about the biological or physiological processes of an individual to him or her, with the objective of empowering the individual to make conscious changes in the processes being monitored; it can be instrumental (using devices that monitor physiological or biological processes) or noninstrumental (using bodily sensations).

bipolar disorders: mood disorders characterized by significant swings in mood from depression to persistent feelings of elation; also known as manic-depressive illness.

brainstem: the region between the brain and spinal cord that controls vital functions such as breathing and heart rate.

bursitis: inflammation of the sac of lubricating fluid located between joints.

calculus: an abnormal crystalline formation of a mineral salt; also called a stone.

cannabinoid: one of a class of diverse chemical compounds that acts on cannabinoid receptors, which are part of the endocannabinoid system found in cells that alter neurotransmitter release in the brain.

cannula: a tube or hypodermic needle implanted in the body to introduce or extract substances.

cartilage: flexible connective tissue between bones.

central nervous system: comprised of the brain and spinal cord; controls thoughts, emotions and actions by electrical signals traveling though neural pathways.

cerebral cortex: the outer covering of the brain that is comprised of neurons and glia cells.

cervical vertebrae: the first seven bones of the spinal column, located in the neck.

cholecystectomy: the removal of a diseased gallbladder or one that contains many gallstones.

cholelithiasis: the formation of gallstones in the gallbladder or the ducts that connect the gallbladder to the liver or small intestine.

colorectal: refers to cancers of the lower digestive tract consisting of the colon and the rectum.

commissurotomy: the severing of the corpus callosum, the fiber tract joining the two cerebral hemispheres.

conditioning: the process of training or accustoming a person or animal to behave in a certain way or to accept certain circumstances.

contraindication: a condition that makes a particular treatment not advisable; contraindications may be absolute (should never be used) or relative (should be used only with caution when the benefits outweigh the potential problems).

convulsion: an instance of high-frequency and amplitude-random electrical activity in the brain; electroconvulsive therapy causes a convulsion in the brain, which is believed to be related to its mechanism of action.

corpus cavernosum: spongy tissue which runs along both sides of the penis and fills with blood to produce an erection.

countertransference: the emotional reaction of the analyst to the subject's contribution.

COX-1 AND COX-2: cyclooxygenase 1 and 2 (COX-1 and COX-2) are important enzymes in the function of the human body; they both convert arachidonic acid to prostaglandins, and are implicated in pain, inflammation, cell multiplication, and other key biologic responses.

cross-cultural medicine: the ability of providers and organizations to effectively deliver health care services that meet the social, cultural, and linguistic needs of patients.

cryotherapy: the therapeutic use of cold.

death anxiety: also known as thanatophobia, a form of anxiety characterized by a fear of one's own death or the process of dying.

deep-tissue massage: a massage technique that's mainly used to treat musculoskeletal issues, such as strains and sports injuries; it involves applying sustained pressure using slow, deep strokes to target the inner layers of muscles and connective tissues.

dependence: a craving for a drug.

depolarization: the first part of an action potential during which there is less negative charge inside the cell, resulting in a more positive membrane potential.

depression: a mood disorder characterized by loss of energy, depressed mood, diminished interest in pleasurable activities, feelings of worthlessness, and difficulty in concentrating.

discontinuation syndrome: a condition caused by the abrupt discontinuation of antidepressant or antipsychotic medications.

disk prolapse: the protrusion (herniation) of intervertebral disk material, which may press on spinal nerves.

dopamine: a neurotransmitter that helps send electrical signals for emotion, movement, and other processes.

durable power of attorney: designation of a person who will have legal authority to make health care decisions if the patient becomes incapable of making decisions for himself or herself.

dyspepsia: upset stomach/indigestion .

dystonia: prolonged periods of unusual muscle contractions exhibiting as limb twistings, repetitive movements, abnormal postures, or rhythmic jerks.

effleurage: a series of massage strokes used in Swedish massage to warm up the muscle before deep tissue work.

electroacupuncture: a procedure in which pulses of weak electrical current are sent through acupuncture needles into acupuncture points in the skin.

electrocardiogram: a recording of the electrical activity of the heart; used during electroconvulsive therapy to monitor changes in heart rate, rhythm, and conduction, any or all of which may be temporarily affected by this procedure.

electrodermal response (EDR) biofeedback: the monitoring and displaying of information about the conductivity of the skin; used for anxiety reduction, asthma treatment, and the treatment of sleep disorders.

electroencephalogram: a brain wave trace used to monitor the onset, termination, and duration of the convulsion or seizure.

electroencephalographic (EEG) biofeedback: the monitoring and displaying of brain wave activity; used for the treatment of substance abuse disorders, epilepsy, attention-deficit disorders, and insomnia.

electromyograph (EMG): an instrument that is capable of monitoring and displaying information about electro-chemical activity in a group of muscle fibers.

endogenous: something naturally found in the body, such as neurotransmitters.

epidural: the injection of an anesthetic into the fluid around the spine or into the epidural space in the back.

equine-facilitated learning (EFL): using horses to promote learning experiences that develop skills intended for real-world environments.

equine-facilitated psychotherapy (EFP): follows a psychoanalytic approach by using the human-horse interactions as a tool for a therapist to gauge and discuss about their patients reactions and intentions.

evidence-based medicine: a method of basing clinical medical practice decisions on systematic reviews of published medical studies.

exogenous: something originating outside the body and administered orally or by injection.

expression: the action of cell biochemistry to produce and release a particular hormone in response to a stimulus.

FDA: U.S. Food and Drug Administration, a federal agency that provides safety, efficacy, and protection from biologicals.

Feldenkrais method: a system of gentle movements that promote flexibility, coordination, and self-awareness.

femur: the leg bone extending from the knee to the hip.

fluoxetine: the generic name for the antidepressant commonly called Prozac.

free association: the mental process by which one word or image may spontaneously suggest another without any apparent connection.

functional medicine: a personalized, systems-oriented model that empowers patients and practitioners to achieve the highest expression of health by working in collaboration to address the underlying causes of disease.

gastrointestinal tract: organs which include mouth, esophagus, stomach and intestines.

glutamate: a naturally occurring amino acid that is the most abundant stimulatory neurotransmitter in the nervous system.

glycine: the simplest naturally occurring amino acid that is a constituent of most proteins and one of the two main inhibitory neurotransmitters in the central nervous system, mainly in the spinal cord.

guided imagery: the use of words and music to evoke positive imaginary scenarios in a subject with a view to bringing about some beneficial effect.

heart rate variability: interval of time in-between heart beats that changes correlates to a changes in emotional states.

helicobacter pylori: bacteria capable of causing intestinal damage and related symptoms.

hematoma: a localized collection of clotted blood in an organ or tissue as a result of internal bleeding.

herbology: the study of herbs and their medical properties, especially when combined.

high-velocity, low-amplitude: short, quick thrust over restricted joints with the goal of restoring normal range of motion in the joint.

hippotherapy: using horses for occupational, physical or speech therapy.

homeopathy: the treatment of disease by minute doses of natural substances that in a healthy person would produce symptoms of disease.

hormone replacement therapy: treatment with estrogens with the aim of alleviating menopausal symptoms or osteoporosis.

hormone: a substance made by the body that travels through the bloodstream to reach its target organ and have its effect.

hospice: care designed to give supportive care to people in the final phase of a terminal illness and focus on comfort and quality of life, rather than cure.

hypertension: high blood pressure; above 130 mm Hg (systolic) / 90 mmHg (diastolic).

hypnotic: a medication that brings about a state of partial or complete unconsciousness.

hypotension: low blood pressure; below 120 mm Hg (systolic) / 80 mm Hg (diastolic).

indica: a species of Cannabis with broader leaves that is typically used for relaxation, appetite stimulation, sleep aid, and pain relief.

inflammation: the body's response to injury that may include redness, pain, swelling, and warmth in the affected area.

intercessory prayer: the act of praying to a deity on behalf of others.

interstitial cystitis: chronic inflammation of the bladder and urinary tract.

intervertebral disks: flattened disks of fibrocartilage that separate the vertebrae and allow cushioned flexibility of the spinal column.

ion: an atom or molecule with a net electric charge that results from the loss or gain of one or more electrons.

ischemia: inadequate blood supply to an organ or part of the body.

lesion: a wound or tumor of the brain or spinal cord.

ligand-gated ion channels: transmembrane protein complexes that conduct *ion* flow through a *channel* pore in response to the binding of a neurotransmitter.

living will: a legal document in which the patient states a preference regarding life-prolonging treatment in the event that he or she cannot choose.

lobectomy: the removal of a lobe of the brain, or a major part of a lobe.

lobotomy: the separation of either an entire lobe or a major part of a lobe from the rest of the brain.

local anesthesia: anesthesia produced by injecting a local anesthetic solution directly into the tissues; also known as local block.

locus coeruleus: a cluster of neurons in the pons of the brainstem involved with physiological responses to stress and panic.

low level laser therapy: form of medicine that applies low-level (low-power) lasers or light-emitting diodes (LEDs) to the surface of the body.

low-velocity, high-amplitude: slow, long thrusts to carry a dysfunctional joint through its full range of motion, with the therapeutic goal of increasing range of motion.

lumbar vertebrae: the five bones of the spinal column in the lower back, which experience the greatest stress in the spine.

major depressive disorder: mental health disorder characterized by persistent depressed mood and loss in interest of social activities.

manual therapy: the skilled application of passive movement to a joint either within or beyond its active range of movement.

MAOI inhibitors: class of drugs that stop the activity of monoamine oxidase enzymes, and includes such antidepressants such as selegiline (**Eldepry**, **Emsam**, **Zelapar**), phenelzine (**Nardil**), isocarboxazid (**Marplan**), tranylcypromine (**Parnate**).

membrane potential: a difference in electrical potential across the cell membrane that results from a disparity in the concentration of ions on either side of the cell membrane.

meridians: each of a set of pathways in the body along which vital energy is said to flow; there are twelve such pathways associated with specific organs.

methemoglobinemia: a condition where there is an elevated blood level of methhemoglobin where the iron is in a state which cannot carry oxygen.

mind/body therapy: techniques designed to enhance the mind's positive impact on the body.

monoamine oxidase inhibitors (MAOIs): a class of drugs that relieve the symptoms of depression by inhibiting the enzyme that deactivates the brain chemical monoamine oxidase.

mood disorders: any of a number of mental conditions characterized by a primary disturbance of mood as distinct from thinking or behavior.

moxibustion: a type of heat therapy in which an herb is burned on or above the skin to warm and stimulate an acupuncture point or affected area.

multidisciplinary care: A comprehensive care provided by professionals from different disciplines, including doctors, nurses, pharmacists, social workers, and many others.

muscle relaxant: any of a number of medications used to paralyze the muscles of the patient temporarily before delivering the electrical stimulus; the main medication used for this purpose is succinylcholine.

nerve impulse: signals transmitted along nerve fibers that consist of a wave of electrical depolarization that reverses the charge differential across the nerve cell membranes.

neuromuscular massage: targets the neurological system and the muscles related to it, addressing trigger points on the body that affect mood and neurological function.

neuromuscular rehabilitation: the process of employing electromyographic biofeedback to correct physiological disorders that have both muscular and neurological components, such as the effects of strokes and fibromyalgia; also called myoneural rehabilitation.

neurons: highly specialized cell found in the nervous system that produces an electrical signal to transmit information.

neurotransmitter: a chemical substance released by one nerve cell to stimulate or inhibit the function of an adjacent nerve cell; a chemical message released from a neuron.

neurotransmitter: small molecules released by neurons to either activate or inhibit neighboring neurons.

NMDA receptor: glutamate-gated cation channels that are highly permeable to calcium ions and play several important roles in the neurobiology of animals.

nonvoluntary euthanasia: a decision to terminate life made by another when the patient is incapable of making a decision for himself or herself.

norepinephrine reuptake transporter: a protein embedded in the membrane of the axon terminus of a presynaptic neuron that decreases the concentration of norepinephrine in the synaptic cleft by effecting norepinephrine reuptake in the presynaptic neuron.

norepinephrine: a hormone released by the adrenal glands; a neurotransmitter released by sympathetic nerves in response to stress, and by clusters of neurons in the brain to enhance alertness, attention, memory formation and retrieval, processing of sensory inputs, and adaptation to changing environments .

NSAIDs: nonsteroidal anti-inflammatory drugs (NSAIDs) are medications that are used to control pain and inflammation in the body.

obsessive-compulsive disorder: a psychiatric disorder that causes a person to ruminate on a particular thought and then act out a ritualistic behavior.

off-label prescribing: when a health provider prescribes a drug that the U.S. Food and Drug Administration (FDA) approved to treat a condition different from your condition.

operationalization: a process of defining the measurement of a phenomenon that is not directly measurable, though its existence is inferred by other phenomena.

opiates: drugs made from the opium flower, such as opium, morphine, and codeine.

opioids: endogenous or exogenous substances (opiates) that relieve pain and cause euphoria.

organic brain syndrome (organicity): changes in memory, orientation, and perception that occur as a side effect of electroconvulsive therapy.

orthopedics: a medical specialty emphasizing the prevention and correction of skeletal deformities.

osteoarthritis: a progressive disorder of the joints caused by gradual loss of cartilage that can result in the development of bone spurs and cysts at the margins of joints.

overdetermination: the idea that a single observed effect is determined by multiple causes at once (any one of which alone might be enough to account for the effect).

pain management: A treatment to control pain and reduce suffering using pharmacological and/or non-pharmacological methods. The goal is to improve quality of life.

palliative care: a specialized medical care that focuses on providing patients relief from pain and other symptoms of a serious illness, no matter the diagnosis or stage of disease.

passive euthanasia: ending life by refusing or withdrawing life-sustaining medical treatment.

patella: the flat, triangular bone in the front of the knee; also called the kneecap.

peptides: short chains of amino acids that, when released, carry out functions in other areas of the body.

peripheral nervous system: refers to all of the neurons in the body located outside the brain and spinal cord.

physiological autoregulation: the process by which an individual utilizes information about a physiological activity to effect changes in that activity in a direction that contributes to normal (or desirable) functioning.

Pilates: system of physical conditioning involving low-impact exercises and stretches designed to strengthen muscles of the torso and often performed with specialized equipment.

placebo effect: phenomenon in which a placebo (a fake treatment, an inactive substance like sugar, distilled water, saline solution, etc.) can sometimes improve a patient's condition simply because the person has the expectation that it will be helpful.

positive symptoms: symptoms of schizophrenia that involve the production of an abnormal behavior.

pranayama: (in Sanskrit prana = energy + yama = control); type of meditation technique that involves various ways of controlling the breathing, with the goal being to withdraw ones senses from the outside world.

pressure points: a point on the surface of the body sensitive to pressure.

priapism: a prolonged and painful erection.

primary dysmenorrhea: pelvic pain which occurs with any underlying infection, condition, or syndrome.

prostaglandins: a large group of biologically active unsaturated, twenty-carbon fatty acids that represent some of the metabolites of arachidonic acid.

psychic healing: the process of sending healing energy by one or more persons to another person in order to re-energize him or her.

psychosis: a mental disorder in which one's emotions and thoughts are impaired, causing a person to lose touch with reality. Primarily characterized by experience of delusions, personality shifts, discontinuous thought patterns and speech, and unrefined social behavior.

psychotic disorder: a psychiatric condition in which an individual's mental state is out of touch with reality, as displayed by abnormal and bizarre perceptions, thoughts, behavior, judgment, and reasoning.

psychotropic: a drug that affects psychic function, behavior, or experience.

pulsed electromagnetic field therapy: uses electromagnetic fields in an attempt to heal non-union fractures and depression.

qi: the circulating life energy that in Chinese philosophy is thought to be inherent in all things; in traditional Chinese medicine the balance of negative and positive forms in the body is believed to be essential for good health.

qigong: a Chinese system of breathing exercises, body postures and movements, and mental concentration, intended to maintain good health and control the flow of vital energy.

reflexology: a system of massage used to relieve tension and treat illness, based on the theory that there are reflex points on the feet, hands, and head linked to every part of the body.

regional anesthesia: insensibility caused by the interruption of nerve conduction in a region of the body.

reinforcer: a stimulus (such as a reward or the removal of an electric shock) that increases the probability of a desired response in operant conditioning by being applied or effected following the desired response.

repetitive transcranial magnet therapy: a form of brain stimulation therapy used to treat depression and anxiety.

repolarization: the second part of an action potential, after depolarization, in which positive potassium ions leave the cell and the membrane potential is returned to a negative value.

resistance exercise: exercise that causes the muscles to contract against an external resistance with the expectation of increases in strength, tone, mass, and/or endurance.

Reye syndrome: a rare but serious disease that most often affects children ages 6 to 12 years old; can cause brain swelling and liver damage; may be related to using aspirin to treat viral infections.

rheumatoid arthritis: a long-term autoimmune disorder that primarily affects joints resulting in warm, swollen, and painful joints.

salicylates: a group of drugs (including aspirin) derived from salicylic acid, used to relieve pain, reduce inflammation, and lower fever.

sativa: a species of Cannabis with taller plants with narrower leaves that is typically used for increased energy and its uplifting and euphoric effects.

schizophrenia: a type of psychotic disorder involving a detachment among one's thoughts, emotions and behaviors.

sciatica: pain affecting the back, hip, and outer side of the leg, caused by compression of a spinal nerve root in the lower back.

sedative: a medication that has a soothing or tranquilizing effect.

selective serotonin reuptake inhibitors (SSRIs): a class of antidepressant drugs, first introduced in 1987, that work by inhibiting the reuptake of the neurotransmitter serotonin, thus making more of it available to brain cells.

self-diagnosis: determining the nature of an ailment and the method of treating it without the aid of a physician; should always be based on sound experience and education rather than on hearsay and guesswork.

self-healing: the process of recovery (generally from psychological disturbances, trauma, etc.), motivated by and directed by the patient, guided often only by instinct.

serotonin reuptake transporter: a protein embedded in the membrane of the axon terminus of a presynaptic neuron that decreases the concentration of serotonin in the synaptic cleft by effecting serotonin reuptake in the presynaptic neuron.

serotonin syndrome: a condition that results from the release of high levels of serotonin into the body, causing agitation, confusion, dilated pupils, and muscle twitching.

serotonin: a neurotransmitter released by neurons in the gastrointestinal tract and central nervous system that regulates appetite, sleep, emotional states, motor function, cognition and many other neurological and physiological functions.

shiatsu: a form of therapy of Japanese origin based on the same principles as acupuncture, in which pressure is applied to certain points on the body using the hands.

signal transduction pathway: A cascade of biochemical reactions inside cells that culminate in a specific cellular response, and are set in motion when a signaling molecule, such as a hormone or growth factor, binds receptors inside the cell or on the cell surface.

spinal anesthesia: anesthesia produced by injecting a local anesthetic around the spinal cord; also known as subarachnoid block.

spinal cord: a column of nervous tissue housed in the vertebral column that carries messages to and from the brain.

static magnets: a magnet that retains its magnetism after being removed from a magnetic field.

steroids: a class of hormones produced by the adrenal glands; can also be made synthetically.

structural integration: a type of bodywork that focuses on the connective tissue, or fascia, of the body; fascia surrounds muscles, groups of muscles, blood vessels, organs, and nerves, binding some structures together while permitting others to slide smoothly over each other.

subluxations: a slight misalignment of the vertebrae, regarded in chiropractic theory as the cause of many health problems.

suppository: a solid, conical-shaped medication preparation designed to be placed into the rectum or vagina and allowed to dissolve to deliver localized medication.

Swedish massage: the most popular type of massage in the United States, it involves the use of hands, forearms or elbows to manipulate the superficial layers of the muscles to improve mental and physical health.

synaptic cleft: the space between neurons at a nerve synapse across which a nerve impulse is transmitted by a neurotransmitter; also called the synaptic gap.

synthetically made neuron: a nerve cell that can conduct electrical impulses from one region of the body to another; it is capable of releasing neurotransmitters.

systemic: affecting the entire body; systemic treatments may be administered orally, directly into a vein, into the muscle, or through mucous membranes.

Tai Chi: a Chinese martial art and form of stylized, meditative exercise, characterized by methodically slow circular and stretching movements and positions of bodily balance.

tendinitis: inflammation of a tendon, a tough band of tissue that connects muscle to bone.

thanatology: the scientific study of death and the practices associated with it, including the study of the needs of the terminally ill and their families.

therapeutic horseback riding: recreational horseback riding for disabled individuals.

thermotherapy: treatment of disease by heat (as by hot air, hot baths, or diathermy).

thromboxane: hormones synthesized by many tissues that are vasoconstrictors and stimulators of platelet aggregation.

tolerance: diminished effect of a drug over time due to its chronic use.

topical: referring to treatments applied directly to the skin or mucous membranes that affect primarily the area in which they are applied.

touch-based therapy: based on the belief that vital energy flows through the human body and can be balanced or made stronger by practitioners who pass their hands over, or gently touch, a patient's body.

traditional Chinese medicine: a branch of traditional medicine that is said to be based on more than 3,500 years of Chinese medical practice that includes various forms of herbal medicine, acupuncture, cupping therapy, gua sha, massage (tui na), bonesetter (die-da), exercise (qigong), and dietary therapy.

Trager approach: a combination of hands-on tissue mobilization, relaxation, and movement reeducation called Mentastics.

transference: a patient's displacement or projection onto the analyst of those unconscious feelings and wishes originally directed toward important individuals, such as parents, in the patient's childhood.

trephination: the opening of a hole in the skull with an instrument called a trephine.

tricyclics: antidepressant drugs that interfere with several neurotransmitters, making more of them available to the brain.

unipolar magnets: magnets with north on one side and south on the other; the north (or negative) side is typically applied to the skin.

upper respiratory tract: the nose, sinuses, throat, ears, Eustachian tubes, and trachea.

ureterolithotomy: the surgical removal of a stone in the ureter.

ureters: the two muscular tubes that connect the kidneys to the urinary bladder and that serve as conduits for urine.

urolithiasis: the formation of stones in the urinary tract.

vasoconstriction: narrowing of blood vessels (arteries and veins).

vasodilation: the dilatation of blood vessels, which decreases blood pressure.

vinyasa: (in Sanskrit vi = special + nyasa = to place) movement between poses in yoga, typically accompanied by regulated breathing.

virilization: the acquisition of physical characteristics typical of males.

viscosupplementation injections: injections to add lubrication into the joint to make joint movement less painful.

voltage-gated ion channels: a class of transmembrane proteins that form ion channels that open or close in response to changes in the membrane potential near the channel.

voluntary euthanasia: a patient's consent to a decision which results in the shortening of his or her life.

weight training: a system of conditioning involving lifting weights especially for strength and endurance.

Western herbal medicine: a clinical practice of healing using naturally occurring plant material or plants with little or no industrial processing.

withdrawal: the body's response, both physical and mental, when an addictive substance is reduced or not given to the body.

yin and yang: a concept of dualism in ancient Chinese philosophy, describing how seemingly opposite or contrary forces may actually be complementary, interconnected, and interdependent in the natural world, and how they may give rise to each other as they interrelate to one another.

yoga: comes from a Sanskrit word meaning "union;" yoga combines physical exercises, mental meditation, and breathing techniques to strengthen the muscles and relieve stress.

Organizations

Agency for Healthcare Research and Quality
5600 Fishers Lane
Rockville, MD 20857
https://www.ahrq.gov/
(301) 427-1364

American Academy of Allergy, Asthma & Immunology
555 East Wells Street, Suite 1100
Milwaukee, WI 53202-3823
https://www.aaaai.org/
(414) 272-6071
info@aaaai.org

American Academy of Craniofacial Pain
11130 Sunrise Valley Drive, Suite 350
Reston, VA 20191
https://www.aacfp.org/
(703) 234-4087
central@aacfp.org

American Academy of Hospice and Palliative Medicine
8735 W Higgins Rd, Ste 300
Chicago, IL 60631-2738
http://aahpm.org/
(847) 375-4712
info@aahpm.org

American Academy of Medical Acupuncture
2512 Artesia Blvd, Ste 200
Redondo Beach, CA 90278
https://www.medicalacupuncture.org/
(310) 379-8261
info@medicalacupuncture.org

American Academy of Orofacial Pain
174 S. New York Ave.; P.O. Box 478
Oceanville, NJ 08231
https://aaop.clubexpress.com/
(609) 504-1311

American Academy of Pain Medicine
8735 W Higgins Rd, Ste 300
Chicago, IL 60631-2738
https://painmed.org/
(847) 375-4731
info@painmed.org

American Association of Acupuncture and Oriental Medicine
PO Box 96503 #44114
Washington DC 20090-6503
https://www.aaaomonline.org/
admin@aaaomonline.org

American Board of Pain Medicine
85 W. Algonquin Rd, #550
Arlington Heights, IL 60005
http://www.abpm.org/
(847) 981-8905
info@abpm.org

American Chiropractic Association
1701 Clarendon Blvd, Suite 200 -
Arlington, VA 22209
https://www.acatoday.org/
(703) 276-8800
memberinfo@acatoday.org

American Chronic Pain Association
P.O. Box 850
Rocklin, CA 95677
https://www.theacpa.org/
(800) 533-3231
ACPA@theacpa.org

American College of Gastroenterology
6400 Goldsboro Rd
Bethesda, MD 20817
https://gi.org/
(301) 263-9000

American College of Obstetricians and Gynecologists
PO Box 96920
Washington, DC 20024-9998
https://www.acog.org/
(202) 638-5577

American Counseling Association
6101 Stevenson Ave.
Alexandria, VA 22304
https://www.counseling.org/
(703) 823-9800

American Headache Society
19 Mantua Rd.
Mount Royal, NJ 08061
https://americanheadachesociety.org/
(856) 423-0043
ahshq@talley.com

American Herbalists Guild
P.O. Box 3076
Asheville, NC 28802-3076
www.americanherbalistsguild.com/
617.520.4372
office@americanherbalistsguild.com

American Medical Marijuana Physicians Association
PO Box 266
Oakland, FL 34760
https://ammpa.net/ | (321) 917-3212

American Massage Therapy Association
500 Davis Street; Suite 900
Evanston, IL 60201
https://www.amtamassage.org/
877-905-2700
info@amtamassage.org

American Migraine Foundation
19 Mantua Road
Mt. Royal, NJ 08061
https://americanmigrainefoundation.org/
(856) 423-0258
achehq@talley.com

American Pain Association
2 Bala Plaza, Suite PL 50
Bala Cynwyd, PA 19004
http://painassociation.org/
(484) 483-3131
info@painassociation.org

American Pharmacists Association
2215 Constitution Avenue NW
Washington, DC 20037
https://www.pharmacist.com/
(202) 628-4410
infocenter@aphanet.org

American Physical Therapy Association
1111 North Fairfax Street
Alexandria, VA 22314-1488
http://www.apta.org/
(703) 684-2782

American Podiatric Medical Association
9312 Old Georgetown Road
Bethesda, MD 20814-1621
https://www.apma.org/
(301) 581-9200

American Society of Anesthesiologists
1061 American Lane
Schaumburg, IL 60173-4973
https://www.asahq.org/
(847) 825-5586
info@asahq.org

American Society of Pain Management Nursing
4400 College Blvd Suite 220
Overland Park, KS 66211
http://www.aspmn.org/
(913) 222-8666
ASPMN@kellencompany.com

American Society of Interventional Pain Physicians
81 Lakeview Drive
Paducah, KY 42001
https://www.asipp.org/
(270) 554-9412
asipp@asipp.org

American Society of PeriAnesthesia Nurses
90 Frontage Road
Cherry Hill, NJ 08034-1424
https://www.aspan.org/
(877) 737-9696
aspan@aspan.org

American Society of Regional Anesthesia and Pain Medicine
3 Penn Center West, Suite 224
Pittsburgh, PA 15276
https://www.asra.com/
(412) 471-2718
asraassistant@asra.com

American Tai Chi and Qigong Association
2465 J-17 Centreville Road, #150
Herndon, VA 20171

http://www.americantaichi.org/
TC@AmericanTaiChi.net

Association for Behavioral and Cognitive Therapies
305 7th Avenue, 16th Fl.
New York, NY 10001
http://www.abct.org/
(212) 647-1890

Biofeedback Certification International Alliance
5310 Ward Road, Suite 201
Arvada CO 80002
https://www.bcia.org/
(720) 502-5829
info@bcia.org

Center to Advance Palliative Care
55 West 125th Street, Suite 1302
New York, NY 10027
https://www.capc.org/
(212) 201-2670

Chronic Illness Advocacy & Awareness Group, Inc.
P.O. Box 1203
Worcester, Massachusetts 01613
https://www.ciaag.net/
(774) 262-6671
info@ciaag.net

Chronic Pain Research Alliance
P.O. Box 26770
Milwaukee, WI 53226
http://www.cpralliance.org/
(262) 432-0350
info@CPRAlliance.org

City of Hope Pain Resource Center
1500 East Duarte Road
Duarte, CA 91010
https://prc.coh.org/
prc@coh.org

The Coalition Against Pediatric Pain
Po Box 1433
Marshfield, Ma 02050
https://tcapp.org/
info@tcapp.org

Defense & Veterans Center for Integrative Pain Management
11300 Rockville Pike Suite 709
Rockville, MD 20852
http://www.dvcipm.org/
(301) 816-4723

Facial Pain Association
22 SE Fifth Ave., Suite D
Gainesville, FL 32601
https://fpa-support.org/
(352) 384-3600
info@tna-support.org

Foundation for Physical Therapy
1111 N. Fairfax St.
Alexandria, VA 22314
https://foundation4pt.org/
(800) 875-1378
info@foundation4pt.org

Global Pain Initiative
14828 W 6 Ave. Ste 16-B Room 1
Golden, CO 80401-5000
https://www.globalpaininitiative.org/

Institute for the Study and Treatment of Pain
5655 Cambie Street, Suite #280
Vancouver, B.C. Canada V5Z 3A4
www.istop.org
(604) 264-7867

International Association for the Study of Pain
1510 H Street NW, Suite 600
Washington, DC 20005-1020
https://www.iasp-pain.org/
(202) 856-7400
IASPdesk@iasp-pain.org

International Association of Yoga Therapists
PO Box 251563
Little Rock, AR 72225
https://www.iayt.org/
928-541-0004

International Foundation for Gastrointestinal Disorders
PO Box 170864
Milwaukee, WI 53217
https://www.iffgd.org/
(414) 964-1799

The Joint Commission
1 Renaissance Blvd.
Oakbrook Terrace, IL 60181
https://www.jointcommission.org/

(630) 792-5000
customerservice@jointcommission.org

Juvenile Arthritis Association
8549 Wilshire Blvd. Suite #103
Beverly Hills, CA 90211
http://www.juvenilearthritis.org/
info@juvenilearthritis.org

Marijuana Policy Project
P.O. Box 21824
Washington, D.C. 20009
https://www.mpp.org/
(202) 462-5747
info@mpp.org

Migraine Research Foundation
300 East 75th Street, Suite 3K
New York, NY 10021
https://migraineresearchfoundation.org/
(212) 249-5402

National Association of Drug Diversion Investigators
1810 York Road #435
Lutherville, MD 21093
https://www.naddi.org/

National Cancer Institute
BG 9609 MSC 9760
9609 Medical Center Drive
Bethesda, MD 20892-9760
https://www.cancer.gov/
(800) 422-6237
NCIinfo@nih.gov

National Center for Complementary and Integrative Health
9000 Rockville Pike
Bethesda, Maryland 20892
https://nccih.nih.gov/
(888) 644-6226
info@nccih.nih.gov

National Coalition of Chronic Pain Providers and Professionals
670 Newfield St # 2
Middletown, CT 06457
http://www.nccppp.org/
(800) 910-0664

National Institute of Allergy and Infectious Disease
5601 Fishers Lane, MSC 9806
Bethesda, MD 20892-9806
https://www.niaid.nih.gov/
(301) 496-5717
ocpostoffice@niaid.nih.gov

National Institute of Arthritis and Musculoskeletal and Skin Diseases
9000 Rockville Pike
Bethesda, Maryland 20892
https://www.niams.nih.gov/
(301) 565-2966
NIAMSinfo@mail.nih.gov

National Institute of General Medical Sciences
45 Center Drive MSC 6200
Bethesda, MD 20892-6200
https://www.nigms.nih.gov/
(301) 496-7301
info@nigms.nih.gov

National Institute of Mental Health
6001 Executive Boulevard
Room 6200, MSC 9663
Bethesda, MD 20892-9663
https://www.nimh.nih.gov/
(301) 443-8431
nimhinfo@nih.gov

National Institute of Neurological Disorders and Stroke
P.O. Box 5801
Bethesda, MD 20824
https://www.ninds.nih.gov/
(800) 352-9424

National Institute on Aging
Building 31, Room 5C27
31 Center Drive, MSC 2292
Bethesda, MD 20892
https://www.nia.nih.gov/
(800) 222-2225
niaic@nia.nih.gov

National Institute on Drug Abuse
6001 Executive Boulevard
Room 5213, MSC 9561
Bethesda, Maryland 20892
https://www.drugabuse.gov/
(301) 443-1124

National Headache Foundation
820 N. Orleans, Suite 201

Chicago, IL 60610-3131
https://headaches.org/
(312) 274-2650
info@headaches.org

National Hospice and Palliative Care Organization
1731 King Street
Alexandria, Virginia 22314
https://www.nhpco.org/
(703) 837-1500

National Organization of Rare Disorders
55 Kenosia Avenue
Danbury, CT 06810
https://rarediseases.org/
(203) 744-0100

National Vulvodynia Association
PO Box 4491
Silver Spring, MD 20914-4491
https://www.nva.org/
(301) 299-0775

Peripheral Nerve Society
5841 Cedar Lake Road, Suite 2014
Minneapolis, MN 55416 USA
https://www.pnsociety.com/
(952) 545-6284
info@PNSociety.com

Providers Clinical Support System
400 Massasoit Avenue
Suite # 307 – 2nd Floor
East Providence, RI 02914
https://pcssnow.org/
(855) 227-2776
pcss@aaap.org

Society for Acupuncture Research
130 Cloverhurst Court
Winston Salem, NC 27103
https://sar.memberclicks.net/
info@acupunctureresearch.org

Society for Pediatric Pain Medicine
2209 Dickens Street
Richmond, VA 23230-2005
https://www.pedspainmedicine.org/
(804) 282-9780
sppm@societyhq.com

U.S. Pain Foundation
670 Newfield Street, Suite B
Middletown, CT 06457
https://uspainfoundation.org/
(800) 910-2462
contact@uspainfoundation.org

World Allergy Alliance
555 East Wells Street, Suite 1100
Milwaukee, WI 53202-3823
https://www.worldallergy.org/
(414) 276 1791
info@worldallergy.org

World Institute of Pain
150 Kimel Park Drive, Suite 100-A
Winston-Salem, NC 27103-6992
http://wip.agoria.co.uk/
(336) 760-2933
wip@worldinstituteofpain.org

Yoga Alliance
1560 Wilson Blvd #700
Arlington, VA 22209
https://www.yogaalliance.org/
(888) 921-9642
info@yogaalliance.org

INDEXES

Category Index

Addiction
Anesthesia misuse, 313
Benzodiazepine misuse, 314
Narcotics and opioid misuse, 318
Prescription drug misuse, 321
Sedative-hypnotic misuse, 325

Addiction Risk
Carisoprodol, 25
Codeine, 26
Dextromethorphan, 32
Fentanyl, 33
Hydrocodone, 37
Ketamine, 278
Kratom, 170
Marijuana, 185
Methadone, 39
Morphine, 41
Opium, 54
Oxycodone, 62
Tramadol, 70
Valium, 71
Vicodin and Norco, 72

Analgesic
Capsaicin, 145
Nitrous oxide, 48

Anesthetic
Ketamine, 278

Antibacterial
Eucalyptus, 149
Oregano oil, 190

Anticonvulsant
Carbamazepine, 21
Pregabalin, 66

Antidepressant
Bupropion, 248
Ketamine, 278
Mirtazapine, 285

Antiemetic
Ginger, 159
Mirtazapine, 285

Anti-inflammatory
Boswellia, 141
Bromelain, 143
Capsaicin, 145
Comfrey, 146
Corticosteroids, 27
Devil's claw, 147
Eucalyptus, 149
Oregano oil, 190
Peppermint, 192
Prescription NSAIDs, 67
Turmeric, 196
White willow, 202
Witch hazel, 204

Anxiolytic
Mirtazapine, 285
Nitrous oxide, 48
Valium, 71

Class of Drug
Alpha-2 adrenergic agonists, 2
Analgesic, 5
Anesthesia, 7
Antianxiety medications, 231
Antidepressants, 233
Anti-inflammatory drugs, 14
Anti-nausea medications, 15
Antipsychotics, 235
Barbiturates, 240
Benzodiazepines, 246
Corticosteroids, 27
Decongestants, 30
Gabapentin, 34
Medications for carpal tunnel syndrome, 329
Medications for foot pain, 334
Medications for headache, 344
Medications for low back pain and sciatica, 352
Medications for menopause, 361
Medications for osteoarthritis, 367

Medications for sinusitis, 375
Narcotics, 42
NMDA receptor antagonists, 49
Non-steroidal anti-inflammatory drugs (NSAIDs), 51
Serotonin-norepinephrine reuptake inhibitors, 303

Decongestant
Dextromethorphan, 32

Functional Food
Flaxseed, 152
Garlic, 155
Ginger, 159
Oregano oil, 190
Peppermint, 192
Rosemary, 195
Turmeric, 196

Herbs and Supplements
Boswellia, 141
Bromelain, 143
Comfrey, 146
Devil's claw, 147
Eucalyptus, 149
Feverfew, 151
Flaxseed, 152
Garlic, 155
Ginger, 159
Kratom, 170
Lavender, 171
Magnesium, 173
Marijuana, 185
Medical marijuana, 188
Oregano oil, 190
Other treatments for menopause, 366
Peppermint, 192
Rosemary, 195
Turmeric, 196
Valerian, 198
White willow, 202
Witch hazel, 204

Muscle relaxant
Baclofen, 19
Benzodiazepines, 246
Carisoprodol, 25
Valium, 71

Narcotic
Pentazocine, butorphanol, nalbuphine, 65

NSAID
Acetaminophen, 1
Aspirin, 17
Cyclooxygenase-2 (COX-2) inhibitors, 29
Prescription NSAIDs, 67

Opioid
Codeine, 26
Fentanyl, 33
Hydrocodone, 37
Methadone, 39
Morphine, 41
Opium, 54
Oxycodone, 62
Pentazocine, butorphanol, nalbuphine, 65
Tramadol, 70
Vicodin and Norco, 72

Over-the-Counter
Acetaminophen, 1
Aspirin, 17
Bismuth subsalicylate, 20
Over-the-counter (OTC) drugs: Cautions and precautions, 60

Physiotherapy
Astym® therapy, 77
Chiropractic, 82
Chronic pain management: psychological impact, 249
Equine-assisted therapy, 269
Exercise, 94
Exercise-based therapies, 96
Hydrotherapy, 100
Lifestyle changes to manage foot pain, 336
Lifestyle changes to manage headache, 346
Lifestyle changes to manage low back pain and sciatica, 354
Lifestyle changes to manage menopause, 365
Lifestyle changes to manage osteoarthritis, 370
Massage therapy, 102
Music, dance, and theater therapy, 287
Other treatments for carpal tunnel syndrome, 333
Other treatments for foot pain, 340
Other treatments for headache, 350
Other treatments for low back pain and sciatica, 358
Other treatments for osteoarthritis, 372

Progressive muscle relaxation, 110
TENS machines, 115
Yoga, 205

Prevention
Companionship, 257
Exercise, 94
Exercise-based therapies, 96
Yoga, 205

Procedure
Arthroplasty, 75
Cervical epidural injection, 80
Disk removal, 89
Epidural anesthesia in childbirth, 92
Euthanasia, 215
Other treatments for low back pain and sciatica, 358
Neurosurgery, 105
Stone removal, 113
Surgical procedures for carpal tunnel syndrome, 332
Surgical procedures for foot pain, 338
Surgical procedures for headache, 349
Surgical procedures for low back pain and sciatica, 356
Surgical procedures for sinusitis, 377
Tooth extraction, 117
Transcranial magnetic stimulation (TMS), 309

Psychological
Coping with a terminal illness, 211

Psychotherapy
Assimilative family therapy model, 237
Behavioral family therapy, 243
Chronic pain management: psychological impact, 249
Cognitive behavior therapy (CBT), 253
Coping strategies, 258
Couples therapy, 262
Dialectical behavioral therapy, 266
Equine-assisted therapy, 269
Group therapy, 274
Group therapy, 274
Lifestyle changes to manage low back pain and sciatica, 354
Lifestyle changes to manage osteoarthritis, 370
Music, dance, and theater therapy, 287
Other treatments for headache, 350
Other treatments for low back pain and sciatica, 358

Play therapy, 293
Psychoanalysis, 297
Reminiscence therapy, 301
Shock therapy, 305

Salicylates
Bismuth subsalicylate, 20

Sedative
Benzodiazepines, 246
Mirtazapine, 285
Valium, 71
Valerian, 198

Therapy or Technique
Astym® therapy, 77
Acupressure, 119
Acupuncture, 121
Assimilative family therapy model, 237
Behavioral family therapy, 243
Biofeedback, 136
Center for Substance Abuse Treatment (CSAT), 317
Chiropractic, 82
Cognitive behavior therapy (CBT), 253
Companionship, 257
Coping strategies, 258
Coping with a terminal illness, 211
Couples therapy, 262
Deep brain stimulation, 88
Dialectical behavioral therapy, 266
Equine-assisted therapy, 269
Exercise, 94
Exercise-based therapies, 96
Faith healing, 273
Group therapy, 274
Heat and cold therapy, 99
Herbal medicine, 162
Hospice, 220
Hydrotherapy, 100
Hypnotherapy, 164
Integrative medicine, 166
Lifestyle changes to manage menopause, 365
Lifestyle changes to manage sinusitis, 377
Light therapy, 279
Magnet therapy, 176
Massage therapy, 102
Meditation and relaxation, 280
Music, dance, and theater therapy, 287
Other treatments for carpal tunnel syndrome, 333
Other treatments for low back pain and sciatica, 358

Other treatments for sinusitis, 378
Pain management during gestation, 109
Palliative care, 224
Palliative medicine, 226
Pet therapy, 291
Play therapy, 293
Progressive muscle relaxation, 110
Psychoanalysis, 297

Reminiscence therapy, 301
Shock therapy, 305
TENS machines, 115
Yoga, 205

Vasodilator
Sildenafi, 68

Subject Index

acathisia, 15, 17
acetabulum, 75, 76
acetaminophen, 1–2, 6, 7, 33, 39, 56, 64, 72–73, 148, 163, 228, 323, 336, 345, 354, 368, 369, 376
acquired immunodeficiency syndrome (AIDS), 225
activator, 82, 83, 87
acupressure, 102, 104, 119–121, 125–127, 129–131, 133, 134, 179, 252
acupuncture, 44, 84, 86, 102–104, 110, 119–135, 168, 169, 177, 179, 181, 252, 350, 373
addiction, 4, 6, 7, 19, 20, 26, 38–40, 47, 55, 64, 65, 70, 73, 88, 120, 128, 164, 165, 170, 185, 189, 211, 221, 229, 232, 240, 247, 313–322, 324, 325, 327
adjunctive, 30, 31
Advil, 14, 56, 59, 67, 376
aerobic exercise, 94, 95, 359
agonist, 4, 39, 42, 43, 46, 48, 65
alcoholism, 139, 169, 283, 325
Aleve, 14, 67
Alexander technique, 96–99
alfentanil, 33, 46
allicin, 158
Almotriptan, 344
alprazolam, 22, 232, 315–317, 326
alternating pole devices, 176, 177
Alzheimer's disease, 22, 24, 88, 163, 168, 174, 197, 279, 290
amiloride, 176
amnesia, 7, 17, 25, 66, 71, 247, 308
Amoxicillin, 143, 347, 375
amygdala, 284, 292
Amyotrophic lateral sclerosis, 177, 183, 221
analgesic, 1, 2, 4–7, 10, 13, 17, 33, 41, 43–48, 56, 59, 66, 67, 70, 90, 107, 110, 114, 116, 117, 144, 145, 217, 241, 286, 318, 345
anesthesia, 4, 5, 7–13, 32, 33, 43, 45, 46, 65, 76, 81, 90, 92–93, 106, 107, 114, 123, 125, 131, 201, 232, 235, 241, 306, 307, 313–314, 332, 333
anesthesiology, 33, 75, 226
anesthetic, 3, 4, 7–13, 33, 48, 50, 76, 80, 81, 93, 117, 125, 131, 192, 278, 305, 313, 314, 325, 358
aneurysm, 105, 107
angina, 80, 173, 175, 344

antagonist, 16, 17, 27, 32, 42, 43, 46, 48, 49–50, 65, 216, 286, 303, 319
anti-anxiety, 22, 187, 247, 248, 314, 317
anticonvulsant, 21–24, 66, 240, 241, 246, 247, 325
antidepressant, 31, 132, 182, 231–235, 248, 249, 278, 286, 303, 304, 307, 346, 353, 368
antidiarrheal medications, 56, 59
antiemetic, 15, 16
anti-inflammatory, 5, 6, 14–15, 18, 25, 56, 67, 76, 129, 141, 148, 152, 170, 195–197, 202, 203, 205, 333, 335
antipsychotic, 73, 235–237, 249, 303
antipyretic, 1, 2, 17, 170
anxiety, 15, 20, 22, 34, 36, 37, 39, 45, 48, 54, 55, 66, 70, 71, 73, 98, 101, 104, 111, 112, 120, 128, 132, 136, 137, 164, 165, 168, 170, 171, 187–189, 195, 199, 200, 206, 207, 211, 213, 214, 216, 220, 221, 227, 228, 231–235, 238–240, 242, 247, 248, 250, 251, 254–256, 259, 262, 270, 276, 283, 284, 286, 287, 289–292, 297, 298, 301, 303, 304, 315–317, 319, 324–327, 343, 365
anxiolytic, 16, 25, 48, 231, 232, 286
arthritis, 14, 15, 18, 28, 29, 67, 77, 87, 97, 100, 115, 120, 124, 141, 148, 161, 184, 196, 334, 336, 351
arthroscope, 76, 333
asana, 205, 207
aspirin, 2, 6, 7, 14, 15, 17–19, 51–53, 56, 60, 62, 67, 68, 152, 159, 161, 202, 203, 251, 330, 335, 345
assimilative family therapy, 237–240
asthma, 6, 14, 15, 28, 86, 95, 97, 103, 104, 111, 133, 136, 137, 139, 141, 142, 149, 150, 165, 168, 174, 191, 207, 208, 283
Astym®, 77–80
ataxia, 32, 35, 66, 71
Ativan, 232, 314, 317
autonomic nervous system, 12, 110, 112, 137, 139, 269, 282
autoregulation, 136, 139
Ayurveda, 162, 166, 167, 196

baclofen, 19–20
barbiturate, 8, 71, 218, 240–242, 325–327
behavioral medicine, 110, 112, 137–139
Bell's palsy, 28, 131

benzamides, 16
Benzocaine, 10
beta-blockers, 345
Betamethasone, 28
biodisplay, 136, 137
biofeedback, 111, 136–141, 169, 252, 282, 283, 350, 359, 365
bipolar disorder, 21, 66, 233, 235, 257, 268
blood pressure, 3–5, 7, 14, 15, 27, 28, 30, 31, 33, 45, 46, 50–53, 68, 73, 81, 87, 92, 95, 97, 99, 106, 110–112, 133, 137, 138, 144, 156, 157, 159, 165, 173–175, 208, 232, 234, 258, 278, 282, 283, 291, 292, 304, 333, 344, 345, 364, 367
boswellia, 141–142
botulinum toxin, 346
brain, 3, 4, 6, 7, 9, 12–14, 22, 25, 26, 32, 38, 39, 42–47, 51, 55, 59, 64–66, 70, 71, 78, 83, 89, 90, 105–108, 135–137, 140, 141, 160, 164, 177, 182, 183, 185, 187, 189, 199, 218, 231–233, 235–237, 241, 247, 253, 272, 280, 284, 285, 287, 292, 303, 305–310, 313, 343, 344, 350, 361, 365
brainstem, 3, 17, 42, 44–46
bromelain, 143–145
Bronchial inflammation, 28
bruise, 143, 146
Budesonide, 28, 376
bunion, 338, 339, 341
Bupivacaine, 10, 93
buprenorphine, 39, 321, 324
bursitis, 14, 28, 120, 141, 202, 339, 341
butyrophenones, 16, 17

calcium, 23–24, 28, 35, 36, 49, 50, 65, 66, 96, 102, 113, 114, 173, 175, 303, 365, 366
calculus, 113
cannabinoids, 15–17, 185, 187–190
cannabis, 15, 32, 36, 185–186, 188
cannula, 105, 106
Carbatrol, 21
Carbocaine, 10
carbon dioxide, 45, 151
cardiovascular disease, 52, 68
carisoprodol, 25–26
Carpal tunnel syndrome, 78, 79, 180, 208, 329–334
Celecoxib, 30, 67, 68, 330, 335, 353, 368
Center for Substance Abuse Treatment, 317–318
central nervous system, 1, 3, 5, 9, 10, 15, 16, 19, 31, 33, 41, 42, 45, 48, 49, 59, 65, 66, 83, 88, 108, 109, 185, 188, 198, 232, 235, 240, 246, 303, 309, 314, 318

central nervous system depressant, 27, 40, 66, 73, 201, 231, 242, 325
cervical, 80, 81, 89, 90, 181
cervical epidural injection, 80–82
Charaxine, 10
childbirth, 92–94, 101, 104, 143, 151, 165, 172
China white, 33
chiropractic, 82–88, 115, 129, 252
Chloroprocaine, 10
cholecystectomy, 113–115
cholelithiasis, 113
cholesterol, 22, 95, 114, 153, 154, 156, 157, 160, 174, 197, 283
chronic illness, 167
chronic pain, 6, 12, 33, 45, 48, 54, 67, 69, 99, 103, 116, 139, 145, 183, 249–252, 286, 292, 303, 304, 322, 359, 368
Chronic pain syndromes, 183, 303
circulatory system, 30, 31, 185, 188, 195
citalopram, 232
clonazepam, 232, 315, 317
cluster headache, 343, 344, 346, 348–350
cocaine, 13, 33, 41, 59, 128, 185, 240, 278, 315, 321, 322, 326
Codeine, 1, 26–27, 32, 36, 41, 43, 45–47, 54, 62, 64, 228, 353
cognitive behavior therapy, 253–257, 266
common cold, 31, 61, 150, 374, 378
complex seizure, 21, 182
conditioning, 94, 96, 98, 243–244, 253, 256, 257, 264
confusion, 7, 17, 21, 32, 34, 50, 59, 65, 66, 164, 170, 232, 279, 286, 308, 315, 316, 319, 326
constipation, 5, 7, 17, 20, 27, 39, 46, 55, 64–67, 70, 152, 153, 170, 227, 232, 234, 248, 286, 304, 319, 354
contraindication, 30, 69, 78, 100, 120, 286–287
convulsion, 21, 22, 31, 108, 242, 246, 305–306, 319
corticosteroids, 14–17, 27–29, 330, 371, 375
Cortisone, 27–29, 76, 330, 335
countertransference, 297, 300
COX-1, 1, 14, 18, 30, 51, 67
COX-2, 1, 14, 18, 29–30, 51, 67, 68, 368
critical care, 7, 224
Crohn's disease, 28, 141, 142
curcumin, 196–198
cyclooxygenase, 1, 17, 18, 30, 67

dance therapy, 288–290
death anxiety, 211, 213

decongestant, 30–32, 56, 62, 347
deep-tissue massage, 102
Demerol, 323
dentistry, 7, 117
dependence, 19, 25, 38–42, 50, 57, 65, 70–73, 99, 101, 170, 187, 214, 219, 231, 232, 236, 241–242, 247, 276, 283, 315–317, 321–325, 327, 368
depolarization, 3, 35, 36
depression, 4, 12, 22, 25, 27, 34, 36, 37, 39–41, 46, 49, 50, 55, 64–66, 73, 88, 95, 97, 104, 105, 109, 111, 120, 128, 132, 160, 163, 168, 170–172, 177, 182, 184, 188, 189, 206–208, 213, 214, 224, 227, 228, 231–235, 238, 239, 242, 247, 250, 251, 253, 255–257, 262, 268, 270, 278, 279, 284, 286, 287, 292, 298, 301, 303, 304, 306, 307, 327, 343, 348, 370
Dermatitis, 28, 116
Desflurane, 8
detoxification, 4, 55, 128, 321, 324, 327
Dexamethadone, 28
Dexamethasone, 17, 28, 330
Dexmedetomindine, 8
dextromethorphan, 32–33, 46, 49, 50, 59, 62
diabetes, 14, 15, 26, 29, 31, 36, 53, 66, 76, 80, 81, 94, 97, 100, 101, 103, 104, 106, 135, 155, 156, 168, 173, 174–176, 179, 183, 196, 249–251, 334, 338, 340, 341
Diabetic retinopathy, 28
dialectical behavioral therapy, 266–269
diarrhea, 4, 17, 20, 26, 42, 43, 45–47, 65, 141, 150, 159, 160, 170, 174, 204, 227, 234, 241, 304, 353, 368, 375
Diazepam, 8, 71, 232, 247, 315, 317, 325, 326, 353
diclofenac, 6, 14, 51, 68, 203, 335, 353, 368
Dihydrocodeinone, 37
discectomy, 90, 356, 357
disk herniation, 90
dizziness, 5, 7, 14, 17, 19, 20, 27, 31, 37, 39, 50, 64, 65–67, 70, 73, 108, 159, 170, 188, 232, 249, 304, 315, 326
dopamine, 16, 17, 64, 88, 109, 235–237, 292, 303
downer, 240, 246
Doxycycline, 375
drama therapy, 288–289, 291
duloxetine, 232, 304, 353, 368
dura, 12, 80, 89
dysmenorrhea, 23, 68, 69, 87, 143, 173, 175, 202
dyspepsia, 68, 69, 192, 193, 195, 197, 198
dysphoria, 17, 34, 45, 65, 313
dystonia, 15, 88

Eczema, 28, 103, 104, 171, 204, 205
effleurage, 102, 104
electroacupuncture, 121, 125–130, 133, 134
electrocardiogram, 305, 327
electroencephalogram, 305
electroencephalograph, 136, 137, 308
electromyograph, 136, 137
emergency medicine, 7, 48, 188, 226
endorphins, 43, 44, 123, 318
endoscope, 76, 377, 378
Enflurane, 8
enkephalins, 43, 44
epidural, 7, 10, 12, 13, 48, 75, 76, 80, 81, 92, 93, 359
epilepsy, 14, 19, 21–23, 105, 108, 116, 133, 136–139, 177, 182, 184, 208, 305, 306
epinephrine, 9, 11, 31, 292, 303
equine-facilitated learning, 269, 271–272
equine-facilitated psychotherapy, 269, 270–271
Erectile dysfunction, 52, 68, 69, 181, 232
escitalopram, 232
estrogen, 94, 154, 155, 173, 196, 361–364, 366
estrogen replacement therapy, 176, 361, 362
etodolac, 14, 68, 335
Etomidate, 8, 305
euphoria, 32, 34, 37, 39, 41, 43, 45, 46, 50, 64, 65, 70, 170, 187, 188, 240, 241, 247, 318, 319, 325, 326
euthanasia, 215–220, 241, 242
evidence-based medicine, 31, 32
Excedrin Migraine, 345

family medicine, 14, 30, 51, 136, 226, 231, 233
FDA, 30, 35, 53, 56, 58, 60–62, 66, 67, 72, 88, 145, 170, 171, 190, 200, 285, 286, 304, 345, 366
Feldenkrais method, 96–99
fentanyl, 33–34, 44, 46, 313, 368
fibromyalgia, 35, 37, 66, 95, 101, 103, 104, 132, 136, 137, 139, 165, 174, 179, 183, 184, 250, 251, 286, 292, 303, 304, 351
5-hydroxytryptamine, 43, 231, 303
fluoxetine, 132, 231, 233, 234, 353, 364
flurbiprofen, 14, 51
fluvoxamine, 231
folate, 23
Fospropofol, 8
free association, 259, 297
"Freud, Sigmund," 259, 263, 296–299
Frovatriptan, 344
functional food, 152, 155, 159, 190, 192, 195, 196
functional medicine, 166

gabapentin, 34–37, 317, 346, 364
gamma-aminobutyric acid, 9, 25, 43, 71, 241, 314, 325
gastrointestinal, 1, 2, 4, 7, 14–17, 20, 26, 30, 39, 52, 57, 65, 67, 68, 73, 97, 120, 141, 144, 148, 149, 152, 159, 168, 185, 188, 192, 195, 196, 201, 286, 303, 319, 345, 353, 354, 364
gestation, 109–110
ginger, 159–162
ginkgo, 22, 159, 163, 168
Glucocorticoids, 27, 28, 330, 335
glutamine, 22, 237
group therapy, 234, 264, 265, 274–277, 321

hallucinations, 7, 17, 20, 25, 31, 32, 34, 50, 65, 70, 71, 170, 182, 183, 188, 189, 236, 237, 242, 249, 278, 324
Halothane, 8
headache, 5, 12–14, 17, 18, 39, 51, 55–58, 66, 67, 69, 70, 80, 81, 83, 85–87, 91, 92, 104, 108, 111, 120, 128, 135, 137, 138, 150–152, 159, 160, 166, 171, 173, 174, 181, 184, 190, 192, 195, 202, 208, 232, 248–251, 282, 283, 304, 305, 323, 343–351, 362, 363
heart rate variability, 137, 269
heel spurs, 339, 342
hematoma, 105, 106
herbalists, 151, 160, 162
herbal medicine, 119, 122, 141, 162–164, 196
herniation, 87, 89, 90, 106
heroin, 33, 34, 39, 41, 43, 44, 46, 54, 55, 59, 62–64, 128, 278, 318, 322
"high-velocity, low-amplitude," 82, 83, 85
hippotherapy, 269, 272
homeopathy, 166–168
homeostasis, 27
hormone, 14, 18, 23, 27–30, 42, 49, 51, 101, 111, 154, 155, 175, 247, 282, 284, 291, 292, 303, 360, 361, 363
hormone replacement therapy, 94, 95, 153, 361–363
hospice, 55, 211–214, 220–226
human immunodeficiency virus (HIV), 103, 104, 133, 159, 191, 225
hydrocodone, 37–39, 41, 64, 72–73, 323, 368
Hydrocortisone, 14, 28, 29
hydrotherapy, 100–101, 167
hypertension, 3, 5, 28, 32, 52, 56, 68, 76, 98, 109, 120, 138, 157, 167, 174, 175, 255, 304
hypnosis, 164–166

hypnotherapy, 164–166
hypnotic, 164, 166, 232, 246, 247, 315, 326
hypoallergenic, 116
hypotension, 3, 5, 13, 17, 28, 40, 65, 188, 232, 242
ibuprofen, 6, 7, 14, 19, 51, 52, 59, 67, 87, 110, 148, 197, 228, 330, 335, 345, 353, 368, 376

IgE-mediated allergies, 28
indica, 185
inflammation, 1, 4–6, 14, 15, 17, 18, 20, 27, 28, 30, 51, 53, 65, 67, 68, 79, 80, 91, 100, 115, 141, 143, 144, 152, 153, 175, 178, 188, 197, 204, 329, 330, 334, 335, 342, 353, 359, 367–369, 371, 373, 374
influenza, 19, 46, 284
insomnia, 17, 22, 31, 55, 66, 96–98, 111, 120, 130, 136, 137, 159, 165, 172, 174, 184, 187, 198–200, 232, 241, 247, 249, 279, 282, 286, 304, 316, 317, 319, 325–327, 335, 365, 368
integrative medicine, 166–170
intercessory prayer, 273
internal medicine, 14, 51, 136, 188, 224, 226, 231
intervertebral disks, 89–91, 105, 106
intravenous, 4, 8, 10, 11, 13, 16, 33, 41, 42, 55, 65, 69, 106, 174, 218, 232
ion, 3, 9, 27, 35, 36, 303
ischemia, 68, 69
isocaine, 10
Isoflurane, 8

joint pain, 51, 67, 75–77, 115, 131, 148, 171, 195, 250, 367, 368, 370, 371

kava, 22, 168, 169, 247, 248
ketamine, 8, 49–50, 278, 313
"Kevorkian, Jack," 216, 218
kidneys, 6, 7, 45, 52–53, 57, 66–68, 113
Klonopin, 232, 314, 317
kratom, 170–171

laminectomy, 90, 106, 356, 357
lean syrup, 26
learning theory, 140, 243–245, 253, 256
lethargy, 22, 26, 32, 187, 319, 327
Levobupivacaine, 10
Levofloxacin, 375
Lidocaine, 10–12
light therapy, 279–280
linseed, 152, 154
Lioresal, 19
Lithium, 195, 196, 346

lobectomy, 105
lobotomy, 105, 106
locus coeruleus, 3
lorazepam, 8, 16, 17, 232, 315, 317, 326
"low-velocity, high-amplitude," 82, 83
lumbar, 11–13, 90, 91, 351, 355

major depressive disorder, 132, 285, 286, 292
MAOI inhibitors, 286
Marcaine, 10
massage, 79, 84–87, 102–105, 120, 124, 128, 129, 162, 168, 252, 331, 341, 348, 350, 358, 373
meditation, 96–98, 119, 167, 168, 205, 207, 260, 280–285, 355, 365, 370
Meloxicam, 51, 67, 68, 335, 353, 368
membrane potential, 34–35, 50
meninges, 91
menopause, 35, 37, 98, 131, 153, 154, 168, 360–366
mental health, 112, 137, 138, 187, 226, 228, 231, 239, 251, 256, 270, 280, 282, 285, 287, 301, 303, 359
Mepivacaine, 10
meridians, 119, 121, 122
methadone, 4, 39–40, 44, 49, 50, 128, 315, 321, 322, 324, 368
methadose, 39
methamphetamine, 41, 59, 62, 321
methemoglobinemia, 1, 2
Methohexital, 8, 305
Methylprednisolone, 17, 28
Midazolam, 8, 313, 317
migraine, 66, 86, 104, 115, 128, 137, 138, 151–152, 160, 168, 171, 173–175, 181, 202, 208, 241, 251, 279, 283, 343–346, 348, 350, 362
mind/body, 166–169, 273
monoamine oxidase inhibitors, 233, 234
morbidity, 13, 232
morphine, 6, 26, 33, 41–43, 45–48, 54, 55, 62, 64, 70, 123, 130, 185, 213, 228, 318, 323, 368
motion sickness, 16, 56, 126, 160, 161
Motrin, 14, 56, 59, 67, 345, 376
moxibustion, 119, 127, 130, 131, 134
Moxifloxacin, 375
multiple sclerosis, 168, 181, 188, 197, 218, 272
muscle relaxant, 19, 25, 71, 85, 90, 246, 247, 305–307, 353
muscle spasm, 71, 115, 353, 359
musculoskeletal system, 1, 7, 19, 25, 71, 72, 75, 77, 82, 99, 110, 115, 141, 145–147, 190, 195, 196, 202, 313
music therapy, 288–290, 302

nabumetone, 14, 51, 68, 335
naltrexone, 39, 46, 313
naproxen, 6, 14, 51, 67, 110, 130, 330, 335, 345, 353, 368
Naratriptan, 344
nasal irrigation, 349, 379
Nasal polyposis, 28
nasal polyps, 53, 377
nasal spray, 349, 376, 379
nasopharynx, 10
nausea, 4, 5, 14–17, 20, 27, 37, 39, 42, 45, 46, 50, 52, 55, 57, 58, 64, 65, 67, 70, 73, 93, 104, 125, 126, 135, 150, 152, 159–161, 165, 168, 170, 171, 179, 188, 189, 192, 194, 197, 227, 232, 235, 241, 249, 278, 304, 316, 319, 327, 344–346, 353, 362, 368, 375
nerve block, 9–11, 251, 332
nerve impulse, 3, 7, 9, 10, 35
nervous system, 1, 2, 7, 17, 21, 26, 27, 32–34, 36–39, 41–46, 49, 55–56, 66, 70–73, 78, 80, 83, 88, 89, 97, 105, 108–110, 112, 137, 139, 145, 150, 170, 171, 185, 188, 194, 198, 201, 231–235, 240, 242, 246, 269, 278, 279, 282, 285, 286, 291, 303, 305, 309, 327, 343
neuroendocrine system, 279
neurology, 7, 88, 89, 105, 115, 136, 188, 226, 233, 235, 305, 309
neuroma, 339, 341
neuromuscular massage, 102
neurosurgery, 88, 105–109
neurotransmitter, 3, 4, 9, 16, 22, 32, 35, 36, 42, 43, 45, 46, 49, 64, 66, 70, 71, 109, 185, 232–235, 237, 241, 279, 286, 292, 303, 304, 306, 314, 325, 326
nitrous oxide, 8, 48–49, 313
Noninfectious rhinitis, 28
Nonprescription, 60–62, 315, 366
nonsteroidal anti-inflammatory drugs, 1, 14, 51–53, 67, 87, 110, 152, 228, 330, 335–336, 341, 345, 353–354, 367–368
norco, 72–74
norepinephrine, 3, 4, 70, 123, 231, 232, 234, 286, 292, 303
Novocain, 10

Obsessive-compulsive disorder, 177, 183, 208, 231, 233, 235
occupational health, 136
operationalization, 243
ophthalmology, 7, 14, 279

447

opiate, 1, 3, 41, 43, 45–47, 54, 55, 59, 64, 70, 170, 322, 326
opioid, 4, 6, 7, 19, 25, 26, 32–48, 50, 54, 55, 62, 64, 65, 70, 72, 73, 93, 99, 110, 116, 130, 170, 186, 228, 229, 292, 313, 315, 318–322, 324, 326, 350, 353, 368
opium, 6, 26, 41, 43, 46, 47, 54–55, 185
oral surgeon, 117
orthopedics, 14, 75, 89, 115
osteoarthritis, 1, 14, 51, 53, 75, 76, 94, 95, 127, 141–143, 145, 146, 148, 151, 160, 161, 180, 181, 197, 202, 203, 208, 304, 334, 366–374
overdetermination, 297, 298
overdose, 19, 31, 33, 34, 39, 41, 44–46, 50, 54, 55, 61, 73, 170, 201, 218, 231, 232, 234, 242, 249, 315, 316, 319, 325, 326
over-the-counter, 1, 6, 16, 17, 20, 32, 50, 52, 53, 55–62, 67, 86, 197, 327, 330, 331, 335–336, 338, 340, 353, 354, 364, 366, 369, 376
oxycodone, 25, 41, 62–64, 72, 228, 323, 353, 368
OxyContin, 63, 64, 322, 323
oxygen therapy, 346

painkiller, 5, 10, 14, 27, 34, 41, 47, 56, 58, 59, 70, 72, 73, 107, 117, 251, 326
palliative care, 54, 211–214, 221, 223–228
Papaver somniferum, 43, 47
paracetamol, 1, 2, 6, 72
Parkinson's disease, 14, 88, 106, 108, 109, 133, 168, 177, 183, 237, 303
paroxetine, 232, 364
partial seizure, 21
Percocet, 64, 72, 323
perimenopause, 361, 366
peripheral nerves, 42, 43, 116, 318
peripheral nervous system, 5, 15, 16, 26, 56, 108, 109, 309
Peripheral neuropathy, 36, 133, 179, 183, 184, 303
pharmaceutical, 38, 56, 67, 70, 77, 100, 142, 150, 156, 167, 168, 172, 278, 291, 293
pharmacist, 47, 61, 62, 224, 225, 324, 327, 331, 336, 347, 354, 364, 369, 376
pharmacology, 42, 231
phenobarbital, 21, 23, 24, 240, 242
phenothiazines, 16, 17, 236, 345
phototherapy, 279
physical therapy, 75–77, 80, 84, 85, 89, 90, 97, 100, 110, 115, 116, 124, 126, 128, 129, 136, 208, 252, 292, 302, 341, 342, 356, 358–359
physiotherapy, 77, 82, 94, 96, 100, 102, 110, 115, 205, 249, 269, 287, 331, 333, 336, 340, 348, 350, 354, 358, 365, 370, 372

Pilates, 96–99
placebo, 84–87, 95, 103, 112, 121, 123–130, 133, 134, 142–144, 146, 148, 150–153, 157, 158, 160, 161, 165, 174–176, 178–181, 192, 193, 197–200, 203, 205, 206, 208
plantar fascia, 339, 342
plantar fasciitis, 339, 341–342
play therapy, 290, 293–297
pneumothorax, 135
polysynaptic, 21
Pontocaine, 10
postmenopause, 361
Post-traumatic stress disorder, 183, 231
Pranayama, 205, 207
Prednisolone, 28, 330, 335
Prednisone, 14, 17, 28, 29, 330, 335, 346
pregnancy, 6, 15, 21, 24, 39, 46, 53, 68, 103, 104, 109–110, 116, 120, 125, 126, 132, 152, 155, 160, 168, 173, 189, 361, 375
premenstrual syndrome, 23, 86, 103, 132, 173, 175
prescription, 2, 6, 14, 15, 26, 31, 41, 44, 47, 53–55, 59, 60, 62–64, 67, 70, 72, 73, 110, 139, 170, 173, 190, 218, 234, 251, 315, 317, 321–325, 327, 330–331, 335, 336, 341, 344, 347, 353, 354, 361, 362, 364, 366, 367–369, 375–376
pressure points, 119
presynaptic, 3, 9, 36, 303
prevention, 1, 12, 15, 16, 30, 73, 75, 91, 94, 96, 97, 151, 153, 156–158, 160, 167, 205, 216, 257, 265, 314, 317, 318, 321, 324, 327
preventive medicine, 136
priapism, 68
Prilocaine, 10
procaine, 10
progressive muscle relaxation, 110–112, 283
prolapse, 89, 90, 174
propofol, 8, 46, 313, 314
prostaglandin, 1, 17, 18, 20, 30, 51, 56, 67, 69, 100, 110, 148, 175
psychic healing, 273
psychoanalysis, 254, 274, 275, 297–301
psychophysiological, 136–138
psychosis, 17, 50, 170, 235–237
psychotherapy, 165, 166, 168, 231, 234, 237, 243, 249, 253, 256, 258, 262, 266–270, 274, 275, 279, 287, 288, 290, 293, 297–301, 305, 350, 354, 358, 370
psychotropic, 17, 246, 247, 305, 308, 315
pulsed electromagnetic therapy, 178
Purdue Pharma, 63

qi, 119, 122, 134
qigong, 96, 97, 99, 119, 162

recreational use, 25, 50, 186, 278, 326
reflexology, 102–104
reinforcer, 243, 245
relaxation, 7, 10, 12, 21, 25, 51, 69, 70, 96, 102, 103, 110–112, 120, 126, 128, 137, 140, 164–170, 173, 185, 207, 238, 240, 241, 252, 254, 255, 260, 280–285, 315, 319, 325–327, 348, 350, 355, 359, 365, 370, 373
repetitive transcranial magnetic stimulation, 177, 182
repolarization, 35
respiratory system, 12, 13, 30, 59, 141, 149, 185, 188, 192
Reye's syndrome, 14, 18, 21, 53, 203
Rheumatoid arthritis, 15, 18, 28, 51, 75, 103, 104, 133, 141–143, 148, 151, 160, 174, 178, 191, 202, 203, 334
Rhinosinusitis, 374
Rizatriptan, 344, 347
Rohypnol, 317, 325, 326
Ropivacaine, 10

Salicylates, 14, 15, 20
Saline, 13, 121, 130, 379
sativa, 185
Schizophrenia, 112, 177, 182, 183, 208, 231, 235–237, 257, 270, 289, 299, 306, 307
sciatica, 82, 85, 351–360
sedation, 3–5, 8, 13, 17, 22, 25, 27, 32, 39, 41, 46, 55, 64, 66, 73, 170, 201, 241, 247, 313, 318, 319, 333
sedative, 3, 4, 8, 16, 22, 41, 45, 47, 57, 71, 144, 172, 198, 199, 201, 217, 232, 240–242, 246, 247, 285, 286, 314, 316, 318, 321, 325, 326
seizure, 4, 19, 21–24, 27, 34, 35, 55, 66, 71, 89, 108, 139, 168, 182, 184, 189, 208, 241, 248, 249, 292, 305, 306, 316, 317, 323, 325, 327
Selective serotonin reuptake inhibitors, 231, 233, 234, 286, 315, 364
self-actualization, 284, 285
self-diagnosis, 55
self-healing, 167
septoplasty, 349
septum, 349, 350
serotonin, 9, 16, 17, 70, 231–234, 237, 286, 287, 303, 304, 344
Serotonin norepinephrine reuptake inhibitors, 232, 286, 303–304

serotonin syndrome, 286, 287
sertraline, 231
shiatsu, 102, 121
shock therapy, 305–309
sinuses, 31, 39, 192, 343, 347, 349, 374, 377–379
sinus headache, 343–344, 346–349
sinusitis, 66, 97, 143, 144, 150, 168, 343, 347, 349, 374–379
soft tissue, 77–79, 85, 115, 148, 339, 359
soma, 25
special K, 278
spinal column, 89–91, 106, 351, 357
spinal fluid, 11, 13, 91
spinal fusion, 355–358
spinal manipulation, 82–87, 129, 358
spinal stenosis, 351, 352, 356
spine, 7, 75, 80, 82, 83, 87, 89–91, 99, 105, 107, 181, 205, 207, 281, 313, 337, 351, 355, 357–359, 366
spondylolisthesis, 351, 356
spondylolysis, 351
sports medicine, 75, 96, 100, 136
sprain, 14, 25, 51, 53, 67, 79, 146, 183, 351
static magnets, 176–180, 184
steroid, 17, 27, 80, 81, 101, 150, 346, 358, 359, 371
stroke, 7, 19, 30, 36, 52, 67, 68, 87, 96, 102, 120, 129, 130, 137, 139, 140, 168, 174, 272, 338, 344, 353, 362, 365, 367, 368
structural integration, 102
subluxations, 82, 83
sufentanil, 33, 46, 93
Sumatriptan, 344, 346
supplements, 23, 24, 28, 29, 62, 83, 87, 141, 143, 146–152, 155–157, 159, 167–171, 173–176, 185, 188, 190, 192, 195, 196, 198, 202, 204, 247, 331, 336, 347, 353, 354, 364–366, 369, 376
suppository, 68, 69
surgery, 7, 8, 12, 13, 15, 28, 33, 45, 46, 51, 75–78, 88–89, 91, 100, 105–109, 113–115, 125, 130, 140, 143, 159–161, 164, 165, 168, 172–174, 179, 182, 192, 193, 201, 226, 227, 251–252, 278, 310, 332, 333, 338–339, 341, 342, 349, 350, 353, 355–358, 372, 377–378
Surgery support, 130, 179
Svoflurane, 8
Swedish massage, 102, 103, 129
synaptic cleft, 3, 36, 303
synthetic, 4, 14, 22, 28, 39, 44, 321, 324, 330, 338, 362, 372
systemic, 10, 11, 14, 31, 101, 143, 190, 334, 344
Systemic lupus erythematosus, 28

449

Tai Chi, 96–99, 119, 206, 281, 373
tendinitis, 14
tendinopathy, 78, 79, 342
tension headache, 85, 86, 128, 137, 138, 166, 192, 202, 343, 348, 351
terminal illness, 211–214, 216, 227, 229
tetanic, 21
Tetracaine, 10
thanatology, 211
Thiopental, 8, 305
thromboxane, 1, 17, 18
tinnitus, 67, 88, 133, 183
tolerance, 6, 7, 16, 17, 27, 39, 43, 44, 46, 55, 73, 78, 116, 175, 242, 315–317, 325, 326
tonic-clonic, 21
tooth extraction, 48, 117
topical, 10, 28, 29, 31, 57, 67, 77, 78, 100, 145–147, 149, 150, 156, 159, 172, 204, 353
Topiramate, 345–346
touch-based therapy, 102, 373
traditional Chinese medicine, 119, 121, 122, 160, 162, 167
Trager approach, 96–99
tramadol, 70, 249, 319
tranquillity, 282
transcranial magnetic stimulation, 309–310
transcutaneous electrical nerve stimulation, 115, 126, 129, 350, 372
transference, 289, 297, 299
trauma, 4, 45, 48, 75, 78, 90, 91, 100, 106, 143, 167, 257, 291, 351, 356
Triamcinolone, 14, 28, 330, 335, 376
tricyclics, 21, 233, 234
tumor, 4, 28, 30, 78, 105–107, 141, 154, 183, 188, 356
Tylenol, 1, 6, 56, 58, 110, 162, 376

Ulcerative colitis, 28, 53, 141–143, 197, 198
Ultrasound, 114, 156, 373
unipolar magnets, 176, 177, 183

upper, 10, 31, 76, 80, 85, 89, 94, 114, 168, 176, 185, 193, 281, 336, 351, 374
ureterolithotomy, 113
urolithiasis, 113

valerian, 22, 169, 198–201, 247
valium, 71–72, 199, 200, 232, 247, 314, 317
valproic acid, 21, 23, 24, 203, 345
varicose veins, 116, 143, 146, 204, 205
vascular medicine, 14, 136
vasoconstriction, 56, 68, 100, 107
vasodilation, 110, 112
venlafaxine, 232, 304, 364
vicodin, 37, 72–74, 323
vinyasa, 205
virilization, 27, 28
Vitamin B_6, 160, 168, 174, 175
Vitamin C, 163
Vitamin D, 24, 28, 168, 365
Vitamin K, 24, 278
Vomiting, 4, 5, 7, 14–17, 20, 27, 39, 45, 46, 50, 52, 55, 57, 64, 65, 67, 70, 73, 125, 126, 135, 150, 152, 159–161, 168, 179, 188, 189, 202, 227, 235, 241, 249, 278, 316, 319, 323, 327, 344, 345, 368

warfarin, 144, 149, 152, 159, 161, 203
withdrawal, 2–4, 6, 19, 20, 25, 26, 35, 36, 39, 40, 42, 43, 46, 50, 64–66, 70, 71, 110, 128, 170, 187, 195, 201, 218, 232, 234, 241, 242, 247, 248, 276, 304, 315–317, 319, 321, 323, 324, 326, 327
wrist splint, 208

Xanax, 22, 25, 232, 247, 314, 316, 317
Xylocaine, 10

yin and yang, 119, 121, 122
yoga, 96–98, 110, 167, 168, 205–209, 280, 281, 355, 365, 370, 373

Zolmitriptan, 344